This Book

was presented to

The E.N.T Department

by R. Chigwila

A.G. Prince

Date 1 July 1980

DG 2107

Scott-Brown's
Diseases of the Ear, Nose and Throat

Volume 4
The Pharynx and Larynx

Titles of other volumes

Scott-Brown's
Diseases of the Ear, Nose and Throat

Fourth Edition

Volume 4

The Pharynx and Larynx

Editors

John Ballantyne, FRCS, HON FRCS (I)
Consultant Ear, Nose and Throat Surgeon,
The Royal Free Hospital and King Edward VII Hospital for Officers, London;
Civilian Consultant in Otolaryngology to the Army

John Groves, MB, BS, FRCS
Consultant Ear, Nose and Throat Surgeon,
The Royal Free Hospital, London

Butterworths
London Boston
Sydney Wellington Durban Toronto

United Kingdom London	**Butterworth & Co (Publishers) Ltd** 88 Kingsway, WC2B 6AB
Australia Sydney	**Butterworths Pty Ltd** 586 Pacific Highway, Chatswood, NSW 2067 Also at Melbourne, Brisbane, Adelaide and Perth
Canada Toronto	**Butterworth & Co (Canada) Ltd** 2265 Midland Avenue, Scarborough, Ontario, M1P 4S1
New Zealand Wellington	**Butterworths of New Zealand Ltd** T & W Young Building, 77–85 Customhouse Quay, 1, CPO Box 472
South Africa Durban	**Butterworth & Co (South Africa) (Pty) Ltd** 152–154 Gale Street
USA Boston	**Butterworth (Publishers) Inc** 10 Tower Office Park, Woburn, Massachusetts 01801

First edition 1952
Second edition 1965
Reprinted 1967
Reprinted 1968
Third edition 1971
Reprinted 1977
Fourth edition 1979

© Butterworth & Co (Publishers) Ltd, 1979

ISBN 0–407–00150–6 Individual volume
ISBN 0–407–00143–3 Set of four volumes

British Library Cataloguing in Publication Data

Scott-Brown, Walter Graham
  Scott-Brown's diseases of the ear, nose and throat. – 4th ed.
  Vol. 4: The pharynx and larynx
  I. Otolaryngology
  I. Ballantyne, John II. Groves, John
  616.2 '1   RF46   79–41008

  ISBN 0–407–00150–6
  ISBN 0–407–00143–3 Set of 4 vols

Phototypeset in Great Britain by
Filmtype Services Limited, Scarborough
Printed and bound by William Clowes & Sons Ltd, Beccles and London

Introduction to the Fourth Edition

Some eight years after the last edition of this work appeared it may now seem to the practising clinician that the present decade has been a relatively quiet one in the history of our specialty. In fact, there has been a steady growth in the scientific foundations upon which an increasing amount of our practice is built, and it is therefore not surprising that the first volume, *Basic Sciences*, has now been considerably enlarged.

There has also been a steady expansion of clinical knowledge, and in planning this new edition we quickly became aware that no single volume from the last edition could stand without revision.

Sadly, the list of authors has been depleted by deaths and retirements of old friends and colleagues, whose contributions to British otolaryngology will never be forgotten. We thank sincerely all our colleagues, both old and new, who have spared no effort in preparing their manuscripts for this new presentation. The connoisseur will notice that a number of distinguished contributors from overseas have again been invited; we hope that this broadening of outlook will be welcomed by readers, and it is in keeping with the concepts of Mr W G Scott-Brown who originated the text nearly 30 years ago and who continues to flourish and to practice.

In some parts of the work, notably in Volume 2 (*The Ear*), advances in academic research have out-paced our ability to classify neatly a plethora of theories, facts (and sometimes fancies) for clinical application. Retaining the clinical approach as far as possible has compelled us, therefore, to commission chapters (for example in the field of sensorineural deafness) which overlap one another very considerably in content, while differing widely in emphasis. We hope that the reader will bear with this, and that the overall presentation will form a wider basis for learning than could be achieved by a more rigidly structured approach.

As far as we could we have used metric and SI units of measurement, even though a sense of humour is needed to accept some of the numerical absurdities which result. We are increasingly aware, too, that the SI system has brought upon us a hybrid and irrational system, heavily be-spattered with eponymously named units, at a time when eponyms are discouraged in the basic scientific disciplines. We are confident that the present generation will continue to honour Eustachius, Morgagni, Paget, Pott, Rosenmüller, and a hundred and one other great names, however the winds of pseudo-change may blow.

It is a great pleasure to thank and acknowledge all those who have helped so much in the preparation of this edition. We are grateful to those many colleagues who have lent us illustrations; to our registrars who have read proofs, criticized, advised and encouraged; and to those artists who have drawn new illustrations. Among the latter we thank especially Mr Frank Price for his unfailing generosity and technical skills. Equally we thank Mr Cedric Gilson and the Photographic Department of the Royal Free Hospital for their tremendous and willing efforts to provide so many of the new photographs.

Finally, our gratitude goes to our publishers, Butterworths, who have done so much to lighten our editorial tasks.

London, 1979
John Ballantyne
John Groves

Introduction to the Third Edition

A radical new departure is made in the presentation of this work in four separately available volumes. This has been done for two main reasons. First, there is a real need, we feel, to recognize the diverse requirements of different readers – the newcomer to the specialty who needs a compact presentation of the special anatomy, physiology and radiology (for preparation for the DLO Part I and Primary FRCS examinations), and the specialist who is more interested in, say, the ear than in the throat. Secondly, advances are more numerous and more rapid in some sub-divisions of the specialty than in others so that it will be advantageous in the future to revise one volume at a time. The reduction in bulk of the individual volumes results, we hope, in easier handling and more pleasant reading.

A consequence of this change in format and policy is that page and chapter cross-references between different volumes cannot be given, nor is it practicable any longer to compile the symptom index featured in the last edition. To offset the former disadvantage some overlapping of subject material has been deliberately introduced wherever it was felt that too frequent referral to another volume would otherwise be necessary. Each volume has its own Table of Contents and Index, the latter compiled on the basis of noun-entries only.

The text throughout has been comprehensively revised. As a matter of general editorial policy, for this and for any subsequent editions which may appear under our direction, we have invited contributions only from those of our colleagues who are still actively engaged in hospital, university or college practice; and it has been our pleasure to welcome several new contributors. By including several new chapters, we have been able to remedy some of the omissions from earlier editions (for example, 'Congenital Diseases of the Larynx'), and also to give due emphasis to such topics as 'Acoustic Trauma' and 'Acoustic Neuroma', each of which now demands a separate chapter. The weights and liquid measures of all drugs, as well as the measures of distance, are all given in the metric system.

We are grateful to all the authors for submitting their work on schedule so that the production can be uniformly up-to-date. We warmly appreciate the efforts and enthusiasm of the Publisher's Editorial Staff, and the kind help we have received from colleagues, artists, and many friends too numerous to be named. It has been a tremendous encouragement to have the continuing interest of Mr W G Scott-Brown, CVO, MD, FRCS, who has read and contributed substantially to the editing of a large part of this edition. We wish to thank him for the honour of his invitation to join in the editorship of this standard textbook, which was established solely by him in the First Edition of 1952. Although he has now handed over completely the pleasant duties of joint Editorship to us and our successors, it remains his book and it retains his name.

London, 1971
John Ballantyne
John Groves

Introduction to the Second Edition

The objects set out in the Introduction to the First Edition have been the guiding principles in the present work. In order to make this new edition authoritative and contemporary in outlook, I asked two of my colleagues to join me as co-editors and I have been most fortunate in having the help and inspiration of John Ballantyne and John Groves. We have together re-cast the main sections, sub-sections and chapters and have given more emphasis to those departments of the specialty which have undergone the greatest changes. We have also made great efforts to have all contributions written and despatched to the printer within one year of starting the project, in order that all the articles shall be finished at the same time and be up-to-date when published. This object has been achieved thanks to the cooperation of our contributors.

It will be seen that the sections on physiology have been extended and improved and the chapters on the ear have been considerably altered and enlarged to include the many fresh ideas and techniques associated with both infective and non-infective ear conditions. The sections on endoscopy have been re-arranged to make the subject as practical as possible for our specialty. It is hoped that the necessary curtailment has not given rise to any major omissions. Neoplasms of the larynx and pharynx have been separated and new chapters on voice and speech have been introduced.

The index has been completely revised, and an innovation in a textbook of this size is an additional index – a symptom index – which is complete for the whole work at the end of each volume. It is hoped that this may be particularly useful to candidates for higher examinations and to general practitioners looking for causes of particular symptoms.

It is a pleasure to acknowledge the generous help which has been given by all the contributors, a number of them new to this book, and to artists and friends, for their kindly and stimulating interest. It is not possible here to record individual acknowledgments, but a special word of thanks must be made to the Editorial Staff of the Publishers.

London, 1965
W G Scott-Brown

Introduction to the First Edition

This work has been compiled with the object of presenting a textbook on Diseases of the Ear, Nose and Throat which would include most of the subject matter required by students and post-graduates with sufficient detail for those taking the higher specialized qualifications. It should also be a suitable reference book for general practice.

To achieve this it was decided to ask a number of teachers, examiners and other well-recognized authorities in the specialty to contribute articles on this general plan while leaving them free to put forward their own views of the particular subject in their own way. This has in some cases meant the presentation of individual preferences, classifications or theories, but as far as possible these have been integrated with the more usual views to give a balanced appreciation of the subject. It is hoped that this individuality of articles will give a more stimulating approach to the subject in spite of some overlapping of subject matter and differences of opinion.

Each section is prefaced by its anatomy and physiology as an essential basis to the understanding of the subject, and also to include in a concise manner the material necessary for the examinee. Methods of examination on the other hand have been cut to a minimum as they can only be learnt by the practical examination of patients. After considerable deliberation it was decided to include a chapter on plastic surgery of the nose and ear which should set out what can be done rather than entering into details of technique which are largely the province of the plastic surgeon.

My thanks are due in the first place to all the contributors who have lightened the editorial burden: they have all been most cooperative and have given freely of their time, knowledge and, in many cases, helpful criticism. Acknowledgment is made in the text for opinions and illustrations used.

I must particularly thank the Publishers' team, all of whom have been not only helpful but also encouraging during the many unavoidable delays and difficulties in the production of a new work.

London, 1952
W G Scott-Brown

Colour plates in this volume

Contributors to this volume

D P Bryce, MD, FRCS(C), FACS (HON), FRCS (ED)
Professor and Chairman, Department of Otolaryngology, University of Toronto; Otolaryngologist-in-Chief, Toronto General Hospital

Stewart W Clarke, MD, FRCP
Consultant Physician, The Royal Free Hospital and The Brompton Hospital, London

F Clifford Rose, FRCP
Physician-in-Charge, Department of Neurology, Charing Cross Hospital; Consultant Neurologist, Medical Ophthalmology Unit, St. Thomas's Hospital, London

David Downton, FDS RCS
Senior Consultant Oral Surgeon, The Royal Free Hospital, London

John Groves, MB, BS, FRCS
Consultant Ear, Nose and Throat Surgeon, The Royal Free Hospital, London

A S Khambata, MB, BS, FRCS
Consultant Ear, Nose and Throat Surgeon, Dartford and Gravesham Group of Hospitals and Queen Mary's Hospital, Sidcup

Stuart R Mawson, MB, FRCS, DLO
Senior Consultant Surgeon, Department of Otolaryngology, King's College Hospital (including Belgrave Hospital for Children), London

Peter McKelvie, MD, CHM, FRCS, DLO
Consultant Ear, Nose and Throat Surgeon, The London Hospital, The Royal National Throat, Nose and Ear Hospital and The Royal Postgraduate Medical School, Hammersmith Hospital, London

R F McNab Jones, FRCS
Surgeon-in-Charge, Ear, Nose and Throat Department, St. Bartholomews Hospital, London; Surgeon, Royal National Throat, Nose and Ear Hospital, London

Gaye Murrills, LCST
Chief Speech Therapist, Charing Cross Hospital, London

R Pracy, MB, BS, FRCS
Consultant Surgeon, The Royal National Throat, Nose and Ear Hospital and The Hospital for Sick Children, Great Ormond Street, London

Sir Douglas Ranger, MB, BS, FRCS
Consultant Otolaryngologist, The Middlesex Hospital and King Edward VII Hospital for Officers, London

Joselen Ransome, MB, BS, FRCS
Consultant Otolaryngologist, Kensington, Chelsea and Westminster Area Health Authority (Teaching)

L F W Salmon, MBE, MS, FRCS
Consultant Surgeon Emeritus, Throat and Ear Department, Guy's Hospital, London

Henry Shaw, VRD, MA, FRCS
Consultant Ear, Nose and Throat Surgeon, The Royal National Throat, Nose and Ear Hospital and Royal Marsden Hospital, London; Honorary Consultant, Ear, Nose and Throat Surgeon, St. Mary's Hospital, London

P M Stell, CHM, FRCS
Professor of Otorhinolaryngology, University of Liverpool

David Wright, MA, MB, BCHIR, FRCS
Consultant Ear, Nose and Throat Surgeon, Royal Surrey County Hospital, Guildford

Contents

1 Methods of examination of the mouth and pharynx
Joselen Ransome

Introduction

Lighting is provided by a concave forehead mirror with a focal length of 23.6 cm (9 in) and a circular aperture of 2 cm ($\frac{3}{4}$ in) in diameter at the centre. Light is reflected from a 'bullseye' lamp, placed just behind the patient. The surgeon looks through the aperture so that his gaze is parallel with the reflected beam of light. Thus, the part under examination is brilliantly illuminated. The diameter of the mirror is 9 cm ($3\frac{1}{2}$ in), so the vision of the other eye is not obscured and binocular vision is retained. The head mirror was invented in the early part of the 19th century and is arguably the most significant advance in otolaryngology ever made, as without it the specialty could not have developed so early.

The bullseye lamp is suspended from a bracket on the wall, or attached to a stand with a heavy base. It is movable from side to side and backwards and forwards so that it may be placed in the proper position, 30 cm (1 ft) behind and to the left of the patient's left ear. This protects the patient from the considerable heat of the lamp and ensures that the beam does not fall directly on the eyes of the examiner, which are protected by the head mirror. An advantage of this form of lighting is that both hands are free to carry out the examination. It is useful to have an extending arm attached just below the bullseye lamp, for easy adjustment to obtain maximal illumination. Movement of the examiner's head is very much restricted, however, as the mirror must be kept in the beam of light. The patient must be moved to bring the part under examination into the appropriate position.

An alternative to the head mirror is a headlight. This may use either a standard battery or mains-operated low-voltage bulb, or may be a fibre-optic light. It is worn on the head with the light as close to the bridge of the nose as possible so that the beam of light coincides as nearly as possible with the line of vision. Illumination by this means is not as perfect as that provided by a head mirror, but the movement of the surgeon's head is not restricted, which is an advantage when operating under general anaesthesia. It is also convenient when visiting patients at home, when it may be run off a dry battery. Whatever form of lighting is used, illumination is greatly improved if the room is darkened.

Examination of the mouth

Lips

First, examine the lips and note whether the mouth is closed during quiet respiration. If it is open, note whether there are prominent upper incisor teeth, and a short upper lip, which may be familial characteristics predisposing to mouth breathing. Nasal or post-nasal obstruction of the airway necessitates mouth breathing, which may persist as a habit after the obstruction has been relieved unless corrected by exercises.

In cases of illness with a high temperature, the lips become dry and cracked. Chapped lips are common in cold weather and may cause a fissure in the middle of the lower lip, which bleeds easily and may lead to a permanent scar. *Angular stomatitis* may be associated with anaemia, as in the case of the Paterson–Brown Kelly (Plummer–Vinson) syndrome. It can also be due to a monilial infection, in turn caused by a slight trickle of saliva due to gaps in the lower dentition. This condition may be pre-cancerous so it is important to recognize and treat it. The upper lip is one of the commoner sites for an extragenital *chancre* of primary syphilis. Owing to the lack of secondary infection, it may remain quite a small lesion and be mistaken for a boil. It is associated with considerable 'rubbery' enlargement of the submandibular and cervical glands, which are distinct from the hard, fixed glands associated with an *epithelioma* which usually occurs on the lower lip. *Herpes simplex* affects the upper lip and is associated with the common cold. It appears as a group of blisters which become dry and cracked, with considerable discomfort and a tendency to bleed. *Harelip* is a cleft in the upper lip due to an incomplete fusion of one maxillary process with the globular process, and a fissure is present between the philtrum and the lateral part of the upper lip. It is frequently associated with a cleft palate. *Congenital haemangioma* may affect the lower lip and cause considerable deformity.

Oral cavity

The mouth is a delicate part of the body and the cooperation of the patient is essential if a satisfactory examination is to be achieved. Difficulty in carrying out the examination may arise because some people are hypersensitive in the mouth and throat to such an extent that they retch when they open their mouths and experience difficulty in cleaning their teeth. In such subjects, if the gag reflex is rather brisk, the examination may be facilitated by the use of lozenges of amethocaine, which the patient can suck quietly whilst another patient is being seen. The patient must be warned that his throat will become numb, as this feeling upsets some people; also, that he should not eat or drink until the effect has worn off, to avoid spill-over into the bronchial tree. Children rarely cause difficulty; if they are treated as adults they will behave like them. Should a child prove fractious, it may have to be restrained. The child is placed on the nurse's right thigh and her legs are crossed over the child's so that it cannot kick. With her left arm and hand she presses the child's arms to its chest, while her other hand is placed on the child's forehead so that its head may be held against her chest. An infant is easily restrained by wrapping it in a blanket, with the arms included.

The normally cooperative patient is instructed to open his mouth and take regular breaths, which should enable him to become perfectly relaxed. The left hand is rested on the patient's head, to place him in the correct position. With his right hand the surgeon places a tongue spatula into the angle of the mouth. This manoeuvre permits inspection of the buccal mucosa, the opening of the parotid duct, the teeth and gums, the tongue and the palate. Furthermore, introducing the spatula in this manner gives the patient confidence that it will not be pushed down his throat.

The buccal mucosa is moist and pink. In cases of *pulmonary tuberculosis* it is strikingly pale, as it is in those suffering from *anaemia*. If there is *stomatitis*, the mucosa is grossly congested and it may become dry, with a varying amount of debris adherent to it; this is common when the mouth has been subjected to a full course of radiotherapy. Thrush, due to infection with *Candida albicans*, was commonly seen in children, but adults taking oral antibiotics may also become infected. It covers considerable areas of the mucosa with milky white patches which are easily removed; examination of a smear taken from the lesion confirms the diagnosis. *Koplik spots* are white lesions, the size of a pin-head, surrounded by an area of erythema, and are diagnostic of measles before the morbilliform rash appears. *Leucoplakia* may affect the buccal mucosa or the 'milky streaks' of *Lichen planus* may be seen. *Bullae* due to pemphigus or erythema multiforme must be distinguished from *pemphigoid*. A *carcinomatous ulcer* has characteristic hard everted edges with a slough in the base, and the regional lymph nodes may by enlarged and hard, and fixed to surrounding structures. In the secondary stage of *syphilis*, there is a generalized upper respiratory infection, and the patient may complain of a 'nasty cold'. The buccal mucosa is congested and the 'snail track ulcers' may affect the cheeks and palate. There is a symmetrical rash on the body and limbs, which also affects the forehead when it is called the 'corona veneris'. There is a generalized lymph node involvement, and examination of a smear from an ulcer under dark-ground illumination reveals the *Treponema pallidum*. In *Addison's disease*, the mucosa is pigmented.

The mouth of the parotid duct is a slit in the mucosa opposite the second upper molar tooth. If there is an infection of the gland, as in epidemic parotitis (*mumps*), the orifice of the duct becomes red and congested, whilst in *suppurative parotitis*, on massaging the gland, pus may be seen coming from it as well. This is often a terminal event in a cachectic patient who has been suffering for a long time from a fatal disease. Rarely, a *calculus* may be present at the opening of the parotid duct. The duct can be palpated bi-manually to exclude a stone along its course, and any swelling of the mucosa of the cheek can be palpated in the same way, to determine its consistency and the nature of its surface and edges. Aphthous ulcers frequently occur on the inner aspect of the lips, and a common site for them is in the gingivolabial fold where they will be overlooked unless a deliberate search is made for them.

Examination of the teeth

The teeth and gums merit close attention. A child has 20 deciduous teeth, two incisors, one canine, and two molars on each side of the upper and lower jaws. Eruption of the deciduous teeth begins at six to nine months of age, the first to appear being the lower central incisors, and is completed by the eruption of the second molars at the age of 20–24 months, but there is considerable variation. The first permanent tooth is the first molar which erupts behind the deciduous molars, which are later replaced by the permanent premolars. It erupts at the age of six years, and is followed by the incisors. The dentition is completed by the eruption of the second molars at the age of 12 or 13 years, with the exception of the third molars, the 'wisdom teeth', which erupt between the ages of 18 and 25 years. In fact, the wisdom teeth may never erupt and instead become impacted. As a result of this a certain amount of pain may arise and this is quite often referred to the ear, causing the patient to consult an otologist. If no local cause for the pain is evident, and particularly if it is said to be in the vicinity of the ear rather than in the ear itself, the teeth must always come under suspicion; similar symptoms may be due to a carious lower molar. When the teeth and gums are heavily infected the tonsils and pharynx may become secondarily infected.

Much can be learned by an inspection of the individual permanent teeth. Ridges on the incisors may indicate a period of malnutrition during childhood, or a severe illness at some time. Congenital syphilis may cause Hutchinson teeth; the permanent incisors are affected. The biting edges are notched and become semilunar, while the teeth are deformed and become peg-shaped. There may be stigmata of the disease elsewhere: saddle-shaped deformity of the bridge of the nose, interstitial keratitis and perceptive deafness. Yellow staining or enamel hypoplasia may be a result of tetracycline therapy in early life.

The bite should be inspected to see that the teeth have a normal articulation or that dentures fit properly. The upper dental arch is somewhat larger than the lower so that the upper incisors overlap the lower when the jaw is closed. The molars of the upper and lower jaws come into exact apposition when the jaw is closed, however, and anything interfering with this arrangement, such as the loss of molar teeth or ill-fitting dentures, may throw the temporomandibular joints out of alignment. This may cause pain in the ear, and may also interfere with the function of the eustachian tube – Costen's syndrome (Costen, 1937).

The roots of the second premolar and first molar are in constant relationship with the floor of the maxillary sinus, and the first premolar and other molars may be related to a well developed sinus. An *apical abscess* may give rise to acute maxillary sinusitis, which is usually associated with a very foul nasal catarrh. Sometimes a root projects into the maxillary sinus, so that when the tooth is extracted an oro-antral fistula may form.

Dental sepsis is the commonest cause of swelling of the tissues of the face, sometimes erroneously thought to be due to acute maxillary sinusitis. This never causes swelling of the face unless it is complicated by osteomyelitis of the maxilla, a rare condition sometimes affecting infants.

Gingivitis, while usually due to local infection, may be a manifestation of some serious general illness. In acute leukaemia the gums become hypertrophied to such an extent that the teeth may be almost completely enveloped; gums in the edentulous are unaffected. Hypertrophied gums also occur in patients taking phenytoin. Scurvy gives rise to spontaneous haemorrhage from the gums which become infected so that the teeth are loosened and may fall out.

The commonest cause of gingivitis is lack of dental hygiene. The teeth should be scaled at regular intervals to remove tartar and they should be brushed regularly, ideally after every meal, to remove food particles. When the gums are infected they become spongy and tend to bleed easily. They may harbour Vincent's organisms, which may affect other parts of the mouth and throat. The tendency to bleed may only be noticed when the teeth are brushed, but some people appear to suck their gums while sleeping and complain of coughing up a little blood in the morning, while it is a well known trick of malingerers to feign haemoptysis. In all such cases it is wise to have a radiograph of the chest to exclude infection there. A blue line on the gum, about 1 mm from its free margin, indicates poisoning by a heavy metal, such as lead.

A complete examination of the dentition before general anaesthesia for tonsillectomy or endoscopy is a wise precaution, and a note should be made of loose teeth, crowns and caries. Such teeth can then be avoided or treated with caution when introducing endoscopes or a gag. A note should also be made of any pre-existing chipped teeth or caries and the patient's attention drawn to these pre-operatively.

Examination of the tongue and floor of the mouth

The patient is instructed to protrude his tongue as far as possible and it is noted whether it is straight or deviated. If the hypoglossal nerve is paralysed, the tongue will deviate towards the affected side and there is hemi-atrophy. Inability to protrude the tongue may be due to tongue-tie or to a neoplasm infiltrating the muscles.

The dorsum of the tongue is dried with a tongue-cloth, which facilitates inspection of the papillae. The patchwork markings of geographical tongue are immediately evident. The markings tend to migrate, making an ever-changing pattern; it is of no significance. A smooth clean tongue devoid of papillae is suggestive of some form of anaemia, often associated with the Paterson–Brown Kelly syndrome, and there may be angular stomatitis as well. In the case of pernicious anaemia, the tongue is red and beefy in contrast to the pallor of the buccal mucosa. In scarlet fever the tongue is at first coated with a yellow fur through which the inflamed papillae project, 'strawberry and cream tongue'; later, the fur disappears and the grossly inflamed organ is described as 'raspberry tongue'. 'Black hairy tongue' is caused by the appearance of long pigmented filaments of keratin on the dorsum of the tongue. It may cause a certain amount of discomfort but is of no significance, tending to clear up spontaneously. *Aphthous ulcers* may affect any part of the tongue; they are small ulcers with clean bases and heal spontaneously. They are extremely painful and cause much distress since they tend to come in crops over a period of weeks.

A *carcinoma* of the tongue may affect any part, and may appear as a lump pushing up the mucous membrane. In this case the movement of the tongue may be severely restricted and it may not be protruded. It may also appear in a patch of leucoplakia on the surface of the tongue, but sooner or later breaks down to form a typical malignant ulcer with hard everted edges and involvement of the cervical lymph nodes. In either case, palpation reveals it as a hard lesion which should lead to a biopsy to establish the diagnosis. *Chronic superficial glossitis* affects the dorsum of the tongue, and may have the appearance of a considerable area of leucoplakia. There are deep fissures on the tongue which may become malignant, and the patient should be under constant supervision so that a timely biopsy can lead to early diagnosis of carcinoma. It is said to be due to smoking, sepsis, syphilis or spirits, and surprisingly its incidence is markedly on the decline.

The tip of the tongue is now grasped with a tongue cloth and moved from side to side so that the edges may be examined. In the case of macroglossia, the edges are scalloped by indentations made by the teeth. The edge of the tongue is a common site for aphthous ulcers or a carcinoma. A dental ulcer lies opposite a jagged tooth, and the cause of the condition may be suggested by the patient. The tooth should receive immediate attention and if the ulcer is not healed within ten days it should be regarded as a carcinoma.

Towards the base of the tongue the vallate papillae may be seen. They are a row of large papillae formed in the shape of a 'V' with its apex at the foramen caecum. A *tumour* at this point in the midline may be an ectopic thyroid gland, or a cyst may form in connection with the thyroglossal duct. Behind the vallate papillae lies the pharyngeal portion of the tongue. The lymphoid deposits are large, and there may be large blood vessels as well. If a patient has cause to look at his tongue and protrudes it far enough to bring this part into view, he may well become alarmed, fearing that he has a neoplasm. This collection of lymphoid tissue is known as the lingual tonsil. It is usually separated from the palatine tonsil by a sulcus, but sometimes there is no clear line of demarcation. The lingual tonsils may become acutely infected, especially when the palatine tonsils have been removed. As with any lymphoid tissue, they may also be the site of lymphomatous or lymphosarcomatous change.

The patient is now told to put the tip of his tongue on his hard palate and the under surface is examined. The frenum can be seen in the midline running down a variable distance behind the tip, to the floor of the mouth. In some cases the frenum extends almost to the tip of the tongue, severely limiting its movement, and thus causing difficulty with speech, a condition called *tongue-tie*. It can be divided if causing symptoms. Abrasions of the frenum are sometimes seen in children suffering from whooping cough, for the tongue is strongly protruded with each cough and the frenum impinges on the lower incisor teeth.

In the floor of the mouth, the submandibular ducts are seen under the mucosa with their orifices on each side of the attachment of the frenum. They may be distended by *calculi*, or a calculus may present at one orifice. Calculi are easily palpated in the duct, and swelling of the submandibular salivary gland is readily identified by bi-manual palpation with one finger on the floor of the mouth and the tips of the fingers of the other hand on the skin of the submandibular triangle of the neck. An enlarged submandibular lymph node cannot be felt in this way because it does not lie in the floor of the mouth. *Ludwig's angina* may complicate dental infection, but it may arise spontaneously. There is cellulitis of the floor of the mouth, extending to the tissues beneath the chin, causing a hard brawny swelling. There may be respiratory embarrassment, and it is a potentially dangerous condition.

In certain cases it is necessary to test the sense of taste. The taste buds of the anterior two-thirds of the tongue are supplied by the chorda tympani, and those on the posterior one-third by the glossopharyngeal nerve. They are capable of appreciating only four basic sensations – sweet, acid, salt and bitter. Sweet and salt are most appreciated at the tip of the tongue, acid along the side, and bitter on the posterior part. Sugar, salt, vinegar and quinine are suitable substances for the test. The major part of the sense of taste is, of course, connected with the sense of smell, and it may be of importance from the medico-legal aspect in establishing the veracity of a man who claims that he has lost his senses of smell and taste as a result of a head injury, but admits that the basic sense is retained.

In electrogustometry a device is used by which a measured current can be applied to either side of the tongue to determine the threshold at which an acid taste is produced. As a quantitative test, the technique can be used in assessment of chorda tympani and facial nerve function.

Examination of the oropharynx and palate

When both sides of the mouth have been examined the spatula is placed on the dorsum of the tongue and depressed to bring the fauces, palatine tonsils, soft palate and oropharynx into view (*Figure 1.1*). The spatula should not encroach on the posterior one-third of the tongue, innervated by the glossopharyngeal nerve, as this induces a gag reflex. If the patient is properly relaxed little pressure is required, but if there is some resistance a firm and gradually increasing pressure may be exerted. Should it be necessary to change the position of the spatula, it should be lifted off the tongue and replaced in the desired position.

The hard palate forms the roof of the mouth and the floor of the nose while the alveolus lies in the base of the maxillary sinus. The soft palate is a muscular curtain which is attached to the posterior margin of the hard palate, from which it extends backwards to the level of the anterior pillar of the fauces with which it is in continuity. In the centre of its free margin there is an appendage of variable length, the uvula. The soft palate is freely mobile and by its elevation together with contraction of the pharyngeal muscles the nose can be completely shut off from the oropharynx during swallowing and speech. This mobility is very important and may be restricted by scarring caused by poor technique in operations for the removal of tonsils and adenoids, or by chronic disease, such as lupus, gummatous ulceration or malignant infiltration; it may also be affected by acute infection, such as quinsy.

Paralysis of the palate may be due to bulbar poliomyelitis, or to diphtheria, in which case it always recovers; or to demyelinating diseases or pseudobulbar palsy, of which it is usually but one manifestation. Unilateral paralysis is demonstrated by making the patient say 'Ah', when the palate is pulled towards the sound side. If both sides are paralysed it may be necessary to make the patient gag to demonstrate it, and paralysis of the pharynx may be noted at the same time. When immobility of the palate is bilateral, there may be serious disability owing to regurgitation of food and fluid through the nose. If the pharynx is involved as well, this may necessitate a tracheostomy and tube feeding. When movement of the palate is restricted by local scarring, the patient may complain of post-nasal drip, for it is by the free movement of the palate that secretions in the nasopharynx are aided in their passage into the oropharynx.

Cleft palate is represented in its least severe form by a bifid uvula, but the soft palate and hard palate may be involved and it may be associated with a hare-lip. These cases require the services of a plastic surgeon.

On the soft palate there may be a unilateral *herpetic eruption* sometimes associated with geniculate herpes, the Ramsay Hunt syndrome. *Herpangina*, due to infection with a Coxsackie A virus, causes lesions resembling aphthous ulcers but rather larger and usually affecting the free margin of the palate. Other parts affected are the pillars of the fauces, the pharyngeal wall and the roof of the mouth. The hard palate is brought into view by tilting the patient's head backwards. A high arch to the palate is associated with a crowded dentition, causing prominence of the upper incisor teeth and a short upper lip predisposing to open mouth. An orthodontist can do much to remedy the condition, which is usually hereditary.

Aphthous ulcers may affect any part of the mouth, but *ulcers* on the palate may occasionally be due to syphilitic or tuberculous infection. Secondary syphilis causes 'snail track' ulcers associated with mucous patches; a gumma forms an ulcer with punched-out edges and a slough in the base. It erodes bone and may cause a perforation of the hard palate; it is relatively painless. Tuberculous ulcers are shallow, with rolled edges, and are extremely painful. Lupus usually affects the soft palate; in some areas there is activity with the formation of 'apple jelly' nodules, while other parts heal with gross scarring causing considerable deformity.

Papilloma is a fairly common tumour on the soft palate, frequently pedunculated and arising near the uvula. Angioma is uncommon unless it is part of a generalized angiomatosis. Torus palatinus is a bony outgrowth in the midline of the hard palate; it is of no consequence unless it interferes with the fitting of a denture, when it should be removed.

A *fibrolipoma* usually occurs in the soft palate; it has a lobulated outline which is easily discernible on palpation.

An *epithelioma* breaks down to form a typical ulcer with hard everted edges and a dirty base; either the soft or hard palate may be involved, and perforation may occur. The cervical lymph nodes may be enlarged, hard, and fixed to surrounding structures. A reticulum-celled sarcoma or fibrosarcoma may also be encountered. Malignant tumours in the nose or antrum may cause depression of the soft palate and even ulcerate through it, causing a perforation. A carcinoma of the maxillary sinus may push the molar or premolar teeth down into the mouth; they become loosened and may fall out. *Tumours of the minor salivary glands* may also occur on the palate, and are more likely to be malignant than tumours of the major salivary glands. A tumour of the *deep lobe of the parotid* may also present as a palatal swelling.

Wounds of the palate may be due to gunshot, sometimes self-inflicted. In children, they may be the result of a fall with something like a pencil in the mouth.

The fauces and palatine tonsils are now examined, with the posterior wall of the oropharynx. The anterior pillar of the fauces is formed by the palatoglossus muscle, and the posterior pillar by the palatopharyngeus muscle. The mucous membrane is pink, like that of the palate. Injection of the vessels in the mucosa of the anterior pillar is suggestive of infection in the tonsils. The tonsils are paired organs which have a remarkable degree of symmetry. Their surfaces are smooth though usually the orifices of the crypts can be seen. Their size is very variable and of no consequence unless they attain such proportions as to interfere with the functions of the alimentary and respiratory tracts, a condition not commonly seen today, but nevertheless potentially dangerous if the possibility of chronic hypoxia is not recognized. The best guide to their condition is provided by the history, but there are certain characteristics which suggest that they are the site of chronic infection.

Chronic infection is suspected when the tonsils appear redder than the buccal mucosa, and oedematous. It is confirmed when pus can be expressed from them. Enlargement of the tonsillar lymph node supports the diagnosis. Asymmetry of the tonsils suggests that one of them is undergoing a pathological process, possibly neoplastic.

Acute pharyngitis may affect both the tonsils and the pharynx. *Acute follicular*

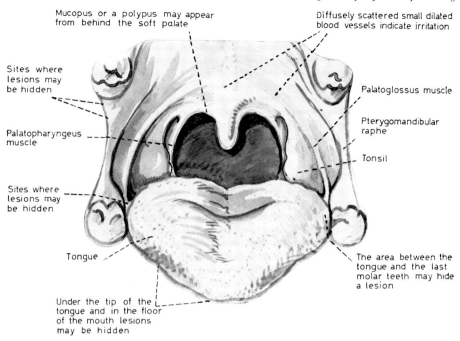

Mucopus or a polypus may appear from behind the soft palate

Diffusely scattered small dilated blood vessels indicate irritation

Sites where lesions may be hidden

Palatoglossus muscle

Pterygomandibular raphe

Palatopharyngeus muscle

Tonsil

Sites where lesions may be hidden

Tongue

The area between the tongue and the last molar teeth may hide a lesion

Under the tip of the tongue and in the floor of the mouth lesions may be hidden

Figure 1.1   Parts of the mouth and pharynx, showing areas of special interest on clinical examination

tonsillitis is characterized by white spots overlying the mouths of the crypts, while *acute parenchymatous tonsillitis* causes acute congestion of the tonsil with some oedema. The membrane of acute *diphtheria* is firmly adherent to the tonsil, and attempts to remove it lead to bleeding; it may also extend over the adjacent palate. This is a potentially lethal disease and it is essential that a throat swab should be taken in every acute throat infection to exclude it from the diagnosis. The anginose form of *glandular fever* resembles it, but this can be diagnosed by means of a blood count or Paul Bunnell reaction. Vincent's infection may occasionally cause considerable destruction of the tonsil, and the membrane appears to be inlaid rather than laid on the surface; the organisms can be identified by examination of a smear taken from the lesion. *Peritonsillar abscess (quinsy)* causes the anterior pillar of the fauces in the region of the upper pole to bulge and the tonsil is displaced medially. It must be distinguished from a *parapharyngeal abscess*, when the whole lateral wall of the pharynx is displaced. Trismus, inability to open the mouth except to a limited extent owing to reflex spasm of the masseter muscle, which can be caused by either a peritonsillar or a parapharyngeal abscess, may make examination and treatment of the patient difficult. Trismus may also be the first manifestation of tetanus.

In acute pharyngitis there may be reddening of the pharyngeal mucosa without involvement of the pharyngeal tonsils, but with reddening and hypertrophy of the lymphoid follicles on the posterior pharyngeal wall. This condition may also occur when the pharyngeal tonsils have been removed. A stream of mucopus trickling down the pharynx may be due to an acute nasal or sinus infection, while hypertrophy of the lateral bands of lymphoid tissue situated between the lateral and posterior walls of the pharynx is suggestive of chronic nasal or sinus infection. *Acute retropharyngeal abscess* occurs in children as a complication of acute infection of the throat or acute otitis media, or it may arise spontaneously. It is due to suppuration in the retropharyngeal lymph nodes which lie to either side of the midline. It presents as a lateral swelling of the posterior wall of the pharynx and may cause difficulty in swallowing and breathing. In infants it is not always easily seen, but can be palpated with the finger. This condition cannot arise in adults, for the retropharyngeal lymph nodes atrophy in early childhood. A midline retropharyngeal abscess may, however, complicate tuberculous infection of the cervical vertebrae, presenting as a bulging of the posterior pharyngeal wall.

Atrophic pharyngitis is often associated with atrophic rhinitis; there is an excessive airway which causes the mucosa to become dry, with destruction of the mucous glands, which aggravates the situation. The process may extend as far as the larynx and trachea. In the pharynx the mucosa is atrophic and thin, so that the pharynx appears large and the outline of the cervical vertebrae may be clearly seen. The diminution of mucous secretion leads to the formation of crusts, with secondary infection and foetor oris.

Keratosis may affect the tonsils, pharynx and tongue, and may even extend to the larynx. There are white keratin processes firmly adherent to the mucosa, which may be mistaken for the follicles of acute tonsillitis. It causes unnecessary alarm, for it is a benign condition which may disappear spontaneously.

Retention cysts in the tonsil appear as yellow smooth tumours and may cause some alarm to the patient; they are easily evacuated after the throat has been sprayed with a local anaesthetic. A *papilloma* may arise from the surface of the tonsil, but otherwise it is rarely affected by simple tumours.

Ulceration of the tonsil is commonly due to an *epithelioma*. It breaks down to form an ulcer with hard everted edges and a slough in the base. The cervical lymph nodes may be involved, and this may be the reason for the patient seeking advice. *Lymphosarcoma* may occur at any age and cause a swelling of the tonsil, but it rarely ulcerates. The cervical nodes may be enlarged but are not very hard. *Syphilis* may cause ulceration of the tonsil. A primary chancre is not unknown, and in the secondary stage there may be ulcers and mucous patches on the surface. A gumma causes considerable destruction of the tonsil, with a punched-out ulcer with clean edges and a slough in the base.

Examination of the nasopharynx

Examination of the nasopharynx is carried out using a post-nasal mirror (*Figure 1.2*). It is warmed by holding it with the glass in the flame of a methylated spirit lamp until it is sufficiently warm to prevent condensation from the patient's breath. The temperature of the mirror is checked by applying it to the hand, and if the patient appears to be apprehensive he may be reassured by placing it on his cheek. The tongue is depressed with a spatula and the patient told to relax and breathe quietly when the soft palate should fall away from the posterior pharyngeal wall to expose the nasopharynx. The mirror is inserted below and behind the free margin of the soft palate. If the uvula is long, it is advisable to insert the mirror on either side of it. The shaft of the instrument may be steadied against the angle of the mouth, but the mirror must not touch the base of the tongue or the posterior pharyngeal wall, which causes retching so that no view can be obtained. The largest mirror which the patient can accommodate should be used, for not only the extent of the view but the brilliance of the illumination depends upon the size of the mirror.

Occasionally, owing to scarring or narrowness of the pharynx, it is impossible to obtain a view of the nasopharynx in this way even in a cooperative adult. The difficulty can usually be overcome in the following way. The oropharynx and one side of the nose are thoroughly prepared with a local anaesthetic, preferably by sucking a benzocaine lozenge and spraying the nose with five per cent cocaine. A small soft rubber or plastic catheter (Jacques type) is passed through the anaesthetized side of the nose until the tip appears in the oropharynx, then this is withdrawn through the mouth leaving the other end hanging out of the nose. Gentle traction by the patient or a nurse on both ends of the catheter will now result in forward retraction of the soft palate, and it will be possible to obtain a good view with a post-nasal mirror. None of this is too cumbersome or time-consuming to carry out in an ordinary clinic and is infinitely preferable to unnecessary admissions for examination under a general anaesthetic. The patient cooperates very well provided care is taken to achieve really good local anaesthesia. It is unfortunate that this examination can rarely be carried out in children. It can give valuable information about the adenoids, but few children are able to cooperate sufficiently and the smallness of the parts militates against it. On no account should the adenoids be palpated in a conscious child. The size of the adenoids and of the airway can be accurately assessed by taking a lateral radiograph of the nasopharynx to show the soft tissues (Zwiefach, 1954).

The first landmark to look for when the mirror is in position is the posterior end of the nasal septum, which is always in the midline. This is followed up to the vault of the

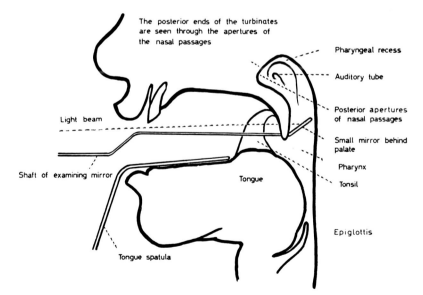

Figure 1.2 Clinical examination of the nasal part of the pharynx; areas of importance on clinical examination

nasopharynx when the adenoids, if present, are brought into view. By turning the mirror slightly to each side both posterior nares may be inspected. The posterior ends of the inferior turbinates can always be seen and usually the posterior ends of the middle turbinates as well. A trickle of pus from the middle meatus is suggestive of infection in the maxillary, ethmoid or frontal sinuses, whereas if it is seen high up in the vault of the nasopharynx the sphenoid is suspect. This emphasizes the importance of this examination in assessing the state of the nose. Nasal secretions are propelled backwards into the nasopharynx by the cilia of the nasal mucosa, so abnormal secretions may first be seen here.

If the nose is full of *polypi* they may be seen protruding from the posterior nares while an antrochoanal polypus, arising in the maxillary sinus and entering the nose through the ostium, is directed backwards to appear in the posterior nares. By turning the mirror a little further to each side, the eustachian cushions are brought into view and conditions such as neoplasm, which may obstruct the tubes, may be seen.

A *carcinoma* is the commonest tumour in the nasopharynx and is seen as an ulcerating mass, either in the roof or on the lateral wall where it may involve the eustachian cushion and cause deafness and earache. There may be an offensive blood-stained nasal discharge. The upper deep cervical lymph nodes are commonly involved and may be hard and fixed to surrounding structures. A *sarcoma* presents a similar appearance. A *plasmacytoma* is a rare tumour resembling a carcinoma, but it does not normally give rise to metastases. A *lymphoepithelioma* differs from other tumours in that the primary growth is very small and may only give the impression that one lateral wall of the nasopharynx is slightly more prominent than the other. There is sometimes involvement of the eustachian tube, but the feature of the condition is the gross enlargement of the upper deep cervical lymph nodes; they are not as hard as those involved by carcinoma. A *fibro-angioma* appears in the roof of the nasopharynx, commonly in youths in their early teens. It is not malignant but may cause a good deal of damage by invasion of neighbouring structures, such as the orbit. A *chondroma* or *myxochondroma* may arise in connection with the eustachian cushion, and a *hamartoma* sometimes occurs in this region.

The nasopharyngoscope (*Figure 1.3*) is similar to a cystoscope with an eyepiece and a light and prism, and a side-window at its distal end. The direction in which the

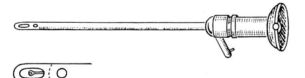

Figure 1.3 An electric naso-pharyngoscope

window is pointing is indicated by a small knob on the eyepiece. It is introduced along the floor of the nose which has first been sprayed with a local anaesthetic. Deformities of the septum, particularly septal spurs, may prevent introduction of the instrument. It gives a rather limited field of view. More recently the introduction of flexible fibre-optic endoscopy has provided the possibility of better inspection by this route, and the facility for biopsy.

Examination of the laryngopharynx

The patient is asked to protrude the tongue as far as possible, and the tip is now grasped with a tongue cloth and pulled gently forward, but not so far as to damage the frenum with the lower incisor teeth, which will be painful and result in loss of cooperation. The patient is made to flex his cervical spine and extend the atlanto-occipital joint so as to bring the mouth and pharynx as nearly as possible into alignment. The patient is now asked to breathe quietly in and out through the mouth,

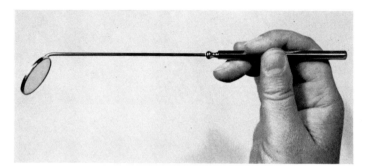

Figure 1.4   Holding the mirror for examination of the lower pharynx

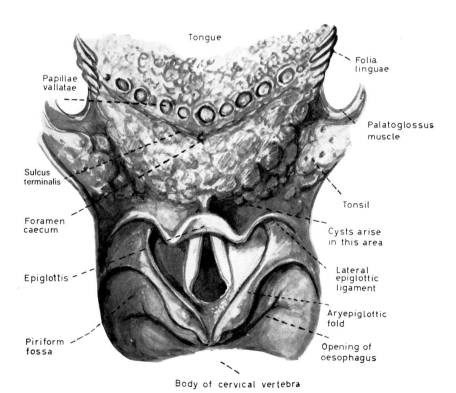

Figure 1.5   The lower pharynx seen in the examining mirror; areas of importance in clinical examination

and to concentrate on breathing, in order to prevent the gag reflex. A laryngeal mirror (*Figure 1.4*), previously warmed by holding the glass over a methylated-spirit lamp, is introduced into the mouth and applied to the soft palate with firm pressure until it is in contact with the posterior pharyngeal wall. The mirror is adjusted to inspect the back of the tongue as far as the base of the epiglottis (*Figure 1.5*). The space in front of the anterior aspect of the epiglottis, the vallecula, is sometimes the site of a *carcinoma*. The base of the tongue and the adjacent pharyngeal walls are carefully examined for any sign of tumour or ulceration. By making the patient say 'E' the aryepiglottic folds are drawn medially and the pyriform fossae are brought into view. They may be ulcerated by carcinoma or *Behçet's disease*. A post-cricoid carcinoma cannot be seen unless it is very advanced, when an ulcerating mass may be seen behind the larynx. However, there may be an accumulation of saliva in the pyriform fossae if there is an obstruction below in the post-cricoid region or upper oesophagus. A useful sign in this condition is the loss of the crepitus, normally elicited by moving the larynx from side to side across the cervical spine, owing to the mass interposed between the structures. The neck should now be palpated for evidence of enlargement of the cervical lymph nodes.

Radiological examination

Radiological examination of every part of the mouth and pharynx can provide essential diagnostic information. The normal radiographic appearances are described in Volume 1.

References

Costen, J. B. (1937). *Mississippi Doctor*, **15**, 33
Zwiefach, E. (1954). *Journal of Laryngology and Otology*, **68**, 758

2 Diseases of the mouth
David Downton

Oral hygiene

On examining the mouth, note must first of all be taken of the general state of
hygiene. Chronic oral sepsis, if severe, can easily mask other pathology. Even in
edentulous mouths ill-fitting and uncleaned dentures can produce chronic irritation.

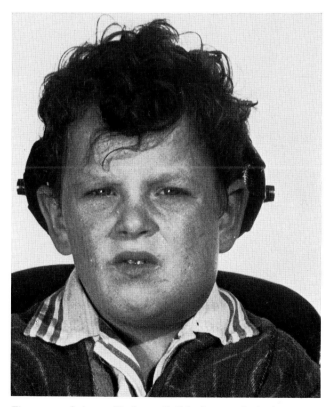

Figure 2.1 Submandibular cellulitis from apical abscess on
mandibular deciduous molar tooth

In cases of neglected oral hygiene, food debris collects around the teeth, and there are heavy deposits of salivary calculus. Irregular teeth, partial dentures, and carious teeth help to make this condition worse, and in the long run gingivitis with periodontal disease will ensue.

Mouth-breathing can cause gingivitis by preventing the normal flow of saliva over the gingivae, which become dry and cracked – secondary infection then follows. With mouth-breathing, even if nasal obstruction is cured, the habit may persist.

During eruption of deciduous teeth the oral mucosa is particularly prone to inflammatory processes, and particular attention should be paid to oral hygiene at this time. Eruption of the permanent teeth usually occurs without complication apart from the third molar, or wisdom tooth. In particular the mandibular wisdom tooth is not infrequently impacted, or there is insufficient space for its normal eruption. A gum flap, therefore, presents over part of the tooth and this can lead to severe acute infection, which may proceed to a *cellulitis* of the face or neck.

One should also bear in mind when examining a mouth, that even when it appears to be well cared for a tooth with a large filling may have an apical infection which can result in abscess formation. *Apical abscesses* usually point into the oral cavity, but may occasionally point extra-orally (*Figure 2.1*). It should not be forgotten that due to the proximity of the apices of upper molars and premolars to the floor of the antrum abscesses on these teeth may point therein and present a picture of maxillary sinusitis.

Pain referred to the ear or face might be due to dental causes, especially with impacted lower wisdom teeth.

In the normal healthy mouth many organisms are found, but when chronic oral sepsis is present their numbers are increased enormously.

With severe oral sepsis infection can spread along the normal anatomical pathways which are connected with the mouth, and when the gingivae and periodontal membrane are involved organisms can enter the systemic circulation.

Congenital and developmental anomalies

Fordyce spots

These present as small elevated yellowish spots on the buccal mucosa. They are due to sebaceous glands and are more apparent in adult life, being present in about 60 per cent of the population.

Malformations of the tongue

Bifid tongue is rare and due to failure of the lateral tubercles of the mandibular arch to coalesce during development.

Macroglossia is uncommon, and usually is seen in association with cretinism, mongolism and acromegaly. A lymphangioma of the tongue can also produce severe enlargement.

The treatment is to remove a wedge-shaped portion of the tongue, but when a *lymphangioma* (*Figure 2.2*) is the cause radiotherapy should be considered.

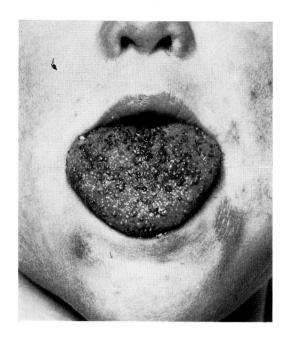

Figure 2.2   Lymphangioma of
the tongue

Microglossia is a smallness or complete absence of the tongue.

Ankyloglossia is tongue-tie, due to maldevelopment of the frenum, or of the anterior two-thirds of the tongue. If severe enough to cause difficulty in articulation, the tongue-tie should be freed surgically before the patient learns to speak.

Median rhomboid 'glossitis' presents as a smooth oval reddish patch in the midline of the dorsum of the tongue anterior to the circumvallate papillae. It is due to the persistence of the tuberculum impar on the tongue's surface.

Furrowed tongue is a congenital fissuring of the dorsum of the tongue and no treatment is indicated unless soreness is produced by particles of food debris collecting and stagnating in the fissures. In such cases regular hygiene of the tongue should be applied.

Accessory thyroid tissue may present as a lingual thyroid at the back of the tongue, as a purplish-red swelling, or may be found deeply placed along the line of the original thyroglossal tract. *Thyroglossal cysts* appear anywhere in this midline tract between the suprasternal notch and the foramen caecum of the tongue.

The treatment of the cysts is by removal. *Lingual thyroid* should be removed only if it causes bleeding, or is so large as to endanger the airway, and it must first be determined whether the gland itself is present and functioning.

See also page 29, 'Congenital telangiectasia'.

Stomatitis

Inflammatory conditions of the oral mucosa can be produced by local or systemic disease. The contents of the oral cavity may be involved as a whole or only by discrete lesions. The tongue (glossitis) and/or gingivae (gingivitis) frequently present lesions when the remainder of the oral mucosa is normal. Clinical diagnosis is frequently possible, but in some cases this is extremely difficult and one may have to resort to haematological, serological, bacteriological and histopathological investigations.

Traumatic injuries to the gingivae and oral mucosa can be caused by very stiff bristles on a toothbrush, or by fish bones becoming detached and embedded in the mucosa. Cheek-biting, ill-fitting dentures and jagged teeth also play their part. These lesions may vary somewhat in appearance but usually the cause can easily be ascertained and when the aetiological factor is removed in the normal healthy individual, healing occurs rapidly.

Severe chronic mucosal damage can be produced by old, ill-fitting and dirty dentures. In the sulci gross hyperplasia may be produced which require surgical removal prior to new dentures being constructed. The mucosa of the dorsum of the tongue may lose its normal papillary appearance and present a smooth shiny surface due to constant trauma against a smooth and dirty palatal surface of a denture.

Thermal injuries from hot foods, or *chemical injuries* following the use of medicaments, may present varied lesions but the history will frequently give the diagnosis. Healing may take from several days to several weeks according to the severity of the damage.

Tobacco smoking may well have an effect on the mucosa, varying from an inflamed patch to one of excessively keratinized epithelium possibly leading to leucoplakia. The treatment will depend on the severity of the lesion. In early cases one should attempt to prevent the patient continuing the habit, but when leucoplakia is present, the treatment may well be surgical (*see* 'Leucoplakia', p. 26).

Radiotherapy produces an inflammatory reaction in the skin and mucosa. The tongue frequently becomes smooth, with atrophy of the papillae. Dryness of the oral mucosa is apparent when the salivary glands have been affected. The dryness of the mouth is extremely unpleasant and may make the wearing of dentures very difficult or even impossible. The mucosa frequently cracks and ulcerates. At this stage the topical use of an antibiotic with hydrocortisone may be helpful. The patient must be instructed in strict oral hygiene. The coating of the lips and mucosa with a lubricant, such as liquid paraffin, may prove beneficial, especially when applied last thing at night.

Avitaminosis

Deficiency of the vitamin B_2 complex

In severe deficiencies of riboflavin and nicotinic acid, pellagra is the end-result. This condition is rarely found in civilized countries, although milder degrees of the deficiency can be found among old people who live alone and neglect their diet. The milder degrees of the deficiency have a less severe clinical picture than pellagra, the lips becoming red, swollen, painful and cracked, especially at the angles of the mouth. There is a painful glossitis, the tongue becoming inflamed and fissured.

Deficiency of vitamin C

Deficiency of vitamin C produces scurvy. This is uncommon today in civilized countries, but it may occur in elderly people living alone. When the teeth are present the gingivae become hyperaemic and swollen, and haemorrhagic when ulceration occurs.

Stomatitis associated with specific micro-organisms

Acute coccal stomatitis presents as an acute gingivitis which is often superimposed upon a pre-existing chronic inflammatory condition of the gingivae. The gingival margins are inflamed and may be painful and ulcerated. A false membrane appearing greyish-white may form on the gingivae, and when detached it leaves a raw bleeding area. In severe cases the patient may have a pyrexia and a local adenitis. The condition may sometimes be mistaken for Vincent's infection, but lacks the typical halitosis associated with this disease. Diagnosis can be confirmed and clarified by smear examination.

The treatment is strict attention to oral hygiene, and systemic antibiotic therapy may be necessary in severe cases.

Acute ulcerative stomatitis (Vincent's angina). It has been suggested that a virus is the actual exciting cause for this condition with the true Vincent's organisms being secondary invaders. However, these organisms are always present in the fully developed clinical condition. Vincent's stomatitis showed a marked increase during the two World Wars and in World War I was so prevalent in the trenches that it was called 'trench mouth'. These facts lead one to think that it is more likely to appear when there is a low general resistance to infection together with a deficiency of certain vitamins and when the oral hygiene of the individual has been neglected.

A marked foetor is present and the ulceration commences on the gingival margins, usually between the teeth, spreading and coalescing to involve the rest of the gingivae. The soft palate, tonsils and faucial pillars can also be affected (Vincent's angina).

The condition is painful and a lymphadenitis is usually present. In severe cases the pyrexia and malaise may be well marked.

In severe cases systemic antibiotic therapy may be necessary; metronidazole by mouth is an excellent antibiotic for this condition. Daily treatment by a dental surgeon is initially essential, all calculus being removed from the teeth and the oral hygiene restored. The local application of 10 vol/vol hydrogen peroxide followed by gentle atomizing or rinsing is of value.

After the acute phase has passed, the teeth and gingivae must be treated, otherwise a chronic Vincent's infection will remain with a tendency to acute exacerbations.

Tuberculosis in the oral cavity. A primary lesion in the mouth is extremely rare but it may be seen as a single painful ulcer on the gingivae, tongue or buccal mucosa. Biopsy will give the diagnosis.

Syphilis may present in the mouth in any of its stages. *Primary chancre* may occur on the tongue or lips. *Secondary syphilis* occurs on the oral mucosa and palate as snail track ulcers while mucous patches may also appear on the tongue. *Gumma* may occur in the tertiary stage of the disease usually on the palate or tongue, in the midline.

Fungal infections of the mouth

Monilia (thrush) is the commonest and is due to *Candida albicans*. The lesions occur on the oral mucosa and tongue. It is more frequently found in infants or debilitated adults. The lesions appear as white or greyish papules which frequently coalesce to form a membrane which is surrounded by a slight erythema. The membrane can be removed leaving a raw area.

Nystatin used locally in tablet form is curative in many cases and the local application of a two per cent solution of gentian violet may be helpful with infants. Good nursing is important. Angular cheilitis is not infrequently described as one of the lesions produced by monilia, but in the vast majority of these cases the causal agent is faulty dentures which do not support the soft tissues sufficiently, and drooping at the angles of the mouth occurs. This results in cracking of the skin and mucosa in this region and monilia are secondary invaders. It is, therefore, essential to exclude faulty dentures prior to any other treatment.

Actinomycosis, blastomycosis and *histoplasmosis* also occur within the oral cavity, but are extremely rare.

Scarlet fever and diphtheria also have their own oral lesions but can be diagnosed from the general signs and symptoms of the patient.

Stomatitis associated with virus diseases

Many well known virus diseases such as measles and chicken-pox have oral lesions, but there are several that may have oral lesions alone.

Catarrhal stomatitis

This usually arises in conjunction with coryza, pharyngeal infection or one of the exanthemata.

The oral cavity shows signs of inflammation similar to those found in the pharynx. Lack of oral hygiene is always a contributory factor.

Herpes

Herpes simplex
In this condition, small vesicles appear which break down to form shallow painful ulcers. The margins of the ulcers are hyperaemic and they may be found in any part of the oral mucosa. One of the diagnostic points is that they are commonly seen in the hard palate, especially round the palatal gingivae when teeth are present.

Recurrent herpetic stomatitis
This may appear in an herpetic subject following quite mild trauma by a toothbrush or the injection of a local anaesthetic. The lesions are similar to those found in herpes simplex.

Recurrent herpes labialis
A well-known lesion frequently referred to as a 'cold sore'. The initial symptom is a

burning feeling in the lip, followed by vesicle formation which finally breaks down to form a crust. This separates after several days, leaving an erythematous area which disappears a few days later. The lesion occurs on the skin at its junction with the oral mucosa.

For typical herpetic stomatitis a mouth-wash of two per cent aureomycin can be used. This in no way treats the herpes, but it deals with the secondary infection and removes a considerable amount of discomfort.

Herpes zoster

Whereas in herpes simplex the causal agent is the herpes simplex virus, in zoster it is thought the causal agent is the virus responsible for chicken-pox. The oral lesions which occur in herpes zoster are clinically indistinguishable from those of herpes simplex.

Coxsackie virus infections

These include herpangina, hand-foot-and-mouth disease and acute nodular meningitis. These infections have oral lesions similar to those found on the fauces and oropharynx.

Allergic stomatitis

This often occurs as part of a generalized allergic reaction to certain foodstuffs.

Chemical or contact allergy

Lipstick is a well-known cause of cheilitis and glossitis, and reaction in the buccal mucosa might follow the use of certain antiseptics in mouth-washes or toothpastes. Aspirin, iodine and acriflavin are some examples of drugs that may produce such a reaction.

Dental materials, especially acrylic resins used in dentures, are very rarely the cause of an allergic reaction.

Stomatitis due to metals and drugs

Metals

Mercury and bismuth

Stomatitis may occur when these metals are used medicinally and is not uncommon in workers handling them. The gingivae become red and swollen and if left untreated the periodontal membrane and alveolar bone become involved. A black or purplish line appears around the gingival margin due to the fact that the soluble salts circulating in the blood come into contact with hydrogen sulphide formed during the decomposition of debris around the teeth. The insoluble sulphide of the metal is then deposited in the gingivae. If untreated the condition is progressive and may lead to necrosis of the jaws and involvement of the salivary glands.

Lead
The lesions are similar to those produced by bismuth and may occur in painters, lead metal workers and small children.

Gold
Still occasionally used for the treatment of certain arthritic conditions and may produce a gingivitis.

Drugs

Epanutin
Used in treatment of epilepsy may produce a considerable gingival hyperplasia which in some cases covers the teeth. Inflammation is not a primary effect of the drug but where present, it has arisen from other sources. The drug should be stopped if possible and a gingivectomy may be necessary. If the drug is continued after a gingivectomy is performed the condition will recur.

Antidepressants
Certain of these drugs produce oral symptoms, usually associated with a dry mouth which may be severe.

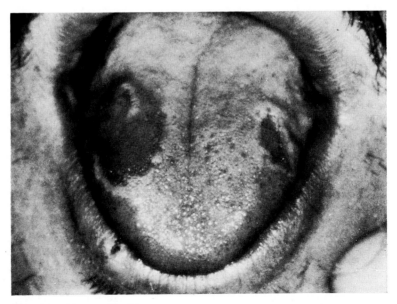

Figure 2.3   Geographical tongue

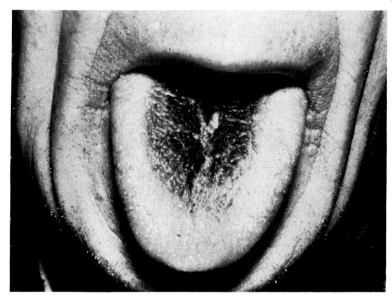

Figure 2.4   Black hairy tongue

Stomatitis and oral lesions of obscure aetiology

Geographical tongue (erythema migrans linguae) (Figure 2.3) presents as reddish patches surrounded by yellow elevated borders. It occurs on the dorsum of the tongue and frequently several patches may develop and coalesce. The characteristic feature of this condition is that the configuration changes from time to time. The filiform papillae have disappeared from the red areas, but at the borders they have become more prolific producing the typical appearance. The condition may start in childhood and continue throughout life, or it may remit spontaneously.

The aetiology is unknown and it rarely gives rise to symptoms.

Hairy tongue (Figure 2.4) presents on the dorsum of the tongue as a profusion of fine 'hairs' usually black or brown in colour. These hairs are produced by an overgrowth of the filiform papillae and can be as much as 1.25 cm in length. The discolouration is possibly due to chromogenic bacteria, tobacco smoking or medicaments.

The aetiology is not understood but it has been noticed to follow the local application of antibiotics or oxidizing antiseptics, especially if they have been used for some time.

The treatment is the removal of the filaments by gentle scraping and the patient is then instructed to brush the tongue twice a day with a soft brush using a weak solution of bicarbonate of soda.

Recurrent ulcerative (aphthous) stomatitis

This is a common condition which can occur in varying degrees of severity. There is no definite known cause. Viruses, psychogenic and endocrine disturbances, and the anaemias have all been said to play a part, but more recent work indicates the condition is probably the result of an auto-immune reaction.

Small vesicles are the earliest sign to appear but may not be noticed. Ulceration soon occurs, leaving an ulcer which varies in size from that of a pin-head to one 2–3 cm. There may be a single lesion or several occurring in all parts of the oral cavity. The ulcers have a sloughing base and a marked area of hyperaemia around the edge. They are usually extremely painful and may last for several days. Healing is usually complete in 14 days although occasionally they have been known to last for some weeks. In patients suffering from this condition mild trauma may bring on an ulcer.

Every effort should be made to discover in these patients if there is any underlying general condition such as nutritional deficiency or anaemia. Small isolated lesions may require no more treatment than re-assurance. In more severe cases hydrocortisone lozenges have been used with reported success. Strict attention to oral hygiene is important and in the isolated lesion the single application of a caustic such as phenol or silver nitrate shortens the duration and removes the pain.

Behçet's syndrome

The cause of this disease is not known. The ulceration that occurs in the mouth is of the aphthous type and there are also ulceration of the external genitalia and lesions on the eyes. Neurological manifestations may appear after a delay of two to five years and resemble an encephalitis or an acute lesion of the brain stem. Blindness may result from the ocular lesions.

The treatment is non-specific but steroids have been tried and are perhaps the drugs of choice at present.

Reiter's syndrome

This is a severe and rare disease, the cause of which is obscure, but bacteriologically the micro-organisms found are similar to those in Vincent's stomatitis. Severe

Gangrenous stomatitis (cancrum oris)

This is a severe and rare disease the cause of which is obscure, but bacteriologically the micro-organisms found are similar to those in Vincent's stomatitis. Severe malnutrition is the real predisposing cause, the condition being found more commonly in the underdeveloped and starving countries.

Stomatitis is usually the first sign of this disease with ulceration rapidly occurring, followed by gangrene. This causes the destruction of whole areas of the cheeks with involvement of the maxilla and mandible. Foetor is intense and the patient extremely ill.

The use of systemic penicillin has revolutionized the treatment of this condition, but the affected areas should be cleaned with five per cent solution of sodium bicarbonate and attention to oral hygiene is of first importance. An increasing number of these patients now survive and plastic surgery is frequently necessary for the repair of the defects produced.

Pemphigus

Pemphigus is a rare condition and may occur in acute or chronic form. It is characterized by the formation of bullous lesions on the skin and oral mucosa. Its origin is not known.

Several types of pemphigus have been described and classification of these has been attempted.

Pemphigus vulgaris is the more common form and is characterized by the formation of large flaccid bullae which rupture easily, leaving a denuded area which tends to increase in size by progressive detachment of the epidermis. Extensive oral lesions are not infrequently the first sign of the disease. In the days before cortisone therapy the lesions often failed to heal and death resulted within several months. Slight friction of the mucosa produces separation of the superficial from the deep layers of the epithelium (Nikolsky's sign) which means that the wearing of dentures and even normal oral hygiene is impossible. There are variations of pemphigus vulgaris but the signs and symptoms described are similar in them all.

Benign mucous membrane pemphigoid

In this condition there is formation of bullae in the mucosa similar to those found in pemphigus vulgaris, and the eyes may also be involved. The condition runs a chronic benign course but severe scarring may result and if the eyes are involved blindness might follow. The diagnosis and the differentiation between pemphigoid and pemphigus vulgaris rest on the biopsy of the bullae.

The steroid drugs have revolutionized the treatment and prognosis of all forms of pemphigus and pemphigoid, but very large doses may be necessary to bring the condition under control.

Erythema multiforme (Stevens–Johnson syndrome)

This may occur in a major or a minor form. The patient is normally a child or young adult and in the major variety the patient becomes severely ill with skin eruptions (so-called 'Iris' target lesions). Conjunctivitis and stomatitis are also present.

The oral lesions present as small vesicles which coalesce to give widespread erosions which bleed freely. The lips are usually severely involved with crusting.

In the minor form there is little or no systemic involvement and the lesions may occur in the mouth only.

It is now thought that this and some of the other conditions described above may be manifestations of auto-immunity.

Lichen planus

Lichen planus is an inflammatory condition of the skin and mucous membranes. The aetiology is not known. On the skin it presents as pinkish patches which are irritable, and there may be lesions on the oral mucosa. It must be noted that skin and oral mucosa lesions may appear separately or together.

In the mouth the condition may be symptomless, but it presents as glistening white papules which form varied patterns. Sometimes they may be plaque-like or arranged in lines giving a lace-like appearance. Hyperkeratosis may be present in varying degrees. Although the patient may in some cases be unaware of the condition, there are occasions when the lesions erode and ulcerate giving rise to severe pain. The wearing of dentures may then become very difficult.

This condition must always be differentiated from leucoplakia and a biopsy is generally necessary. Even histologically the distinction may not be easy.

The only treatment required in many cases is reassurance but oral hygiene is important especially if ulceration occurs. Certain authorities advocate the intra-mucosal injection or systemic use of steroid drugs. Occasionally spontaneous remissions occur.

Leucoplakia (*Figure 2.5*)

This is a clinical term meaning literally a *white patch*. There are many diseases in which white patches appear in the mouth. They may appear in scleroderma, they may be seen with a white spongy naevus, and monilia can also give this appearance.

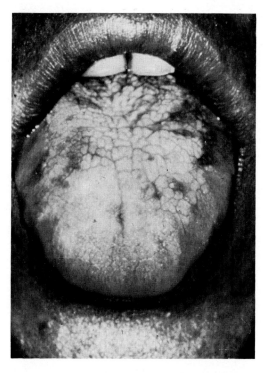

Figure 2.5   Leucoplakia of the tongue

Biopsy or excision biopsy is usually necessary and the term leucoplakia is now generally reserved for those cases where no other diagnosis can be made.

A simple hyperkeratosis can be associated with local irritation and if (when the irritation is removed) the mucosa returns to normal, this should not be regarded as true leucoplakia. If, however, hyperkeratosis becomes irreversible it should be regarded in that light. Chronic irritation whether from a tooth, smoking, strong alcohol or spiced foods, is undoubtedly of some aetiological significance.

This condition should be regarded as pre-cancerous and where possible excision should be carried out.

There may be no symptoms in the early stages when the appearance is usually that of several raised, rather hard plaques which may coalesce. On the dorsum of the tongue there may be isolated white patches and on the cheeks there may be several whitish bands which can give the appearance of lichen planus. In the severe case the normal mucosa may disappear completely. Pain follows when these plaques crack and ulcerate.

When the leucoplakia appears on a very inflamed area (erythroplakia) it must be regarded as very far advanced, with malignant change already having occurred.

The treatment is to remove any source of chronic irritation, excise the lesion completely if possible, and observe at regular intervals post-operatively. Cryosurgery has also been used.

Xerostomia

Dry mouth is a symptom which may be associated with a stomatitis but is frequently a complaint even when the oral mucosa is normal.

The causes are numerous e.g. mouth breathing, diseases of the salivary glands, certain drugs such as some tranquillizers, diuretics etc., diabetes and following radiotherapy. When the cause can be eliminated normal salivary flow will return but when the salivary gland tissue is permanently damaged e.g. in Sjögren's syndrome or after radiotherapy, treatment is palliative and often not effective. A one per cent solution of methyl cellulose mouth-wash and lubrication of the oral mucosa at night with liquid paraffin may be helpful.

Oral manifestations of diseases of the blood

Anaemias

Occasionally the oral lesions of the anaemias are the first to appear, as extreme pallor of the lips and oral mucosa and glossitis. The tongue is red and sore and in the typical Hunter's glossitis, which may well be the first sign of pernicious anaemia; it is also smooth.

Polycythaemia

In this condition there is a bluish-red discoloration of the oral mucosa, and glossitis and/or cheilitis may be present in varying degrees.

Infectious mononucleosis (glandular fever)

The cause of this disease is a virus. There is a considerable increase in the total number of white cells and a relatively great increase in the number of large mononuclear cells.

Frequently there are no oral lesions but the uvula may be swollen and oedematous, and an inflammatory reaction in the buccopharyngeal mucosa together with sore throat may occur. In about 20 per cent of all cases there are petechial spots on the palate.

The submandibular and cervical lymph nodes are enlarged but are part of the general symptoms and usually occur without any oral signs being present.

Besides the increase in the white cell count, the Paul Bunnell test usually becomes positive five days after the onset of symptoms.

There is no specific treatment for this condition.

Agranulocytosis

This is caused by sensitivity to drugs containing the benzene ring, especially amidopyrine, the sulphonamides and more recently the cytotoxic agents. There is a marked reduction in the neutrophil polymorphs.

Agranulocytosis is a severe disorder and frequently fatal. There is a sore throat of sudden onset and ulceration of the tongue, buccal mucosa and pharynx occurs, together with false membrane formation. Pyrexia is high and the patient is extremely ill. Diagnosis is confirmed by a typical blood and marrow picture. The treatment should consist of the withdrawal of any causal drug, while antibiotics, steroids and vitamin B_{12} therapy are instituted, with blood transfusion as required.

The leukaemias

Acute lymphatic leukaemia is the commonest form, and occurs chiefly in children. The first signs may well be enlargement of, and bleeding from the gingival margin, rapidly worsening with severe ulceration ensuing. Leucocytosis may be in the region of 100 000 cells/mm^3 and immature cells are always present in relatively large numbers.

In the chronic leukaemias, the oral lesions are not nearly as well marked and in many cases do not appear at all.

The diagnosis is always made from the blood picture.

Disorders of the temporomandibular joint

Costen was the first to draw attention to dysfunction of this joint as a cause of earache. Clicking noises from the joint are not always significant. They may be produced voluntarily without pain or restriction of movement, and they may also disappear spontaneously. The condition can, however, present as clicking of the jaw with restricted movement, with or without pain. There may be a complaint of earache or facial pain not associated necessarily with clicking. The pain in the ear is due to a referred otalgia while that in the face is frequently due to spasm of the associated muscles. Conductive deafness which is usually slight may result from dysfunction of the eustachian tube. Loss of mobility or stiffness in mandibular movement, especially on wakening, is also a common symptom.

The onset of symptoms may be associated with a blow, yawning, or following dental treatment, although frequently there is no such history. The main cause is malocclusion. The condition is more common in young women.

Radiography is usually negative unless osteoarthritic changes have occurred.

In the treatment and management of these patients exercises can be of value where the patient has produced 'a bite of convenience'. The patient can frequently be shown how to relax the muscles of mastication, to open the jaw without deviation and to masticate on both sides. If the occlusion is definitely deranged a bite plate should be made in the first instance to restore the occlusion and in some cases, where bruxism occurs and might well be the main aetiological factor, the plate can be worn at night only. The correction of the occlusion should aim at restoration of the vertical dimension, replacement of missing teeth, and correction of dentures if already worn. The aim should be to allow free sliding movements of the mandible in mastication so that there is minimal cuspal interference. In cases of sudden onset, such as following acute trauma, intra-articular hydrocortisone injection is of value, but thereafter the joint must be rested for a minimum of 14 days. If malocclusion is present this must be treated after the rest period. The operations of condylectomy or condylotomy may become necessary in those cases which do not respond to treatment, but they are usually only advisable if osteoarthritic changes have occurred.

Cysts of the mouth

Developmental cysts

Medial group

These cysts are situated in the line of fusion of the two maxillae and are usually symptomless unless they become infected. They are frequently found on routine dental radiographs. The nasopalatine cyst, also in the midline, arises from tissue in the incisive canal or cell rests in the incisive papillae and presents usually in the palate or occasionally in the floor of the nose.

Lateral group

The lateral group of developmental cysts occur in the line of fusion of the maxillary and premaxillary elements of the palate and may cause separation of the canine and lateral incisor teeth.

Congenital telangiectasia

These are multiple lesions and seen on the skin and mucous membranes. They can occur in the mucosa of the mouth and may produce haemorrhage, which at times can be severe and require the application of cautery to the bleeding point.

Cysts of dental origin

These are derived from the epithelium that has been associated with the development of the tooth concerned.

The primordial cyst arises from the epithelium of the enamel organ before the formation of the dental tissues. The most common site is in the third molar region of the mandible and that tooth will of course be absent.

Cysts of eruption occur over a tooth that has not yet erupted and arise from the epithelial remains of the dental lamina. They are found in young people and may occur over deciduous or permanent teeth. They appear as small bluish fluctuant swellings and usually an elliptical incision is sufficient for the cyst to be removed and the underlying tooth to erupt.

The dentigerous cyst (*Figure 2.6*) arises from the follicle around an unerupted tooth, the tooth projecting into the cyst cavity.

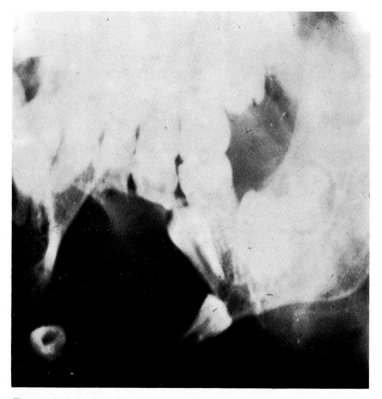

Figure 2.6   Dentigerous cyst of mandible

The dental cyst arises from epithelial remains in the periodontal membrane and is the most common cyst to occur in the jaws. Chronically infected dead teeth or roots produce a granulomatous reaction at the apex. This granuloma contains epithelium which proliferates initially to produce the cyst lining. It is, therefore, common to find a dead tooth or root in conjunction with a cyst. Occasionally teeth or roots might have been removed and the cyst left behind (residual cyst).

Most of these cysts are symptomless unless they become infected. Many are found on routine radiographs, or it might be noticed that a tooth is missing, or the patient may simply complain of a swelling of the jaw. Fluctuation does not occur until the cyst has perforated the outer or inner alveolar plate.

In the maxilla a dental cyst arising from a premolar or molar tooth might easily invade the antrum and in some cases completely fill it.

X-ray examination is essential for diagnosis of cysts in the hard tissue and the important point is that they show, as a rule, a very clear outline. When there is a multilocular radiolucent area in the jaws or the outline is not clear, a differential diagnosis must be made from metastases or endosteal tumours. It must be remembered that the brown tumour of hyperparathyroidism is sometimes the first sign of this disease and the jaws are not an uncommon site for its appearance.

Retention cysts

These are not uncommonly found in the oral cavity, palate and buccal mucosa. They are due to occlusion of the mucous glands present there. In the floor of the mouth such a retention cyst can progress to a very large size, lifting the oral mucosa and base of the tongue (Ranula).

Odontomes

Several different types of odontome are described and they should be regarded as developmental anomalies. They arise from epithelial and mesenchymal parts of the tooth germ and consist of a number of tooth-like structures surrounded by a capsule or a cyst, while others are merely calcified masses.

Clinically one or two normal teeth are missing and frequently a hard swelling is noticed at this site. They rarely give rise to pain unless infection occurs.

Radiographic examination is necessary and the treatment is by surgical removal.

Tumours of the jaws and oral cavity

The most common tumour-like lesions that appear in the oral cavity arising from soft tissues are probably due to an inflammatory reaction. They are fibrous epulis, the giant-celled epulis and the fibro-epithelial polyp. Although not true tumours they are usually treated as such.

The great majority of tumours that occur in various parts of the body may also occur in the oral cavity and therefore there are many types to be considered. Always the most important consideration is whether the lesion is benign or malignant. It must be remembered that the mouth may be invaded by tumours arising from the nose, pharynx and other related structures in the neck. Furthermore, the mandible or maxilla may be the site of a metastasis.

Benign epithelial tumours

Papilloma is not uncommon and may present as a pedunculated or sessile tumour in any part of the oral cavity. Its treatment is by excision.

Adenoma occurs rarely in the mouth but the most common site is in the palate. It is frequently one of the varieties of the so-called mixed salivary tumour. This can be a most unpleasant tumour and while not invariably malignant has the tendency to become so. It should be removed completely and even then close follow-up is essential for a long time.

Benign connective tissue tumours

Fibroma

Fibroma is not an uncommon tumour in the mouth and may be found in any site, not infrequently on the buccal mucosa when it may become painful if ulcerated by the teeth. It can be pedunculated or sessile and should be removed completely.

Fibrous epulis

'Epulis' means *on the gums*, and therefore any lump on the gum may be referred to as an epulis with the descriptive adjective immediately before it. Fibrous epulis is pedunculated and attached to the gum, and is usually situated between two teeth. The colour is similar to that of the normal gum although if inflamed it might appear much redder. The size can vary from 0.5 cm to 3 cm or more in diameter, and it may occur at any age. This epulis probably arises initially through an inflammatory response to irritation and on histological examination it is sometimes noticed that there has been an abscess formation and then the epulis may be referred to as a granuloma pyogenicum.

The treatment is by complete surgical excision, extraction of the associated teeth being unnecessary in the first instance.

Giant-cell epulis (*Figure 2.7*)

This is occasionally referred to as a peripheral osteoclastoma or even a myeloid epulis but it is almost certainly not a true osteoclastoma. It consists of multinucleated giant cells in a fibrous matrix and in appearance it is much more purple in colour than the fibrous epulis, and bleeds easily. Histologically two types are sometimes described: the first type, where many spindle cells can be seen in which multinucleated giant cells are embedded, and the second, the vascular type, where the connective tissue matrix is much looser in structure, many giant cells are present and the vascularity is increased. The treatment is by complete excision. There is a tendency to recurrence and in such cases the adjacent teeth must be extracted.

With these giant-cell lesions it is always advisable to have the serum electrolytes estimated with a view to eliminating the possibility of hyperparathyroidism.

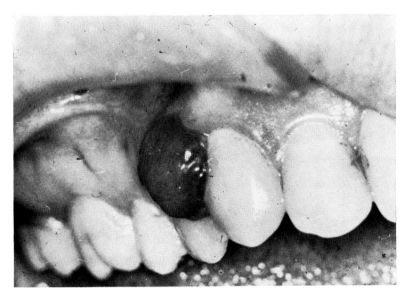

Figure 2.7   Giant-cell epulis

Pregnancy tumour

This is not a true tumour, but is included as an 'epulis'. During pregnancy there is a period of disturbance in the endocrine secretions and subacute gingivitis may occur. This may appear as a generalized gingival inflammation with hypertrophy, but occasionally it may be localized on the gingivae between one or two teeth producing a tumour, which clinically is an epulis. Histologically it is very vascular.

Lipoma

This tumour may be found in the floor of the mouth, lips or tongue, and should be excised.

Muscle tumours

Muscle tumours may be found in the tongue and oral cavity but they, like the myxomata, are only rarely found in this situation.

Haemangiomatous formations

Scattered telangiectiases, and cavernous and capillary haemangiomata, may be found in the oral cavity, as indeed may some of the rarer tumours that are found in other parts of the body.

Osteoma

True compact or cancellous osteoma may be found in either jaw, but not commonly. A more frequent bony abnormality which is sometimes given the name of an osteoma may appear in the hard palate, the so-called *torus palatinus*, or on the lingual side of the mandible in the premolar region, the so-called *torus mandibularis*. These latter are usually bilateral.

Torus palatinus (*Figure 2.8*)

This is not a true tumour, but is an overgrowth or exostosis in the midline of the hard palate. It is bony hard and is usually bilateral, involving both the palatine processes though they may not be equally affected. The shape and size vary from a small and flat elevation to a larger mass, and the surface may be fissured or smooth.

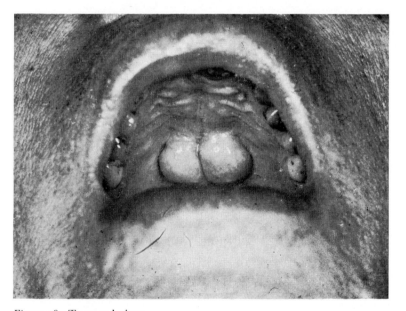

Figure 2.8   Torus palatinus

In slight cases no treatment is necessary but if very large and causing discomfort or interfering with a denture then this overgrowth should be removed.

Torus mandibularis

The cause is not known but these bony protruberances can be extremely large on the lingual side of the mandible. If they make the fitting of a denture impossible they should be removed.

Benign reparative giant-cell granuloma

It is more commonly found in females and may affect either jaw. Microscopically many giant cells are seen in a fibrous matrix and are evenly distributed, the tumour grows slowly and deformity is caused by size. Egg-shell crackling may be present when a considerable amount of bone has been resorbed. Radiographs show a soap-bubble trabeculation within a partial or complete boundary wall, but without erosion of other parts of the jaw. The treatment is by radical excision. In the past this granuloma has been frequently referred to as an osteoclastoma. The latter is a rare tumour in the jaws and when it does occur its behaviour is similar to osteoclastoma in any other situation.

Plasmacytoma

This may occur anywhere in the mouth but occasionally presents as an epulis; hence the importance of sending such tumours that are excised for histological examination. The plasmacytoma tends to recur and multiple myelomatosis may follow.

Ameloblastomas

These are sometimes classified as odontomes. They have been known previously as adamantinomata, or multilocular cysts. The tumour, however, does not contain enamel, it is not necessarily multiloculated and may not even be cystic. It may arise from any part of the epithelium responsible for tooth formation.

The tumour increases in size slowly and invades the bone which may become completely resorbed and it will progress, unless treated, to a large mass. It may be monocystic or polycystic. This is why even apparently simple dental cysts should be sent for histological examination. Some of these tumours may remain solid and microscopically there are masses of cells arranged in palisaded groups separated by connective tissue. In many instances they appear histologically rather like a basal cell carcinoma. It is in this solid mass of cells that cystic degeneration may occur.

Clinically these tumours occur more commonly in young adults and the mandible is more frequently affected than the maxilla. In the first instance they present as an expansion of the jaw but when the bone has been destroyed the tumour feels firm or fluctuant according to its type. The teeth in the region of the lesion become loosened and occasionally their roots resorb. In very large tumours which perforate the oral cavity, ulceration occurs.

The radiographic appearance is that of a multilocular cyst or occasionally even a radicular or dentigerous cyst.

These tumours must be regarded as locally malignant and radical excision is therefore necessary. In very large lesions resection of considerable parts of the mandible may be necessary, followed by bone grafting. If the lesion is small it is sometimes possible to leave the lower border of the jaw as sufficient tissue can be removed from around the tumour.

Malignant epithelial tumours

By far the most frequent carcinoma is the squamous cell carcinoma but occasionally adenocarcinoma or the mixed salivary type of tumour may occur in the palate, floor of the mouth and buccal mucosa, arising from the mucous glands and occasionally from aberrant salivary tissue.

Carcinoma of the anterior two-thirds of the tongue

This is more frequent in men than in women and occurs mainly in middle and old age. It varies from a highly keratinized to an anaplastic tumour.

Hyperkeratosis may be a precursor. It is certain that chronic irritation plays a part and syphilis may also be a contributory factor.

In the initial stages it may vary clinically. It may appear as a small warty growth or papilloma. Ulceration may occur in leucoplakia, the base of the ulcer being indurated and sloughing with an everted edge.

Pain is common in the later stages, foetor is frequently marked and the tongue becomes fixed on the side of the lesion.

Lymph node metastases are common and if the lesion is at the tip of the tongue the submental nodes are usually the first to be involved.

Any doubtful lesion should be subjected to a biopsy (excision if possible) and one should remember that cytological examination can be useful in this area.

Cancer of the tongue may be treated by excision or radiotherapy or by a combination of these methods. With the advances in radiotherapeutic equipment and techniques this is becoming the method of choice, in preference to mutilating surgery. The cytotoxic drugs have also been used in these cases and in the advanced case where metastases into the cervical lymph nodes have occurred a block dissection of the neck and hemiresection of the mandible may be necessary. Some authorities advocate so-called 'prophylactic' neck dissection. Oral hygiene is of the utmost importance.

Carcinoma of the buccal mucosa and floor of the mouth (*Figure 2.9*)

This presents similar clinical features to carcinoma of the tongue. Primary growths may occur in any part of the mouth, especially in the region of the opening of the submandibular ducts. The oral mucosa may also be affected by spread from carcinoma of the tongue or alveolus. The principles of diagnosis and management are similar to those outlined above for carcinoma of the tongue.

Carcinoma of the lip

This has a more favourable prognosis than the other oral lesions. Surgical excision with plastic reconstruction is giving way to radiotherapy, especially in the more advanced cases. Lymph node metastases require block dissection.

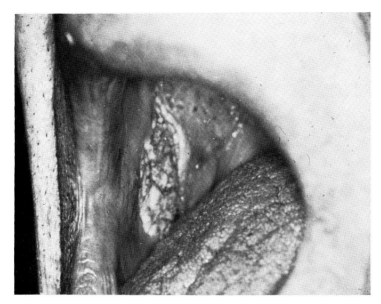

Figure 2.9   Carcinoma in leucoplakia of buccal mucosa

Melanoma

Pigmented tumours, both benign and malignant, may occur on the lips and within the oral cavity. They are extremely rare and the majority of malignant melanomata reported have occurred in the maxilla. It must be remembered that melanine spots may occur, rather like freckles, on the lips in cases of intestinal polyposis, and melanin deposits are not uncommon in the oral cavity in certain races. Addison's disease not infrequently causes melanin deposits on the gingivae and a differential diagnosis must be made before treatment is planned.

Malignant connective tissue tumours

Sarcoma of the tongue and jaws is very rare and frequently fatal. Various types, such as fibrosarcoma, lymphosarcoma, osteogenic sarcoma and the reticulum-cell sarcoma have all been reported. Radical excision followed by irradiation is necessary, but even in the early stages the chances of recovery are very small.

For further reading

Farmer, E. D. and Lawton, F. E. (Eds) (1966). *Stones' Oral and Dental Diseases* (5th edn), Livingstone; Edinburgh

Gayford, J. J. and Haskell, R. (1971). *Clinical*

Oral Medicine, Staples Press; London

Shafer, W. G., Hine, M. K. and Levy, B. M. (1974). *A Textbook of Oral Pathology* (3rd edn), Saunders; London

3 Diseases of the salivary glands
Douglas Ranger

It is customary to divide the salivary glands into two main groups – the major and the minor. The sublingual glands are commonly grouped in the major category, together with the parotid and submandibular, but they more closely resemble and are more easily considered with the other minor glands which are scattered widely throughout the pharyngeal and oral mucosa including the lips.

Although they will not be considered here it is worth noting that similar glands with comparable secretions are found in the nose, sinuses, post-nasal space, larynx, trachea and bronchi. The lacrimal gland is of the same general type and may (rarely) be the site of tumours identical with those arising in the salivary glands.

Surgical anatomy

Parotid glands

The parotid glands are the largest of the salivary glands and in the adult each gland weighs on average 20–25 g. Patey and Ranger (1957) showed that in 25 subjects in whom the gland was removed *post-mortem* the weight of the gland varied from 11 g to 30 g, and that the lower weights were found in subjects who were elderly or emaciated.

The gland is enclosed in and adherent to a well-defined fibrous capsule derived from the deep cervical fascia. A particularly thickened part of this fascia forms the stylomandibular ligament which supports the gland antero-inferiorly and separates it from the submandibular gland.

The parotid gland forms a somewhat irregular mass, roughly triangular on horizontal section, with its base externally and its apex projecting into the space between the mandible in front and the mastoid process and sternomastoid muscle behind. These structures groove the antero-medial and postero-medial surfaces. Superficially the gland extends forwards over the masseter muscle. It is from this part of the gland that the parotid duct, about 5 cm long, emerges to curve around the anterior border of the masseter muscle and open into the mouth opposite the second upper molar tooth. The direction of the duct is indicated by a line drawn from the tragus to the midpoint of the upper lip.

The deep aspect of the parotid gland is related to the upper portion of the posterior belly of the digastric muscle and to the styloid process, stylohyoid and stylomandibular ligaments and the stylohyoid, styloglossus and stylopharyngeus muscles. These structures separate the gland from the carotid sheath and related nerves and more anteriorly from the parapharyngeal space. As a result of this relationship a small proportion of tumours arising in the deep portion of the parotid gland may present as a swelling of the faucial region and soft palate.

A number of structures traverse the parotid gland or are closely applied to it and have relationships of considerable surgical significance. They will be considered in the order of their depth from the surface.

The great auricular nerve arises from the second and third cervical nerves and curves around the posterior border of the sternomastoid muscle near its centre, pierces the deep fascia and ascends across that muscle running with the external jugular vein deep to the platysma muscle. It reaches the postero-inferior portion of the parotid gland and then runs upwards on the capsule or in the most superficial part of the gland before dividing into an anterior branch which supplies the skin over the angle of the jaw and a posterior branch which supplies sensation to the lobe of the ear.

The facial nerve traverses the gland in a postero-anterior direction deep to the great auricular nerve and immediately superficial to the veins. After emerging from the stylomastoid foramen, about 7 mm deep to the tympanomastoid suture, the facial nerve runs forward 4–5 mm below the bony external auditory meatus to enter the posterior surface of the parotid gland accompanied by a branch of the stylomastoid artery which runs just below it. Within the substance of the gland 1–2 cm from its point of entry the nerve nearly always divides into two main divisions, temporofacial and cervicofacial, and these soon divide into a number of terminal branches which spread out to supply the muscles of facial expression including the buccinator. These branches emerge from the gland on its deep surface near its anterior margin and cross the surface of the masseter muscle to their destinations. There are usually a number of filamentous communications between adjacent branches. They are inconstant and cannot be assumed to be present but in some patients they may allow a main branch to be cut without paralysis developing. However, the uppermost branch, to the frontalis, and the lowermost, the cervical branch, only exceptionally have connections with adjacent branches and as a result damage to these branches nearly always leads to paralysis. Occasionally there are two cervical branches – a smaller superficial one and a larger deep branch.

The plane of the facial nerve divides the gland artificially into superficial and deep portions. There is no anatomical separation of the two parts into separate lobes but the gland can be divided surgically in the plane of the nerve and as a result it is possible to resect the whole parotid gland while preserving the facial nerve intact.

Immediately deep to the facial nerve lies a plexus of veins draining into the posterior facial vein running from above downwards in the same plane. This vein originates by the union of the superficial temporal and maxillary veins and at the lower part of the parotid it divides into an anterior division which joins the anterior facial vein to form the common facial vein, and a posterior division which becomes the external jugular vein after being joined by the posterior auricular vein. Very occasionally the posterior facial vein runs between the lower branches of the facial nerve lying immediately superficial, instead of deep, to the lowest one or two branches of the nerve.

Just above the posterior belly of the digastric muscle the external carotid artery enters the deep aspect of the parotid gland and at this point is separated from the veins by a moderate amount of gland tissue. As the artery travels upwards it becomes more and more superficial until at the upper pole the arteries and veins lie together. In the parotid gland the external carotid artery divides into the maxillary and superficial temporal arteries.

The auriculotemporal nerve arising from the mandibular division of the trigeminal nerve passes backwards on the surface of the tensor palati muscle deep to the lateral pterygoid muscle and then between the neck of the mandible and sphenomandibular ligament just above the maxillary artery. The nerve then turns laterally to the deep aspect of the upper part of the parotid gland behind the neck of the mandible. Passing around the upper pole of the parotid gland the auriculotemporal nerve emerges just behind the superficial temporal vessels at the condyle of the mandible. It then turns upwards with the vessels to cross the zygomatic arch before dividing into superficial temporal branches.

It is the auriculotemporal nerve which is generally considered to carry the parasympathetic secretomotor fibres to the parotid gland. Reaching the glossopharyngeal nerve from the inferior salivary nucleus the fibres run in the lesser superficial petrosal nerve to emerge from the skull through the foramen ovale (or the foramen innominatum) and relay in the otic ganglion before joining the auriculotemporal nerve. However, clinical observations in patients after intracranial division of the glossopharyngeal nerve and in other patients with gustatory sweating suggest the possibility that secretomotor fibres to the parotid gland may also be supplied through the chorda tympani nerve; Diamant (1958) considers that there is this dual parasympathetic supply. The sympathetic supply to the parotid glands is derived from the plexus around the external carotid artery after relay in the superior cervical ganglion.

The relative importance of the parasympathetic and sympathetic nerves in producing secretion of saliva is not known with certainty. In the past it has been customary to regard the parasympathetic nerves as having the dominant secretomotor role and the sympathetic as supplying the blood vessels and possibly also the myoepithelial cells in the ducts. However, studies by Eneroth, Hokfelt and Norberg (1969) using catecholamine fluorescence, choline esterase staining and electron microscopy suggest that the human parotid and submandibular glands are supplied by fairly equal numbers of sympathetic and parasympathetic nerves and that both sets of fibres innervate parenchymal cells. It has not yet been established to what extent sympathetic activity can produce a secretion of saliva but some clinical observations are certainly in keeping with the suggestion that the sympathetic nerves to the salivary glands have at least some secretomotor activity.

The parotid gland contains a considerable amount of lymphoid tissue. Some of this is aggregated into discrete lymph nodes under the capsule or within the substance of the gland while in other areas masses of lymphocytes surround acini and ducts without having any nodal pattern.

Submandibular glands

The submandibular glands lie beneath the floor of the mouth on each side deep to the body of the mandible and extending below it in the submandibular triangle. Like the parotid the submandibular gland also has a well-defined capsule derived from the deep cervical fascia but in contrast it is not normally adherent to it and it is possible to excise the submandibular gland by intracapsular dissection unless inflammatory or other conditions have rendered it abnormally adherent.

The larger part of the submandibular gland lies superficial to the mylohyoid muscle extending as far forwards as the anterior belly of the digastric muscle covered by skin, platysma and fascia in the lower part and also by the mandible and medial pterygoid muscle in the upper part. Around the posterior border of the mylohyoid muscle the superficial portion of the gland becomes continuous with the deep portion lying on the hyoglossus and styloglossus muscles and extending forwards deep to the mylohyoid muscle.

The lingual and hypoglossal nerves cross the hyoglossus deep to the gland – the lingual above and the hypoglossal below. The submandibular duct emerges from the deep part of the gland between the lingual and hypoglossal nerves and runs forwards and upwards to open into the mouth just to the side of the frenum of the tongue. The lingual nerve first descends across the lateral side of the duct and then curves upwards and forwards medial to it. The duct thus passes upwards, inwards and forwards through a loop in the nerve.

The facial artery usually enters the postero-inferior part of the deep lobe of the gland and after traversing the gland at a variable depth emerges from the upper surface to cross the body of the mandible just in front of the origin of the masseter muscle where it is readily located. Anatomically the facial artery is merely embedded in the gland and sometimes its groove is so shallow that the artery is readily separated from the surface of the gland and can be preserved without difficulty during excision of the submandibular gland. The artery is accompanied by veins lying superficially to it.

Just deep to the mandible the artery and veins are crossed superficially by the cervical branch of the facial nerve which can be found at the junction of the planes of the lower border of the mandible and the facial artery by reflecting the platysma upwards. As the submandibular gland can be excised, for non-neoplastic conditions, by intracapsular dissection the nerve can best be safeguarded by opening the capsule well below the mandible.

The parasympathetic nerve supply to the submandibular gland travels from the superior salivary nucleus in the nervus intermedius, and then in the chorda tympani to join the lingual nerve. The fibres leave the lingual nerve to relay in the submandibular ganglion lying on the hyoglossus muscle just below the lingual nerve at the upper portion of the deep lobe of the gland. Just as it has been postulated that the parotid has a double parasympathetic nerve supply there is also the possibility of a dual supply to the submandibular gland from the tympanic branch of the glossopharyngeal nerve and lesser superficial petrosal nerve as well as from the chorda tympani. The sympathetic nerve supply is derived from the carotid plexus along fibres accompanying the facial artery.

Some lymph nodes lie within the capsule of the submandibular gland but lymphoid tissue is not normally found scattered in the substance of the gland itself.

Both the parotid and submandibular glands are compound racemose glands with a single duct dividing into multiple branches arranged into lobes and lobules and ending terminally in alveoli enclosed in a basement membrane continuous with that of the duct. Almost all the alveolar cells of the parotid produce a serous secretion but there are usually a few cells in the alveoli which secrete mucus and there are nearly always a number of mucus-secreting goblet cells opening into the ducts. The submandibular gland contains a roughly equal proportion of mucous and serous alveolar cells.

Minor salivary glands

The minor salivary glands are widely scattered through the oral and pharyngeal mucosa. Although separate groups are described according to their anatomical situation there is little to be gained by detailed description. The sublingual glands lying just to the side of the lingual frenum, are the largest of the minor glands and open into the floor of the mouth and into the submandibular duct through several small ducts. The palatal glands are the most numerous and there are some 400 glands distributed over the hard and soft palates and the uvula (*Figure 3.1*). Their

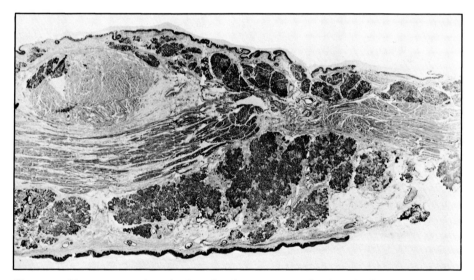

Figure 3.1   Transverse section of palate showing numerous glands on both upper and lower aspects

distribution is often readily assessed by the beads of secretion to be seen on the palate after the administration of drugs with cholinergic activity used during the course of anaesthesia.

The secretions of the minor salivary glands may be serous or mucous but the term 'mucous gland' is commonly used to designate the minor salivary and other glands of similar type whatever may be the type of secretion.

General clinical considerations

The salivary glands have such a large reserve capacity for producing saliva to aid chewing and swallowing that diminution of secretion is not noticeable unless it is severe, as occurs in widespread interference with salivary secretory activity. It is not uncommon for patients to have both submandibular glands removed and some patients may have both parotids excised but such a loss does not produce any noticeable disability as far as the secretion of saliva is concerned. However, patients do have great difficulty with mastication when there is extensive interference with the activity of the salivary glands, as may occur in association with the irradiation of malignant neoplasms in the region of the mouth and pharynx or in certain disorders of the glands constituting the sicca syndrome.

Dryness of the mouth in itself does not act as a stimulus to secretion of saliva as is well shown in patients with nasal obstruction who are forced to breathe through the mouth.

In most patients palpation does not give any clear indication of the size or outline of the parotid gland because it has much the same consistency as the surrounding tissues. However, in some people the parotid is distinguishable and appears enlarged without there being any other indication of abnormality. Some of these patients whose glands have been explored have been found on biopsy to have merely a generalized increase of interlobular fat.

The submandibular gland is often palpable externally and can usually be felt easily on bi-manual palpation with one finger in the mouth and the fingers of the other hand under the mandible. In some patients the submandibular gland lies unduly low in the neck and can be readily seen and felt below the mandible.

The minor salivary glands are not normally distinguishable through the intact mucosa of the mouth or pharynx but are often encountered in operations on these regions and should not be confused with aggregations of lymphoid tissue.

Examination and investigations

Most patients with lesions of the salivary glands present with a swelling and unless this is intermittent, as occurs for example with a submandibular calculus, the swelling will be evident on inspection and on palpation. Small parotid tumours may become more obvious on turning the head to the opposite side. The orifices of the parotid and submandibular ducts should be examined. Palpation of the parotid and submandibular areas should be carried out both from in front of and from behind the patient. For lesions in the submandibular area, floor of mouth, in the palate and peritonsillar region and also for examining the parotid and submandibular ducts, bi-manual palpation with one finger in the mouth and the fingers of the other hand over the skin in the appropriate area allows more accurate assessment than each method used independently. For swellings which are intermittent and occur at meal times the simplest method for promoting secretion is to give the patient a slice of freshly cut lemon or a boiled sweet of the 'acid drop' variety to suck.

Plain radiographs of the submandibular areas, which should include intra-oral films, will usually show any calculi which are present but in the parotid region plain films are not so valuable because of underlying bony shadows and the small size of many parotid calculi. Multiple calcified thrombi may be evident in plain radiographs of some haemangiomas.

The duct systems of the parotid and submandibular salivary glands can be demonstrated by contrast sialography after injection of an oily radio-opaque dye. Not more than 0.5 ml should be injected in order to avoid rupture of any of the ducts. Sialography should not be undertaken during episodes of acute inflammation and if preliminary plain films demonstrate an opaque calculus little of value will be gained. In patients with tumours sialography is unlikely to demonstrate more than the size and site of the tumour within the gland.

Gamma-emission radiosialography following the intravenous injection of Technetium, as the pertechnetate, can also be used to demonstrate the outline of masses within the salivary glands. While the outlines of benign tumours as cold nodules tend to be sharper and smoother than with malignant tumours the diagnosis cannot be made with sufficient certainty to affect the management in the way which will be described subsequently. 'Hot' nodules can occur in oncocytic tumours and are a reliable indicator of their nature.

Both contrast sialography and emission radiosialography have a limited value in the investigation of salivary gland disorders. Contrast sialography can help in the diagnosis and management of inflammatory and obstructive conditions and can be of use in demonstrating whether a mass is within the gland and demonstrate its size and position. This is of greater importance with lesions in the deep lobe of the parotid than with those in the superficial lobe or submandibular gland. Radiosialography has little value in inflammatory lesions and has only a minor role in the management of tumours. Perhaps its main contribution is that the demonstration of a hot nodule can provide a diagnosis of a benign oncocytic tumour and allow operation to be deferred.

Retention cysts

Obstruction of the parotid duct usually leads to suppression of the secretion from the serous alveoli and a tendency to recurrent infection. However, secretion of mucus is not inhibited in the same way and obstruction of the submandibular duct leads to swelling of the gland when secretion of saliva is stimulated by eating. Because the gland is enclosed in a firm fascial capsule this swelling produces a considerable increase in pressure and this is accompanied by pain.

Similar obstruction of the opening of a minor salivary gland usually leads to the development of a thin-walled cyst which is painless because there is no firm capsule surrounding it and the overlying mucosa stretches easily. The condition presents as a smooth painless swelling covered by thin mucosa and the cystic nature of the swelling is usually obvious on inspection and palpation.

Such cysts may occur in any part of the mouth or pharynx. When they occur on the lips they are readily noticed by the patient and his relatives and when they occur on the buccal surface of the cheek they tend to interfere with the closure of the teeth. In those situations, therefore, they are unlikely to become very large before advice is sought. However, when they occur in the floor of the mouth they may enlarge to a considerable size before causing any discomfort or disability and for that reason have tended to be given a separate name – *ranula*. In some instances the cyst wall is so thin that it ruptures and the contents extravasate into the tissues as was shown by Bhaskar, Bolden and Weinmann (1956). This explains the extent of some of these ranulae and the difficulty of their complete eradication in some instances. When the extravasation has extended widely through the tissue planes the term sometimes applied to the condition is 'burrowing ranula'.

Treatment of retention cysts generally presents no problems. Excision can be carried out immediately outside the cyst wall, which usually separates easily from the surrounding tissues unless there has been previous infection. In the floor of the mouth care must be taken to avoid damage to the lingual nerve and submandibular duct. In patients with burrowing ranulae the essential aspect of the operation is to remove the gland from which the mucoid secretion is arising by adequate excision of the mucosa forming the wall.

Salivary fistulae

Parotid fistulae occasionally occur from the cut surface of the gland when it is damaged in accidental injuries or surgical incisions. Such fistulae may (rarely) develop in the post-auricular region after mastoidectomy or on the cheek after drainage of an abscess or other operation or injury there. In spite of the large area of cut surface of the parotid which is left exposed after partial parotidectomy it is very rare for a fistula to develop. Provided the parotid duct is normal and provided there is no neoplasm such glandular fistulae present no special problems. If they persist after the rest of the incision has healed they can be dealt with simply by ligating and excising the fistulous track a short distance from the surface and suturing the skin without drainage.

Injuries to the parotid duct, on the other hand, are more difficult to deal with. The first principle of treatment is to try to establish free drainage into the mouth. In any recent injury if there is reason to suppose that the parotid duct might have been injured because of the position of the wound then the duct should be identified and examined. If it is found to be divided or injured the cut ends should be identified and a fine polyethylene catheter inserted as far as possible into the posterior part of the duct after being passed through the natural opening of the duct and along the remaining anterior portion. If the two cut ends can then be approximated without tension this is done, but if not the catheter is left to bridge the gap. The catheter is sutured to the buccal mucosa and left in position for three weeks before being removed. If the natural opening of the parotid duct is involved in the injury then the catheter is brought into the mouth through a stab wound at an appropriate point.

If a salivary fistula has developed on the cheek from a previous injury then a similar method is employed and is usually successful. Even if the duct cannot be identified because of scar tissue but there is a cavity containing saliva associated with the fistula then drainage of this cavity into the mouth with a catheter may well succeed in establishing adequate drainage into the mouth and healing of the fistula. Morel and Firestein (1963) report such a result in a patient explored six weeks after a knife wound and at follow-up 15 months later there was free flow of saliva through the surgically-created buccal opening. Such methods are much simpler and probably more effective than attempts to construct a new portion of duct from oral mucosa.

Abolition of salivary secretion by radiotherapy is a procedure which has been used in patients with parotid fistulae but a full tumour dose may be necessary and even this cannot be guaranteed to prove effective. Such dosage has considerable disadvantages and if all attempts at repairing the fistula should fail, conservative parotidectomy with preservation of the facial nerve can be carried out with less hazard than with radiotherapy.

Submandibular salivary fistulae are uncommon and when they do occur they are not difficult to control because of the comparative simplicity of excising the submandibular gland.

Salivary calculi

Calculi sometimes form in the salivary glands. Over 90 per cent occur in association with the submandibular gland and only rarely are they found in the sublingual gland. The calculi consist of an organic matrix similar to that found in urinary calculi but with somewhat less tendency to form concentric laminations (Harrill, King and Boyce, 1959). The main inorganic constituent is calcium in the form of calcium phosphate but there are usually also traces of magnesium. These inorganic constituents account for the almost invariable opacity of salivary calculi on x-ray examination but small calculi in the parotid gland may be obscured by overlying bony shadows. In both the submandibular and parotid regions intra-oral films may show calculi which would otherwise be missed.

Calculi in the submandibular gland are usually larger than in the parotid and are less likely to be multiple. The calculi may be situated anywhere in the course of the ducts. Sometimes the calculus ulcerates through the duct wall and is extruded into the mouth or into an abscess cavity in the tissues surrounding the duct. In either case the obstruction will be relieved at least temporarily although a stricture may form subsequently at the site of ulceration. The symptoms produced by the presence of salivary calculi will depend on the site and degree of obstruction, on the effect of the obstruction on salivary secretion and on whether or not there is infection present. Glands which secrete mucus are capable of functioning against considerable resistance and mucoceles may develop in many parts of the body when drainage of mucous glands is obstructed in the absence of any infection. On the other hand serous glands cease to function early in the presence of obstruction.

Because there are large numbers of mucus-secreting alveoli in the submandibular gland, secretions continue to be produced even if the duct is completely occluded and as a result the usual symptom produced by a calculus in the submandibular duct is recurrent swelling of the gland in association with meals. Infection may occur but is not common. On the other hand calculi in the parotid duct lead to a greatly diminished secretion of saliva from the gland and infection is much more likely to develop. As a result of this the common effect produced by parotid calculi is the occurrence of repeated attacks of acute parotitis.

The treatment of salivary calculi will depend on the symptoms produced and these will be determined largely by the site. In the parotid gland the problem is usually one of recurrent infections and is more conveniently dealt with under that heading in the next section.

In the submandibular gland the common symptom is recurrent swelling and pain in the submandibular region on eating. Stimulation of salivary activity by lemon juice or a sweet containing fruit juice usually produces a demonstrable enlargement of the submandibular gland. A calculus may be felt on bi-manual palpation of the duct and gland. Calculi in the submandibular gland or duct are almost invariably opaque to x-rays and are revealed on plain x-rays provided intra-oral views are taken. If the calculus is situated in the duct itself it is usually a simple matter to remove it by an incision through the oral mucosa and a substantial proportion of patients treated in this way have no further trouble. If the calculus recurs, or if it is situated in the gland itself so that it cannot be removed via the duct, then excision of the submandibular gland is required.

Infections

Non-suppurative infections of the salivary glands may occur in mumps and there is usually little difficulty in diagnosis except when the condition is unilateral or involves only the submandibular glands without the parotids being affected. A blood count shows no leucocytosis and in any cases of doubt estimations of antibody titres provide conclusive diagnostic evidence. Occasionally non-suppurative infection may occur in the course of glandular fever.

As with other systems in the body bacterial infection is more common in the presence of obstruction. In the salivary glands this may be caused by the presence of a foreign body in the form of a calculus or by a stricture of the duct. The obstruction may block the main duct in which case the whole gland is involved, or one of the minor ducts when the process will be confined to only a lobe or a lobule of the gland. Reduced salivary secretion such as occurs in dehydrated states and in some pathological conditions of the glands may also be a factor in the aetiology. Infection itself is liable to reduce salivary secretion by damaging or destroying acinar cells and may also lead to strictures of the ducts. Both of these processes increase the likelihood of further infection developing later. Oral sepsis increases the chances of infection spreading along the ducts but glands which are secreting normally and are not obstructed are remarkably resistant to even gross infections in the mouth.

Acute bacterial infection of the salivary glands is normally not difficult to diagnose. The condition follows the general course of such infections elsewhere in the body and is characterized by the rapid development of pain and tenderness in the gland with a variable but usually slight degree of systemic effects and there are usually inflammatory changes evident in the opening of the duct. There is usually a purulent exudate which discharges from the duct spontaneously or in response to pressure. The common organism is a streptococcus but sometimes mixed flora are responsible. If the condition is untreated a tense abscess may develop and this will tend to rupture. In the case of the parotid gland rupture may occur into the external auditory meatus. In the submandibular gland rupture into the floor of the mouth is most likely. However, most of these infections respond rapidly to antibiotics and abscess formation is unusual in any patient so treated. Swabs should be taken from the pus expressed from the duct but while the result of this is awaited ampicillin is probably the antibiotic of choice.

Although a single attack of acute infection may occur in a previously normal gland chronic and recurrent infections of the salivary glands are nearly always associated with obstruction or with diseases in which there is reduced salivary secretion. In the submandibular gland the problem of chronic or recurrent infection is not a difficult one because the offending gland can be removed easily and safely. It is in the parotid gland where operation carries the risk, however slight, of a permanent facial paralysis that recurrent infections present difficulties in management.

As has been mentioned already acute attacks of bacterial parotitis usually respond to antibiotics and some will settle even without them, often with a sudden gush of purulent mucoid material from the duct into the mouth. Initial attacks are often diagnosed as mumps and second attacks may also be so regarded in spite of the fact that such an event must be exceptionally rare if it occurs at all.

The investigation of a patient who has had recurrent attacks of parotitis involves plain x-rays of the region including intra-oral films. Parotid calculi are often very small and there are other shadows in the area which may obscure the calculi. Contrast radiography to outline the duct system with an opaque material is a valuable diagnostic measure but must be done with care. Thackray (1955) has shown that duct walls which have been damaged by inflammatory changes are liable to rupture easily under pressure and that saccular or globular opacities seen on the x-rays after injection of an opaque material into the duct represent extravasated material in the substance of the gland. The appearance of fusiform sialectasis seen in some films indicates a true dilatation of the ducts with the epithelial lining remaining intact, while the appearance of sialectasis in any form indicates the presence of chronic infection of the gland. Thackray provided pathological evidence that extravasation produces a marked fibrous reaction and this may prevent resolution of the existing infection as well as predisposing to further infection and rendering surgical excision more difficult with the possible consequence of damage to the facial nerve during operation. Once a duct has ruptured injection of any more material tends to increase the extravasation and is of no further value in outlining the duct system. In an experimental study Ian Ranger (1957) showed that in 20 parotid glands and 20 submandibular glands removed *post-mortem* from adults a complete duct pattern was seen in all cases when 0.5 ml of neo-hydriol was injected and that the injection of further material tended to obscure the duct pattern by acinar filling and by duct rupture in the case of the parotid gland. Pattinson (1969) has advised that initial injection of the parotid duct should be limited to 0.5 ml in adults or 0.25 ml in children and further injection made only if required after inspection of the original films. In the submandibular gland amounts of 1.5 ml may be used.

The treatment of an acute bacterial parotitis has already been considered. The management of patients who have recurrent or chronic parotitis will depend on the result of the investigations just mentioned.

If x-rays show a single calculus in the main parotid duct then dilatation of the orifice of the duct may result in passage of the stone. Incision of the duct through the mouth or through an incision in the cheek to remove the calculus is often not the simple operation it might seem in that there is nearly always considerable surrounding fibrosis and the procedure is likely to be followed by stricture formation.

If there is a stricture of the main duct intermittent dilatation with bougies may succeed. Insertion of a small polyethylene catheter if possible and suture to the buccal aspect of the cheek to retain it in position for a period of three weeks (based on experience of injuries to the duct) is a technique of value in some patients but even after the passage of bougies it is not always possible to insert a catheter.

If investigations do not show any obstruction in the ducts and if secretion is within normal limits then there is a good chance that the attacks will subside. Any oral sepsis is dealt with and steps taken to ensure that the patient does not become dehydrated at any time.

If x-rays show multiple calculi or obstruction of the ducts which is not amenable to treatment or if treatment of the obstruction fails, or if there is greatly diminished secretion, then the likely course of events is that attacks of parotitis will recur with increasing frequency as each attack produces further damage and predisposes to further infections. In this situation parotidectomy may be the only means of ensuring a cure but other methods mentioned below may be successful and are worth trying if otherwise parotidectomy would be advocated.

Intra-oral ligation of the parotid duct as described by Laage-Helman (1955) and by Diamant (1958) may be successful in a large proportion of patients. Diamant found that six out of his seven patients were cured by the procedure, combined with pre-operative radiotherapy, and Maynard (1965) reported 73 per cent successful results in a series followed up for one year. Although Diamant advised pre-operative radiotherapy the possible disadvantages of this, especially in young people, are such that some workers would regard it as unjustifiable. An alternative method of temporarily reducing parotid secretion in the immediate post-operative period is to perform a tympanotomy and divide the tympanic branch of the glossopharyngeal nerve on the promontory of the middle ear and also the chorda tympani. These intratympanic procedures in themselves do not seem adequate to cure recurrent parotitis but seem to reduce parotid secretion temporarily and appear to be a reasonable and less damaging alternative to radiotherapy as an adjunct to ligation of the parotid duct. The problem about ligation of the duct arises from the fact that the mucous elements in the gland may continue to secrete and as a result the condition may be made worse and parotidectomy become essential. Accordingly the treatment can be carried out only on patients who have accepted this risk and in centres which are prepared to undertake parotidectomy for this condition if it is needed.

The indications for parotidectomy, because of recurrent parotitis, will depend on the frequency and severity of the attacks and the acceptance by the patient of the risk of a facial paralysis. This risk must be very slight with surgeons who have considerable experience of parotid surgery and although Patey (1965a) reported that temporary functional facial paralysis is commoner after operations for parotitis than for tumours all his patients had recovered full facial movements.

Specific infections of the salivary glands are uncommon. Tuberculosis may occur in the gland substance but is more likely to develop in a lymph node within the capsule. In the parotid the condition presents as a parotid 'tumour' and there are no particular features to distinguish it from a true neoplasm. In the submandibular gland the condition is even more uncommon and again is more likely to be diagnosed as a tumour than an infection. In either, gland excision is usually undertaken before the diagnosis is apparent. In a patient treated by the author the histological and cultural findings provided conclusive evidence of tuberculosis even though a pre-operative Mantoux test was negative.

Sarcoidosis occasionally involves the parotid glands and rarely the submandibular glands. Unlike tuberculosis, it generally produces a diffuse enlargement of the gland and is usually bilateral. The condition is part of a generalized disease and occurs in about five per cent of patients with sarcoidosis. In the great majority of patients, a radiograph of the chest shows either hilar lymphadenopathy or pulmonary infiltration or both. The Kveim test is positive in about 80 per cent of the patients and there is usually enlargement of peripheral lymph nodes, commonly including the epitrochlear nodes. In about one-third of patients with parotid sarcoidosis, there is an associated uveitis and ophthalmic examination is necessary whenever sarcoidosis of the salivary glands is suspected. Peripheral neuritis, especially of the cranial nerves, is not uncommon and when the facial nerve is involved it is natural to associate it directly with the parotid enlargement. However, Pennell (1951) and later Höök (1954) showed that facial paralysis occurs no more commonly in sarcoidosis with parotid involvement than in sarcoidosis generally and concluded that pressure from the enlarged parotid gland is not the cause of the paralysis. This view has been supported by others having considerable experience of sarcoidosis, such as Greenberg *et al.* (1964).

In most patients with sarcoidosis of the salivary glands, the presenting symptom is usually a swelling of the glands and some patients also notice some dryness of the mouth. In a few patients, ocular symptoms occur first. The activity of the process varies considerably and in a proportion of patients, there is a persistent low-grade fever – the 'febris uveoparotidea subchronica' described by Heerfordt (1909) in his classical paper of the syndrome. In about half the patients, the salivary glands return to normal within six months. In the others, resolution may take up to three years. Corticosteroids reduce the size of the glands in the more acute conditions, but seem to have little influence on the overall course of the disease and are usually not indicated.

Actinomycosis is very uncommon in this country now and syphilis rarely involves the salivary glands.

Other conditions

Enlargement of the parotid glands, usually bilateral, as a result of increase of the intraglandular fat has already been mentioned. It is of no consequence and requires no treatment but may cause confusion in diagnosis. Sialography and secretion are normal. Differential diagnosis includes hypertrophy of the masseter muscles but this is unlikely to cause difficulty provided the possibility is considered.

Enlargement of the parotid occasionally occurs in patients receiving treatment with thiouracil. Barbero and Sibinga (1962) reported that 92 per cent of patients with mucoviscidosis had significant enlargement of the submandibular glands but the parotids seem to escape.

In a few patients the lymphoid tissue in the parotid or submandibular glands is involved in a reticulosis and sometimes this can be difficult to distinguish clinically and histologically from a sialoadenitis when it is the presenting symptom and when there is no evidence of other lymphoid tissue being involved.

Enlargement of the parotids and sometimes the submandibular glands with diminished secretion also occurs in an ill-understood group of conditions which, for this reason, are described under various names. In 1888 at a meeting in Königsberg, Mikulicz described a patient with swelling of the lacrimal, submandibular and parotid glands and this was reported in 1892. Since then the term 'Mikulicz Disease' or 'Mikulicz Syndrome' has been used as an eponymous title and other names such as

Gougerot (1926) and Sjögren (1933) have been added by some people. More recently the term 'sicca syndrome' has been used as a descriptive title to emphasize one of the main features of the disorder.

Histological evidence shows that the gland is infiltrated by lymphocytes and plasma cells leading to fibrosis. Patey and Thackray (1955) also reported atrophy of acinar cells with squamous epithelial proliferation of the ducts and multiple minute calculi. Sialography shows a picture of punctate sialectasis and Jones (1958) reported 50 per cent of patients with a significantly raised γ-globulin. Some patients have other diseases such as rheumatoid arthritis or dermatomyositis and in some antinuclear factors have been demonstrated in the blood suggesting an auto-immune process. In a few patients the changes in lymphoid elements in the gland have made it difficult to distinguish the condition from an adenolymphoma.

Whatever the aetiology of the condition, or group of conditions, the clinical features which present problems are the liability to recurrent infection, the enlargement of the gland suggesting a diagnosis of neoplasm and last, but often the most important to the patient, the associated xerostomia. If the lacrimal glands are also involved there will be diminished tear formation and a tendency to kerato-conjunctivitis. The problem of infection has been referred to already and neoplasia will be considered in the next section. Symptomatic relief of xerostomia is never satisfactory but patients sometimes obtain some relief from glycerin.

Pain in the parotid region in association with eating may develop in patients who have had the superior cervical ganglion excised. The symptom is usually not very troublesome but in one patient in whom the author had resected a neurofibroma involving the ganglion this complication was severe. Gardner and Abdullah (1955) have ascribed the pain to sudden excessive vasodilatation within the parotid as a result of the unopposed parasympathetic activity after post-ganglionic neuronal degeneration has occurred. This explanation appears to be physiologically sound and to fit the clinical facts.

Neoplasms

Although tumours arising from the lymphoid or supporting connective tissues may occur in the salivary glands they are rare, as also are secondary malignant neoplasms, and most of the tumours found in the salivary glands arise from the specialized epithelial cells of the ducts or acini. They form only two to three per cent of all tumours but are of particular significance because of the special features which they exhibit and the consequent difficulty in classification and terminology. Rewell (1963) has aptly remarked that 'in this field terminology has proliferated madly enough to be termed "malignant"'.

Although salivary tumours of almost any type may occur in any of the glands there is considerable variation in the frequency with which different types of tumour occur in individual glands and in the proportional distribution of benign and malignant tumours, not only between the major and minor glands but also between different groups of minor glands. Approximately 80 per cent of the tumours are situated in the parotid gland, ten per cent in the submandibular gland and ten per cent in the minor salivary glands. This distribution does not correspond with the relative weights of the glandular tissue and among the minor glands the frequency in different sites is not related to the number of glands in a particular area.

Classification

No system of classification so far devised has received universal acceptance but the publication by Thackray and Sobin (1972) has provided an authoritative and official scheme. It has not ended all controversy but it has done much to dispel a lot of doubt and confusion which has occurred in the past. It may also help to stop the publication of long lists of so-called synonyms which in many cases are not true synonyms at all.

The primary classification of salivary gland tumours, shown in *Table 3.1*, is into the epithelial, non-epithelial and unclassified tumours. The epithelial tumours are by far the commonest in adults, in whom they account for over 95 per cent of the total, but in children approximately 60 per cent of tumours are non-epithelial in origin – mainly haemangiomas, lymphangiomas and neurofibromas. The unclassified group is self-explanatory and includes the rare examples of metastases from neoplasms elsewhere. Some of these metastases, such as those from clear cell carcinomas of the kidney, may give rise to difficulty in differentiation from some of the primary salivary tumours.

Table 3.1   Histological typing of salivary gland tumours

I. EPITHELIAL TUMOURS

    A. ADENOMAS
        (1) Pleomorphic adenoma (mixed tumour)
        (2) Monomorphic adenomas
           (a) Adenolymphoma
           (b) Oxyphilic adenoma
           (c) Other types
    B. MUCO-EPIDERMOID TUMOUR
    C. ACINIC CELL TUMOUR
    D. CARCINOMAS
        (1) Adenoid cystic carcinoma
        (2) Adenocarcinoma
        (3) Epidermoid carcinoma
        (4) Undifferentiated carcinoma
        (5) Carcinoma in pleomorphic adenoma
           (malignant mixed tumour)

II. NON-EPITHELIAL TUMOURS

III. UNCLASSIFIED TUMOURS

The distribution of the main types of tumours is shown for the different sites in *Table 3.2* which has been compiled from the comprehensive detailed figures given by Bardwil, Luna and Healey (1967); Eneroth (1964); Eneroth, Hjertman and Moberger (1967); Farr (1967); Foote and Frazell (1954); Harrison (1956); Naunton Morgan and Mackenzie (1968); Patey (1965b); Patey, Thackray and Keeling (1965); Ranger, Thackray and Lucas (1956); Thackray (1961).

Table 3.2   Distribution of main types of tumour occurring in different salivary glands expressed as an approximate percentage of the total

Type of tumour	Parotid gland	Sub-mandibular gland	Lip and cheek	Palate	Floor of mouth and tongue	Peri-tonsillar area	Total
Pleomorphic adenoma	61	4	1	2.7		1	69.7
Muco-epidermoid tumour	3.5	1		0.7			5.2
Adenoid cystic carcinoma	1.5	1.5	0.4	1.2	1.3	0.2	6.1
Other types of carcinoma	11	2.5	0.1	0.4			14
Miscellaneous	5						5
Total	82	9	1.5	5	1.3	1.2	100

Note: This table refers only to those glands which can properly be classed as 'salivary' glands, major or minor, and does not include similar tumours found in the nose, sinuses, larynx, trachea, bronchi, etc.

The main types of salivary tumour will now be considered in more detail and then their management will be discussed in relation to the site of origin.

Pleomorphic adenoma

For many years these tumours have been referred to as 'mixed' tumours on account of their histological appearance. They are the commonest of all the salivary tumours and occur more than twice as frequently as all the other types combined. The tumours are essentially benign but may recur locally if removal is incomplete and a small proportion (less than five per cent) undergo malignant change, sometimes after a very long interval. Patey, Thackray and Keeling (1965) report such a change in a woman whose history went back 46 years.

These tumours occur most commonly in young adults, the majority developing before the age of 40. Males and females are almost equally affected. The parotid gland is by far the commonest site and nearly 90 per cent of all salivary pleomorphic adenomas occur in that gland.

Macroscopically the tumour is firm and usually lobulated with a well-defined capsule surrounding it. However, histologically it can be seen that portions of tumour frequently extend through the capsule. In single sections these outgrowths may appear to be detached from the main tumour (*Figure 3.2*) but as has been demonstrated by Patey and Thackray (1953), serial sections show that there is always a projection through the capsule although the strand may be quite slender. As any tumour may have several such outgrowths, the strands of which are easily torn across if the tumour is enucleated, recurrences are usually multicentric in type and serial sections of recurrent neoplasms show connecting strands between the different recurrent tumours which are growing apparently as one mass.

A pleomorphic adenoma has a slowly progressive rate of growth and if left

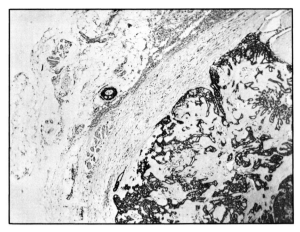

Figure 3.2 Pleomorphic adenoma with a well-defined capsule and an extension of neoplasm outside the capsule. In this single section the nodule appears to be separate from the main mass of tumour but serial sections showed that the two were connected by a fine strand penetrating the capsule. (× 35) (From Ranger, Thackray and Lucas [1956], reproduced by courtesy of the Editor of *British Journal of Cancer*)

untreated may come to weigh as much as 2 or 3 kg. Frylinck (1953) has reported a tumour in a patient whose religion prevented her having any operation until her life was threatened with haemorrhage from a surface vessel. The tumour had then been growing for 30 years and after removal it weighed over 27 kg and contained more than 15 litres of turbid fluid in its necrotic centre.

Rarely, metastases may appear in distant parts of the body (*Figure 3.3*).

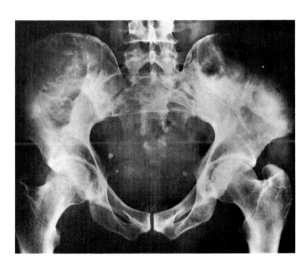

Figure 3.3 Metastatic tumour of ilium from a pleomorphic adenoma of the parotid. The metastasis, from which a biopsy was taken in 1942, showed the histological features of a typical pleomorphic adenoma identical in appearance with a parotid tumour removed in 1919

Microscopically the tumour consists of epithelial cells in a hyaline stroma having a chondroid appearance and it was this that led to the original description of 'mixed' tumour. However, it is now believed that the stroma is a secretion but there is still considerable difference of opinion about its exact origin and significance. The amount of matrix present varies considerably from one tumour to another and even in different areas of the same tumour.

Other types of adenomas

About two per cent of the salivary adenomas do not have the specific features indicative of adenolymphomas or oxyphilic adenomas and yet do not exhibit the heterogeneous histologic appearances characteristic of pleomorphic adenomas. The histological pattern is much more uniform in each tumour although different types occur. Clear cell adenoma, basal cell adenoma, tubular adenoma, trabecular adenoma, sebaceous adenoma and sebaceous lymphadenoma have been described. Clinically and on naked-eye examination these tumours cannot be differentiated from pleomorphic adenomas and the treatment is identical.

Muco-epidermoid tumours

Muco-epidermoid tumours form about five per cent of parotid tumours and are also occasionally found in the submandibular gland and in the palate but are very rare elsewhere. When these tumours were first clearly described by Stewart, Foote and Becker (1945) and later by Linell (1948) they were considered to include both benign and malignant varieties. However, it is now generally accepted that none can be regarded as truly benign although the degree of malignancy is variable.

Histologically these tumours contain varying proportions of epidermoid cells, mucus-secreting cells and intermediate cells and as a result the cut surface of the tumour may appear to be a solid mass or collection of mucous cysts.

Although some of these tumours may be of high-grade malignancy the prognosis is generally better than with other types of malignant salivary tumours. There is evidence that at least some of these tumours are radio-sensitive.

Adenoid cystic carcinoma

These tumours are frequently referred to by other names such as cylindroma or basalioma. These terms serve to describe two of the characteristic features of the pathology but fail to include the predominant concept of malignancy and therefore fail to distinguish them adequately from 'mixed' tumours with a cylindromatous appearance. For this reason the term 'adenoid cystic carcinoma' has come to be used increasingly throughout the literature on salivary tumours.

In the parotid gland adenoid cystic carcinomas form only a small proportion of the total tumours (less than two per cent) but in the palate they form a much higher proportion (about 30 per cent) and in the tongue and floor of mouth virtually all the salivary gland tumours are of this type.

These tumours are invasive and often infiltrate along tissue planes, particularly in perineural and perivascular spaces. Although malignant, their rate of growth is usually slow and it may be several years before they reach appreciable size or recur after removal. Occasionally the presenting symptom may be facial paralysis without there being any evidence of tumour on inspection or palpation. They are liable to metastasize widely, especially after local recurrences have developed but the metastases usually grow slowly and patients with metastases may continue to live for several years in a generally fit state.

Histologically the tumours are characterized by the occurrence of masses of cells around cystic or alveolar spaces in a scanty connective tissue stroma but in some instances the cells occur in solid sheets without any cystic spaces.

Acinic cell tumours

These are malignant tumours with a distinctive histological appearance of masses of uniform acinic cells with a well-marked cell membrane and small deeply-staining nucleus. The cells are usually arranged in solid masses but sometimes exhibit a micro-cystic or papillary cystic form. They occur predominantly in women and almost entirely in the parotid gland. A small proportion of the tumours are painful.

The acinic cell tumours are malignant but appear to have a better prognosis than the other malignant neoplasms.

Other carcinomas

In addition to the muco-epidermoid tumours, acinic cell tumours and adenoid cystic carcinomas which have been described already, other malignant tumours are found in the salivary glands. The commonest of these is the spheroidal cell carcinoma without any recognizable glandular elements and with masses of undifferentiated rounded cells. Some of these tumours arise *de novo* but from 30 to 40 per cent develop in glands which have previously been the site of a pleomorphic adenoma. The next most common type is the adenocarcinoma and in approximately 50 per cent of these there is also evidence of a pre-existing pleomorphic adenoma. Histologically these tumours have obvious tubule formation of frankly malignant type but without the special features found in the adenoid cystic tumours. About 50 per cent of spindle cell carcinomas arise in pleomorphic adenomas and occasionally they have been found in association with adenoid cystic carcinoma. They are characterized by masses of spindle-shaped cells without any glandular structure. Squamous cell carcinomas with varying degrees of keratinization are sometimes found in the parotid and may occur in the minor salivary glands as well but in those sites it is impossible to distinguish them from squamous cell carcinomas arising from the mucosa of the area.

Secondary tumours

Occasionally secondary tumours may be found in the parotid gland and even more rarely in the submandibular gland, although of course either may be secondarily involved by direct extension of malignant neoplasms occurring in the neighbourhood.

Melanomata of the face and scalp may give rise to a metastatic lymph node in the parotid without the primary lesion being obvious and the patients may be regarded as having a primary parotid tumour. Blood-borne metastases have also occurred from carcinoma in such distant sites as bronchus, breast, kidney, stomach, pancreas, etc.

Connective tissue tumours

Connective tissue tumours are not common in the salivary glands but in children they form more than half the total because of the numbers of haemangiomas and also some lymphangiomas. Other connective tissue tumours found in the salivary glands include neurinomas, neurofibromas and plexiform neurofibromas. Lipomas are rare. Sarcomas may occur but are uncommon.

The management of salivary tumours

Although the behaviour of any salivary neoplasm is largely determined by its pathological type, the diagnosis and treatment will depend on its site of origin and its relationship to adjacent anatomical structures as well as its histological classification. In view of this it is convenient to discuss the management of tumours according to the gland which is affected.

Parotid tumours

In the parotid gland more than three-quarters of the neoplasms are benign and in addition some inflammatory lesions present as painless tumours indistinguishable from neoplastic conditions. The frequency of various types of parotid tumour encountered in a series of 651 parotid tumours treated in the Middlesex Hospital is shown in *Table 3.3* (Thackray and Lucas, 1974).

Table 3.3

Parotid tumours	*Percentage incidence*	
Adenomas	83.4	
Pleomorphic adenoma		72.0
Monomorphic adenoma		
Adenolymphoma		9.0
Oxyphilic adenoma		0.6
Other types of adenoma		1.8
Muco-epidermoid tumours	2.3	
Acinic cell tumours	1.2	
Carcinomas	13.1	
Adenoid cystic carcinoma		3.3
Adenocarcinoma		1.0
Epidermoid carcinoma		1.0
Undifferentiated carcinoma		3.7
Carcinoma in pleomorphic adenoma		4.1

Only very few parotid tumours, e.g. haemangiomas, have special features which enable a pathological diagnosis to be made pre-operatively on clinical and radiographic evidence. Most tumours present as painless swellings without any particular distinguishing features. Although evidence of involvement of the facial nerve is an indication of malignancy the majority of malignant tumours are not associated with any facial weakness when the patient is first seen.

Biopsy of parotid tumours leads to spillage of cells and may well lead to the development of tumour in the scar. *Figure 3.4* shows a typical example. Because of this

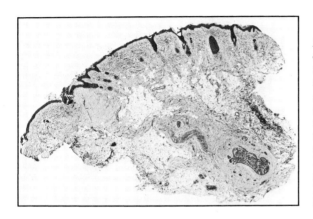

Figure 3.4 Adenoid cystic carcinoma in a parotid scar. Histology of the excised scar showed active viable cystic carcinoma after a radical course of radiotherapy administered before total radical parotidectomy with excision of the scar. (Photomicrograph by Mr. D. Bishop, Ferens Institute of Otolaryngology, from a slide provided by Professor A. C. Thackray, Bland Sutton Institute of Pathology)

it is inadvisable to perform a preliminary biopsy of any parotid tumour and biopsy at the time of operation is indicated only in particularly difficult cases. Cytological examination of material obtained by aspiration biopsy is a method which is used in some centres but the results are unlikely to provide a certain anwer on which treatment can be soundly based. Eneroth, Franzen and Zajicek (1966) were able to confirm the presence of a tumour in 92 per cent of cases, but this degree of probability is no greater than that resulting from simple clinical examination. More particularly, in only about 50 per cent of cases could the question of malignancy be correctly evaluated. Few people can have had such extensive experience as these workers and in less skilled hands the figures would be even less favourable.

Surgical exploration remains the most certain way of determining the correct diagnosis of any swelling in the parotid gland and of assessing the most appropriate form of management. The passage of the facial nerve through the parotid gland dominates the anatomical features and the relationship of the tumour to the nerve can be determined precisely only at operation. As a result of the types of operation which have been developed over the years by Redon (1965) and others the plane of the facial nerve can be defined with exactitude and the superficial portion or the deep portion of the gland can be removed with any contained tumour. If the pathological nature of the condition requires it the superficial and deep portions can both be excised with preservation of the facial nerve. Clinical experience and pathological studies have shown that in a large number of tumours enucleation from within any capsule which is present is liable to leave residual small nodules of tumour which lead to multicentric recurrences although the rate of growth of many tumours is such that this may not be obvious for some years. When there is no connective tissue capsule and the tumour is contained merely within a surrounding area of compressed normal gland tissue then clearly any attempt at enucleation in this plane must be surgically unsound.

The common tumours of the parotid gland are not radio-sensitive and radio-therapy is not an alternative to surgical excision although some people regard it as an adjuvant to be used in conjunction with enucleation of the tumour. Excision of the tumour with a surrounding area of normal parotid gland is preferred by most surgeons and Morrison (1966) has described the indications for radiotherapy in the management of pleomorphic adenomas of the parotid as being confined to those cases in which the capsule of the tumour ruptures at operation or, exceptionally, the tumour is large and for some reason is inoperable.

A small proportion of patients with parotid tumours arising in the deep lobe of the gland present with a mass in the parapharyngeal space. These will be considered in more detail later under the heading of peritonsillar tumours but, in general, the principles of management are the same as with other parotid tumours although some modification of technique may be required at operation.

In a small number of patients with parotid tumours there will be clear pre-operative indications of malignancy and in them a biopsy will be required to determine the precise type of malignant tumour. After histological confirmation of the malignancy most of these patients are best treated with a course of radiotherapy followed, if operable, by radical excision but even so the prognosis is very poor.

Operative technique

In a very large majority of patients with parotid tumours there are no pre-operative signs to suggest malignancy and therefore in most patients the operation starts with a vertical incision in front of the ear, in a pre-auricular skin crease, extended in a wide 'S'-shaped curve below the ear and then prolonged forwards in an upper cervical skin crease to the level of the tip of the greater cornu of the hyoid bone. The incision is extended through superficial and deep fascia exposing the sternomastoid muscle with the external jugular vein and great auricular nerve crossing it obliquely. These are preserved at this stage and the deep fascia dissected off the muscle to its anterior edge, dividing in the process any posterior fibres of the platysma which are in the way. The muscle is cleared posteriorly as far back as the mastoid process and the greater auricular nerve is now exposed with the posterior fibres running to the lobe of the ear. These fibres can usually be preserved intact unless there is a tumour situated in the posterior part of the gland.

Unless there is a very large tumour posteriorly, dissection then proceeds in the interval between the anterior border of the base of the mastoid process and the mandible by division of the fascia extending from the parotid to be firmly attached to the cartilage of the external auditory meatus. The upper part of the sternomastoid muscle is retracted backwards and the stylohyoid muscle and posterior belly of the digastric exposed and identified. The main trunk of the facial nerve is then located by blunt dissection after it has emerged from the stylomastoid foramen and is running forwards in the angle between the external auditory meatus and the digastric muscle to enter the posterior surface of the parotid. Although the cartilage of the external auditory meatus often provides a pointer to the nerve the most certain landmark is the tympano-mastoid suture. In adults the nerve constantly emerges 6–8 mm deep to the suture. A small artery accompanies the nerve, usually lying just below it, and if this can be safeguarded it will reduce the risk of a temporary facial weakness.

Once the nerve has been identified it can be followed forwards into the gland where it soon divides into its main upper and lower divisions. At this point an assessment is made of the site of the tumour in relation to the nerve and of any infiltration which may be present. In most instances the tumour will be entirely superficial to the plane of the facial nerve and in that case the treatment of choice is a resection of the superficial portion of the gland with preservation of the nerve. If the tumour lies deep to the nerve then the deep portion of the gland should be removed; to allow this, in some instances the superficial portion need only be reflected upwards with the nerve, but in other patients adequate access to the deep lobe may be obtained only after resecting the superficial part of the gland.

The post-operative complication most feared after parotidectomy is, of course, facial paralysis but with the development of the technique of precise identification of the nerve any permanent paralysis can be avoided except when it is necessary deliberately to sacrifice the nerve.

The most frequent post-operative complication is gustatory sweating – sweating of the side of the face on eating – shown by Glaister and his colleagues (1958) to be the result of divided parasympathetic secretomotor fibres coming to activate sweat glands in the area. Although this seems to be the explanation of the phenomenon, treatment by intratympanic division of the parasympathetic nerves has not always been effective in curing the condition in those few patients in whom the condition is a considerable disability. Patey (1968) has referred to one such patient treated in conjunction with the author. Fortunately in most patients the complication amounts to only a minor nuisance.

Salivary fistula after parotidectomy is rare and has been referred to already under 'Salivary Fistulae', p. 46. It usually presents no difficulty in management.

In the patients in whom at operation the tumour appears to be malignant, as judged by infiltration of the facial nerve or diffuse spread within the gland, a biopsy should be taken and submitted to frozen section. If there is undoubted evidence of malignancy on frozen section then radical excision should be undertaken including not only the facial nerve but also the ascending ramus of the mandible and associated muscles of mastication unless the tumour is very superficial. Post-operative radio-therapy would also be appropriate.

If the frozen section shows a benign tumour without any evidence of malignancy the excision should be as indicated previously. If the definitive histology confirms that the tumour is benign then nothing further needs to be done. If the definitive histology shows evidence of malignancy, possibly in part of a benign tumour, then further treatment will depend on the precise histological findings and on the exact re-lationship of the malignant portion to the tissue already excised. In many instances it will be considered necessary to proceed to radiotherapy followed by radical excision.

Submandibular tumours

In the submandibular gland most swellings are associated with an obstruction of the duct, usually by a calculus, and neoplasms are uncommon. Of the neoplasms a significant proportion are malignant. Among 187 primary tumours of the submandibular gland Eneroth, Hjertman and Moberger (1967) found that one-third were malignant and this figure is lower than that in many other series. As is seen in *Table 3.2* the composite figures obtained from many different series show that more than one-half of the sub-mandibular neoplasms are malignant.

In the management of submandibular tumours the first essential is to suspect the condition. In patients with a swelling of the gland the majority will have a history of recurrent swelling with meals and clinical or radiological evidence of a calculus in the gland or the duct. If neither of these features is present then a neoplastic condition must be suspected as a possibility.

As the parotid gland, treatment consists essentially of excision but in this case there are no important anatomical structures to interfere with complete removal of the gland. If subsequent histological examination of the gland shows that the tumour is malignant then post-operative radiotherapy is indicated.

Operative technique

The operation of excision of the submandibular gland starts with an incision in the upper skin crease of the neck extending from a point opposite the angle of the jaw almost to the midline of the neck. In excision of the gland for inflammatory conditions and to deal with the problems of calculi the fascial capsule of the gland can be opened immediately and all subsequent dissection carried out in that plane to avoid the risk of damage to the mandibular branch of the facial nerve supplying the muscles of the lower lip at the corner of the mouth; the facial artery and veins can also be ligated and divided close to the gland and, on the deep surface of the gland, the lingual nerve above and hypoglossal nerve below can be identified lying on the hyoglossus muscle and are preserved carefully while the duct is divided as it runs forwards and inwards in the loop of the lingual nerve. However, in suspected neoplasms, as in the parotid gland, at an early stage of the operation there must be a careful assessment of the nature of the lesion and the degree of any infiltration of surrounding structures. If the tumour is malignant excision will need to be radical and to include nerves and muscles and, in most instances, a portion of the mandible.

Minor salivary glands

In the *lip* it is almost exclusively the upper lip which is likely to be the site of salivary tumours (*Figure 3.5*) and here, as in the cheek, the tumour is unlikely to be malignant. The differentiation from a retention cyst is usually easy on palpation and because of their situation such tumours are easily excised with a surrounding area of soft tissue. If the histology of the resected tissue shows that the tumour is malignant then post-operative radiotherapy should be given to the area but such an event is a rarity.

In the *palate* the tumours are often neglected and may become large before the patient seeks medical advice. A typical palatal salivary tumour is shown in *Figure 3.6* while an unusually large one is shown on a lateral x-ray film in *Figure 3.7*. In approximately half the patients the tumour is malignant, commonly an adenoid cystic carcinoma, and the bone of the palate may be involved without there being any evidence of this until the bone is removed and examined histologically (*Figure 3.8*). If

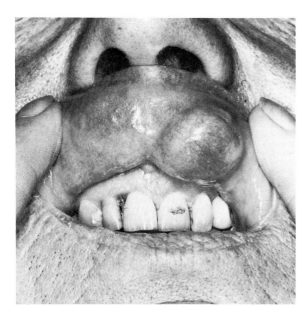

Figure 3.5 Typical pleomorphic adenoma of the upper lip

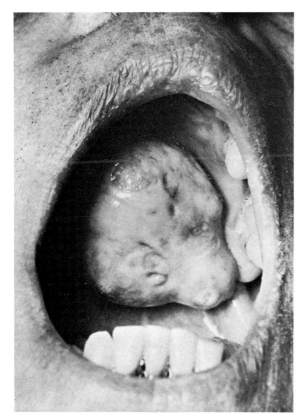

Figure 3.6 Typical pleomorphic adenoma of the hard palate. (From Ranger, Thackray and Lucas [1956], reproduced by courtesy of the Editor of *British Journal of Cancer*)

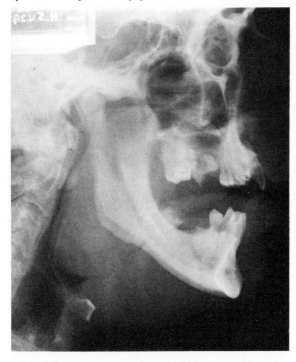

Figure 3.7 Lateral radiograph showing the extent of a very large pleomorphic adenoma arising in the palate. The patient was aged 30 and the tumour had first been noticed at the age of 19. (From Ranger, Thackray and Lucas [1956], reproduced by courtesy of the Editor of *British Journal of Cancer*)

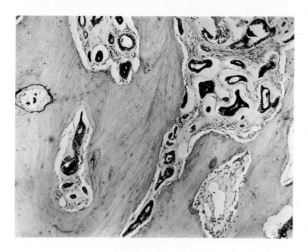

Figure 3.8 Adenoid cystic carcinoma in the hard palate. There is extensive spread of tumour throughout the Haversian system without any destruction of bone and therefore without any clinical, radiological or operative evidence of involvement of bone. (× 70) (From Ranger, Thackray and Lucas [1956], reproduced by courtesy of the Editor of *British Journal of Cancer*)

such tumours are not adequately removed they extend upwards and eventually may invade the middle cranial fossa (*Figure 3.9*).

Because of their situation in relation to bone, salivary tumours arising in the area of the hard palate are most easily removed by simple enucleation off the bone and undoubtedly this fact has contributed largely to the high recurrence rate of even pleomorphic adenomas in this situation as stressed by Ranger, Thackray and Lucas (1956). As has been mentioned already, enucleation of almost any salivary tumour is liable to leave behind residual neoplastic areas and in addition statistics show that in the palate approximately half the tumours are malignant. For these reasons it is

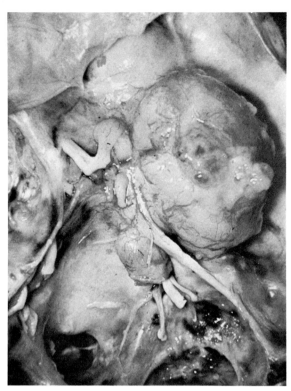

Figure 3.9 Adenoid cystic carcinoma invading the middle cranial fossa. The patient presented with a tumour of the palate which had been present for four years. Treatment was by excision followed by radiotherapy. Multiple pulmonary metastases developed six years later and death occurred from the intracranial extension after a further two years

considered that the treatment of choice for palatal tumours is to remove the tumour by excising the area of palate to which it is attached and this applies whether the tumour is situated in the hard or soft palate. The resulting defect can be closed by an obturator and the defect to be covered in this way will be smaller than any deficiency resulting from attempts to treat multicentric recurrences. Furthermore, operation for eradication of recurrence is unlikely to be successful.

In the *floor of the mouth* and *tongue* salivary tumours are almost invariably malignant and are clinically similar to squamous cell carcinomas invading that area of the mouth. Also in this area surgical excision of malignant tumours may require extensive resection of tissues including possibly the mandible. For these reasons this is one situation in which it is considered that the management of salivary tumours is governed by the fact that they are not clearly distinguishable from other malignant tumours occurring in the same area and as a result biopsy will be the initial requirement. In the light of the histological evidence the decision will rest between primary excision and primary radiotherapy.

In the *peritonsillar region*, in striking contrast with the floor of the mouth, most salivary tumours are of the pleomorphic adenoma type and in the author's experience the majority of them arise from the deep portion of the parotid gland. Occasionally tumours develop in a peritonsillar mucous gland and these appear localized to the soft palate and fauces. Tumours arising in the deep portion of the parotid are likely to be larger and may present with a tumour visible externally as well as in the peritonsillar area (*Figure 3.10*).

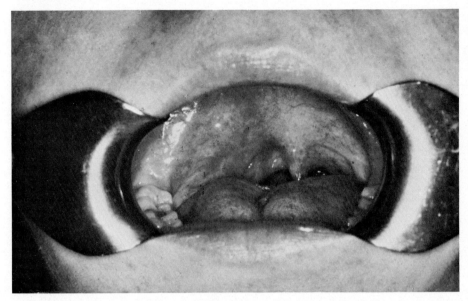

Figure 3.10   Pleomorphic adenoma of the deep lobe of the parotid presenting in the soft palate and peritonsillar region. There was also an obvious swelling externally in the parotid area

While it may be possible to excise a tumour arising from a peritonsillar mucous gland by an incision through the pharyngeal mucosa, those arising in the deep lobe of the parotid can be excised safely only by an external approach and removal of the whole of the deep lobe after defining the plane of the facial nerve with exactitude. The author has found that in some instances the facial nerve has run within a few millimetres of the external aspect of the tumour.

Preliminary biopsy of a tumour bulging into the pharynx, although a technically simple procedure, is inadvisable. Once a biopsy has been taken in this way tumour cells are spilled into the tissues and the scar becomes adherent to the tumour. As a result excision of this area of mucosa is necessary and makes the excisive procedure more hazardous when an external operation is required. In any event if it is not possible to remove the tumour via a pharyngeal incision then an external operation will be required whether the biopsy shows that the tumour is a pleomorphic adenoma or, much more uncommonly, a parapharyngeal neurofibroma or some other tumour. If it is considered possible to excise the tumour through a pharyngeal approach then a preliminary biopsy is not needed.

The removal of a tumour of the deep lobe of the parotid presenting in the parapharyngeal region follows the same lines as has already been described in the account of parotidectomy but there are added difficulties because of the large mass lying deeply in the space between the styloid process and the mandible. Division of the stylomandibular ligament and fracturing of the styloid process as advocated by Patey and Thackray (1957) improves the access but in some large tumours even this is inadequate and considerable help can be obtained by division of the mandible with retraction of the ramus forwards and upwards (*Figure 3.11*). Cook and Ranger (1969) reported that in six patients such a procedure made removal very much easier and had no troublesome post-operative sequelae. The loss of lip sensation gradually

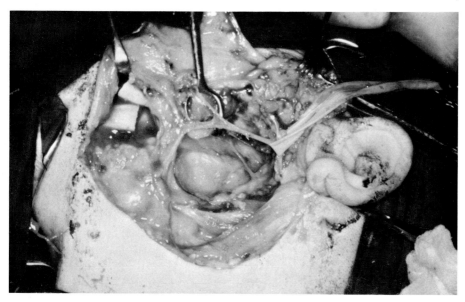

Figure 3.11 Exposure of the deep parotid area. The body of the mandible has been divided in the region of the second premolar tooth and a retractor placed around the angle of the mandible retracts the ramus forwards, upwards and outwards. The facial nerve is retracted with thin latex. (From Cook and Ranger [1969], reproduced by courtesy of the Editor of *Journal of Laryngology and Otology*)

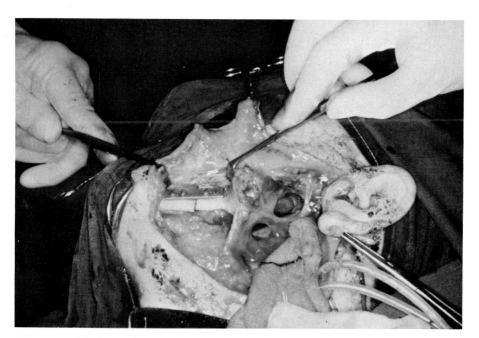

Figure 3.12 Method of fixation of the divided mandible by means of a Vitallium Venables fracture plate. (From Cook and Ranger [1969], reproduced by courtesy of the Editor of *Journal of Laryngology and Otology*)

improved and in most patients returned to normal. They advocated repairing the mandible with a small Vitallium (chrome cobalt) Venables fracture plate to allow immediate mobilization (*Figure 3.12*). Berdal and Hall (1970), in the six patients in whom they found it necessary to divide the mandible, fixed the bone afterwards with stainless steel wire and found satisfactory healing per primam.

References

Barbero, G. J. and Sibinga, M. S. (1962). 'Enlargement of the submaxillary glands in cystic fibrosis', *Paediatrics*, **29**, 788–793

Bardwil, J. M., Luna, M. A. and Healey, J. E. Jnr. (1967). *Cancer of the Head and Neck* (Eds W. S. Maccomb and G. H. Fletcher); Williams and Wilkins, Baltimore

Berdal, P. and Hall, J. G. (1970). 'Parapharyngeal growth of parotid tumours', *Acta Otolaryngologica Stockholm*, Suppl., **263**, 164–166

Bhaskar, S. N., Bolden, T. E. and Weinmann, J. P. (1956). 'Experimental obstructive adenitis in the mouse', *Journal of Dental Research*, **35**, 852–862

Cook, H. P. and Ranger, D. (1969). 'A technique for excision of parapharyngeal tumours', *Journal of Laryngology and Otology*, **83**, 863–871

Diamant, H. (1958). 'Ligation of the parotid duct in chronic recurrent parotitis', *Acta Otolaryngologica Stockholm*, **49**, 375–380

Diamant, H. and Wiberg, A. (1965). 'Does the chorda tympani in Man contain secretory fibres?', *Acta Otolaryngologica Stockholm*, **60**, 255–264

Eneroth, C. M. (1964). 'Histological and clinical aspects of parotid tumours', *Acta Otolaryngologica Stockholm*, Suppl., **191**, 6–99

Eneroth, C. M., Franzen, S. and Zajicek, J. (1966). 'Cytologic diagnosis on aspirate from 1000 salivary gland tumours', *Acta Otolaryngologica Stockholm*, Suppl., **224**, 168–171

Eneroth, C. M., Hjertman, L. and Moberger, G. (1967). 'Malignant tumours of the submandibular glands', *Acta Otolaryngologica Stockholm*, **64**, 514–536

Eneroth, C. M., Hokfelt, T. and Norberg, K. A. (1969). 'The role of the parasympathetic and sympathetic innervation for the secretion of human parotid and submandibular glands', *Acta Otolaryngologica Stockholm*, **68**, 369–375

Farr, H. W. (1967). 'Tumours of the parotid gland', in: *Proceedings of the International Workshop on Cancer of the Head and Neck* (Ed. J. Conley), pp. 542–549; Butterworths, London and Boston

Foote, F. W. and Frazell, E. L. (1954). 'Tumours of the major salivary glands', in: *Atlas of Tumour Pathology* (Sect. IV; Fasc. II); Armed Forces Institute of Pathology, Washington DC

Frylinck, J. R. (1953). 'An unusual tumour', *South African Medical Journal*, **30**, 479

Gardner, W. J. and Abdullah, A. F. (1955). 'Parotid pain following superior cervical ganglionectomy: A clinical example of the antagonistic action of parasympathetic and sympathetic systems', *American Journal of Medical Science*, **230**, 65–68

Glaister, D. H., Hearnshaw, J. R., Heffron, P. F. and Peck, A. W. (1958). 'Mechanism of post-parotidectomy gustatory sweating', *British Medical Journal*, **2**, 942–946

Gougerot, H. (1926). 'Atrophe des glandes salivaires et muqueses de la bouche, des conjonctives (et parfois des muqueses nasale, laryngee, vulvaire, séche resse de la bouche, des conjonctives, etc.)', *Bulletin de Medecin, Paris*, **40**, 360–368

Greenberg, G., Anderson, R., Sharpstone, P. and James D. G. (1964). 'Enlargement of parotid glands due to sarcoidosis', *British Medical Journal*, **2**, 861–862

Harrill, J. A., King, J. S. Jnr. and Boyce, W. H. (1959). 'Structure and composition of salivary calculi', *Laryngoscope*, **69**, 481–492

Harrison, K. (1956). 'A study of ectopic mixed salivary tumours', *Annals of the Royal College of Surgeons of England*, **18**, 99–122

Heerfordt, C. F. (1909). 'Über eine "Febris uveo-parotidea subchronica", an der Glandula Parotis und der Uvea des Aeges lokalisiert und haufig mit paresen cerebrospinaler Nerven kompliziert', *Albrecht v. Graefe's Archiven der Ophthalmology*, **70**, 254–273

Höök, O. (1954). 'Sarcoidosis with involvement of the nervous system', *Archives of Neurological Psychiatry, Chicago*, **71**, 554–575

Jones, B. R. (1958). 'Lacrimal and salivary precipitating antibodies in Sjögren's syndrome', *Lancet*, **2**, 773–776

Laage-Hellman, J. E. (1955). 'Ligatur Av ductus stenoni som terapeutisk Åtgärd', *Svenska Läk-Tidn.*, **52**, 3150–3153

Linell, F. (1948). 'Mucus-secreting and cystic epidermoid carcinomas of mucous and salivary glands', *Acta Pathology and Microbiology Scandinavia*, **25**, 801–828

Maynard, J. D. (1965). 'Recurrent parotid enlargement', *British Journal of Surgery*, **52**, 784–789

Mikulicz, J. von (1892). 'Über eine eigenartige symmetrische Erkrankung der Tränen-und Mundspeicheldrüsen', *Beiträge zur Chirurgie, Festschrift*, 610–630

Morel, A. S. and Firestein, A. (1963). 'Repair of traumatic fistulas of the parotid duct', *Archives of Surgery*, **87,** 623–636

Morrison, R. (1966). 'Tumours of the parotid gland'. *Proceedings of the Royal Society of Medicine*, **59,** 429–437

Naunton Morgan, M. and MacKenzie, D. H. (1968). 'Tumours of salivary glands. A review of 204 cases with 5-year follow-up', *British Journal of Surgery*, **55,** 284–288

Patey, D. H. (1965a). 'Inflammation of the salivary glands with particular reference to chronic and recurrent parotitis', *Annals of the Royal College of Surgeons of England*, **36,** 26–44

Patey, D. H. (1965b). 'Diseases of the salivary glands', in: *Clinical Surgery* (Vol. 9): *Head and Neck* (Ed. C. Rob and R. Smith), ch. 3, pp. 37–61; Butterworths, London and Boston

Patey, D. H. (1968). 'Tumours and other diseases of the salivary glands in relation to general physiology and pathology', *Journal of Laryngology and Otology*, **82,** 853–866

Patey, D. H. and Ranger, I. (1957). 'Some points in the surgical anatomy of the parotid gland', *British Journal of Surgery*, **45,** 250–258

Patey, D. H. and Thackray, A. C. (1953). 'Salivary gland tumours', *Annual Report of the British Empirical Cancer Campaign*, **31,** 74–75

Patey, D. H. and Thackray, A. C. (1955). 'Chronic "Sialectatic" parotitis in the light of pathological studies on parotidectomy material', *British Journal of Surgery*, **43,** 43–50

Patey, D. H. and Thackray, A. C. (1957). 'The pathological anatomy and treatment of parotid tumours with retropharyngeal extension (dumb-bell tumours)', *British Journal of Surgery*, **44,** 352–358

Patey, D. H. and Thackray, A. C. and Keeling, D. H. (1965). 'Malignant disease of the parotid'. *British Journal of Cancer*, **19,** 712–737

Pattinson, J. N. (1969). 'Head and neck lymph nodes', in: *Operative Surgery* (Vol. 6): (Eds C. Rob, R. Smith and M. Ewing), pp. 167–171; Butterworths, London and Boston

Pennell, W. H. (1951). 'Boeck's sarcoid with involvement of central nervous system', *Archives of Neurological Psychiatry, Chicago*, **66,** 728–737

Ranger, D., Thackray, A. C. and Lucas, R. B. (1956). 'Mucous gland tumours', *British Journal of Cancer*, **10,** 1–16

Ranger, I. (1957). 'An experimental study of sialography and its correlation with histological appearances in normal parotid and submandibular glands', *British Journal of Surgery*, **44,** 415–418

Redon, H. (1965). *Chirurgie des Glandes Salivaires*; Masson, Paris

Rewell, R. E. (1963). *Pathology of the Upper Respiratory Tract*; Livingstone, Edinburgh

Sjögren, H. (1933). 'Zur Kenntnis der Keratoconjunctivitis sica (Keratoconjunctivitis Filiformis bei Hypofunktion der Tränendrüsen)', *Acta Ophthalmologica*, Suppl., **2,** 1–151

Stewart, F. W., Foote, F. W. and Becker, W. F. (1945). 'Muco-epidermoid tumours of salivary glands', *Annals of Surgery*, **122,** 820–844

Thackray, A. C. (1955). 'Sialectasis', *Archives of the Middlesex Hospital*, **5,** 151–159

Thackray, A. C. (1961). 'Mucous gland tumours', *Clinical Radiology*, **12,** 241–245

Thackray, A. C. and Lucas, R. B. (1974). *Tumours of the Major Salivary Glands*; Armed Forces Institute of Pathology, Washington DC

Thackray, A. C. and Sobin, L. H. (1972). *Histological Typing of Salivary Gland Tumours*, Series of the International Histological Classification of Tumours, No. 7; World Health Organisation, Geneva

4 Pharyngitis – acute and chronic
Joselen Ransome

Inflammation of the pharynx is frequently limited to the oropharynx, but all three parts of the pharynx may be involved, together or separately. Inflammation of the hypopharynx (Paterson–Brown Kelly syndrome) is described in the next chapter.

Nasopharyngitis

Acute nasopharyngitis may be caused by viruses or bacteria. It may be the first sign of a cold or attack of influenza, when it is described as a raw, hot feeling 'behind the nose'. It may also occur as a secondary infection in acute sinusitis and rhinitis, especially when the posterior group of sinuses is involved; and very rarely secondary to acute suppurative otitis media, due to pus escaping from the eustachian tube.

Apart from discomfort behind the nose, the only symptom is post-nasal discharge.

Examination with a post-nasal mirror reveals reddening of the mucous membrane, and discharge which may be mucoid or mucopurulent.

Treatment need only be symptomatic when the condition is obviously only part of a self-limiting upper respiratory virus infection. Antibiotics may be required for a bacterial infection, plus routine treatment of sinusitis if present.

Chronic non-specific nasopharyngitis is almost invariably secondary to chronic rhinitis and sinusitis, or due to excessive exposure to dust. Treatment is that of the underlying cause.

Atrophic nasopharyngitis occurs as an extension of atrophic rhinitis, and the patient may be conscious of crusting behind the nose. Examination with a post-nasal mirror shows dry crusts adhering to a dry-looking mucous membrane. Treatment is that of the nasal condition.

Chronic specific nasopharyngitis

Syphilitic lesions are hardly ever seen in the nasopharynx.

Tuberculous deposits may occur in miliary spread.

Scleroma spreads into the nasopharynx from the nasal cavities. It is a rare disease in western Europe (*see also* under 'Oropharynx') but in affected subjects the naso-pharynx is often involved. The sites of predilection are the posterior end of the septum and the eustachian cushions (Zwiefach, 1955). After initial catarrhal and granulomatous stages, dense scar tissue forms, which may also affect the soft palate, retracting it upwards to form the so-called 'gothic palate'. The nasopharynx becomes almost closed off with scar tissue. Treatment is with systemic tetracyclines or streptomycin.

Oropharyngitis – acute non-specific

Aetiology

Up to 50 per cent of cases are caused by viruses (Rowson, 1973), mainly influenza, para-influenza, enterovirus, rhinovirus and adenovirus. The rest are mainly caused by haemolytic streptococci, and this organism accounts for most of the more serious cases. Pharyngitis can also be caused by *Streptococcus pneumoniae* and by *Haemophilus influenzae*. There may also be a mixed infection, or virus–pyococcal sequence. Gonococcal pharyngitis may also occur.

It is not possible to distinguish viral from bacterial infections on clinical grounds, and as far as respiratory viruses are concerned, each is capable of producing a wide range of clinical syndromes; sometimes oropharyngitis may be associated with rhinitis and nasopharyngitis, at other times with conjunctivitis, cervical adenitis or bronchitis. It follows that any of these syndromes may be due to a number of different organisms.

Symptoms

The disease may be trivial, with a slight sore throat lasting for a few days, a little malaise and a mild degree of pyrexia. In this form the disease often occurs in epidemics. In more severe cases there may be intense sore throat with toxaemia, fever and headache. The patient looks ill and may have difficulty in swallowing his saliva. When the palate is oedematous there may be an irritating cough caused by the elongated uvula touching the back of the tongue.

Signs

Local

In mild cases the pharynx may be uniformly injected, or redness may be confined to the pillars of the fauces. In severe cases the pharynx is grossly injected, particularly in the region of the lateral bands. The mucosa is oedematous, often involving the palate and uvula. The lymphoid follicles on the posterior pharyngeal wall stand out and may be covered with sloughs, and the lingual tonsils may be similarly affected. The tonsils are injected and there may be exudate on their surface, or a peritonsillar abscess may have formed. The regional lymph nodes may be enlarged and tender.

In very severe cases examination of the pharynx may be difficult owing to trismus: the breath is foul and the mouth is full of saliva.

General

In mild cases there are no general signs. In severe cases, as with any infection, there may be a high temperature and tachycardia.

Diagnosis

In mild infections diagnosis presents no difficulties, but when exudate is present diphtheria and Vincent's angina must be excluded. Culture of a throat swab establishes the diagnosis, but treatment must rely on clinical judgment. In diphtheria the degree of toxaemia is usually out of proportion to the rise in temperature, but the pulse rate is unduly raised (*see below*). Although there is exudate on the tonsils, the inflammatory reaction of the pharynx is not, as a rule, as marked as it is in the case of streptococcal infection. The exudate is firmly adherent and may extend to the soft palate: its removal leaves a bleeding area. Diphtheria antitoxin and penicillin should be given without delay. In all cases of sore throat a swab should be taken and the result will act as a guide to the correct antibiotic therapy (if any). It must be remembered that the condition may be the prodromal stage of other acute specific fevers, besides diphtheria.

Complications

Local

Direct spread of infection inferiorly may reach the larynx and produce *oedema of the glottis* and the risk of respiratory obstruction. Direct spread anteriorly into the floor of the mouth produces a brawny cellulitis known as *Ludwig's angina*. Direct spread postero-laterally into the parapharyngeal space may lead to a *parapharyngeal abscess* which presents as pain and swelling in the lateral wall of the oropharynx, sometimes with marked swelling in the neck as well.

Spread via lymphatics gives rise to *cervical adenitis*, affecting mainly the upper deep cervical group of nodes in the anterior triangle. Occasionally the inflammatory process in an affected node proceeds to suppuration, and a *cervical abscess* is formed.

General

As with severe infections elsewhere, toxaemia, bacteraemia, septicaemia and pyaemia may all occur, especially in streptococcal pharyngitis; and in patients with valvular heart disease there is a risk of subacute bacterial endocarditis.

Treatment

Treatment of the disease

Mild cases without fever or malaise either require no treatment, or need only soluble aspirin for symptomatic relief.

More severe cases with fever and general malaise require bed rest and systemic antibiotics, usually a penicillin. This treatment can be carried out at home. Treatment is given on the assumption that there is up to a 50 per cent chance that the infection is caused by a penicillin-sensitive organism. It is not practicable to await the results of virus culture and in any case no curative treatment for virus infections is available.

Very severe cases with high temperature and severe pain require admission to the side ward of an ENT unit, especially if there has been no immediate response to antibiotics begun at home, because of the risk of complications.

These cases are rare nowadays but require the following regimen immediately. On arrival the patient, who is confined to bed, is put on a four-hourly observation chart and a fluid balance record. A throat swab is taken but, without waiting for the result, the patient is given two mega-units of crystalline penicillin intramuscularly and then one mega-unit intramuscularly six-hourly. (After 24–48 hours the patient's clinical response and swab result can be reviewed, and the antibiotic changed if appropriate.) If the patient has severe throat pain he may not be able to swallow enough liquid to replace his inevitable losses, in which case parenteral fluid administration will be required. Analgesics should be given, but sedation is best avoided.

If the patient appears to be developing the slightest degree of respiratory obstruction, as indicated by the development of inspiratory stridor and a rising pulse rate, he will require oxygen and humidification, together with intramuscular injections of hydrocortisone, in the hope of averting a tracheostomy. Suction, suction catheters, and a laryngotomy or tracheostomy set should be available at the bedside. The patient should be on a half-hourly pulse chart. The operating theatre and anaesthetist should be alerted to the possibility of an elective tracheostomy. The patient is given nothing by mouth in case an anaesthetic is required.

In the vast majority of patients medical treatment will ensure rapid recovery within a few days.

Treatment of the complications

Respiratory obstruction
Respiratory obstruction – usually due to spread of inflammatory oedema to the glottis but occasionally caused by massive oedema of the oropharynx – is the most alarming

complication of acute pharyngitis, and fortunately nowadays is rare in countries where primary medical care is available to the mass of the population. The treatment is initially medical as above, and often nothing further is required. However, if stridor persists for some hours or worsens, and especially if the pulse rate is rising (in the absence of a matching rise in temperature), this indicates that the patient is not holding his own and elective tracheostomy in the operating theatre must be carried out.

This is best done with a general anaesthetic and endotracheal tube; however, it requires an experienced and skilled anaesthetist because of the glottic oedema. The chances of success in intubation must be weighed against the fact that injecting local anaesthetic into the soft tissues of the neck is undesirable because of the risk of further spreading the infection. The patient should be anaesthetized in the theatre with the otolaryngologist standing by, prepared to proceed at once to tracheostomy in case of difficulty.

Ludwig's angina
This, also, is rare nowadays. The cellulitis of the floor of the mouth, readily palpated bi-manually, is extremely tender, and tongue movements and swallowing are very painful. The victim may therefore become depleted of fluids, and also the cellulitis may spread, with risk of respiratory obstruction.

Initially, treatment is the same as for severe pharyngitis. If the condition fails to respond to antibiotics, incision and drainage under a general anaesthetic are performed, using a midline incision from the chin above to the level of the thyroid cartilage below.

Parapharyngeal abscess
The dangers of this complication can be deduced from *Figure 4.1*: there is no anatomical barrier to prevent infection from spreading upwards to the base of the skull and downwards to the superior mediastinum.

The treatment is the same as for severe pharyngitis initially. The swelling may resolve completely on antibiotic therapy. Occasionally, antibiotics limit the spread of inflammation, but suppuration occurs resulting in a fluctuant abscess. This will require incision and drainage, either through the mouth, or externally through the neck, according to where the maximum swelling lies. If the former route is chosen, reference to *Figure 4.1* will indicate the anatomical dangers of this procedure, because of the proximity of the carotid arteries and internal jugular vein, as well as the smaller ascending pharyngeal and ascending palatine vessels. However, incising over the most fluctuant area, making sure there is no pulsation, and incising only very superficially with a knife and then using sinus forceps, ensures a relatively risk-free procedure. It should be done under a general anaesthetic given by an experienced anaesthetist, using a cuffed endotracheal tube, and with a Boyle–Davis gag in position, suction ready, and the operating table with a head-down tilt.

Cervical adenitis and cervical abscess
Cervical adenitis is a common complication of pharyngitis, and normally resolves with the pharyngitis. Treatment is that of the primary condition. Occasionally suppuration occurs leading to an abscess in a lymph node: this too may respond to antibiotics, but if not it will require incision and drainage, or excision of the whole

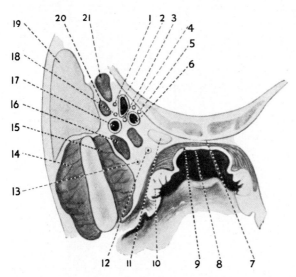

Figure 4.1   Transverse section at the level of the tonsil to illustrate the parapharyngeal space. (From St. Clair Thomson, Negus and Bateman [1955], *Diseases of the Nose and Throat*, page 401, Figure 167, Cassell, London; after Cunningham)

1 Spinal accessory nerve	12 Ascending pharyngeal artery
2 Internal jugular vein	13 Ascending palatine artery
3 Hypoglossal nerve	14 Masseter muscle
4 Vagus nerve	15 Medial pterygoid muscle
5 Sympathetic nerve	16 Styloglossus
6 Internal carotid artery	17 External carotid artery
7 Prevertebral fascia	18 Glosso-pharyngeal nerve
8 Aponeurosis of pharynx	19 Parotid gland
9 Superior constrictor muscle	20 Stylohyoid
10 Tonsil	21 Digastric muscle
11 Post-pharyngeal lymphatic gland	

node, if it is freely mobile and can obviously be excised without difficulty (this has the advantage that the histology can be checked when doubtful).

Acute aphthous ulceration of the mouth and pharynx constitutes an acute form of pharyngitis of unknown aetiology. It is described in Chapter 2.

Oropharyngitis – acute specific

This occurs in several conditions, some of which are described in detail below.

The infectious fevers

It would be out of place here to give a full account of the specific fevers but, as many of them exhibit lesions in the mouth or pharynx, they must be considered in the differential diagnosis of acute infection in this region.

Diphtheria

Aetiology

Diphtheria is caused by *Corynebacterium diphtheriae*, a thin-beaded Gram-positive bacillus containing metachromatic granules demonstrable by special staining techniques. Although growing mainly in the pharynx (including tonsils), nose and larynx, it produces its most serious effect by wide diffusion of the diphtheria toxin, which can cause myocarditis and neuritis.

Pathology

The lesion is usually confined to the pharynx, but may occur in the nose, larynx or elsewhere. The tonsils are commonly affected, and there is superficial ulceration, with the formation of a false membrane which may spread to the soft palate and the uvula. The exudate is grey-white, firmly adherent, and appears to have been laid on the surface rather than inlaid, as in the case of Vincent's infection; its removal is difficult and leaves a bleeding area. There is relatively little reaction in the surrounding parts although, in severe cases, there may be oedema of the palate and uvula.

The disease is usually spread by exposure of susceptible subjects to those suffering from the disease or incubating it, but individuals may carry infection and infect others without showing any evidence of disease themselves. These 'carriers' may have had the disease, but some have never shown any clinical signs of it. Many suspected carriers are harbouring organisms which prove, on biological examination, to be avirulent, and others respond to treatment with penicillin.

Symptoms

Children are commonly affected, and the disease starts with general malaise, headache, vomiting, and sore throat. There is not a marked degree of pyrexia, but the pulse rate is unduly raised. The breath is foul, with a sweetish odour, which is regarded as an important diagnostic feature. The regional lymph nodes are enlarged and tender, and may be grossly affected as in the classical 'bull neck'. In cases in which the nose is involved, constitutional symptoms are not severe, and bleeding from the nose, with purulent nasal discharge, often unilateral, is frequently associated with 'impetigo' of the upper lip. In laryngeal cases, respiratory obstruction is the presenting feature, and life is very often threatened.

Complications

Complications may arise from the spread of infection, causing respiratory obstruction or pneumonia, and also from the action of the toxin, which has an affinity for neuromuscular junctions and the myocardium; for this reason early diagnosis and treatment are of the greatest importance.

Diagnosis

The condition must be differentiated from acute streptococcal infection, Vincent's infection, and other forms of acute ulceration in the pharynx. In nasal cases, the presence of a foreign body may be suspected.

The organism can be identified by culture, but many hours must elapse before the diagnosis can be established by this means, so one must rely on clinical acumen if the treatment is not to be delayed; examination of direct smears and other rapid bacteriological methods are unreliable. When in doubt, it is better to treat a suspected case as one of diphtheria and to administer adequate doses of antitoxin until the diagnosis is established by bacteriological examination.

Treatment
Prophylactic. Much can be done to prevent the disease by active immunization. Susceptibility can be determined by the Schick test, and if this is positive, immunization can be induced by graduated doses of toxoid. An attack of the disease usually confers immunity, but if antitoxin has been given early in the disease, permanent immunity may not be acquired, so a history of a previous attack does not necessarily exclude the possibility of a further infection.

Passive immunity can be produced by prophylactic injection of 16 000 units of antitoxin, and it is justifiable to do this in the case of one who has been seriously ill and has been inadvertently exposed to infection. In the case of healthy individuals exposed to infection, it is better to keep them under close observation than to induce passive immunity, because a carrier state may be produced in this way.

Curative. The most important measure is the administration of adequate doses of antitoxin intramuscularly, or intravenously if necessary. The initial dose should never be less than 16 000 units, and as much as 72 000 units intravenously may be indicated. The patient must be kept absolutely at rest, and complications must be dealt with as necessary. Antibiotics are indicated, and a throat swab must be taken before they are administered. The importance of this was illustrated in a recent epidemic of diphtheria among children attending the same school. They were treated as cases of acute streptococcal tonsillitis and the nature of the infection was only suspected when one of them died of myocarditis. Since they had all been treated with penicillin, it was impossible to confirm the diagnosis by taking throat swabs. However, a routine swabbing of the pupils unaffected by the disease revealed a number of carriers of *Corynebacterium diphtheriae*. Another disturbing revelation was that a number of those affected by the disease had previously received active immunization with toxoid.

Scarlet fever (*Scarlatina*)

Aetiology
Scarlet fever is caused by the spread of toxin from a streptococcal infection of the pharynx and tonsils. The incubation period is from two to seven days.

Clinical picture
The onset is sudden, with a rise of temperature, malaise and shivering; headache is a feature, and vomiting may be pronounced. The throat is sore and the regional lymph nodes are enlarged and tender. In the early stage the pharynx may be red, or there may be a yellow slough on the tonsils; this can be easily wiped from them. The tongue undergoes characteristic changes, being first covered with a yellow fur through which the papillae project, 'strawberry-and-cream tongue', becoming later 'strawberry tongue' or 'raspberry tongue' as the fur disappears. Within two days of the onset of the disease an erythematous rash appears on the trunk and limbs, but rarely on the face, which is flushed save for an area of circumoral pallor.

Complications

Fortunately the disease runs a relatively mild course at the present time, but in the past the mortality rate was high. Acute otitis media, sinusitis, nephritis and pneumonia are frequent complications, and many who have recovered from the disease become carriers. The patient must be bacteriologically free from infection before he is released from isolation, and surgical measures may be necessary for the throat, ear or sinuses in order to eliminate the infection. Antibiotics, usually penicillin, are given in all cases.

Measles

Aetiology

Measles is caused by a virus infection, and occurs in epidemics; the incubation period is 10–12 days. It is a serious disease, particularly in the young, because of the possible development of pneumonia, which may be viral or bacterial.

Symptoms

The prodromal stage lasts for three or four days, when the symptoms are those of severe coryza with conjunctivitis, nasal catarrh, diarrhoea and vomiting. Laryngitis (measles croup) may be pronounced and may lead to a mistaken diagnosis of laryngeal diphtheria unless the nature of the disease is recognized.

Signs

Diagnosis may be made at this stage by inspection of the buccal mucosa; this is injected and, scattered over its surface particularly in the region of the molars, are small white spots (Koplik's spots) about the size of a pin-head, surrounded by an area of erythema. After four or five days the typical morbilliform rash appears and Koplik's spots fade. Membranous pharyngitis may occur.

Complications

Acute otitis media, mastoiditis, bronchitis, and pneumonia may complicate the condition, but since the introduction of antibiotics and chemotherapy they may be largely prevented by prophylactic treatment. In ill-nourished children infection can lead to gangrene of the mouth (cancrum oris) or of the vulva (noma vulvae), but such cases are rarely seen now.

Chicken-pox

Aetiology

Chicken-pox is due to a virus infection and the incubation period is 14–21 days.

Symptoms and signs

There is a short prodromal period with a feeling of general malaise, followed by the eruption of macules or maculopapules. They are centripetal in distribution, which serves to differentiate them from the lesions of smallpox. The eruption takes place over a period of two or three days, so that fresh lesions are appearing while the older ones become superficial vesicles or pustules. The scab separates with, in some cases, ulceration which may give rise to pock marks. The lesions may affect the buccal and pharyngeal mucosa early in the disease and may be confused with the vesicles of herpes. The conjunctivae may also be affected, but only with superficial lesions which leave no permanent effects unless secondary infection occurs.

Relation to herpes zoster. The virus responsible for chicken-pox is also responsible for herpes zoster. Many cases of herpes zoster have been recorded among those in contact with chicken-pox.

Infectious mononucleosis (*glandular fever*)

This may occur in the pharynx, giving rise to small vesicles, which then rupture to Chapter 6.

Vincent's angina

This condition affects the tonsillar, pharyngeal and buccal mucosa, and is described in Chapter 2.

While not truly an infectious fever – occurring more in poor conditions rather than being passed from patient to patient – it is an acute specific infection and must not be forgotten when considering other infections of the pharynx.

Herpetic lesions of the pharynx

Herpes simplex

This may occur in the pharynx, giving rise to small vesicles, which then rupture to form small shallow painful ulcers. The condition is self-limiting and of short duration.

Herpes zoster

This occasionally affects the pharynx in the distribution of the 9th and 10th cranial nerves. Vesicles appear unilaterally and are intensely painful.

Treatment
Recently some success is claimed for the application of idoxuridine five per cent (in dimethyl sulphoxide) ('Herpid') solution applied to the lesions four times daily for four days.

Gonococcal pharyngitis and tonsillitis

Nowadays these are not rare, and must be borne in mind when dealing with any acute pharyngitis, as gonococcal pharyngitis cannot be distinguished from other infections on clinical grounds.

Oropharyngitis – chronic non-specific

Aetiology

Chronic pharyngitis may be due to a primary infection in the pharyngeal tissues but more commonly the pharynx becomes infected as a result of disease in other parts of the upper respiratory tract or other systems.

Rhinitis and sinusitis

In some cases, inspection of the oropharynx reveals mucopus festooned over the posterior pharyngeal wall, and it is evident that a quantity of infected material is passing from the nose into the pharynx. In other cases, examination with a post-nasal mirror shows a thin stream of mucopus coming from the posterior end of the middle meatus and tracking down the lateral pharyngeal wall. Evidence of its passage is seen in the hypertrophied and inflamed lymphoid tissue of the lateral columns of the pharynx.

Since mucus is normally passed backwards from the nose into the nasopharynx, infection in the nose or paranasal sinuses may not lead to any nasal symptoms and, indeed, many patients deny excessive use of the handkerchief, even when there is clear evidence of post-nasal catarrh. Unless a careful examination of the nasopharynx is made, therefore, the cause of the pharyngeal condition may be overlooked. Even if the nose and nasopharynx appear healthy, infection in the paranasal sinuses cannot be excluded on clinical grounds only, and x-rays of the sinuses will be required.

The mouth

Teeth

A number of patients consult laryngologists for conditions which are greatly aggravated by dental sepsis, even if not directly attributable to it. One has only to observe the improvement in the state of carcinomatous ulcer in the pharynx after dental sepsis has been corrected to realize the importance of this source of infection. Chronic pharyngitis is common where dental sepsis prevails, and tonsillitis and laryngitis may also occur.

Tonsils

Chronic infection in the tonsils naturally exerts an unfavourable effect on the condition of the pharynx, and if the primary focus of infection lies here, tonsillectomy should benefit the patient. If the focus of infection is elsewhere, however, the tonsils may be merely the site of secondary infection and their removal cannot improve the pharyngeal condition.

Mouth-breathing

When the air is breathed in through the mouth, it is not subjected to the humidification, warming and cleansing which normally take place during its passage over the nasal mucosa. Consequently, the pharynx becomes dry and is subjected to an abnormal degree of infection. The cause of mouth-breathing may be any of the following.

Nasopharyngeal

The most common cause of mouth-breathing in the young is obstruction due to excessive adenoid tissue. In older subjects, tumours of the nasopharynx or antro-choanal polypi are found.

Nasal

Nasal obstruction may be due to maldevelopment, congenital atresia of the posterior choanae, or to structural defects, e.g. deflection of the nasal septum or large turbinates. Inflammatory conditions, such as acute or chronic rhinitis, may cause thickening of the nasal mucosa, as also may allergic states. Nasal polypi or, more rarely, tumours may cause complete obstruction, or the nasal airway may be narrowed by scarring after acute infections, syphilis, lupus or leprosy.

Dental

Protruding teeth prevent the lips coming into apposition, and consequently there is a tendency for mouth-breathing to occur. This prevents the normal development of the alveolus and palate, with aggravation of the dental condition.

Habitual

Some people breathe through their mouths habitually, even though their nasal airways are free. This is particularly the case in those in whom an organic nasal obstruction has been relieved. It is important, after the removal of the adenoids, to ensure that nasal respiration is established and breathing exercises may be necessary.

Pharynx

Excessive scarring of the pharynx for any reason, including poor technique at tonsillectomy, may be a contributory factor in oropharyngitis.

Faulty voice production

The pharynx plays an important part in the production of the voice, because not only does it regulate the flow of air through the nose during speech, but by contraction of its muscles it regulates the size of the lumen of the pharynx to effect a change in resonance. Excessive use of the voice, particularly should voice production be faulty, predisposes to chronic pharyngitis.

External conditions

Living in industrial areas, where the atmosphere is laden with smoke and other waste products of industry, undoubtedly predisposes to chronic pharyngitis, and in the past many people in the course of their duties were exposed without adequate protection from the harmful gases. Although much has been done to purify the atmosphere and to provide protection against irritant fumes, some subjects appear to be unduly sensitive to such agents and consequently develop pharyngitis when others would suffer no inconvenience.

Smoking

Smoking is a common cause of pharyngitis, and few heavy smokers do not show some evidence of it.

Digestive disorders

Since the pharynx is part of the alimentary tract, pharyngitis may be a manifestation of disorders of digestion. In addition, dyspeptics may refer to the pharynx symptoms due to gastritis, water-brash or eructations after aerophagy.

Those who indulge excessively in alcohol, especially spirits, usually suffer from some degree of pharyngitis, and the habitual use of condiments and highly-spiced foods is an aggravating factor.

Pulmonary conditions

In cases of chronic bronchitis and bronchiectasis, heavily infected sputum is constantly passing into the pharynx and exerting an adverse influence there.

General conditions

It is important to consider the general condition of the patient, lest one's attention be concentrated on what amounts to no more than an insignificant complication of a grave disease.

Symptoms

The symptoms experienced by people who suffer from chronic pharyngitis vary considerably and seem to bear little relationship to the pathological changes in the pharynx. Thus a man who indulges freely in alcohol and tobacco may have a pharynx which would be expected to cause acute discomfort and yet he is free from symptoms, whereas an introspective individual may complain bitterly of pharyngeal symptoms when his pharynx may well appear normal. The most constant symptom is discomfort in the throat, which may amount to actual pain, especially early in the morning; or there may be a sensation of a foreign body in the throat. There is undue irritability, and spasms of coughing and retching may be induced by factors which would leave most people undisturbed.

Once the dryness and discomfort experienced on waking, often due to mouth-breathing during sleep, have passed off, the throat is more comfortable until later in the day, when the symptoms return owing to the strain of talking and exposure to irritating agents. Indeed, in some cases the only complaint is that of 'tiredness of the voice' while the patient is conscious of the undue effort required in speaking; this, of course, is an aggravating factor.

The voice may lose its quality and singers become uncertain of getting the correct note, or the voice may crack with the production of a sound akin to 'falsetto'. For this the blame may be wrongly laid upon the larynx.

Owing to the constant discomfort in the throat, there is a tendency to cough or to clear the throat, or to interrupt speech in order to swallow.

Signs

Chronic catarrhal pharyngitis

In chronic catarrhal pharyngitis there is congestion of the pharynx with engorgement of the vessels, which may be seen coursing across the posterior pharyngeal wall. The pillars of the fauces may appear somewhat thickened. There is increased secretion of mucus, and the walls of the pharynx may be covered with frothy fluid.

The condition may persist for some time, or it may pass gradually into one of the other forms of chronic pharyngitis.

Chronic hypertrophic pharyngitis

In this form of the disease there is considerable hypertrophy of the pharyngeal mucosa. The tonsils and adenoids may be similarly affected, but hypertrophic pharyngitis may arise after these organs have been removed. The whole of the pharyngeal wall may be involved, or hypertrophy may be limited to the lateral bands of lymphoid tissue. This hypertrophy may also extend to the muscular coat in this region, and the masses may attain proportions which lead to their being mistaken for faucial tonsils, when these have been removed.

At first there is excessive secretion of mucus, but later the mucous glands may become obstructed by hypertrophied lymph nodules and there may be a little sticky secretion on the pharyngeal wall; this causes the patient to make repeated attempts to swallow and so further aggravates the disease. The pharynx is engorged and large vessels may be seen running over its surface. The palate is injected, and the uvula may be elongated and may appear almost oedematous, or it may be short and thickened. The pharyngeal wall may appear granular because of hypertrophy of the lymphoid follicles which may coalesce to form large masses. Granulations may form round the openings of the mucous glands and obstruct them, causing them to become distended and adding to the general thickening of the pharyngeal wall. This form of pharyngitis is often seen in those who use their voices excessively, particularly when voice production is faulty; hence the name 'clergyman's throat'.

Treatment

Rest is the most important factor for treating chronic pharyngitis, and much can be done to secure rest by explaining exactly the cause of the symptoms to the patient. He must be told that it is detrimental to swallow repeatedly in order to remove the 'crumb' or 'lump' in the throat because, in fact, none is there; he must be forbidden to clear his throat, hawk, or perform any of the pharyngeal contortions which he has devised; his cough must be suppressed. He must rest his voice, and in the case of a patient whose work demands the use of his voice, a long holiday is advisable; a course of instruction in voice production will do much to help.

Assistance can be given by prescribing applications to reduce the discomfort in the throat. Gargles of hot saline solution, Glycothymoline brand solution, or potassium chlorate and phenol should be used on rising, or a steam inhalation of compound tincture of benzoin or of menthol may be preferred. Mandl's paint may be applied with a camel-hair brush, and lozenges of potassium chlorate, formalin, or glycerin and blackcurrant may be sucked during the day. Temporary relief may be obtained by the use of a spray containing the following:

Tincture of ferric chloride	4 ml
Stovaine	300 mg
Menthol	300 mg
Spiritus vinus rectus	12 ml
Glycerine	12 ml
Aqua	30 ml

The nasal cavities may be used as a reservoir for pharyngeal applications, since any substance placed there is slowly passed into the pharynx, and the use of a bland oil containing white soft paraffin (one part) and liquid paraffin (three parts), warmed before use, can give relief for considerable periods. A potent linctus, such as linctus codeine, should be given in doses sufficient to suppress the cough, especially at night.

In cases in which hypertrophy is marked, the lymphoid tissue may be cauterized with ten per cent silver nitrate used sparingly on a probe, or with the electric cautery, but it is doubtful whether symptoms are relieved by this and the procedure may serve only to fix the patient's attention more firmly on his throat. Cryosurgery, however, may sometimes be helpful.

In the case of secondary pharyngitis, the primary cause must receive appropriate treatment. The nose and sinuses must be restored to health, and the teeth and tonsils must receive attention. The patient's diet and habits must be regulated, and he should be removed from unsuitable surroundings, at least for a reasonable period. The pharynx must receive treatment as well, however, because once the pharyngitis has become established, it may persist after the cause has been removed, owing to the faulty habits the patient has developed.

Chronic atrophic pharyngitis

Aetiology

Chronic atrophic pharyngitis is usually associated with atrophic rhinitis, and perhaps with laryngitis as well. It may be of a secondary nature, but most often is regarded as a direct extension of disease from the nose. In its mild form, sometimes known as pharyngitis sicca, it may follow granular pharyngitis, or conditions which lead to mouth-breathing. It is sometimes associated with diabetes mellitus or gout, or with some other constitutional disorder.

Symptoms

The symptoms are similar to those in other forms of chronic pharyngitis, but dryness of the throat is very marked and may cause great discomfort. The patient may find relief in taking sips of water. Talking aggravates the condition, and the presence of crusts may cause constant hawking and coughing.

Signs

There is atrophy of the pharyngeal mucosa and of the mucous glands in particular, so that the pharynx assumes a dry parchment-like appearance. The surface appears glazed and becomes wrinkled when the muscles contract. Absence of mucus leads to the formation of crusts, which favour secondary infection; this causes foetor oris. The lumen of the pharynx appears large and, owing to the thinning of the walls, the **outline** of the cervical spine is clearly visible.

Treatment

Causes for the condition must be sought in the nose or elsewhere and must be appropriately treated. This form of pharyngitis also calls for special forms of local treatment to prevent the formation of crusts, or to remove them when they have been formed. Alkaline lotions should be sprayed on to the pharynx as often as the severity of the case demands, but not less than three times a day. Ten per cent glucose in glycerin as a nasal application improves the condition of the nose, and also trickles into the pharynx; or an oily preparation may be indicated. Crusts must be removed, and this is facilitated by the use of an oily application, or by hydrogen peroxide; it is important to prevent the formation of crusts, however, because in their removal, the surface epithelium is damaged and infection perpetuated. Potassium iodide administered in 325 mg doses promotes secretion of mucus and may give relief, but it should be prescribed only for short periods. 'Airbron' spray effectively loosens crusts and assists in their removal.

The regimen advised for chronic pharyngitis should be followed.

Oropharyngitis – chronic specific

Syphilis

Syphilitic lesions in the pharynx may occur at any stage of the disease, but it is in the secondary stage, when spirochaetes are most widely distributed throughout the body, that manifestations are most regularly seen.

Primary syphilis

Probably the most common site for an extragenital chancre is the lip or the mouth. The lesion may be mistaken for a boil on the lip, or impetigo, but the characteristic rubbery feel of the enlarged regional lymph nodes should suggest its nature and lead to further investigation. The lesion presents the typical features of a primary chancre, with the 'cartilaginous' base and ulceration with a dirty slough, but it may remain small owing to the relative absence of secondary infection. In other cases, the chancre may be situated on the tonsil, or cheek, when it may be mistaken for a carcinoma or Vincent's infection. In the early stages, the Wasserman reaction may be negative, but examination under dark-ground illumination of a smear taken from the lesion reveals *Treponema pallidum*, which has to be distinguished from the spirochaetes which normally inhabit the mouth (Vincent's organisms).

Secondary syphilis

In the secondary stage of the disease, which usually arises in 6–8 weeks, the spirochaetes are widely distributed throughout the body, and the mucous membranes are partially affected. There is some degree of sore throat, which may cause acute discomfort, or merely the symptoms associated with a bad cold. When the disease is florid, there may be a rash symmetrically distributed over the body, and of a colour likened to that of raw ham; when the forehead is involved, it is called corona veneris. There is associated anaemia, the hair tends to fall out, and there is a general enlargement of the lymph nodes. The pharynx is uniformly injected, and on the fauces and palate there are mucous patches and snail track ulcers symmetrically placed, with the characteristic lymphadenitis of syphilis. The disease is now in its most infective state and an early diagnosis is important; serological tests are probably positive, and the spirochaetes can be seen in smears taken from the mucous patches and ulcers.

Tertiary syphilis

By now the invasive stage of the disease has been overcome, but localized activity continues and the manifestations may occur almost coincidentally with the secondary stage, or many years later. The typical lesion is a gumma, which is formed as a result of chronic infection of the tissues, with endarteritis of the arterioles and necrosis in the area of their distribution. Secondary infection leads to the formation of a punched-out ulcer with a wash-leather slough at the base. Bone is commonly involved, thus there may be perforation of the hard palate, but the soft tissues are also affected and ulceration of the tonsil and pharynx is often seen. Since the nerve endings are destroyed early in the disease, there is little pain, and ulceration of the palate and fauces may have progressed to a remarkable extent before the patient seeks advice. The regional lymph nodes become affected owing to secondary infection.

Congenital syphilis

In congenital syphilis the pharynx may be involved in gummatous infiltration owing to infection acquired *in utero*. The lesions resemble those seen in tertiary syphilis but progress more slowly, with considerable scarring in consequence. There may be perforation of the palate.

The permanent teeth, particularly the upper central incisors, may be affected and show the well-known deformity described by Hutchinson. The cutting edges are eroded and tend to become semilunar, while the whole tooth is malformed and shaped like a peg.

Differential diagnosis

The ulcer may be confused with that due to tuberculous infection, but in this condition there is a shallow ulcer with undermined edges; there is much pain and there is evidence of pulmonary involvement; nevertheless, large terminal pharyngeal tuberculous ulcers may be painless.

In the case of epithelioma, the ulcer is hard with everted edges, and the regional lymph nodes, if involved, are hard and may be attached to the surrounding tissues. Vincent's ulceration may resemble either secondary or tertiary syphilis, but pain is more severe, and direct examination of the exudate and serological tests should establish the diagnosis.

Treatment

Cases should immediately be referred to a venereologist for treatment and observation. Early treatment is important to arrest the progress of the disease.

Tuberculosis

Tuberculosis is seen in the pharynx in three forms: acute miliary tuberculosis; chronic tuberculous ulceration; and lupus vulgaris.

Acute miliary tuberculosis

This manifestation of the disease is associated with spread of tubercle bacilli by the blood stream. There is an eruption of tubercles on the fauces, soft palate, base of the tongue or buccal mucosa. There is some discomfort at this stage, but when the tubercles break down to form ulcers, there is acute pain and dysphagia. There is a tendency to bleed and to excessive salivation; mucus adheres to the ulcerated area. There is considerable constitutional disturbance, with high temperature, and the general condition of the patient deteriorates rapidly.

Chronic ulcerating tuberculosis

Chronic ulcerating tuberculosis is always associated with advanced pulmonary tuberculosis, and the sputum is laden with tubercle bacilli. There is ulceration in the pharynx and on the tongue, where the ulcers are usually situated at the tip. The ulcers are shallow, with undermined edges and relatively clean bases; their progress is indolent. The nerve endings are intact, so there is much pain with all the symptoms associated with acute dysphagia.

Treatment

There is great improvement in tuberculous ulceration of the upper respiratory tract when treatment of the pulmonary lesion is instituted. There may be little change in the appearance of the lesion for a few weeks, but pain is rapidly relieved and the lesions eventually heal. If there are bacilli in the sputum, a culture should be made and sensitivity tests carried out.

A wide range of anti-tuberculous drugs is now available, but the treatment protocol is best left to the respiratory physician treating the pulmonary condition, and he will prescribe combinations or sequences of drugs according to the sensitivities of the organism. Nowadays treatment is usually so effective that local treatment is not required, other than mouth-washes and analgesics, until healing begins.

The otolaryngologist should keep the pharyngeal lesions under observation during treatment, and should also observe the patient's auditory and vestibular function, if potentially ototoxic drugs have been selected. Treatment is usually continued for 18–24 months.

Lupus vulgaris

Pathology

Lupus vulgaris is essentially a cutaneous manifestation of tuberculosis, and perhaps the most benign. The favourite site in the upper respiratory tract is the anterior end of the nasal septum and the inferior turbinate, whence the disease may spread to the face or the pharynx.

In the pharynx, the soft palate and fauces may be affected, but rarely the tonsils. There is often associated disease in the nose, larynx or, infrequently, the chest; occasionally, however, the pharyngeal lesion is the sole manifestation of the disease.

There is an eruption of 'apple jelly nodules' which soon become grey and appear more solid; microscopically they resemble tubercles. The mucosa becomes hard and loses its mobility; the nodules break down and the surface of the mucosa is destroyed, with exposure of a granular area. Both sides of the soft palate may be involved, but perforation does not occur. In the rare cases in which the hard palate is affected, bone may be exposed but is not involved in the disease process. The disease runs a very chronic course, with a tendency to heal in parts while activity continues elsewhere; consequently there is considerable scarring, involving the palate, and the uvula may be reduced or may vanish.

Symptoms

In the early stages, or when the disease resumes activity, there is a burning sensation and a slight degree of sore throat. Later, the quality of the voice may change owing to a fixation of the palate, and there may be some dysphagia, but it is only in very advanced cases that regurgitation of fluids through the nose occurs.

Diagnosis

The lesion may be confused with syphilis; in syphilis, however, the disease runs a much more rapid course with greater destruction of tissue, and serology is positive. A diagnosis of lupus vulgaris may be confirmed by biopsy.

Treatment

As for pharyngeal lesions associated with pulmonary tuberculosis, treatment consists of systemic administration of appropriate anti-tuberculous drugs for 18–24 months.
    The patient should be kept under observation for many years, however, owing to the remittent nature of the disease. Nothing can be done to prevent the gross scarring which is a feature of the disease.

Fungal infections

Monilia (thrush)

Many small white patches develop on the buccal and pharyngeal mucosa, caused by *Candida albicans*. It occurs chiefly in debilitated patients, especially after courses of broad-spectrum antibiotics, or prolonged use of topical antibiotics in the form of lozenges. The condition may be symptomless, or may give slight discomfort or considerable soreness.

Treatment

Nystatin suspension 1 ml is held in the mouth in contact with the lesions as long as possible. This treatment is carried out four times daily and continued for 48 hours after clinical cure. Systemic nystatin may be required if the infection involves other organs.

Actinomycosis

This rarely occurs in the pharynx. As elsewhere, deep ulcers and sinuses occur containing 'sulphur granules'. If these are seen it is essential to trap them and send them to the laboratory, as they contain the actinomyces colonies, and without them diagnosis is difficult.

Treatment is initially a long course of large doses of penicillin, continuing treatment for at least two months after clinical cure.

Blastomycosis

This is a very rare but serious fungal infection which may involve the pharynx, with formation of shallow granulating ulcers.

Treatment is with amphotericin suspension 1 ml four times daily held in contact with the lesions. Systemic treatment may be required if other areas are involved.

Scleroma

This chronic inflammatory disease occurs mainly in parts of Eastern Europe, North Africa and Central America. The causal organism, described by Frisch, is the *Klebsiella scleromatis*. The disease usually begins in the nose, spreading from there to the nasopharynx, pharynx and larynx. A full description of the pathology and clinical picture is given in Volume 3.

Treatment is with systemic tetracyclines or streptomycin.

Leprosy

This also is a chronic inflammatory disease, caused by *Mycobacterium leprae*, with a site of predilection in the nose (Barton, 1975). Eventually the disease may involve skin and peripheral nerves as well as mucous membranes. In the early stages of nasal infection, there is copious mucoid discharge containing huge numbers of *M. leprae*. Besides being a means of transmitting the disease, this highly infected discharge is passed into the pharynx where further leprous lesions can occur. The nodules become ulcerated, then heal leaving a stellate scar. The lesions are painless.

Treatment is with courses of dapsone. Rifampicin has also been found to be effective (Barton, 1975).

Keratosis pharyngis

Keratosis pharyngis (*Figure 4.2*) is a condition of unknown origin, and one which may cause much needless distress because the appearance of the throat suggests some serious lesion, whereas in fact the disease runs a singularly benign course, tending to undergo spontaneous resolution in a matter of months. Symptoms are negligible, amounting to no more than slight discomfort, but the patient may be prompted to examine his throat. The lesions appear in the throat as grey-white or yellow horny

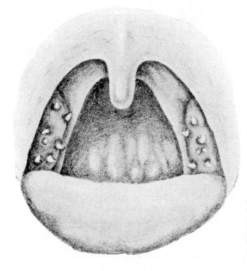

Figure 4.2   Keratosis pharyngis. (From St. Clair Thomson, Negus and Bateman [1955], *Diseases of the Nose and Throat*, page 471, Figure 204, Cassell, London; after Cunningham)

outgrowths; they are in fact formed by hypertrophy and keratinization of the epithelium. They are firmly adherent and can be removed only with difficulty. The tonsillar crypts are most frequently involved, but the lesion may be scattered over the pharynx, and the lingual tonsils seldom escape. The lesions may extend to the hypopharynx and larynx. Swabs taken from the lesions show a variety of organisms and fungi, but there is no evidence that they are in any way responsible for the condition. The disease has been likened to black hairy tongue, since in this case the 'hairs' consist of keratinized epithelium.

When the lesions are plentiful, diagnosis should present no difficulty, but when they are confined to the faucial tonsils they may be mistaken for acute follicular tonsillitis; there is, however, no acute pharyngitis or constitutional disturbance. They may be mistaken for collections of debris in the tonsillar crypts, but these are cheesy and yellow and may be expressed with a spatula.

The disease does not require treatment, but the patient may be assured that no harm will result even should the lesions persist, while it is likely that they will disappear spontaneously in the course of time.

Stenosis of the pharynx

Aetiology

Stenosis of the pharynx is due to scar tissue. This may follow acute infections, such as scarlet fever or gangrenous tonsillitis. Chronic disease, notably syphilis or lupus vulgaris, may be followed by extensive scarring, with narrowing of the pharynx or fixation of the palate. Operative measures for neoplastic disease, or removal of tonsils and adenoids, may also cause a narrowing of the pharynx. Other cases are due to wounds, or the swallowing of corrosives.

Symptoms and signs

Usually the upper parts of the oropharynx and nasopharynx are involved, with resulting obstruction to nasal respiration. The voice may be altered so that the patient speaks with rhinolalia clausa. Examination of the pharynx immediately reveals the state of affairs, with gross scarring of the palate and pharynx.

Treatment

Treatment is unnecessary except in the most severe cases. Dilatation with bougies may be successful, but if there is no relief, surgical intervention is necessary. Division of adhesions and mobilization of the palate are doomed to failure unless a Thiersch graft is inserted to prevent further scarring. The graft, which should be taken from a hairless area of the body, should be held in position for a week or two by a stent mould, and a similarly shaped obturator should be prepared for insertion after the mould has been removed. This obturator must be worn for 6–12 weeks to prevent the contraction of scar tissue that will otherwise take place.

The results of these operations are often unsatisfactory but it is nearly always possible to give some nasopharyngeal opening that allows nasal breathing. Operation should be reserved for severe stenosis.

References

Barton, R. P. E. (1975). *Annals of the Royal College of Surgeons of England*, **57**, 309
Rowson, K. E. K. (1973). In: *Recent Advances in Otolaryngology 1973* (Eds J. Ransome, H. Holden and T. R. Bull); Churchill-Livingstone, Edinburgh and London
Zweifach, E. (1955). *Journal of Laryngology and Otology*, **69**, 321

5 Pharyngeal lesions associated with general diseases
Joselen Ransome

Introduction

Lesions of the pharynx not infrequently occur as the presenting symptoms of, or in the course of, general diseases. In some of these, early diagnosis is of great importance, and therefore the otolaryngologist needs to develop an awareness of the full spectrum of general diseases affecting this area.

Trauma

Corrosives

Ingestion of strong acids or alkalis causes destruction of the tissues of the mouth, pharynx, oesophagus and stomach. The presenting symptoms vary from mild to severe: there may be only a burning sensation confined to the mouth and pharynx associated with dysphagia, or in addition there may be severe substernal and epigastric pain, abdominal distension, vomiting, and shock with feeble pulse. The presence of sloughing burns in and around the mouth and pharynx, even when general symptoms are absent, should alert the surgeon to the possibility of corrosive poisoning, especially in young children. According to Rosenow and Bernatz (1974) nearly 50 per cent of patients with oral burns have also sustained corrosive burns of the oesophagus, and this must be borne in mind even when symptoms appear to be confined to the mouth and pharynx. The incidence of corrosive poisoning appears to be increasing in Denmark, where in a recent series of 68 cases 80 per cent were children, and 62 per cent were children under two years (Winther, 1978). Treatment is described in Chapter 9.

Inflammatory lesions

Recurrent acute pharyngitis (non-specific)

This tends to occur in any patient with a *defective host defence mechanism,* for instance: in immunoglobulin deficiency (primary and secondary); in haemopoietic diseases; in all conditions leading to neutropenia (*see below*); in any of the chronic debilitating diseases (such as diabetes and chronic nephritis); in chronic inflammatory conditions such as syphilis; in malnutrition; and in addiction to drugs and alcohol.

Acute specific pharyngitis

The reader is referred to Chapter 4 for an account of the pharyngeal lesions in diphtheria, scarlet fever, measles, chicken-pox, herpes zoster, Vincent's angina, and gonorrhoea, and to Chapter 6 for an account of infectious mononucleosis.

Chronic specific pharyngitis

The reader is referred to Chapter 4 for an account of the pharyngeal lesions in syphilis, tuberculosis, fungal infections, leprosy, and scleroma.

Generalized neoplastic diseases affecting the pharynx

Benign

A *neurofibroma* may occasionally occur in the pharynx in patients with generalized neurofibromatosis (Von Recklinghausen's disease).

Malignant: the reticuloses

Since nearly all the reticuloses may affect the pharynx by one mechanism or another, an outline of this important group of diseases is given, following the classification of Dameshek and Gunz (1964) which is summarized below.

The diseases in Group A affect the pharynx because they cause proneness to infections, while some of those in Group B may present with swelling of the lymphoid tissue in the pharynx.

Group A. Primary malignant diseases of bone marrow (myeloproliferative diseases)

Acute
(1) Acute leukaemia:
   Myeloblastic.
   Lymphoblastic.
   Monoblastic.
(2) Acute erythraemia.
Chronic
(3) *a.* Chronic granulocytic leukaemia.
    b. Chronic lymphocytic leukaemia.
(4) Polycythaemia vera.
(5) Essential thrombocythaemia.
(6) Myelofibrosis.

Group B. Primary malignant diseases of lymphoid tissue

(1) Hodgkin's disease.
(2) Reticulum cell sarcoma.
(3) Giant follicular lymphoma.
(4) Lymphosarcoma.
(5) Burkitt's lymphoma.
(6) Myelomatosis.

To these should be added:

(7) 'Hairy-cell' leukaemia (leukaemic reticuloendotheliosis).

Group A

Acute leukaemia

Definition. An acute proliferative disease of the bone marrow characterized by infiltration with blast cells. There are three forms: lymphoblastic, myeloblastic and monoblastic; the clinical features of all three are the same.
   Aetiology. In animals viruses have been proved to be causal agents but this has not been proved in man. Previous irradiation, however, is a factor.
   Clinical picture. The symptoms, which develop rapidly, are due to failure of the bone marrow to produce the normal elements of blood. Thus there are:

(1) Anaemia (with *pallor of mucous membranes* including the pharynx).
(2) Thrombocytopenia, giving rise to a *haemorrhagic state*, with purpuric spots (which may occur in the pharynx) and haemorrhage from mucous membranes, including the gums and pharynx.

(3) Neutrophil leucopenia leading to *infections* including pharyngitis, with sloughing ulcers.

In the lymphoblastic form there may also be local or general lymphadenopathy. The spleen may be enlarged.

Diagnosis. The presence of anaemia, haemorrhages and infection, with or without splenomegaly and lymphadenopathy, strongly suggests leukaemia. Confirmation is obtained from the blood and bone marrow.

Treatment is best carried out in special units, and consists of prednisone with various cytotoxic chemotherapeutic agents in various combinations and sequences. In the lymphoblastic form, occurring mainly in children, complete remissions can be obtained in 95 per cent of cases; however, despite maintenance therapy relapses occur and life expectancy is short. In the myeloblastic form, which occurs throughout the life-span, results of treatment are worse and only 50 per cent obtain complete remission. Supporting treatment consists of red-cell and platelet transfusions, and antibiotics for infections.

Acute erythraemia

In this condition there is infiltration of the bone marrow and blood with primitive normoblasts. It presents in the same way as acute leukaemia. The response to treatment and the prognosis are poor. The treatment is as for acute myeloblastic leukaemia.

Chronic granulocytic leukaemia

Definition. A proliferative disease of bone marrow involving mainly developing cells of the granulocyte series.

Aetiology. Previous irradiation is the only proven factor; 70 per cent of cases occur in the 30–60 year age group.

Clinical picture. The patient presents with any or all of the following: general malaise, lassitude, weight loss, pallor, and purpura (which may involve the pharynx). Examination reveals splenomegaly and signs of anaemia and/or a haemorrhagic state. Occasionally there is priapism, and bone and skin lesions.

Diagnosis is confirmed by examination of the blood and bone marrow.

Treatment consists of cytotoxic chemotherapy plus supportive measures.

Prognosis. The condition is invariably fatal within 2–3 years. Treatment does not prolong life, but improves the quality of life until the acute terminal phase begins; this phase resembles acute myeloblastic leukaemia.

Chronic lymphocytic leukaemia

Definition. Proliferation of lymphocytes infiltrating the bone marrow and blood.

Aetiology. Irradiation is *not* a factor. Eighty per cent of cases occur in the 40–70 year age group. The disease is fairly common in Europe and North America, and more common in Jews, but very rare in China, Japan and the West Pacific sea borders.

Clinical picture. There may be local or general lymphadenopathy. There is great proneness to infections (including pharyngitis) because of the lack of antibodies. Other symptoms include malaise, lassitude, anaemia and purpura. The disease does not become acute, and the terminal phase is due to infections, infiltration of other organs, haemolysis, and associated carcinomas to which these patients are very prone.

Diagnosis is confirmed by the presence of persistent lymphocytosis in the blood and/or bone marrow. In the majority of cases there is also hypogamma-globulinaemia.

Treatment consists of radiotherapy, cytotoxics and steroids, plus the usual supportive measures (transfusions, antibiotics, and if necessary gammaglobulins).

Prognosis is variable. The median survival time is five years, though 15 per cent survive to ten years.

Polycythaemia vera

Definition. A primary proliferative disease of the red cell series mainly, but frequently including granulocytes and platelets.

Aetiology. The cause is unknown. The disease occurs in the later decades.

Clinical picture. The presenting features are mainly vascular because of the increased viscosity of the blood, and include symptoms of disturbed cerebral circulation such as headache, vertigo, visual disturbances, dysphagia and hemiplegia. There may also be a *haemorrhagic* tendency because of abnormal platelets. The appearance of the patient is plethoric and there may be splenomegaly. The condition may end up as myelofibrosis (*see below*), or may become frankly leukaemic.

Diagnosis. The condition is strongly suggested by the above features and is confirmed by finding excessive numbers of the red cell series, and often granulocytes and platelets, in the blood and bone marrow.

Treatment. The red cell volume can be controlled by venesection and the platelet count by ^{32}P. However, the latter can cause acute leukaemia so the smallest possible effective dose is used. Chemotherapy is held in reserve. The disease may end up as myelofibrosis (*see below*).

Prognosis. Treatment has lengthened survival time from about 18 months to about 12 years.

Essential thrombocythaemia

In this condition there is gross proliferation of platelets, but as the platelets are abnormal, a *haemorrhagic state* develops. The diagnosis is suggested (among other conditions) by the presence of a haemorrhagic state and splenomegaly, and is confirmed by the blood count. Treatment is with ^{32}P. The course is similar to polycythaemia vera and, like it, may end with myelofibrosis (*see below*).

Myelofibrosis

This is a proliferation of the connective tissue of the marrow. It may follow polycythaemia vera or essential thrombocythaemia, but otherwise the cause is unknown. It is a disease of middle age.

It presents with *anaemia* and splenomegaly, and may lead to aplasia of the marrow, or may pass into acute leukaemia.

Treatment consists of transfusion and splenectomy. Androgens may sometimes stimulate the bone marrow when there is aplasia.

Group B

Hodgkin's disease (lymphadenoma)

Pathology. A primary malignant disease of lymphoreticular tissue in which there is proliferation of reticulum cells, which are transformed into the characteristic Reed–Sternberg giant cells.

Aetiology. The disease is more common in males and can occur throughout adult life, though there are two peaks of incidence: at ages 25 and 70 years.

Clinical picture. Characteristically the disease presents with painless enlargement of a lymph node, usually in the neck, but it may also be in the axillae, inguinal region, chest or abdomen. The *tonsil* may also be the primary site, as may the spleen or liver. Later the disease may spread to involve almost any organ, particularly bone, the nervous system, and skin. Lymph nodes are at first firm, rubbery and discrete, but later may become matted together. There may be severe pain in affected structures on taking alcohol. If the disease progresses there will be general malaise, loss of weight, anaemia, and the Pel–Ebstein type of fever.

Diagnosis is only made by finding Reed–Sternberg cells in biopsy material, usually taken from a lymph node.

Management. After biopsy has confirmed the presence of the disease, its extent is estimated by some or all of the following methods: clinical examination, tomography of the hilar regions, lymphangiography, liver function tests, liver and spleen scans, and bone marrow biopsy. The disease can then be staged as follows:

Stage I   Limited to lymph nodes of one anatomical region.
Stage II   Limited to lymph nodes on one side of the diaphragm.
Stage III Disease present on both sides of the diaphragm, but limited to lymph nodes and the spleen.
Stage IV   Other tissues apart from lymph nodes and the spleen are involved.

For Stages I and II, radiotherapy is given to the involved and adjacent lymph nodes. Chemotherapy is used as adjuvant therapy only if urgent reduction in tumour size is required, e.g. if there is a mass compressing a bronchus.

Stage III cases are treated by chemotherapy only, or a combination of chemotherapy, plus radiotherapy to all lymph nodes both above and below the diaphragm.

Stage IV cases can only be treated with chemotherapy.

Reticulum cell sarcoma

Definition. Proliferation of reticulum cells of lymphoreticular tissue.

Aetiology. The cause is unknown. The disease may occur at any age but is more common in middle and later life.

Clinical features. Like Hodgkin's disease, there may first be enlargement of lymph nodes or the spleen, but the disease can also begin in the tonsil or other lymphoid tissue of the pharynx. The disease may spread rapidly to involve other organs, including the alimentary tract, lungs, pleura, peritoneum, meninges and central nervous system. As it disseminates the patient becomes anaemic and prone to infections.

Diagnosis is made by biopsy.

Treatment is similar to Hodgkin's disease.

Prognosis is poor and may be only 2–3 years. If the disease is localized when it first presents the outlook is more favourable.

Giant follicular lymphoma

Definition. Proliferation in lymph nodes or spleen resulting in the formation of giant pseudofollicles.

Aetiology. The cause is unknown. It is more common in middle and later life.

Clinical features. The commonest presenting symptoms are local or general lymphadenopathy with or without splenomegaly. Occasionally the lymphoid tissues of the pharynx are involved. Sometimes there is only splenomegaly.

Diagnosis depends on biopsy, usually of a lymph node. Occasionally the spleen has to be removed to reach a diagnosis.

Treatment. Radiotherapy is the treatment of choice if the disease is well localized. If it is generalized, chemotherapy is given. If the disease appears to be confined to the spleen, splenectomy alone may suffice.

Prognosis is variable. Some run a rapid course, while others appear to be cured by splenectomy. About 40 per cent of cases are alive at five years.

Lymphosarcoma

Definition. Infiltration of lymph nodes, spleen, and other organs with lymphoblasts or lymphocytes.

Aetiology. The cause is unknown. The disease affects all age groups.

Clinical features. The presentation may resemble that of reticulum cell sarcoma and, as in that condition, may involve the lymphoid tissues of the pharynx. Sometimes the blood and bone marrow are infiltrated, when the condition may resemble acute or chronic lymphatic leukaemia.

Diagnosis is made by biopsy.

Treatment is as for reticulum cell sarcoma or lymphatic leukaemia.

Prognosis is very variable. Most cases survive only two or three years, although occasional long-term survivals have been recorded.

Burkitt's lymphoma

Definition. A particular form of lymphosarcoma with a distinctive histological appearance and anatomical distribution.

Aetiology. The Epstein–Barr virus is probably a causal factor. The disease occurs chiefly in the malarious areas of Africa, and mainly in children.

Clinical features. The disease most commonly presents as a tumour of the upper jaw. Sometimes the lower jaw of the same side is also affected resulting in a massive tumour of the face and palate, sometimes extending as far back as the pharynx. Other areas frequently involved are: kidneys, ovaries, retro-peritoneal tissue, and other bones. The disease may become generally invasive or may enter a leukaemic phase.

Diagnosis depends on biopsy, when lymphoid cells surrounded by phagocytes giving the typical 'starry-sky' appearance are found.

Treatment. The disease is extremely sensitive to cytotoxic agents, and often there is a dramatic response to a single injection. However, after disappearance of the mass relapses may occur if maintenance therapy is not given.

Prognosis is very variable depending on the stage at which the case presents, but many seem curable.

Myelomatosis

Definition. Malignant proliferation of plasma cells in the bone marrow, associated with excessive production of immunoglobulins G, A, D and E.

Aetiology. The cause is unknown. Eighty per cent of cases are over 50 years of age.

Clinical features. The disease may begin as a solitary extramedullary plasmacytoma, sometimes in the upper respiratory or alimentary tracts. At this stage there is no change in the plasma proteins. These may metastasize to lymph nodes, or multiple myelomatosis may follow, sometimes after some years, but this course is not inevitable.

If the disease is generalized on presenting, any or all of the following features may be present:

(1) Painful osteolytic bone lesions.
(2) Anaemia, leucopenia and thrombocytopenia due to bone marrow infiltration (and therefore proneness to infections and haemorrhagic state).
(3) Renal failure.
(4) Hypercalcaemia (due to excess re-absorption of calcium from bone).

Diagnosis is by biopsy.

Treatment of a solitary plasmacytoma, after excluding generalized myelomatosis, is by radiotherapy, wide excision, or a combination of both. For myelomatosis chemotherapy, or a combination of radiotherapy and chemotherapy, is used.

Hairy-cell leukaemia (reticuloendotheliosis)

This was first described as a separate entity by Bouroncle, Wiseman and Doan (1958), and it accounts for two per cent of all leukaemias.

The characteristic cells, which infiltrate the blood and bone marrow, have long cytoplastic villi, giving a 'hairy' appearance. The nature and origin of these cells is still controversial.

Clinically the disease presents in the second half of life with *infections* or a *haemorrhagic state*, due to leucopenia and thrombocytopenia. There is usually also anaemia. It runs a chronic course, with a median survival time of 3–5 years. Survival times of over ten years have been reported. The disease is said not to respond to chemotherapy, but chlorambucil may be tried.

Anaemias

Definition. Anaemia is a condition of diminished oxygen-carrying capacity of the blood, due to a reduction in the numbers of red cells, or in their content of haemoglobin, or both.

All anaemias give pallor of the mucous membrane of the pharynx. It is customary to inspect the conjunctival sac to estimate the haemoglobin level clinically, but the pharyngeal mucosa is just as good an indicator. Symptoms include fatigue, shortness of breath, headache and palpitations. The anaemias command the attention of the pharyngologist by a number of mechanisms.

Iron-deficiency anaemia

Definition. A form of anaemia in which lack of iron leads to shortage of haemoglobin, though the production of red cell envelopes is normal. Less haemoglobin is deposited into each red cell resulting in small-sized hypochromic red cells.

Aetiology. The cause is either excessive loss of iron (as after haemorrhage), deficient iron intake in the diet, or impaired absorption (e.g. in the malabsorption syndrome).

Clinical features. In addition to the usual features of anaemia, there may be koilonychia, angular stomatitis and atrophic glossitis. If to these are added *atrophic hypopharyngitis* and a web in the post-cricoid region resulting in dysphagia, the sufferer, almost invariably female, has developed the Paterson–Brown Kelly syndrome, which must be regarded as a pre-malignant condition.

Diagnosis depends on the blood count and estimations of the serum iron and the iron-binding capacity of the serum.

Treatment. First, the underlying cause is sought and corrected. To correct the iron deficiency, iron is given orally as ferrous sulphate 200 mg four times daily after meals, or ferrous gluconate 600 mg four times daily after meals. Parenteral therapy is occasionally indicated.

Dysphagia in the Paterson–Brown Kelly syndrome is often reversible when iron deficiency is corrected. Endoscopic dilatation of the post-cricoid region may be required on occasions. Careful follow-up is required because of the pre-malignant nature of the atrophic hypopharyngitis.

Anaemias due to vitamin B₁₂ or folic acid deficiency

Definition. In these anaemias haemoglobin synthesis is normal but red cell synthesis is affected resulting in a reduction in the red cell count with large hyperchromic cells. Production of white cells and platelets may also be affected, resulting in neutropenia and thrombocytopenia.

Aetiology:

(1) *Inadequate intake of vitamin B₁₂* is excessively rare and almost confined to rigid vegetarians. Folic acid deficiency is less rare and is found in the elderly poor due to lack of fresh vegetables.

(2) *Inadequate absorption* of vitamin B₁₂ occurs in *pernicious anaemia*, in which there is failure to synthesize Castle's intrinsic factor, produced by the stomach, which is necessary for vitamin B₁₂ absorption. Total gastrectomy may give the same result. Folic acid is poorly absorbed in lesions or excision of the jejunum.

(3) *Increased demand* as in pregnancy, or in conditions of increased haemopoiesis.

(4) *Inability to utilize folic acid* as with the administration of some drugs, including methotrexate, phenytoin and trimethoprim.

Clinical features. These are the same as for all anaemias, but in addition there is a tendency to *infections* (including pharyngitis) *and haemorrhages* (due to neutropenia and thrombocytopenia). In true pernicious anaemia only, subacute combined degeneration of the spinal cord is a serious complication, which may be reversible in the early stages, making early diagnosis and treatment imperative.

Diagnosis. Examination of the blood and bone marrow shows a macrocytic anaemia. Estimations of serum folate and vitamin B₁₂, together with tests of vitamin B₁₂ absorption, and of folic acid deficiency, show which kind.

Treatment is with vitamin B₁₂ by intramuscular injection or folic acid by mouth.

Aplastic anaemia

Definition. Failure of the bone marrow to produce red cells, white cells, and platelets. Occasionally only the neutrophil series is affected leading to agranulocytosis.

Aetiology. A long list of drugs and industrial poisons may affect the bone marrow, as may excessive exposure to irradiation (*see also* under 'neutropenia', below). The condition may also be idiopathic.

Clinical features:

(1) Symptoms and signs of all anaemias.

(2) *Painful sloughing ulcers of the mouth and pharynx* due to agranulocytosis.

(3) Purpura, and haemorrhages from mucous membranes, due to thrombocytopenia.

Diagnosis depends on examination of the blood and bone marrow.

Treatment consists of removing the cause if found. Androgens and steroids may stimulate the bone marrow and produce remissions. Supporting treatment consists of fresh blood transfusions, and antibiotics to control infections.

Haemolytic anaemias

In these there is an abnormally rapid breakdown of red cells in the circulation, resulting in a rise in serum bilirubin, causing latent or overt jaundice.

Excessive haemolysis may be hereditary or acquired: the acquired form may be caused by incompatible blood transfusion or by infections.

Hereditary forms

The pharyngologist needs to be aware of these as they constitute a hazard to tonsillectomy (or any operation), anaesthesia for which may cause a haemolytic crisis.

(1) *Acholuric jaundice* need not be considered, as it would usually be cured by splenectomy before a case presents to an otolaryngologist.

(2) *Sickle-cell anaemia* is almost confined to negroes, and is inherited as a Mendelian dominant. The red cells contain abnormal haemoglobin which causes the cells to become sickle-shaped if oxygen tension is low. The abnormal shape leads to increased blood viscosity and capillary thrombosis, as well as to haemolysis.

Anaesthesia may bring about a severe and dangerous crisis and therefore every negro patient in whom surgery is contemplated needs to have a sickle-cell test. If positive the reasons for surgery would have to be very compelling. There is no treatment apart from transfusion for severe anaemia.

(3) *Thalassaemia major* (Cooley's anaemia) is found in races bordering the Mediterranean and is due to an inherited (homozygous) metabolic fault leading to production of the fetal type of haemoglobin. This usually leads to death in childhood from haemolysis.

(4) *Thalassaemia minor*, due to heterozygous inheritance of the same gene is usually symptomless and is only detected on routine blood examination. It is not a deterrent to surgery.

(5) *Glucose-6-phosphate dehydrogenase deficiency* (G6PD). This rare red cell enzyme abnormality renders the red cells unduly prone to haemolysis especially on administration of many drugs including most antibiotics. It is principally on account of the latter that the condition is of interest to the otolaryngologist, who must exercise great care in the management of upper respiratory infections. There is no contra-indication to surgery and anaesthetic agents do not precipitate haemolysis, but aspirin and many analgesics do, so that postoperative control of soreness after tonsillectomy or other operations is difficult.

Acquired haemolytic anaemia

The principal cause is incompatible blood transfusion, and since the pharyngologist may on occasions need to transfuse patients, he must familiarize himself with the theory and practice of blood transfusion and its alternatives, cultivate the habit of consulting with the Haematology Department, and discipline his own staff regarding safeguards against a mis-matched transfusion.

Very rarely haemolysis may complicate a severe streptococcal or staphylococcal infection, or result from drug idiosyncrasy.

Neutropenia

The word means that the neutrophil count is below the lower limit of normality (normal range 2500–7500/mm³). The term *agranulocytosis* is reserved for extreme leucopenia, in which the neutrophil count is below 1000/mm³. Whatever the cause, such cases are naturally very prone to infections including pharyngitis, and in agranulocytosis, to painful sloughing ulcers of the pharynx. The causes are many and some have been referred to already. They can be summarized as follows:

(1) Overwhelming infections.
(2) Haemopoietic diseases.
(3) Poisoning with chemicals and drugs, such as benzene, amidopyrine, sulphon-amides, thiouracil, arsenic, gold, nitrogen mustards.
(4) Excessive irradiation.
(5) Chronic debilitating diseases.
(6) Anaphylactic shock.
(7) Miscellaneous diseases, including disseminated lupus erythematosis, myx-oedema, hypopituitarism, cirrhosis of the liver, and secondary carcinomatosis of bone marrow.
(8) Idiopathic.

Haemorrhagic disorders

These are of interest to the pharyngologist because:

(1) They may cause petechiae and purpuric spots in the upper respiratory tract including the pharynx.
(2) They may give rise to massive bleeding into the mucous membrane of the pharynx and larynx leading to respiratory obstruction.
(3) If undiagnosed pre-operatively they may cause excessive or prolonged bleeding after tonsillectomy or other pharyngeal operations, rendering the procedure hazardous if not fatal.

If discovered pre-operatively, the indication for surgery should be reviewed, and if absolutely compelling, close cooperation is required with the haematologist. The otolaryngologist should have some acquaintance with the problems involved.

Mechanisms

A tendency to abnormal bleeding may result from:

(1) A *coagulation defect*, due to lack of one of the substances required for the formation of a firm blood clot. The factors involved in clotting are summarized in *Table 5.1.*
(2) *Thrombocytopenia* ⎫
(3) *Capillary abnormality* ⎭ the purpuras.

Table 5.1 Summary of the mechanism of clotting of blood

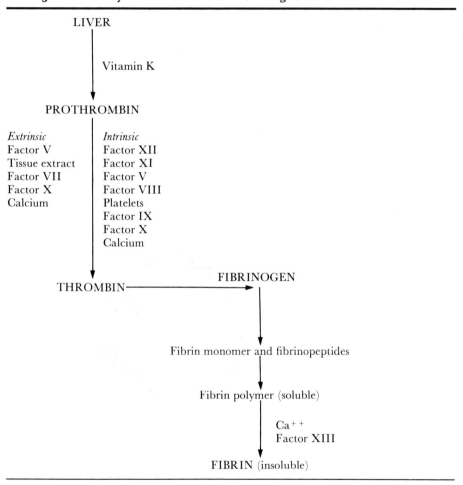

LIVER

Vitamin K

PROTHROMBIN

Extrinsic	*Intrinsic*
Factor V	Factor XII
Tissue extract	Factor XI
Factor VII	Factor V
Factor X	Factor VIII
Calcium	Platelets
	Factor IX
	Factor X
	Calcium

THROMBIN———————→ FIBRINOGEN

Fibrin monomer and fibrinopeptides

Fibrin polymer (soluble)

Ca^{++}
Factor XIII

FIBRIN (insoluble)

Coagulation defects

Hereditary

Haemophilia and Christmas disease
These are due to deficiencies of Factor VIII and Factor IX respectively, which

influence the conversion of prothrombin to thrombin. During bleeding episodes these cases are transfused with fresh frozen plasma, or with whole blood if the blood loss justifies this. Before elective surgery a good supply of human Factor VIII is obtained, so that the plasma Factor VIII level can be maintained at least to 50 per cent of the normal level for two weeks post-operatively.

Von Willebrand's disease

In this there is a prolonged bleeding time and a Factor VIII deficiency, plus some other factor, as treatment with whole blood transfusion is more effective than purified Factor VIII. The disease gives rise to bleeding from mucous membranes.

Hereditary telangiectasia (Osler–Rendu–Weber syndrome)

In this condition the nose, mouth, pharynx, lips, face, fingers and alimentary tract show areas of telangiectatic vessels presenting as multiple small purplish swellings in the skin and mucous membranes (*Plate 1a, facing page 112*). These are very susceptible to trauma. Those in the pharynx are less likely to give troublesome bleeding than elsewhere. If there is persistent bleeding from one site in the pharynx, electrical cautery can be tried but the results are not always satisfactory.

Deficiencies of Factors V, VII, IX, X, XII and XIII

Such deficiencies can occur separately or in combination. Treatment is to supply the missing factor.

Acquired

Administration of anticoagulants

This is the most obvious iatrogenic cause. Such patients are always precariously balanced and slight trauma may result in haemorrhage into the tissues, which in the neck is potentially life-threatening as the airway may rapidly become obstructed. The haemorrhage into the mucosa and pharynx shown in *Plate 1b, facing page 112* occurred in a patient being treated with warfarin. She also had bruising of the neck and complained of dysphagia. (Exactly the same symptoms and signs could occur in any type of coagulation defect.)

Advanced liver disease and uraemia

This may also induce a haemorrhagic state.

The purpuras

These are defined as multiple spontaneous capillary haemorrhages into the skin and mucous membranes.

Vascular (non-thrombocytopenic) purpuras

Drugs. Carbromal, penicillin, sulphonamides, salicylates, barbiturates, meprobamate and iodides may all increase capillary fragility.

Scurvy. Vitamin C deficiency also causes changes in capillary walls.

Dysproteinaemias. Abnormal increase in plasma globulins may lead to purpura although the mechanism is obscure.

Thrombocytopenic purpura

Failure of platelet production occurs in *aplastic* anaemia from any cause (*see above*) and in *neoplasias* of the bone marrow (reticuloses, secondary carcinomatosis, macrocytic anaemias).

Excessive destruction of circulating platelets occurs in the condition known as idiopathic thrombocytopenic purpura, in acute infections, and in treatment with some drugs (particularly salicylates and phenylbutazone). Other causes are disseminated lupus erythematosus, burns, heat stroke, and the defibrination syndrome.

Pharyngeal lesions due to nerve dysfunction

Functional disorder

Emotion causes a variety of sensations in the pharynx and larynx, so it is natural that people who are emotionally unstable should refer symptoms to this region.

'Globus hystericus'

Globus hystericus is a condition in which a patient, often a middle-aged woman, complains of the sensation of a lump in the throat, usually in the region of the thyroid cartilage. There may be other symptoms suggestive of a functional state, and the patient may admit that a relative or friend has recently succumbed to 'cancer of the throat'. The patient makes repeated attempts to swallow the lump which aggravate the symptoms and may lead to aerophagy and gastric discomfort. There is, however, no true dysphagia and the symptoms disappear on, or are improved by, taking a meal. Examination of the pharynx and larynx shows no evidence of disease. The condition may be confused with the Paterson–Brown Kelly syndrome, but clinical and blood examination should exclude these.

Re-assurance may relieve the patient, but sedatives should be prescribed if necessary. It is usually advisable, however, to arrange a barium-swallow and, if the symptom persists, to perform direct endoscopy, as it is only by these means that an early organic lesion in the oesophagus can be excluded. Sometimes the barium-swallow will show spasm of the cricopharyngeus; this is a reflex result of stimulation of the vagus by lesions at the lower end of the oesophagus or in the stomach, such as carcinoma, achalasia, or hiatus hernia. It is important that a barium meal as well as swallow should be performed to exclude these conditions.

Neurotrophic conditions

Herpes

Herpetic eruptions may occur anywhere in the mouth or pharynx, but the soft palate is commonly involved. The lesion may occur by itself or it may complicate eruptions elsewhere, such as geniculate herpes (Ramsay Hunt's syndrome). This is a herpes zoster involvement of the spheno-palatine ganglion, and not to be confused with a local virus infection such as herpangina.

The throat is sore for a few hours before a vesicular eruption appears. The vescicles break down to form shallow ulcers similar to those seen in aphthous stomatitis. Pain is severe, and may persist after the lesions have healed. There is little constitutional disturbance save that which usually accompanies a painful lesion in the throat, leading to interrupted sleep and disinclination to take food.

Local treatment must be employed to keep the mouth clean, and local analgesics should be given before meals to ensure adequate nourishment. Analgesics are necessary to relieve the pain.

Neuralgia

Glossopharyngeal neuralgia is a rare condition similar to trigeminal neuralgia, save in the distribution of pain. There are agonizing stabs of pain, which start in the region of the tonsil and radiate towards the ear; in other cases, the pain is situated in the ear or just below it, between the angle of the jaw and the mastoid process.

The attacks are precipitated by a stimulus in the trigger area. When this is situated in the throat, pain may be brought on by swallowing; temporary relief may be obtained by the application of cocaine to the posterior third of the tongue and the lateral pharyngeal wall. When the symptoms are confined to the ear, external stimulation on the ear or skin may cause an attack.

The attacks may be relieved by the administration of sedatives but, if these prove ineffectual, operation on the nerve may be necessary. The nerve may be approached within the skull, at the base of the skull, or at its periphery where it comes into relation with the tonsillar fossa.

Within the skull the nerve fibres can be divided soon after their emergence from the medulla, ensuring the relief of symptoms over the area of distribution of the nerve and its connections, notably that with the tympanic plexus. It is a formidable procedure, but with modern neurosurgical techniques there is no undue risk.

Approach to the nerve at the base of the skull is difficult. The nerve is small and is lying at a considerable depth in relation to important structures. It leaves the cranium through the middle compartment of the jugular foramen lying in front of, and medial to, the vagus and accessory nerves. It passes between the internal jugular vein and internal carotid artery, crossing the latter obliquely, and passing beneath the styloid process to reach the posterior border of the stylopharyngeus muscle. When the nerve has been found it must be avulsed to remove the jugular and petrosal ganglia, otherwise the connections with the tympanic plexus remain intact, and symptoms referred to the ear are not relieved. The results of this operation are not as certain as are those of intracranial section, and there is sometimes recurrence of symptoms.

Wilson has approached the nerve through the tonsillar fossa, where the nerve can be found lying on the stylopharyngeus muscle (Wilson and McAlpine, 1946). By dividing the nerve he relieved a patient whose symptoms were confined to the throat, but he claimed that it would be possible to follow the nerve to the base of the skull. Sometimes the neuralgia is associated with an abnormally long styloid process. This may be removed through the pharyngeal wall after tonsillectomy.

Paralysis of the palate and pharynx

Aetiology

Any lesion affecting the vagus nerve trunks or nuclei can cause unilateral or bilateral paralysis of the pharynx, often associated with palatal paralysis, and paralysis of the larynx and cricopharyngeus.

The nucleus ambiguus may be involved in postero-inferior cerebellar artery thrombosis, tumours of the medulla, bulbar palsy, syringobulbia, motor neurone disease, encephalitis, poliomyelitis, rabies and Landry's paralysis.

Posterior fossa lesions may involve the vagus nerve trunks as they emerge from the brain stem but before leaving the skull. Usually the ninth, eleventh, and twelfth cranial nerves are also involved. Tumours, syphilitic meningitis, and lesions of the jugular foramen such as glomus jugulare tumour can affect the nerve at this site.

Extracranial nerve trunk lesions occur as a result of tumours or penetrating injuries of the neck.

The nerve endings are affected by the diphtheria toxin which has an affinity for neuromuscular junctions.

Symptoms

When the palate is paralysed, the nasopharynx cannot be shut off from the rest of the pharynx and the flow of air through the nose cannot therefore be controlled during speech. This causes the form of speech heard in cases of cleft palate (rhinolalia aperta) although the disability is not usually so marked. During deglutition, fluids and even solids may regurgitate through the nose. In spite of this, however, the patient is usually able to swallow sufficient for his needs unless the pharynx is also involved. In this case the condition is much more serious, since it is almost impossible for the patient to swallow, and also because he loses control of secretions in the pharynx, which may enter the larynx and cause inhalation pneumonia. Any attempt at swallowing results in a spasm of coughing, particularly when fluids are taken.

Signs

When the paralysis is bilateral the palate remains immobile during phonation. It may be difficult to decide whether there is any movement, but if the patient is made to gag, it is at once apparent that the palate is paralysed. The patient is unable to comply with the request to blow up a balloon or to whistle.

In cases in which the paralysis is unilateral, the symptoms are not so marked, but when the patient phonates or is made to gag, the palate is drawn up to one side like a curtain, and the uvula is displaced with it.

Diagnosis

Paralysis of the palate must be distinguished from local fixation. Scarring after syphilis, lupus vulgaris or scarlet fever, or after operation for the removal of tonsils and adenoids or new growth, may also reduce the mobility of the palate.

Sometimes cases of palatal paralysis are referred to laryngologists because the symptoms are attributed to the presence of adenoids. In the case of nasal obstruction the speech defect, rhinolalia clausa, is entirely different and should not be confused, while regurgitation of fluids does not occur.

Treatment

Treatment is dictated by the cause of the condition, and a paralysis of the palate is unlikely to call for any special measures, but if regurgitation is marked, swallowing may be facilitated by holding the nose during the act. When the condition is associated with pharyngeal paralysis, the passing of a stomach tube may become necessary to ensure adequate nourishment, and a sucker should be used to keep the pharynx free from secretions. Despite this, repeated inhalation of secretions may occur, and it may be necessary to carry out a tracheostomy and insert a cuffed tracheostomy tube. When no recovery of the paralysis can be expected, long-term management is difficult, and section of the cricopharyngeus muscle assists some patients to swallow their saliva. Various surgical techniques have been tried to close the glottis but none is entirely satisfactory and occasionally laryngectomy may have to be resorted to, if the patient's life expectancy is good, because of the complications of long-term use of cuffed tubes (infection, necrosis and stenosis of the tracheal wall).

Diphtheritic paralysis of the palate and pharynx

Pathology

Diphtheritic paralysis of the palate and pharynx is due to the action of toxin on the neuromuscular junctions. The toxin may reach the nerve endings by the blood stream, but it is possible that in cases of faucial diphtheria access is gained locally.

Paralysis occurs three or four weeks after the onset of the disease, but may occur earlier in severe cases. It may be associated with other forms of paralysis but is often the only manifestation of neuritis. It is a complication which may be expected in severe cases, but it often occurs after a mild infection, when the patient is ambulant and presents himself because of regurgitation of fluids and alteration in his speech. On questioning the mother of such a case, it was found that the patient had recently had a

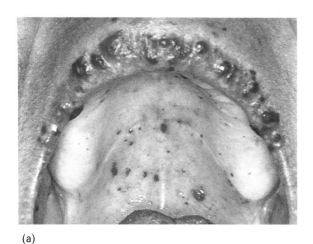

(a)

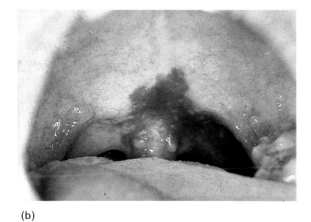

(b)

Plate 1 (a) Hereditary telangiectasis; (b) haemorrhage into the palate and pharynx of a 63-year-old patient being treated with warfarin

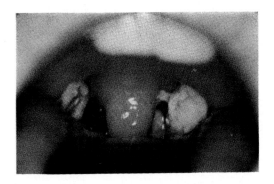

Plate 2   Tonsillar involvement in infectious
mononucleosis

sore throat and that his brother was 'in a fever hospital with diphtheria and a paralysed palate'.

Pharyngeal paralysis usually occurs rather later than palatal paralysis. It is a serious complication because swallowing becomes almost impossible and there is a risk of inhalation pneumonia. It complicates grave cases, and there may be respiratory paralysis as well.

Diagnosis

The diagnosis presents no difficulty when the subject is known to be suffering from diphtheria, since the paralysis is a complication which may be expected. In ambulant cases, a history of recent sore throat can usually be obtained, but the possibility of the membrane being situated elsewhere, in the nose or in a wound, must be remembered.

Treatment

Palatal paralysis calls for no treatment other than that dictated by the general condition of the patient. In cases in which the diagnosis has not already been made, the throat should be swabbed and the patient isolated until three negative results have been obtained. It is advisable to administer diphtheria antitoxin although, since the paralysis occurs late in the disease, the attack must have been mild to escape detection. Nevertheless, the patient must be kept in bed completely at rest.

When the pharynx is involved, active treatment is required to secure adequate nourishment and also to prevent inhalation pneumonia. If necessary, a stomach tube must be passed through the nose; this may be left *in situ* to avoid disturbing the patient who is likely to be desperately ill and to require absolute rest. A sucker may be used to remove pharyngeal secretions and prevent their entry into the larynx. Diphtheria antitoxin is required in doses of up to 200 000 units/day, by the intravenous route if necessary. Tracheostomy with a cuffed tube may be necessary.

Although the paralysis always recovers spontaneously, the restoration of movement may be hastened by exercises, and the patient should be encouraged to whistle or to blow up balloons.

Prognosis

This is largely dependent upon the general condition of the patient. When the palate alone is involved, the prognosis is not unduly affected, but in the case of pharyngeal paralysis, which often occurs in grave cases, the risk of inhalation pneumonia and difficulty in feeding render recovery less certain.

Should the patient survive, the paralysis always recovers sooner or later.

Myasthenia gravis

Myasthenia gravis occurs in persons of all ages, but is usually seen in adolescents; they are sometimes referred for the removal of the adenoids, when the pharynx is involved.

There is a defect at the neuromuscular junction, which is believed to be due to destruction of acetylcholine, depriving the junction of its activating substances. The result is a gradual loss of power in the affected muscles. Any group of muscles may be involved, commonly those in the lower limb, but occasionally the lesion is restricted to the muscles of the mouth and pharynx. There is dysarthria and dysphagia, with regurgitation of fluid through the nose, and movements of the tongue, palate and pharynx are sluggish. Disability is minimal after a night's rest, but increases as the day passes.

The cause of the condition is unknown and treatment must be symptomatic. Many patients are able to live a restricted life on neostigmine or pyridostigmine taken orally. In selected cases thymectomy (Keynes, 1949) may be beneficial.

Acute anterior poliomyelitis

This disease is of interest to the laryngologist because, when the medullary nuclei are affected (the bulbar type of acute anterior poliomyelitis), paralysis of the pharynx and larynx may occur.

Aetiology

The disease is due to a virus of which three principal strains have been identified. It may occur in epidemics, or sporadically. Epidemics commonly occur in hot weather, starting in midsummer and reaching their height in the autumn. Infection may be spread by people who are in the early stages of infection, or by healthy carriers who are infective for a few days. The disease is spread by faecal contamination, the portal of entry being the intestinal epithelium; at least one epidemic has been ascribed to the ingestion of infected milk.

Study of the epidemiology of the disease is difficult, because many cases do not progress to the stage at which the diagnosis is certain and, in the absence of an epidemic, cases must occur in which the true nature of the condition is not recognized. The disease occurs most regularly in children, but in the post-war epidemic in Great Britain adults formed a large proportion of the victims. The relative immunity of the adult population is probably conferred by previous unrecognized infection.

Motor, sensory and sympathetic axons may all be invaded by the poliomyelitis virus. The virus does not multiply in the axons but does so when it reaches the anterior horn cells. The cells invaded bear no anatomical relation to the site of inoculation, but certain groups of cells, those involved in maintaining decerebrate rigidity, appear to be more sensitive than others.

Pathology

Once the virus has gained access to the central nervous system it becomes widely disseminated throughout the brain stem and anterior horn cells of the spinal cord.

The cortex and sympathetic ganglia are less severely affected. The first changes which occur are round-cell and lymphocyte collections round the vessels in relation to the nerve cells. This does not occur when the cells are degenerate, and it is assumed that this reaction is the result of the action of the virus on healthy nerve cells. Nerve cells are destroyed early in the disease, certainly within three days, and no further destruction occurs. The destroyed cells are rapidly removed by neurophages, leaving no trace. Other cells show evidence of damage by loss of Nissl granules, but these are likely to recover later. Clinical signs of paralysis are not noticeable until probably at least one-third of the cells are destroyed, and paralysis is complete, when only one-tenth remain. It is very unusual for all the cells to be destroyed.

Symptoms and signs

When the disease runs its full course, there are three distinct phases.

In the first stage, there is general malaise, with either gastro-intestinal disorder or upper respiratory infection. Symptoms may be severe, with pyrexia, or so mild as to escape notice except during an epidemic. The patient is ill for a few days and then recovers; in abortive cases, health is restored and further symptoms do not appear. Within 48 hours of apparent recovery, the second stage of meningitic involvement is entered. Symptoms may be severe, with headache and neck rigidity, or they may be mild.

This stage is of short duration and the disease may be arrested or it may pass into the third stage, in which sudden paralysis of groups of muscles occurs. This is due to involvement of the anterior horn cells in the spinal cord, or more rarely of the medullary nuclei. There is pain and tenderness in the affected muscles, and although at first the paralysis may be widespread, a variable degree of recovery may be expected. The lower limb is usually involved, but the upper limb and respiratory muscles may be affected. In the bulbar type of infection, the larynx and pharynx may be paralysed; these are severe cases and the prognosis is not good.

Diagnosis

In the first stage the disease resembles a minor gastro-intestinal upset, or a mild upper respiratory infection, and it is unlikely that the correct diagnosis will be made except in the presence of an epidemic. In the second phase, of meningitic involvement, the diagnosis can be made with certainty by examination of the cerebrospinal fluid, which contains an increased number of cells, chiefly lymphocytes, and raised protein, but normal glucose and chloride concentrations. In the third stage, the sudden onset of widespread paralysis presents little difficulty in diagnosis.

Treatment

It would be out of place to discuss the treatment of all aspects of the disease, but pharyngeal and respiratory paralysis may demand the attention of the otolaryngologist. In pharyngeal paralysis the main dangers are respiratory infection due to inhalation of food and secretions, and lack of nourishment; and in laryngeal paralysis, asphyxia owing to respiratory obstruction. These are treated by tracheostomy with a cuffed tube and the passage of a Ryle's tube into the stomach. This ensures adequate nourishment while the lower respiratory passages are protected and an adequate airway obtained. Secretions in the bronchial tree may be aspirated as often as necessary, and if the muscles of respiration are paralysed a positive-pressure respirator may be employed.

Once the extent of the paralysis, which comes on over a period of some hours, has been established, the condition of the patient remains unchanged for a variable period, which may amount to weeks. Sooner or later, however, a period of recovery sets in which may continue for some weeks. Many are able to discard their tracheostomy tubes and regain their powers of swallowing and speech, although there may be some permanent residual paralysis. The less fortunate may be condemned to a life made possible only by the continued use of a respirator.

Immunization

Although the existence of a virus was demonstrated many years ago by its passage through filters, which prevented the passage of bacteria, and the production of disease by the filtrate, it is so small that it could not be observed with the aid of the most powerful magnification at that time. Its precise form and mode of life was a mystery until the invention of the electron microscope, when it could be observed. The viruses were observed and cultured, and various strains recognized. The production of vaccines followed, and in no field have the results been more dramatic than that of acute anterior poliomyelitis. It was found that three strains of virus were responsible for the disease and Salk introduced the first vaccine by killing the three strains of virus with formalin and injecting the products of destruction systemically. Apart from one tragic episode when, owing to faulty technique, a batch of vaccine containing live virus was released, with consequent infection of a number of people, the method proved satisfactory. It is thought that the antigen forms a coating over the cells of the body which prevents invasion by the virus. More recently, this method has been superseded by the oral administration of attenuated live virus. It is thought that the intestinal cells are protected from invasion by the virus, but that with large doses a certain amount of antigen is absorbed into the circulation. In this method of immunization it is realized that attenuated virus is excreted in the faeces and that other individuals may become infected, but where the immunization of a community is the aim this is an advantage rather than a risk. It is not known for how long immunity is conferred by either method. There is no doubt, however, of the success of immunization since no epidemic has occurred among immunized communities since its introduction.

Spasm of the pharynx

This is a rare condition and consequently may present some difficulty in diagnosis. Frequently it is one of the signs of a well-established neurological condition, but occasionally it is the presenting feature.

frequent small haemorrhages from mucous membranes after trivial trauma, such as brushing the teeth. In severe cases there may be haemorrhages into muscles and joints. There is also a proneness to infections including dental infections and pharyngitis.

Vitamin K

This vitamin is essential for the liver to form prothrombin. It is hardly ever deficient in the diet, and can be synthesized by bacteria in the gut, but it is not absorbed if there is an absence of bile from the alimentary tract. Deficiency therefore occurs in obstructive jaundice, and may lead to a haemorrhagic state. Treatment is to give the vitamin by injection.

Miscellaneous conditions

Behçet's syndrome

This disease was first described by Behçet in 1937; the *aetiology* has since been extensively investigated but is still not clearly understood. However, some predisposing factors have recently come to light. As with other forms of aphthous ulceration, immunological factors are involved, and levamisole therapy resulted in improvement in some patients (Lehner, Wilton and Ivanyi, 1976). In another survey, deficiencies of iron, folate and vitamin B_{12} were found in a higher percentage of patients with aphthous ulcers than in matched controls (Wray *et al.*, 1975), and when these deficiencies were corrected, the ulcers were controlled. Underlying coeliac disease has also been reported with remission of ulcers on a gluten-free diet; however, gluten may of itself be toxic to oral mucosa in these patients and a gluten-free diet may improve the oral condition even in patients with no coeliac disease (Walker *et al.*, 1978).

Pathology and clinical features

The disease runs a protracted course with periods of remission and acute relapse, when there is pyrexia, leucocytosis and raised sedimentation rate in the blood.

The disease is characterized by massive and indolent ulceration of the mucous membranes and, sometimes, the skin. The anogenital region is commonly affected, the labia minora and cervix in women, and the urethra, glans penis and scrotum in men. There is an associated inflammation of the eye. Iritis with hypopion, conjunctivitis, choroiditis, retinitis or retinal haemorrhages are encountered. In the mouth, the manifestation consists of aphthous ulcers, rather larger and more persistent than those normally seen. Lesions in the pharynx may resemble leucoplakia, or even carcinoma. Skin lesions may resemble pemphigus or lichen planus. The central nervous system may be involved, and acute encephalitis with raised lymphocyte count and protein content of the cerebrospinal fluid may be simulated. There may be acute lesions of the brain stem or pyramidal tracts, and dementia may set in. Lesions affecting the central nervous system usually arise after several years and indicate a poor prognosis. Pain is a marked feature of the lesions, and loss of weight may be considerable. The lesions heal with gross scarring, and complications such as vesico-vaginal fistula may arise.

Investigation and diagnosis

The disease resembles any condition giving rise to ulceration in the areas referred to: syphilis, tuberculosis, carcinoma, leucoplakia, agranulocytosis and malignant granuloma, to mention a few. These may be excluded by serological tests, blood count, examination of smears from the lesion, or biopsy. In Behçet's disease these investigations do not yield any specific information, and it is usually considered that the diagnosis is confirmed when any two of the sites usually involved are affected. However, the blood count may reveal anaemia, and estimations of serum iron, folate and vitamin B_{12} should also be carried out and may reveal deficiencies. Immunoglobulin abnormalities may also be present.

Treatment

This consists of finding and treating any underlying deficiencies. Since the aetiology of the disease in many cases cannot be identified, the exhibition of steroids may be required and usually leads to an improvement in the lesions. In the mouth and pharynx, ulceration may be controlled by topical administration in the form of trochiscus hydrocortisone hemisuccinate 2.5 mg six-hourly, but sooner or later systemic administration becomes necessary, at least 20 mg of prednisone daily being required. Occasionally a gluten-free diet may be tried. The patient may survive for a number of years, but a complete cure is unlikely.

Wegener's granulomatosis

The condition may present in the pharynx, though more rarely than in the nose. It may begin on the anterior pillar as a painless but progressive ulcer. For an account of the diagnosis and management of this disease the reader is referred to Volume 3, and to page 417 in this volume.

References

Behçet, H. (1937). *Dermatologische Wochenschrift*, **105,** 1152
Behçet, H. (1938). *Bulletin de la Société française de dermatologie et de syphiligraphie*, **45,** 420
Behçet, H. (1939). *Bulletin de la Société française de dermatologie et de syphiligraphie*, **46,** 674
Bouroncle, B. A., Wiseman, B. K., and Doan, C. A. (1958). *Blood*, **13,** 609

Dameshek, W. and Gunz, F. (1964). *Leukaemia*, 2nd edn; Grune and Stratton, New York
Keynes, G. (1949). *British Medical Journal*, **2,** 611
Lehner, T., Wilton, J. M. A. and Ivanyi, L. (1976). *Lancet*, **ii,** 926
Rosenow, E. C. and Bernatz, P. E. (1974). *The Esophagus* (Eds W. S. Payne and A. M. Olsen); Lea and Fibiger, Philadelphia

Walker, D. M. , Dolby, A. E., Mead, J.,
Llewelyn, J. and Rhodes, J. (1978).
'International Association for Dental Research
British Division', *Annual Meeting April, 1978,*
Abstr. no. 204
Wilson, C. P. and McAlpine, D. (1946).
Proceedings of the Royal Society of Medicine, **40,** 81

Winther, L. K. (1978). 'Accidental corrosive
burns of the oesophagus', *Journal of Laryngology
and Otology,* **92,** 693
Wray, D., Ferguson, M. M., Mason, D. K.,
Hutcheon, A. W. and Dagg, J. H. (1975).
British Medical Journal, **i,** 490

6 Diseases of the tonsils and adenoids (excluding neoplasms)
Stuart R Mawson

The word tonsil derives from the Latin *tonsilla*, a mooring post, and there are three so-named anatomical structures forming part of Waldeyer's ring of lymphoid tissue encircling the entrance from the mouth and nasal passages to the pharynx; *palatine* (faucial) *tonsil* situated, one on each side, between the folds of the palatopharyngeus and palatoglossus muscles; *lingual tonsil*, one on each side between base of tongue and vallecula; and a single *nasopharyngeal tonsil* (adenoids: Greek *aden*, gland; *eidos*, form) in the roof of the nasopharynx (epipharynx).

The palatine tonsil is a subepithelial lymph node with prominent germinal centres concerned in the production of lymphocytes and plasma cells, penetrated by branching crypts from the medial surface; the lateral surfaces being separated from the pharyngeal wall by a distinct capsule of condensed connective tissue. Surface epithelium and crypt linings are of stratified squamous epithelium. Efferent lymphatics pass to the jugulodigastric lymph node behind the angle of the mandible, and thence to the cervical chain. The lingual tonsils are similar subepithelial nodes but with smaller crypts and without a capsule. The subepithelial nasopharyngeal tonsil has neither crypts nor capsule, but prominent folds lined by respiratory epithelium (for anatomy, *see* Vol. 1).

Nomenclature

In British otolaryngology the word tonsil(s) has long been understood as referring, in practice, exclusively to the palatine (faucial) tonsil(s). The nasopharyngeal tonsil is customarily called (the) adenoids, while the two lingual tonsils retain their full title. This has the merit of avoiding confusion. The traditional terms, tonsils, adenoids and lingual tonsils will therefore be retained and hereafter used in the sense defined.

Function

A summarization (Morag and Ogra, 1975) of numerous investigations into the immunological role of the tonsils and adenoids carried out in recent years suggests that the tonsils are immunologically reactive organs with specific antibody, and

β- and T-cell activity in response to a variety of antigens. Adenoids also appear to be immunologically reactive but less so than the tonsils. Tonsils and, to a small extent, adenoids may contribute to the normal immunological developmental process, and removal during the early growth period may compromise local nasopharyngeal immunological responses and overall immunity against infections in the respiratory tract.

At birth the tonsils are without germinal centres and usually quite small in relation to the oropharyngeal inlet, but coinciding with the loss of maternal source antibody there is an enlargement of the tonsils and adenoids, and to a lesser extent the lingual tonsils, further exacerbated it would seem by the exposure to infection that occurs on entry to nursery school at the age of three and primary school at the age of five. Enlargement of tonsils and adenoids is therefore normal in early childhood and probably an index of immunological activity. There are, however, considerable individual variations within this general trend, often related to familial tendencies or to other factors such as severe respiratory infections in infancy. Occasionally children are born with tonsils and/or adenoids of such size as to constitute an embarrassment to respiration from the start.

At or before the onset of puberty there would appear to be a decline in functional activity accompanied by a marked involution of these organs. While the tonsils and lingual tonsils remain still visible, the adenoids may completely disappear, so that indirect nasopharyngoscopy in the adult commonly reveals a roof as smooth as in those who have had the adenoids removed. In the present state of our knowledge it is generally agreed that, certainly in the early years, the tonsils and adenoids should be conserved as probable immunological assets unless by their size they are causing severe embarrassment to respiration, eustachian tube function, speech or feeding, or unless they have become the seat of a disease the best remedy for which is excision.

Obstructive enlargement

As stated above, children may be born with tonsils and especially adenoids of such a size as already to cause some obstruction to the upper respiratory tract. In the case of adenoids difficulty may very occasionally arise with feeding (as in congenital choanal atresia) and in this event it will be necessary to differentiate between the two conditions by passing a soft rubber catheter through the nose. It is most unusual for such a catheter not to be able to find a way past the adenoids and become visible in the oropharynx. But in cases of doubt a firmer instrument (e.g. eustachian catheter) or instillation of a radio-opaque contrast medium should resolve the problem.

Obstruction of a serious nature, however, seldom occurs much before the end of the first year and is more usually seen between the ages of three to five.

While it is a simple matter to assess the size of the tonsils by direct inspection, it is not so easy clinically to determine the size of the adenoids. The degree of obstruction is related to and may be inferred from the symptoms of mouth-breathing and snoring. Obstruction may also be inferred from the appearance of the tympanic membranes which may be retracted, due to absorption of air, if the tubal orifices are blocked. An attempt should always be made to try to see the adenoids with a nasopharyngeal mirror in any child who can be persuaded to keep the mouth open and tolerate a tongue depressor. Provided the approach is unhurried and careful, a rewarding view may be obtained in a surprising proportion of young patients. Uncertainty as to the size of the adenoids may be resolved by taking a soft-tissue lateral x-ray of the area, when the shadow of the adenoids may be seen in relation to the available airway.

Treatment

Attempts have been made to reduce the size of the adenoids by radiotherapy but this treatment is too uncertain, both in terms of adenoid response and latent effects, to be recommended. When the obstruction is interfering seriously with respiration and feeding especially, or with hearing and speech, then relief by adenoidectomy will come under consideration as the best treatment at present known.

The operation, however, is not without disadvantages, especially in the younger child (*see* 'The operation of adenoidectomy', p. 160).

(1) Risk of haemorrhage. Depletion of blood volume reaches a critical stage more quickly in smaller, younger children.
(2) Risk of recurrence. It is impossible to remove every vestige of adenoid tissue with a curette. The earlier adenoids are removed the more likely are remnants and other subepithelial deposits in the nasopharynx to undergo compensatory hypertrophy, due to the natural tendency towards tonsil tissue hypertrophy in the first five years of life.
(3) Technical difficulty is greater in the very young child.

Thus, unless hypertrophy of adenoids is causing serious retardation of the physiological functions mentioned, it is nearly always better to avoid operation until a child has at least reached the age of two, and preferably postpone it until the fourth year. Very occasionally it will be necessary to accept the disadvantages and operate earlier.

On many occasions it is wise to precede a decision to operate by taking the soft-tissue lateral radiograph of the post-nasal space, already referred to.

The tonsils by size alone seldom give rise to the same degree of obstruction as the adenoids and, again, it is preferable whenever possible to postpone operation until at least the age of four.

Acute tonsillitis

The tonsils, being covered by the mucous membrane common to the oropharynx, may become inflamed as part of a general pharyngitis, usually concurrent with an acute upper respiratory infection. Such an inflammation has, in the past, been called *acute catarrhal* or *superficial tonsillitis*. In these cases there is little or no swelling of the tonsils, the surface merely appearing inflamed in continuity with the rest of the pharyngeal mucosa. Clinically true acute tonsillitis presents in three main forms:

(1) *Acute follicular tonsillitis* (cryptic tonsillitis, lacunar tonsillitis) when inflammatory

exudation from the crypts marks the reddened surface with whitish or yellow spots.

(2) *Acute parenchymatous tonsillitis*, when the whole tonsil is uniformly congested, presenting as a definitely abnormal red swelling – the phlegmon of older textbooks.

(3) *Acute membranous tonsillitis*, in which the exudation from the crypts may coalesce to form a confluent membrane over the surface.

While acute tonsillitis can present in any one of these forms the clinical distinction between them is not of great importance, and is often blurred.

Aetiology

Acute tonsillitis is predominantly a disease of childhood with a peak incidence in the fifth and sixth years of life, but it occurs relatively frequently in adolescence and early adulthood, often as periodic exacerbation of an underlying chronic tonsil infection. It is rare in infancy and after the age of 50.

It may occur as a primary infection, that is to say infection originates with the tonsil, or as a secondary infection derived from a general infection of the upper respiratory tract. In the latter case the initial infecting organism is most likely to be a virus. Important members of the group of viruses responsible for causing local upper respiratory disease by multiplication in the epithelium are the following (Dudgeon, 1969): influenza A, B and C; para-influenza 1, 2, 3, and 4; adenoviruses (over 30 different members identified); respiratory syncitial virus; common cold or rhino-viruses (over 80 varieties classified). Of these the adenoviruses are the most commonly identified in relation to the tonsils.

While an attack of acute tonsillitis may be initiated by a local upper respiratory virus infection the typical follicular, parenchymatous or membranous appearance results from bacterial action. Virus growing in mucous membrane cells quickly renders them liable to secondary invasion by streptococci, straphylococci and pneumococci which can be present in the mouth even in health. These bacteria may be responsible for a primary local acute tonsillitis if the patient's resistance is low or if the tonsils themselves are at a disadvantage through previous infections, accumulation of debris in the crypts or incomplete attempts at removal. However, there is one organism with a predilection for the tonsils and which is cultured in over 50 per cent of throat swabs, namely the haemolytic streptococcus. Most attacks of acute tonsillitis are caused by this agent and the attacks usually present clinically as the acute follicular type of infection. The process of inflammation originating within the tonsil is accompanied by hyperaemia and oedema, with conversion of lymphoid follicles into small abscesses which discharge into the crypts.

Streptococcal tonsillitis occurs in epidemics, especially where spread of infection is encouraged by overcrowding or inadequate ventilation. In institutions, such as hospitals, it may present a quite serious problem of cross-infection. Carriers of the streptococcus may initiate infection in others while remaining symptom-free themselves.

Symptoms and signs

A patient developing acute tonsillitis from an upper respiratory infection may, at first, only complain of the dry throat, general malaise, slight fever and thirst common to the latter. Sore throat is not an invariable symptom, especially in children in whom diagnosis may only be apparent on inspection of the throat during a routine search for the cause of unexplained pyrexia or refusal to eat, or in some cases abdominal pain. But once acute tonsillitis has developed it is usual for sore throat exacerbated on swallowing to be the predominant symptom. A typical primary tonsillitis due to haemolytic streptococcal infection is accompanied by a sense of fullness in the throat, severe dysphagia, often acute, with pain radiating to the ears and anorexia (largely due to the dysphagia). The voice has a plummy quality. There are pains in the neck, which is held stiffly, due to the swelling of regional lymph nodes; headache, and sometimes pains in the back and limbs. The patient feels shivery due to fever, and generally unwell.

On examination there may be some circumoral pallor. The tongue is furred and dry and the breath foetid. The tonsils are swollen and red and spotted with purulent exudate from the crypts or in severe cases covered with a purulent membrane. There is an accumulation of viscid mucus due to the patient's dislike of swallowing. In the parenchymatous type of tonsillitis the livid swellings of the tonsils, accompanied by oedema of the uvula and soft palate, may appear quite to occlude the oropharyngeal inlet, with consequent increase in dysphagia. However, dysphagia severe enough entirely to prevent the patient swallowing his own saliva seldom occurs unless a quinsy (peritonsillar abscess; *see* p. 135) has formed. The jugulodigastric (tonsillar) lymph nodes behind the angles of the mandible are enlarged and tender. The temperature is raised, varying from 37.8°C (100°F) to 40.5°C (105°F).

Differential diagnosis

Acute tonsillitis is a disease of sudden onset with a typical clinical triad of sore throat, fever and malaise running, even if untreated, a relatively benign course within a week to ten days. Response to antibiotic treatment is usually rapid, at times dramatic, and it is rare for the condition of the patient, in uncomplicated cases, to give cause for anxiety. Suspicion of the presence of some other condition will be prompted by departure from this clinical pattern, or by some unusual appearance of the tonsils themselves.

Scarlet fever is a streptococcal tonsillitis with general disturbances due to the production of soluble toxins, one of which causes a punctate erythematous rash in susceptible subjects. Apart from the rash, there is tachycardia out of proportion to the pyrexia, a stippled palate, a 'strawberry tongue', and an intensely red appearance of the tonsils. Sometimes the tonsils are covered with a yellowish exudate which is usually readily removable. The blood picture shows a polymorphonuclear leucocytosis and eosinophilia.

Glandular fever (infectious mononucleosis; *see* p. 166) may be seen in the so-called 'anginose form' as clinically, at least in the initial stages, indistinguishable from a severe attack of acute tonsillitis. It is today not too uncommon and should always be considered whenever an apparent attack of acute tonsillitis, especially in a young adult, persists, with fever, despite antibiotic therapy, with extreme local discomfort and an alarmingly swollen, membrane-covered pair of tonsils.

There is a total lymphocytosis of at least $4500/\text{mm}^3$ in the peripheral blood with at least 51 per cent lymphocytes in the differential leucocyte count, of which a significant number are atypical.

Serum heterophile antibody (sheep's cell agglutinin) titres rise during the first 2–3 weeks in nearly all adult patients. Demonstration of the presence of these antibodies by the Paul Bunnell–Davidson or ox cell haemolysis tests is diagnostically specific for infectious mononucleosis. Other signs of the infection, such as lymph node enlargement elsewhere as well as in the neck, and palpable spleen, should always be looked for.

Vincent's angina (see p. 165). This is essentially a subacute tonsillitis with ulceration. It is of slower onset and accompanied by less sore throat and lower fever than acute tonsillitis. A sloughing membrane forms on the ulcer, and the patient's breath is characteristically foetid. It is rare in children. The characteristic organisms, Vincent's fusiform bacillus and *Spirochaeta denticola*, may be cultured from a throat swab.

Diphtheria, now rare in the United Kingdom, is unlikely to be confused with acute tonsillitis but must be considered whenever there is a membrane on the surface of the tonsil. Diphtheria is slower in onset, and is at first accompanied by less constitutional disturbance and less local discomfort. The membrane, which may extend beyond the surface of the tonsil onto the palate, is dirty grey in colour. It is adherent and removal causes bleeding. The identification of the Klebs–Löffler bacillus in the membrane is diagnostic.

Granulocytopenia and *leukaemia* may be accompanied by necrosing lesions of the tonsils resembling those seen in glandular fever and may present with acute sore throat. Ulceration is usually present elsewhere in the mouth and oropharynx, noticeable for absence of surrounding inflammatory reaction. The obvious severity of the patient's condition in these blood diseases renders them unlikely to be confused with typical tonsillitis.

Treatment

It is a generally accepted principle of medical practice that antibiotics should not be given for minor conditions because of the risk of the development of resistant strains of organisms or of allergic reactions on the part of the patients, which may limit the use of the antibiotic in the possible event of a future major illness. Since many cases of acute tonsillitis naturally run a relatively short, mild course, it is advocated that antibiotics should be withheld in the early stages unless or until it is clear that the patient has a major attack not to be assuaged by symptomatic treatment or is known to have had complications with previous attacks. Successful antibiotic treatment moreover depends on the achievement of adequate concentration, adequately maintained at the site of infection. It is therefore also advocated that if the decision is made to administer antibiotic (and penicillin is the most appropriate in most cases) it should initially be given in relatively high dosage by intramuscular injection, reserving oral therapy for maintenance, which should never be discontinued, even in apparently rapid cure, within less than five days.

The principles of treatment being established the management of acute tonsillitis can be considered as follows.

General and symptomatic

Patients should be put to bed, isolated and encouraged to drink plenty of bland fluids. The temperature and pulse should be recorded every eight hours. If possible, a throat swab should be taken and sent for culture of organisms and antibiotic sensitivity tests. If the patient's disinclination to eat solid food results in constipation a mild aperient may be given but purging, as such, is of no therapeutic value. For the sore throat aspirin taken in soluble form, dissolved as a drink, is preferred, e.g. aspirin soluble tablets BP, 1–3 tablets up to four times daily (one tablet three times daily in children 6–12 years old; half a tablet three times daily if under six years). Lozenges containing antibiotics are of no benefit in true tonsillitis, and only encourage the overgrowth of monilia. Pain in the neck due to tender lymph nodes can to some extent be helped by warmth; a cotton wool collar held in place with a sock or handkerchief is an old-fashioned but comforting remedy.

Antibiotic therapy

If, despite general and symptomatic treatment, the temperature remains high and there is marked toxaemia, and where the exudation from the tonsil crypts or the tonsillar swelling is marked, it is advisable to administer antibiotic, preferably according to laboratory indications. Antibiotic should also be given if previous attacks of tonsillitis have been associated with complications, especially quinsy, rheumatic fever, acute glomerulonephritis or chorea. Since, however, swab results may not be returned for several days and about 40 per cent will be sterile or show only normal commensals it is often necessary to proceed on the assumption that the infection is due to a streptococcus against which penicillin, at the time of writing, remains the most universally effective agent. If the choice, by laboratory test, lies between a new and an old agent, both equally safe and effective, then the old agent should be used. In this way emergence of bacterial resistance to the new agent will be delayed. A short course of a narrow-spectrum agent in a high dosage is better than a prolonged course of a broad-spectrum agent in low dosage. The course of treatment for acute infections should be 5–7 days, depending on the extent and severity of symptoms (British National Formulary, 1968). These considerations endorse the choice of penicillin in acute tonsillitis, which may be administered as follows to patients who have not had allergic reactions to it previously.

Initial

Intramuscular injection of 300 mg (300 000 units) of procaine penicillin combined with 60 mg (100 000 units) of benzylpenicillin (procaine penicillin injection, fortified BP). In severe cases the injection (in all ages over six years) should be repeated in 12 hours; and continued once or twice daily according to age, until the patient is able or willing to take phenoxymethylpenicillin (penicillin V) by mouth every six hours.

Maintenance

Penicillin V is available in tablet, capsule or elixir form. Doses of 250 mg (125 mg in children aged 1–5) every six hours produce adequate blood levels, but it cannot be said too often that success depends on a rigid adherence to the six-hourly regimen, and to the continuance of antibiotic in those cases who really need it for a full week.

As an alternative, for example, if there is strong patient aversion to ingestion, a course of amoxycillin may be effective (dose: in adults 250 mg eight-hourly; in children up to age ten years, 125 mg eight-hourly as elixir). Amoxycillin has the advantage of requiring to be administered only three times in 24 hours and thus allows for an undisturbed night's sleep.

Complications

These are classified as local and systemic.

Local

Chronic tonsillitis (see p. 132). The tonsil does not always return to a state of complete health after an attack of acute tonsillitis, especially after the follicular type where minute abscesses have formed in the lymphoid follicles surrounding the crypts and possibly become walled-off by fibrous tissue. Inadequate antibiotic therapy especially reveals this tendency as following apparent subsidence of an acute attack there may be recurrence after as short a time as ten days, clearly a recrudescence of latent, inextinguished infection rather than fresh infection acquired from an outside source. This process of apparent cure followed by relapse may go on for some weeks; while in other cases the patient settles into a pattern of recurrent acute tonsillitis every 3–4 months, where the frequency of attacks points to some predisposing factor such as chronic tonsil infection or failure of local community.

Quinsy (peritonsillar abscess, paratonsillar abscess; *see* p. 135). Spread of infection from the tonsil with formation of pus in the areolar space between the tonsil capsule and the tonsil bed may occur as a complication of acute tonsillitis, especially in a patient with chronic infection who suffers from repeated acute exacerbation.

Parapharyngeal abscess (see p. 138). Infection may spread from tonsil or quinsy through the superior constrictor muscle and give rise to pus formation between the muscle and deep cervical fascia.

Suppurative cervical adenitis. Occasionally suppuration may occur in the regional lymph nodes (jugulodigastric) as a result of acute infection in the tonsil. This complication is much less commonly seen than in the pre-antibiotic era, and, as in the case of quinsy and parapharyngeal abscess, generally results from infection with a penicillin-resistant *Staphylococcus aureus.*

Acute otitis media. Acute otitis media is a less common complication in acute tonsillitis than the anatomical proximity of the eustachian tube orifice in the pharynx would predict. However, some children appear to have a special susceptibility and suffer a regular sequence of tonsillitis followed by otitis media which, if too often repeated, constitutes one of the accepted indications for prophylactic tonsillectomy.

Systemic

Systemic complications are seen principally in association with Group A beta-haemolytic streptococcal infections, discussed below.

Rheumatic fever. This occurs as frequently in patients who have had their tonsils removed as in those who have not. But the tonsil is undoubtedly the portal of entry in some cases with close incidental association between the onset of acute streptococcal tonsillitis and the rheumatic fever.

Acute glomerulonephritis. Urine is not infrequently scanty, highly coloured and charged with urates but seldom contains albumen during an attack of acute tonsillitis. Albuminuria may presage acute nephritis which, together with all systemic complications, is less commonly seen since the advent of antibiotics.

Chorea. Sydenham's rheumatic chorea may be derived from tonsil infections but is, again, rare.

Subacute bacterial endocarditis. In patients with a pre-existing valvular lesion of the heart, infection of the tonsil with *Streptococcus viridans* may, through systemic infection, initiate an attack of *subacute bacterial endocarditis*. Acute tonsillitis in such at-risk patients should always be treated with antibiotics.

Acute lingual tonsillitis

This is a rare condition arising from the same causal factors as acute tonsillitis. It tends to be unilateral with one-sided dysphagia as the leading symptom. It may otherwise be accompanied by the same symptoms as acute tonsillitis. On examination there is more pain on tongue depression than in the case of acute tonsillitis, and tongue protrusion is more inhibited. A mirror must be used to view the lingual tonsils, which appear swollen and inflamed. The condition may be distinguished from Ludwig's angina by the absence of swelling of the floor of the mouth.

Treatment

As for acute tonsillitis except that antibiotics should be administered immediately on diagnosis.

Complications

Lingual quinsy. Pus formation within the lingual tonsil may call for surgical drainage.

Epiglottitis and laryngitis. These structures are liable to involvement by contiguity of infection. Oedema of epiglottis or larynx may be dangerous.

Acute adenoiditis

Acute superificial adenoiditis may be presumed to occur in every case of acute upper respiratory infection, but acute adenoiditis, as such, does not exist as a clinical diagnosis. 'Infected adenoids' will be considered under the heading 'Chronic adenoiditis' (p. 157).

Chronic tonsillitis (non-specific)

To pass through childhood without an attack of acute tonsillitis is rare. To suffer one or two attacks of acute tonsillitis a year between the ages of four to nine is normal. Undue susceptibility to acute tonsillitis may arise from poor immunological defences or environmental exposure to excessive bacterial populations. But in many cases it arises because local defences are reduced by the establishment of chronic infection in the tonsils themselves.

Aetiology

Following an attack of acute tonsillitis, the tonsil may or may not return to a state of complete health. In the latter event (as shown by post-operative histological studies) minute abscesses, having formed in the lymphoid follicles, may become walled-off by fibrous tissue and surrounded by a zone of inflammatory cells. It is also possible for inflammatory debris to become trapped in crypts by fibrous occlusion of the openings, and for such debris to expand into neighbouring crypts. Germinal centres can become markedly hyperplastic with notable thickening of fibrous septa.

It is possible for these histological changes to be found in tonsils which have not been associated with local symptoms of sore throat, and for there to be no direct relation between polymorphonuclear cell infiltration or fibrosis and the frequency or severity of clinical attacks of sore throat or tonsillitis. But the existence of the histological changes points to chronic infection in the tonsils through lowering of local tissue resistance as a probable cause of unusual susceptibility to acute tonsillitis. That it is indeed a principal cause has been shown by the beneficial results of tonsillectomy in countless well-selected cases.

Chronic tonsillitis is usually a complication of acute tonsillitis, but may also become established more insidiously by subclinical tonsil infections manifested only as sore throat. A 'feed-back' system becomes established until, in severe cases, attacks of acute tonsillitis may occur once every six weeks or so with the throat feeling constantly sore or uncomfortable in between attacks. While chronic tonsillitis, as inferred from the frequency of attacks of sore throat or acute tonsillitis, has its highest incidence in childhood between the ages of five and eight years, it is by no means uncommon in teenagers and young adults. It is rare after the age of 50.

Symptoms and signs

Minor symptoms of chronic tonsillitis are a bad taste in the mouth (cacagus), halitosis and discomfort in the throat, all due to accumulation and discharge of infected cryptic debris. These symptoms alone in some cases have led to the designation of a *chronic follicular (lacunar) tonsillitis* specifically diagnosed by the demonstration of such debris in the crypts on inspection. Similarly, when the tonsils are much enlarged giving rise to a 'thick' voice and some embarrassment of respiration and deglutition, with perhaps snoring and food faddism, the tonsillitis has been called *chronic hypertrophic (parenchematous) tonsillitis*. But at the other end of the scale severe symptoms of sore throat and dysphagia may well be associated with small fibrotic tonsils, harmless in appearance, so-called *chronic fibroid tonsillitis*. None of these definitions has much significance. The symptom *par excellence* of chronic tonsillitis is sore throat, grading from a mild discomfort to the severe dysphagia of acute tonsillitis, and this may occur in relation to tonsils of varying shape, size and appearance; with combined elements of cryptic infection, fibrosis or hypertrophy sometimes occurring in the same case.

Neck tenderness from enlarged regional lymph nodes may be present, and, in children, chronic tonsillitis may be associated with enlargement of mesenteric lymph nodes, the child complaining of recurrent abdominal pain, accompanied perhaps by vomiting. Chronic tonsillitis may occasionally give rise to other distant symptoms, such as headache, muscle and joint pains or dyspepsia. The whole question of secondary effects due to focal infection in the tonsils is considered below under 'Complications'.

There is no definitive appearance of the tonsils on inspection on which to base an unequivocal diagnosis of chronic tonsillitis. As indicated above, the tonsils may be hypertrophic or fibrotic, or there may be debris in the crypts. The latter is a sign of some significance, but size alone is no reliable indication of the health or otherwise of these organs. If chronic infection is present it is usual for the tonsils, and especially the anterior pillars of the fauces, to appear more hyperaemic than the adjacent mucous membrane. The tonsils may also be comparatively tender on finger palpation. One of the most reliable signs of chronic tonsil infection is enlargement of the regional (jugulodigastric) lymph nodes. These become enlarged in association with attacks of acute tonsillitis and do not normally remain palpable once the tonsil has returned to a healthy state. Persistently enlarged regional lymph nodes point, therefore, to a continuance of infection.

The polymorphonuclear white cell count may be raised and the erythrocyte sedimentation rate prolonged.

Diagnosis

Unilateral enlargement is commonly seen in quinsy, but it may, especially in an adult, have other more serious implications, as the first indication of developing malignancy. Lymphosarcoma, in particular, is prone to declare itself as an insidious swelling. Ulceration or membrane formation does not occur in non-specific chronic tonsillitis and will suggest, for example, glandular fever or Vincent's angina. Necrosing lesions of the tonsils may point to granulocytopoenia or leukaemia.

Chronic non-specific tonsillitis is a diagnosis based chiefly on the history of recurrent sore throats or acute tonsillitis. When such a history is accompanied by chronic enlargement of the regional lymph nodes and hyperaemia of the tonsils or anterior pillars of the fauces, and *nothing else* in the upper respiratory tract can be found to account for the symptoms, the diagnosis may be considered well substantiated.

Treatment

At the time of writing there is no medical treatment known that will eradicate chronic tonsillitis. Fibrosis within the tonsil barricades microscopical septic foci against effective concentration of antibiotic. Gargles, mouth-washes and suction of crypts are at best palliative. Acute exacerbations treated with antibiotic fail to sterilize the tonsil for the reason given above. Long-term administration of antibiotic may be helpful in children who for some good reason are not suitable for surgery, but radical enucleation of the tonsils is the only certain cure for chronic tonsillitis and the only certain prophylaxis against recurrent acute tonsillitis. The effectiveness of tonsillectomy in these conditions has been shown in controlled clinical trials (McKee, 1963; Mawson, Adlington and Evans, 1967; Roydhouse, 1969) in which the post-operative attack rate of sore throat has been compared with randomly matched patients whose operation had been postponed. It would hardly seem necessary to substantiate the rationale for operation by these expensive trials, since it is difficult to see how a patient who has had the tonsils properly removed could again suffer from tonsillitis. But the operation has tended at times to fall into disrepute because of bad selection, bad preparation, bad operative techniques and bad post-operative management of some cases (these are considered on pp. 140–156 under 'Tonsillectomy'). The question of operation is best approached from a standpoint of preferential conservancy, modified by knowledge of the undoubted benefit that may be conferred by removal of the tonsils when the indications are favourable.

Indications for tonsillectomy

Chronic infection

(1) Repeated acute tonsillitis, more than three attacks a year.
(2) Repeated sore throats, not necessarily amounting to clinical acute tonsillitis but occurring 4–6 times a year or more.
(3) Chronic enlargement of regional lymph nodes in association with sore throats or acute tonsillitis, the attacks not necessarily being as frequent as in (1) or (2).
(4) Quinsy (*see* p. 135).
(5) Recurrent middle-ear infection in association with sore throats or acute tonsillitis.

(6) Chronic infection with beta-haemolytic streptococci or diphtheria organisms in carriers, not necessarily associated with symptoms.
(7) Secondary effects in other organs. Infected tonsils may occasionally provide a provocative focus from which may be derived inflammatory or allergic reactions in distant organs (*see* 'Complications', *below*). Decision when to remove the tonsils in these cases will depend mainly on whether there is an adequate local basis for a diagnosis of chronic tonsillitis; i.e. history of sore throats, hyperaemia, pus in crypts and enlarged regional glands.
(8) Tuberculous cervical adenitis is adversely affected by superadded chronic infection. Tonsillectomy is generally helpful.

Chronic enlargement
Chronic infection may be associated with gross hypertrophy of the tonsils which, if sufficient to interfere significantly with respiration, swallowing or speaking, may require removal to restore normality of these functions.

Complications

Quinsy (peritonsillar abscess, paratonsillar abscess)

Infection in the tonsil, especially the lacunar type involving the large crypt in the upper pole, may spread through the capsule into the potential space between the tonsil capsule and the tonsil bed. Here pus may quickly form and give rise to a peritonsillar abscess. In 90 per cent of cases the accumulation is antero-superior to the tonsil, so that it lies behind the anterior pillar of the fauces, but pus can also form lateral to the tonsil or posteriorly in relation to the posterior pillar and the lower pole.

While a quinsy rarely if ever arises except as a local complication of tonsil infection it sometimes forms without any preceding symptoms of acute or chronic tonsillitis. As a rule, however, abscess formation is preceded by some indication of active tonsil infection, and is most commonly seen in young adults.

Quinsy (from the older term 'cynanche': Greek *cyon*, dog; *anchein*, throttle) has become less frequent since the use of antibiotics in tonsillitis. But whereas cultures of pus used to grow a mixed bacterial flora of streptococci, staphylococci or pneumococci, the tendency recently is for the appearance of pure growths of *Staphylococcus aureus* (pyogenes) often insensitive to penicillin. Although acute and chronic tonsillitis have their highest incidence in childhood, quinsy is not often seen before the age of 12. Occasionally a latent quinsy is discovered as a symptomless collection of pus during a routine tonsillectomy.

Symptoms and signs
Save in the rare cases of bilateral quinsy, the leading symptom is increasing unilateral pain in the throat developing after a few days of generalized sore throat due to tonsil infection. The pain is severe, maximal behind the angle of the jaw and radiating to the ear; it may be so intense as to prevent the patient swallowing anything at all, including saliva, which accumulates, dribbles out of the mouth, and confers a phlegmy quality upon the speech. Muscle spasm causes trismus and neck fixation

with lateral inclination to the side affected. The patient feels ill, miserable and apprehensive. Dysphagia results in thirst and dehydration, toxaemia, weakness, and, in extreme cases, prostration.

On examination the anxious facies and stiffly held head may be evident. Trismus increases *pari passu* with pus formation so that it may be difficult to look into the mouth. Depression of the dry furred tongue reveals the typical appearance of a manifest quinsy and puts the diagnosis beyond doubt. There is gross, unilateral swelling of the palate and anterior pillar of the fauces. The uvula is displaced across the midline towards the opposite side and the tonsil is displaced downwards and medially, so that the oropharyngeal inlet may be quite occluded. Mucus hangs from the immobile palate which is discoloured an angry dusky red. The cervical lymph nodes on the side affected are large and tender, and the tissues of the neck feel thickened. The pulse rate is increased and temperature raised.

In peritonsillitis, before pus formation, the clinical features are those of severe tonsillitis without trismus and without displacement of the tonsil. Pus formation is associated with increasing oedema of the surrounding soft tissues and in advanced cases the tonsil itself may not be visible.

Treatment

Natural resolution follows spontaneous discharge of pus either through the tonsil or the anterior pillar of the fauces, but such an outcome may take as long as a week or ten days during which time the patient is in extreme pain and some danger. Extension of the infection into the parapharyngeal space can result in thrombosis of the internal jugular vein, or rupture of the vein or one of the carotid arteries with fatal haemorrhage. Prolonged dehydration and toxaemia, if occurring in the elderly, may also prove fatal. Oedema may spread downwards to the supraglottic areas with risk of asphyxia. If the abscess ruptures spontaneously into the mouth during sleep pus may enter the trachea with, again, possible fatal consequences. For these reasons it is necessary to perform a drainage operation as soon as there is reasonable certainty of the presence of pus in the pericapsular space. At the same time, if the patient is seen before pus is thought to have formed, he should be given large doses of penicillin by intramuscular injection in the hope of aborting the abscess. The distinction may be a nice one, but patients generally fall into one of three groups:

(1) Pus is not suspected.
(2) Pus is suspected but the abscess does not look ripe for incision.
(3) The examiner is in little or no doubt that pus is present and should be drained.

For patients in groups (1) and (2), any antibiotics being given by the oral route should be discontinued and benzylpenicillin injection BP 0.6 g (1 mega-unit) should be given intramuscularly every six hours (0.3 g six-hourly in children aged 5–12). Bed rest, analgesics and mouth-washes will be ordered, while the patient will be encouraged to drink as much bland fluid as he will. Progress will be carefully observed. Response to antibiotic will usually be presaged by a gradual fall in temperature. Many patients will then slowly, and some dramatically, improve and become symptom-free. Once response is assured the six-hourly injections may be discontinued and a twice daily injection of procaine penicillin 300 mg (300 000 units) given until the patient has been free of all symptoms and signs for 24 hours. If pus is present in a group (2) patient there may be initial improvement which then ceases. In such a patient abscess tonsillectomy (*see below*) may be considered as a means of treatment.

Incision
When pus is present or believed to be present and accessible for drainage into the pharynx, the safest course to pursue is to make an incision, without general anaesthetic, through the anterior pillar of the fauces. The pain of the quinsy is already intense and pain does not summate so that a sharp stab through the mucosa and muscle is not as brutal as it may seem. The patient sits holding a basin under his chin and his mouth open as far as possible. The most prominent part of the swelling is selected (if this is not obvious a site of selection is chosen half-way between the base of the uvula and the upper third molar tooth) and a pledget of wool moistened with ten per cent cocaine gently applied to the area. While the patient closes his mouth and waits for a few moments the surgeon selects a sharp scalpel (e.g. size 15 Bard–Parker) and leaving 6 mm of the tip only uncovered protects the rest of the blade with adhesive tape. He then takes a tongue depressor, instructs the patient to open his mouth, depresses the tongue and, without more ado, stabs the knife into the chosen site. He then thrusts a pair of sinus forceps through the incision, opens them widely, closes them, withdraws them and tells the patient to spit the pus into the basin. When pus is found the relief is so immediate that any distress occasioned by the operation is soon forgotten.

There is a tendency for quinsy to recur in the same patient. In view of the disagreeable nature of the condition and the risk of possible serious complications it is wise permanently to prevent further attacks by removing the tonsils. An *interval tonsillectomy* is therefore advised and usually performed 6–8 weeks after the resolution of the quinsy.

Abscess tonsillectomy
The tonsil forms the medial wall of a peritonsillar abscess. It has in many cases been separated from its bed by pus except for the mucosal margins and pedicle. It is therefore a reasonable procedure to drain the abscess by removing the tonsil. This has the merit of avoiding the later necessity for an interval tonsillectomy and, being performed under general anaesthesia, of sparing the patient the ordeal of the standard incision.

Logical though this procedure may seem, however, it is not without risk. Criticism has been levelled against it because of a theoretical risk of spread of infection through opening of tissue planes. But the only tissues that need to be incised are the mucosal attachment of the tonsil to the margins of the anterior and posterior pillars of the fauces. The real risk lies elsewhere, in the administration of a general anaesthetic and in the removal of the other tonsil which is nearly always inflamed in these cases. If during the induction of anaesthesia in a semiconscious or unconscious patient the mouth is forced open, as it is likely to be for the purposes of intubation, muscular action may compress the abscess and cause it to burst prematurely into the mouth. There is then a grave risk of the pus being inhaled, giving rise to a lung abscess and a possible fatal outcome. This complication may be avoided by a skilled anaesthetist keeping the patient's head *below* the level of the laryngeal inlet during induction, and an electrical sucker at hand to aspirate pus should the abscess burst. The second tonsil, however, being usually inflamed *may* give rise to excessive haemorrhage during dissection. This is not by any means always the case. But the risk exists and should be recognized.

Abscess tonsillectomy may be of value in selected cases, especially those where pus is suspected, perhaps in relation to the lower pole, where antibiotics have been given with some improvement, and where the chance of finding pus by a standard stab incision does not seem high, that is to say in group (2) cases. But before embarking on this operation, three conditions *must* be fulfilled:

(1) There must be a *reasonable* expectation of finding pus.
(2) The patient must have been on high-dose penicillin by injection for at least 24 hours, and have shown some response (i.e. lowering of temperature).
(3) A skilled anaesthetist must be available, confident in his ability to induce anaesthesia in such a way as to avoid aspiration of pus into the trachea.

Parapharyngeal abscess

This is a rare but serious complication of tonsillitis or quinsy. Pus forms in the deep substance of the neck between the pharyngeal wall (superior constrictor muscle) and the investing layer of the deep cervical fascia, in close proximity to the jugular and carotid blood vessels.

Symptoms and signs
The patient experiences symptoms of pain in the throat and neck, as in quinsy, with marked dysphagia. Toxaemia is more severe and rigors may occur.

On examination there is a diffuse tender swelling of the neck below the angle of the mandible. Inspection of the oropharynx may reveal a quinsy or an apparently localized infection of the tonsil which, however, will be somewhat displaced medially. There is a swinging temperature typical of an abscess, with peaks in the region of 39.4°C (103°F) to 40.5°C (105°F). The patient is obviously ill and in need of hospital treatment.

Treatment
A parapharyngeal abscess is a dangerous condition because, apart from the toxaemia, the inflammatory process may cause thrombosis in the internal jugular vein or necrosis of the wall of the vein or carotid artery with resultant massive fatal haemorrhage. Treatment therefore demands early external drainage of the abscess through an incision in the neck combined with administration of benzylpenicillin by intramuscular injection, 0.6 g (1 mega-unit) four-hourly.

Intratonsillar abscess

This is an uncommon complication of chronic follicular (lacunar) tonsillitis, where communications form between enlarged crypts, and a collection of pus declares its presence by a constant trickle from the surface of the tonsil, sometimes in association with a protruding granulation.

Treatment
The only satisfactory cure for this condition is removal of the tonsils.

Tonsillolith (calculus of the tonsil)

Chronic infection in the tonsil crypts is often accompanied by accumulation of caseous inflammatory debris which may be expressed on swallowing (or with a spatula). On occasion, however, the phosphates or carbonates of calcium and magnesium also become deposited, forming harder chalky concretions. These gradually increase in size and may eventually become quite large, up to 28 g in weight.

The patient generally complains of discomfort in the area, but may seek advice because of having noticed, fortuitously, the appearance of something unusual in the tonsil. The dirty white, hard matter may give rise to suspicion of malignancy but the differential diagnosis is usually resolved by probing.

Treatment
Sometimes the tonsillolith can be hooked out with an instrument and, if other indications are lacking for removal of the tonsils, further calcareous depositions may be discouraged by gargling daily with warm phenol gargle BPC. In cases where the stone has become incarcerated in the substance of the tonsil the only satisfactory treatment is tonsillectomy.

Tonsil cyst

Debris accumulating in the tonsil crypts may become sealed off by fibrous occlusion of the surface openings. This results, in some cases, in the formation of a cyst which presents as a visible white or yellowish swelling on the tonsil. The cysts are often multiple, usually quite small and frequently symptomless. Occasionally a larger cyst may give rise to discomfort due to tension.

Treatment
In the absence of symptoms no treatment is required. Patients with discomfort or who are worried lest they have some serious condition may benefit from incision of the cyst or cysts after topical application of ten per cent cocaine solution to the surface. The contents, expressed with a spatula, are usually sterile on culture.

The cysts have a tendency to recur and, if local incision has failed to relieve the patient of symptoms, the question of tonsillectomy may arise. Since the cysts may be indicative of a low-grade chronic tonsillitis there may be good grounds for advising operation. But in the elderly, in whom the cysts seem more prone to occur, unless the symptoms are marked it is advisable to depend on local incisions, topical applications of iodine paint (Mandl)* and re-assurance.

---

*Mandl's paint: iodi puri 0.4 g; pot. iod. 1.3 g; ol menth pip 0.3 cm³; glycerine 30.0 cm³.

Focal infection

Rheumatic fever and glomerulonephritis. The theory that a septic focus in some part of the body could give rise to disease in a distant part of the body has been substantiated in the past mainly by observing the effects of removing such a suspected focus. As is the tendency in medicine when a new theory seems to offer hope in difficult cases the removal of suspected septic foci, in particular teeth and tonsils, has sometimes been practised in excess of reasonable expectation of benefit and thus fallen into disrepute. But there is evidence that a group A haemolytic streptococcus, which is generally recognized to be the agent of rheumatic fever, causes permanent structural damage to the heart because the streptococcus has certain antigens in common with glyco-proteins from the heart valve. Also, an extract of the cell wall of a nephrotoxic strain of group A streptococcus has been found which shares an antigenic factor in com-mon with human kidney. Antibody–antigen reactions which destroy the glomerular basement membrane are believed to be the probable cause of glomerulonephritis.

That the tonsil can be a source of group A haemolytic streptococcus is certain, and that the two systemic diseases, rheumatic fever and acute glomerulonephritis can result from 'allergic' reactions to the streptococcus from the tonsil seems beyond doubt. If eradication of foci of infection was much overdone in the past there is now some danger that it is being too much neglected.

Tonsillectomy does not help established cases of rheumatic fever or nephritis, but is indicated under antibiotic cover in persistent streptococcal infection of the tonsils of children who have had rheumatic fever, or when attacks of acute nephritis occur with recurrent tonsillitis.

Eye conditions. Episcleritis, recurrent conjunctivitis and choroiditis have been shown to improve after the removal of infected tonsils. Iritis and retrobulbar neuritis have not been favourably influenced.

Skin conditions. Exacerbations of psoriasis occurring in relation to attacks of tonsillitis will almost certainly respond to tonsillectomy. Other conditions which may have a relation to focal sepsis are erythema multiforme, chronic urticaria and purpura.

Other conditions. Apart from rheumatic fever some chronic rheumatic conditions may come under consideration as stemming from a septic focus. But the classification is still very imperfect. Infective arthritis and fibrositis may well benefit from removal of infected tonsils. Rheumatoid arthritis, on the other hand, will not, as irreversible changes have taken place in the joints.

In all cases of suspected focal infection decision to remove the tonsils must be based on an adequate probability of chronic tonsillitis. Unless there have been local symptoms, or there are some signs of chronic infection, or a pathogen such as a haemolytic streptococcus has been cultured from the throat, it is unlikely that operation will prove helpful. Decision should furthermore be jointly taken by surgeon and physician concerned after full discussion of the merits of each case.

The operation of tonsillectomy

In children between the ages of four and eight adenoidectomy is often combined with tonsillectomy, when hypertrophy and chronic infection of these organs tend to coexist. Rather less than 200 000 operations on the tonsils and adenoids, combined or separate, including all ages, are performed in the United Kingdom annually. This is an unnecessarily large number in the opinion of some, and the operation is still currently undergoing criticism as being performed too often without adequate indication and as subjecting too many children to unnecessary risk and suffering.

The figures which the Office of Population Censuses and Surveys have issued as representing the deaths associated with tonsillectomy and/or adenoidectomy are:

1959	20	1964	3	1969	5
1960	16	1965	11	1970	1
1961	12	1966	7	1971	6
1962	21	1967	6	1972	8
1963	13	1968	7	1973	5

The operation figures show, in the comparison of the three five-year periods, that there was a reduction in the annual average number of deaths from a little more than 16 to 5.

In 1968 there were three deaths attributable to disease of the tonsils and adenoids in which no operation had been performed. Two were certified by coroners and the other was certified after a *post-mortem* examination. Of these three deaths one was due to a generalized septicaemia following acute tonsillitis and the other two were due to respiratory obstruction in young children associated with gross hypertrophy of the tonsils and adenoids exacerbated by an acute infection.

It is thus apparent that possession of the tonsils and adenoids is not without risk, and that considerable progress has been made in recent years through improved management in reducing the risk of operation to extremely small proportions.

As to suffering, if an adult is questioned after operation (adults complain more of post-operative pain than children) and asked to compare the soreness of the throat with an attack of acute tonsillitis the answer nearly always is 'about the same'. Certainly the post-operative pain of tonsillectomy does not compare with that of quinsy, and can be rendered quite tolerable with analgesics. It is therefore fair to say that the suffering from operation in terms of physical pain or discomfort is not more than the pain that will be suffered from the next and subsequent attacks of tonsillitis which the operation is calculated to prevent.

Psychological suffering is another matter. Young children especially will feel anxious and insecure if removed from their parents and placed in a hospital without explanation. To those under the age of four it is difficult to give such an explanation. For this reason it is advisable to try to postpone operation until this age, or to arrange for the mother to be admitted to hospital with the child. Skilful anaesthesia with adequate pre-medication is also necessary to ensure that this, often first, experience of surgery does not lay foundations for future fears.

Frequency of operation, in itself, does not merit criticism as long as benefit results. That benefit does result has been shown in the controlled studies already mentioned (p. 134). But the responsibility incurred in operating upon a child is very great. Otolaryngological surgeons with a proper sense of responsibility will not operate unless they are convinced the child's health requires it, and are satisfied that all facilities, such as operating theatre and nursing care, are entirely adequate.

Selection of cases

Having satisfied himself that tonsillectomy is indicated for one or more of the reasons given on p. 134 it then becomes incumbent upon the surgeon to determine whether any contra-indication exists to the performing of this operation. The tonsils should not be removed if the patient is likely to be exposed to greater risk than the really extremely small one normally inseparable from this form of surgery, when carried out by a competent surgeon with the help of a competent anaesthetist in a proper operating theatre on a fit patient with skilled nursing assistance. This is not to say that having recognized a special risk the patient may not come to deferred operation once the necessary steps have been taken to provide against it. Even patients suffering from haemophilia, if there are exceptional reasons for removing the tonsils, may be safely operated upon with the right safeguards (*see below*), but the additional risks *must* be eliminated and these fall into three main categories:

(1) Additional risk from haemorrhage.
(2) Additional risk from anaesthetic.
(3) Additional risk from infection.

Haemorrhage

The average blood volume is about five litres. A close approximation may be calculated from the ratio of 70 ml/kg of body weight. Up to one litre may be lost without serious risk but if more is lost transfusion replacement is required. It is rare for an adult to lose much blood during tonsillectomy as vessels can at once be clamped and tied. The real risk comes in the immediate post-operative period from reactionary haemorrhage when a lot of blood may be lost in a relatively short time.

In a small child, whose total blood volume is proportionally less, rapid blood loss becomes more serious much sooner. His compensatory mechanism is liable to sudden failure and his heart is more susceptible to arrest from anoxia. At King's College Hospital, children are not accepted for routine operation unless they have attained a body weight of 15 kg. It is considered advisable always to transfuse if the blood loss reaches ten per cent of the total volume. The loss of 100 ml is not too exceptional at operation and this represents ten per cent of blood volume in a 15 kg child. It is essential in low-weight children to ensure that operating facilities include availability of cross-matched blood, cannulation of a vein *before* blood loss and compensatory peripheral vasoconstriction make it difficult, and proper provision for resuscitation. If the natural mechanisms of haemostasis or the oxygen-carrying power of the blood are already impaired then the stage is set for disaster. The surgeon must be certain, therefore, that the patient is not suffering from a constitutional haemostatic defect or from anaemia. This necessitates a careful enquiry to exclude bleeding tendencies in patient *and* family, and to discover possible causes of anaemia such as recent blood loss (e.g. epistaxis, menorrhagia) or debilitating or inherited illness. Where these enquiries encounter the slightest suspicion of such tendencies or causes, appropriate blood investigations must be carried out. (Hb, platelets , clotting)

Constitutional haemostatic defects

These fall into two main groups, capillary contraction defects and coagulation defects. If capillary contraction is defective there will be immediate and continuous oozing from the small vessels of the tonsil bed which can be controlled by pressure, provided it is maintained long enough for the clotting mechanism to operate to seal the vessels. On the other hand if there is a coagulation defect, bleeding will occur 2–4 hours after operation when capillary contraction has relaxed, and no amount of pressure will control it. Absence of clot means further bleeding as soon as pressure is again relaxed, while the pressure itself will cause bruising of the tissues and extend the field of bleeding. The management of bleeding which is due to a coagulation defect depends on tracing the missing factor and replacing it, not only at the time of operation but also throughout the period of healing.

If careful enquiry has raised the slightest doubt in the surgeon's mind about the possible existence of a haemostatic defect the following laboratory *screening tests* should be performed:

(1) Bleeding time (Duke's method)   normal: less than 5 minutes.
(2) Platelet count   normal: 200 000–500 000/mm^3.
(3) One-stage prothrombin time   normal: 12–14 seconds (Quick's method).
(4) Partial thromboplastin time   normal: 30–40 seconds.

(The exact figures for normal may vary from laboratory to laboratory.)

If these tests are normal the patient may be considered not to be suffering from a constitutional haemostatic defect. But if the patient fails to pass one of these tests, or if doubt still exists because of a positive personal or family history of bleeding, further laboratory blood tests should be carried out in consultation with a haematologist.

Of patients with coagulation defects 88 per cent are deficient in Factor VIII which is antihaemophilic globulin (AHG) In eight per cent the deficiency is of Factor IX (Christmas disease); the remaining four per cent include all other very rare deficiencies. Von Willebrand's disease is due to a double haemostatic defect with poor capillary contraction *and* a deficiency of Factor VIII. Operation in all these patients is a major undertaking depending entirely for success upon close cooperation between surgeon, haematologist, anaesthetist and physician. The investigation and supervision of the replacement materials and the surgery demand the exceptional facilities of an experienced unit.

Anaemias

Iron deficiency anaemias are not uncommon among children and it is essential to insist on a pre-operative haemoglobin estimation in every case. Allowance must be made for the possibility of haemorrhage, and to start operation with a depleted haemoglobin is an additional, avoidable risk to the patient. Every effort should be made to raise the haemoglobin level to upwards of 11.5 g/100 ml before operation. If anaemia does not respond to simple iron therapy further investigations should be carried out to find the reason.

The sickle trait has a normal haemoglobin and apart from an occasional target cell the peripheral blood film is normal. It can only be detected by a combination of the sickling test and haemoglobin electrophoresis. These patients only suffer from the presence of the abnormal haemoglobin under conditions of low oxygen tension such as may occur in anaesthesia. Therefore steps should be taken to detect such cases before operation. The giving of bicarbonate before and after operation aims to prevent the development of acidosis which tends to increase the risk of intravascular sickling. Special care must be taken during anaesthesia to avoid low oxygen tension at any time.

Hb–S sickle-cell disease presents a more difficult and dangerous problem of operation. Cases with this disease are always anaemic with a haemoglobin level of only 6–8 g/ 100 ml. If it is essential to operate very careful preparation is required. Apart from giving bicarbonate, a transfusion will be necessary. There are two ways of doing this: by repeated small transfusions to raise the haemoglobin level slowly and depress the patient's bone marrow, thereby reducing the proportion of cells capable of sickling in the circulation, or by carrying out some form of exchange transfusion.

HbS–C disease and rarer combinations involving an HbS gene occupy an intermediate position. They usually have some degree of anaemia and may or may not require transfusion.

The sickle trait and sickling diseases occur almost exclusively in patients of African Negro descent. As the sickle-cell trait may appear normal without complete laboratory investigation, any patient of such descent who requires an emergency operation must be assumed to carry the S gene unless already excluded.

Anaesthesia

The anaesthetist should be regarded as the physician to the surgical team. All patients prior to operation should, wherever possible, be examined by the anaesthetist. If this is not practicable, the examination should be delegated to a responsible qualified medical practitioner. The object of such an examination will be to exclude any condition affecting the patient that might, by increasing the risk, contra-indicate the administration of an anaesthetic. Common conditions falling within this category include: (a) cardiac; (b) respiratory; (c) haematological (some already considered above); (d) laryngeal; (e) metabolic.

Infection

(1) A patient with an acute upper respiratory infection is at double risk from operation. First, administration of anaesthetic is accompanied by additional risk of spreading the infection to the lower respiratory tract. Second, there is greater risk of bleeding from acutely inflamed tissues. Thus operation is contra-indicated within at least two weeks of a patient having contracted such an acute upper respiratory infection.

(2) It is also most undesirable for operation to be performed on a patient who has been in contact with one of the infectious diseases of childhood, especially measles. If measles develop in the post-operative period the attack may not only be more severe owing to decreased resistance, but may be a cause of secondary haemorrhage from the tonsil bed.

(3) The bulbar type of poliomyelitis has been observed to occur with relatively

greater frequency in patients who have recently had tonsils removed. It was at one time the practice to cease all such operations during an epidemic of poliomyelitis, and should such an epidemic recur it would be wise to do so again. But some years have passed since the last epidemic occurred in the UK. The question that now commonly arises is in connection with the administration of polio vaccine. In general it is advised that all children should have been immunized before they undergo operation for removal of tonsils (and/or adenoids), and that operation should not be performed within less than six weeks of the last administration of vaccine.

Pregnancy and menstruation

If tonsillectomy must be performed at all in a pregnant patient it should be carried out during the middle trimester, that is between the 13th and 25th weeks. In general it is best to avoid operation as administration of general anaesthesia cannot yet be said to be entirely without risk to the foetus. Menstruation is traditionally thought to be associated with a greater risk of bleeding from the operation site. There is as yet no really convincing evidence that this is true, nor that menstruation need be considered a contra-indication to operation. It may be more convenient and comfortable, however, from the patient's point of view to select the intermenstrual period.

Voice changes

Professional singers may enquire whether removal of the tonsils is likely to alter the voice. Recurrent tonsillitis in itself is associated with a greater risk of laryngitis, while removal of the tonsils, provided the dissection is carried out with meticulous avoidance of damage to the palatal muscles, is not in itself associated with changes in the range and power of the voice. The change that may occur is in quality or timbre and usually this is for the better. Indifferent singers may sometimes seek an excuse for their lack of success and find a recent tonsillectomy a ready one. Intubation anaesthesia carries a recognized risk of vocal cord granuloma and this must be weighed in the anaesthetist's mind against other considerations, such as safety.

Hypernasality may occur in children after removal of adenoids (*see* p. 165).

Preparation of patient

Examination

It is advisable to admit the patient the evening before operation. This allows sufficient time for preliminary examination to be carried out by the anaesthetist or his deputy and for haemoglobin estimates and blood grouping to be performed. It also ensures a good night's rest (with the help of sedatives if necessary) and the opportunity for two preliminary (night and morning) temperature readings. In the event of the examination or the readings being unsatisfactory the surgeon can be informed well in advance, and a decision taken whether operation should be deferred. In the case of a non-lifesaving procedure such as tonsillectomy it is always right to postpone operation if the *slightest* doubt arises as to the patient's fitness.

Apart from a full clinical examination the following check list should be applied and cleared:

(1) No bleeding tendency in patient or family.
(2) No recent (within two weeks) upper respiratory or other infection.
(3) No recent contact with an infectious disease to which the patient is not immune.
(4) Is the patient allergic to any antibiotic?
(5) Has the patient been immunized against anterior poliomyelitis?
(6) Has the patient ever received steroid therapy?

Pre-medication

The purpose of pre-medication is to counteract the rise of metabolic rate associated with fear and apprehension, to help to prevent cardiac inhibition and to suppress the secretory activity of the mucous glands of the upper and lower respiratory tract. Most pre-medications, therefore, are a combination of a sedative drug and a drying agent. Choice and dosage rest with the anaesthetist, who will decide according to the age of the patient the anaesthetic to be administered at operation. To avoid risk of post-anaesthetic inhalation of vomit the patient must have taken nothing by mouth for six hours before the anaesthetic is due to be given.

Induction of general anaesthesia and intubation

This is the province of the anaesthetist, and it is generally agreed that intubation of the trachea is desirable when anaesthetizing a patient for any operation on the head and neck as it gives more certain control of the airway, both with regards to oxygenation and protection against inhalation of blood, mucus, or stomach contents. If the tonsils alone are being removed the tube may conveniently be introduced by the nasal route. But an oral tube may be effectively kept out of the operation field by employing a Doughty fenestrated tongue piece in the conventional Davis gag, and this apparatus is recommended for routine use for the removal of tonsils and adenoids (singly or combined).

From the surgeon's point of view the overriding requirements are an absolutely safe technique; a still, relaxed patient; the minimum of bleeding; and a non-explosive anaesthetic agent.

Local anaesthesia

Local anaesthesia is rarely employed for tonsillectomy in the UK. Patients and surgeons who have had experience of a really good, safe general anaesthetic rarely remain in doubt of its advantage. With local anaesthetic there may be less bleeding at the time of operation but the overall strain on surgeon and patient is much greater. A suitable local anaesthetic is prilocaine hydrochloride o.5 per cent with adrenaline 1 in 250 000. Prior to injection the tonsil areas may be lightly sprayed with a five per cent solution of cocaine hydrochloride (or four per cent lignocaine). The patient lies on the operating table with the head raised. The tongue is depressed and the pillars of

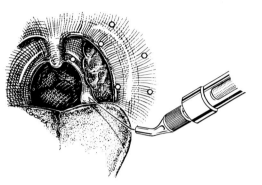

Figure 6.1 Injection sites for local anaesthesia

the fauces and tissues external to the tonsil capsule are infiltrated as shown in *Figure 6.1*, 2 ml into each site. Ten minutes are allowed to elapse before starting the dissection.

Dissection of the tonsils

There are several satisfactory methods employed for removing the tonsils by dissection, each with its own minor variation of technique according to the preference of the individual surgeon. Basically it is necessary:

(1) To divide the mucous membrane where it leaves the margins of the pillars of the fauces to invest the tonsil.
(2) To dissect the areolar tissue off the tonsil capsule by which it is held lightly to the lateral wall of the oropharynx, except near the lower pole where a condensation of fascia, the falciform ligament, attaches it firmly.
(3) To divide the pedicle, or lingual attachment.

In good hands tonsillectomy is a rapid and relatively bloodless procedure that may appear deceptively easy. In the hands of the inexperienced it can be traumatic and bloody, and never should be first attempted except under the tutelage of an expert. It cannot be learned from textbook descriptions. There is no substitute for operating theatre instruction.

The method of removal of the tonsils with the guillotine is not favoured. With it the tonsils can be removed very quickly, but it will not succeed where the tonsils are attached firmly to the lateral oropharyngeal wall by fibrous tissue, as is not infrequently the case where there has been much recurrent tonsillitis. Moreover, since the advantage of speed can only be realized with a light anaesthetic, from which the patient recovers almost at once in order to cough out blood (no ligatures having been applied), there is neither sufficient palatal relaxation nor the time for a careful and unhurried curettage of the adenoids, so often required in children at the same time as the tonsillectomy.

Technique

Stage I – insertion of gag

The patient lies on his back, shoulders slightly raised on a small pillow or sand-bag and the head slightly extended. A Davis gag with Doughty tongue piece of suitable size is inserted, care being taken to avoid damaging the teeth or lips.

When the anaesthetist is satisfied that the anaesthetic tube has not been compressed or displaced and there is full control of the airway, the gag is held open in position by a 'jack' or other device (*Figures 6.2* and *6.3*).

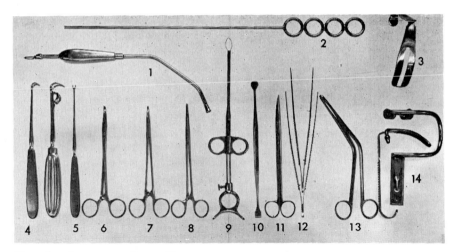

Figure 6.2   Instruments for tonsillectomy

1 Yankauer's tonsil suction tube
2 Draffin suspension apparatus (one of two bipods)
3 Doughty's slotted endotracheal tongue plate
4 St. Clair Thomson adenoid curettes (guarded and unguarded)
5 Negus knot tier and ligature adjuster
6 Negus tonsil artery forceps
7 Birkett's fine tonsil artery forceps (curved)
8 Birkett's fine tonsil artery forceps (straight)
9 Eve's tonsil snare
10 Mollison's semi-sharp enucleator
11 Wilson's tapered and round-ended scissors
12 Waugh's tenaculum dissection forceps
13 Denis Brown's tonsil-holding forceps
14 Davis gag and Boyles's tongue plate

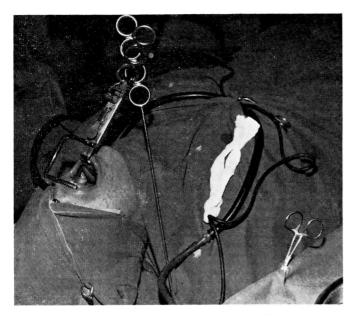

Figure 6.3 Position of Boyle-Davis gag for tonsillectomy under general anaesthesia

Stage II – dissection

(1) The tonsil is grasped firmly with a Denis Browne's tonsil-holding forceps near the upper pole and retracted medially. With the point of a Waugh's tenaculum dissection forceps the mucous membrane is penetrated over the upper pole (*Figure 6.4a*). The closed forceps may then be used to tunnel beneath the membrane, between it and the tonsil capsule, so that a narrow plane of separation is made between the tonsil and margin of each pillar of the fauces as far as the lingual attachment (*Figure 6.4b*). One blade of a pair of Wilson's tapered round-ended scissors is slipped, along each tunnel and the membrane is snipped (*Figure 6.5a*).

(2) Still using the Waugh's forceps, areolar tissue is stripped from the upper pole of the tonsil (*Figure 6.5b*) until it has been freed sufficiently to change the grip of the tonsil-holding forceps so that the upper pole is held between the blades. This grip is then maintained while the fibrous areolar tissue is dissected from the tonsil capsule with Mollison's semi-sharp enucleator (*Figure 6.5c*). Significant bleeding may be encountered at this stage. If profuse, the bleeding point must be picked up with Birkett's fine tonsil artery forceps. If not profuse the blood may be aspirated by an assistant using a Yankauer's tonsil suction tube while the dissection continues.

(3) When the tonsil has been freed from its bed it will then be necessary to divide the pedicle or lingual attachment. The wire loop of an Eve's tonsil snare is slipped over the tonsil (*Figure 6.5d*) and then closed firmly and divided by the crushing action of the snare, and the tonsil is removed (*Figure 6.6*).

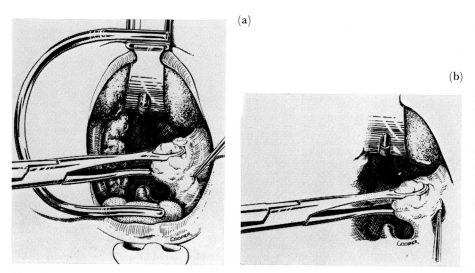

Figure 6.4 Tonsillectomy. (a) First penetration of the mucosa of the anterior pillar; (b) defining the plane of dissection

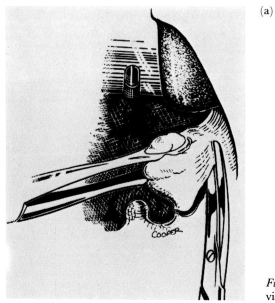

Figure 6.5 Tonsillectomy. (a) Division of mucosal attachments;

(b)

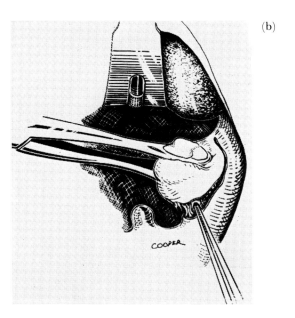

(c)

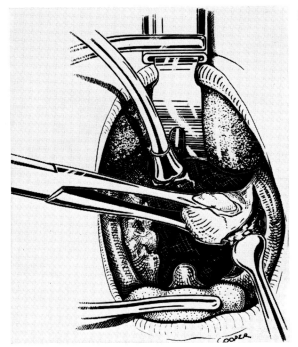

Figure 6.5 (contd) Tonsillectomy. (b) Releasing the upper
pole; (c) blunt dissection frees
the body of the tonsil towards
the lower pole

(d)

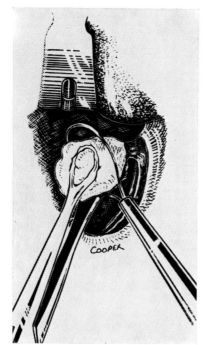

Figure 6.5 (contd) Tonsillectomy. (d) Application of Eve's snare

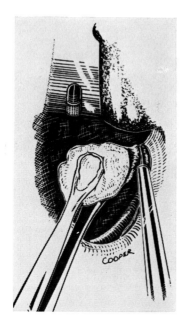

Figure 6.6 Tonsillectomy. Severance of lower pole by closure of snare

Stage III – arrest of haemorrhage

While the second tonsil is being dissected the first fossa is packed with gauze. Unless there is much bleeding from a large vessel this will generally prove sufficient to control bleeding by compression. At the conclusion of the second dissection the first pack is removed and the tonsil bed meticulously examined for bleeding points, using the other, specially designed end, of the Mollison enucleator to retract the anterior pillar of the fauces. Any bleeding point that has not ceased bleeding after ten minutes of packing must be controlled by other means. Small vessels may be coagulated with diathermy, but large vessels, such as the paratonsillar vein, should always be tied. The point is grasped with a Birkett's forceps and lifted slightly to allow the curved blades of a pair of Negus' or Wilson's tonsil artery forceps to be passed between the end of the Birkett's forceps and the tonsil bed and closed on the vessel. Birkett's forceps are then removed and a thread is passed around the tip of the curved forceps and tied, using a Negus knot tier and ligature adjuster (*Figure 6.7*).

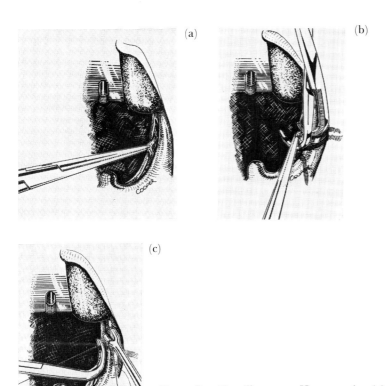

Figure 6.7 Tonsillectomy. Haemostasis: (a) bleeding point taken; (b) application of curved forceps across the tissue to be ligated; (c) ligature of bleeding point with use of Negus ligature adjuster

Stage IV – removal of gag and anaesthetic tube

When the surgeon is satisfied that each tonsil bed is completely dry the nasopharynx will be emptied of blood (which will have accumulated during the operation due to the deliberate positioning of the patient's head to drain blood away from the larynx). This may best be achieved by passing a soft catheter attached to the suction apparatus down one nostril. The gag and tongue piece are then carefully removed and an airway inserted. The patient's mandible, which may have become dislocated by over-opening of the gag, is tested for normal mobility. The anaesthetic tube may then be removed, and the patient turned onto one side, to remain in such a position on table, trolley or bed until return to consciousness.

Post-operative care of the patient

Protection of airway

Retain patient in operating theatre area until conscious.

(1) Until patient has recovered sufficiently to cough spontaneously and protect his own airway, the laryngeal inlet must be kept clear of blood or vomit.
   (a) Turn patient on side immediately after operation without a pillow so that larynx is higher than operation site.
   (b) Insert artificial airway in mouth.
   (c) Hold mandible forwards, closed on airway to keep base of tongue clear of posterior pharyngeal wall.
   (d) Have electrical suction apparatus near patient with catheter that will pass down the artificial airway, together with a Yankauer's suction tube.
(2) Relief of laryngeal spasm. If patient goes into spasm and cyanosis develops:
   (a) Make sure artificial airway is in correct position with mandible held forwards and closed. If this fails:
   (b) Apply oxygen mask and attempt manual inflation with bag. If this fails:
   (c) Insert laryngoscope. Aspirate clot, mucus, or other matter from larynx (usual cause of spasm). If spasm continues inject suxamethonium (10 mg/6.5 kg [1 stone]) intubate and artificially respire with oxygen.

Control of reactionary haemorrhage

Recurrence of bleeding soon after the return of the patient from the operating theatre, although relatively uncommon, may constitute a grave danger if unrecognized. Blood may be swallowed and not dribble, as a warning, from nose or mouth. The utmost skilled nursing vigilance is necessary, with:

(1) Quarter-hourly pulse recording for first two hours. Half-hourly pulse recording for next four hours. Hourly pulse recording for subsequent six hours, and four-hourly pulse recording for following 12 hours. Thereafter the pulse should be taken six-hourly.
   A pulse that remains high or is rising should be regarded as a sign of bleeding until proved otherwise by inspection of pharynx.
(2) Close watch for swallowing movements. A semiconscious patient may betray the presence of bleeding by repeated swallowing movements.
(3) Listen for 'rattle' in the breathing. Air passing in and out through blood in the pharynx cannot have the desirable quiet dry quality.

If bleeding is suspected, the tonsil beds must be properly inspected. A headlight and tongue depressor must always be readily available, together with Luc's forceps (for removing clot) and Birkett's artery forceps. If suspected bleeding is obscured by a blood clot the latter is removed with the Luc's forceps. This alone may allow the tissues to retract and the bleeding to stop spontaneously. If the bleeding continues it may be sufficient to apply pressure with a small gauze roll held in the Birkett's forceps. If the bleeding still continues it is possible for a skilled surgeon to pick up the bleeding point with the Birkett's forceps and ligature the vessel (as described previously under 'Technique'). The tonsil bed is relatively insensitive for a few hours after operation and these measures can be carried out in a cooperative patient without undue discomfort. A slight ooze may not merit such action and may stop if the patient is given ice to suck as a sedative.

If all measures taken to arrest the bleeding prove unavailing it will be necessary to return the patient to the operating theatre and tie off the bleeding point under general anaesthetic. The administration of a second anaesthetic, necessary in these circumstances, demands the service of a skilled and experienced anaesthetist. In the rare event of inability to identify a bleeding point or control the bleeding with ligatures a roll of gauze may be held in the fossa by stitching the pillars of the fauces over it. The stitches and the gauze will need to be removed in 24 hours.

Arranging the return of the patient to the theatre may take time. It should be as short as possible as continuing blood loss is a mounting hazard to life. The patient should, while awaiting removal, be cross-matched for transfusion and a request made for the correct blood. If rising pulse rate indicates failing compensatory mechanism to lowered blood volume an intravenous drip of dextran BP should be set up. If needed, blood can then be readily substituted.

Control of secondary haemorrhage

Secondary haemorrhage generally occurs between the fifth and tenth post-operative day, either associated with separation of ligatures or infection of the tonsil bed with softening of clot, or both. Such bleeding is seldom severe and usually stops if the patient is given ice to suck, a sedative, and injections of penicillin. In very rare cases it may be necessary to tie a bleeding point as in reactionary haemorrhage.

General care

A soft diet, with plenty of fluids, is administered for the first few post-operative days. Pain is controlled by analgesics. A warm phenol gargle BPC every 4–6 hours is soothing and cleansing to the healing areas. Children must not be allowed to become overtired but will often be ready to be got up and dressed on the second post-operative day. Adults require longer to recover from the operation and generally require 5–7 days in hospital before going home.

Other complications of tonsillectomy

Unusual haemorrhage

Alarming harmorrhage may occur through accidental injury of aberrant vessels. This is less likely to occur if a careful method of dissection is employed. The internal carotid artery is mainly at risk and special care must be taken if pulsation is visible behind the posterior pillars of the fauces.

Pulmonary complications

Operation on the tonsils and/or adenoids is nearly always accompanied by inhalation of some blood, despite every precaution taken against it but, although the presence of blood in the lungs can give rise to atelectasis, bronchitis, pneumonia or lung abscess, these complications, with the exception of atelectasis, are extremely rare.

Inhalation of blood is most likely to occur in the immediate post-operative period when the patient is recovering from anaesthesia. Symptoms of atelectasis are cough, dyspnoea, raised respiration rate and, if massive, cyanosis. All patients should have their chests examined post-operatively before discharge from hospital. Abnormal physical signs must receive the appropriate investigations and treatment.

Focal infection

Transient bacteraemia occurs after operation in a high percentage of cases. Serious complications including meningitis, brain abscess and cavernous sinus thrombosis have been reported. Exacerbation of existing infections in the heart, kidney and joints may also occur post-operatively (Gibb, 1969). These complications are, considering the number of operations performed annually, very rare. Patients with such existing infection should have the tonsils removed under antibiotic cover. If the temperature rises post-operatively antibiotic should be administered as a precaution, but it is not considered necessary to perform every operation under an antibiotic umbrella.

Surgical trauma

Lack of skill (preventable by proper training) may result in damage to the uvula, soft palate, tongue, teeth or pharyngeal wall. Accidental breakage of a snare wire may occur at any time but it is usually a simple matter to recover the wire. Not so with the breakage of a needle. If a surgeon decides to undersew a bleeding point and the needle breaks it may prove extremely difficult to find the fragment. It is best to avoid this procedure wherever possible.

Chronic lingual tonsillitis

The pathology of chronic lingual tonsillitis resembles that of chronic tonsillitis. Lingual tonsillitis is, however, comparatively rare but more likely to be encountered in patients who have already had the tonsils removed. The lingual tonsils may undergo compensatory enlargement and come to occupy the lower part of the tonsil fossa, giving an illusion of an incomplete tonsillectomy.

Symptoms

The throat feels 'thick' and uncomfortable but the patients seldom complain of dysphagia to the same extent as in tonsillitis. There is a constant desire to clear the throat and the voice may take on a 'plummy' quality. On inspection with a laryngeal mirror the enlargement of the lingual tonsils is easily seen, sometimes unilateral, and the surface may be covered with exudate. Regional cervical lymph nodes may be palpable.

Treatment

Not infrequently the patients' complaints seem out of proportion to the pathological appearances. Owing to the position of the lingual tonsils it is not an easy matter to remove them surgically and such an operation is seldom undertaken. If surgery should be contemplated due to gross hypertrophy it is best confined to attempts at reduction in size by diathermy coagulation or cryosurgery. Most patients respond to medical treatment with gargles, sprays, throat paints or lozenges.

Chronic adenoiditis

Chronic infection of the adenoids is seen most frequently in children between the ages of three and six years. The adenoids at the same time are usually enlarged and, more often than not, the tonsils in these cases are chronically infected, giving rise to an overall clinical picture of chronic upper respiratory infection and obstruction – which has been called the 'T's and A's syndrome'. While it is frequently necessary to consider removal of the tonsils and adenoids at the same operation, either because of infective symptoms or obstructive symptoms, or both, there are nevertheless, distinctive symptoms and signs of chronic adenoiditis which may point to the advisability of adenoidectomy on its own merits. T's and A's has come to appear on operating lists as a convenient shorthand for tonsillo-adenoidectomy. It should not become a symbol of short thinking about the precise indications for surgical treatment of the tonsils and/or the adenoids in every individual case.

Symptoms and signs

The child with chronic infection of the adenoids *may* exhibit one or more of three classical symptoms:

(1) Post-nasal or anterior nasal catarrhal discharge.
(2) Nocturnal cough.
(3) Headache.

The catarrh takes the form of mucopurulent discharge. Parents often describe it as a cold that has never cleared up. The child is always blowing his nose or sniffing. Sometimes, especially in the mornings, overnight accumulation of discharge in the pharynx causes nausea, even vomiting, and the child has a poor appetite for breakfast. Nocturnal cough results from the chronic post-nasal drip. Headache is presumably due to the infected material in the roof of the nasopharynx. It is frontal in type but at the age when chronic adenoiditis occurs the frontal sinuses have not developed and it is always a mistake to attribute frontal headache in young children to frontal sinusitis. The maxillary sinuses, however, may become chronically infected due to the dam-back effect of the adenoids on ciliary drainage. Chronic infection of these sinuses often coexists with chronic adenoiditis and, especially where catarrhal symptoms are prominent, an x-ray should be taken in case treatment of the sinuses is required at the same time as, or independently of, the adenoids.

Other symptoms of chronic adenoiditis are recurrent earache, mouth-breathing and snoring. These may result more from enlargement of the adenoids than from infection, but where the earaches develop into acute otitis media infection of the adenoids is a likely cause.

Chronic adenoiditis may also be present without giving rise to anything more than an enhanced susceptibility to colds, as evidenced by the diminution in the number of colds that may follow removal of adenoids in some cases. But susceptibility to colds involves immunological factors as yet not fully determined and frequent colds are not to be regarded, *per se*, as symptomatic of chronic adenoiditis or an indication for adenoidectomy.

On examination of the post-nasal space indirectly with a mirror, the adenoids may be seen to be invested with a lacing of mucopus or mucus. Sometimes there is so much of this catarrhal matter as to obscure the view completely. There may be visible enlargement of glands behind the pharyngeal wall on one or both sides of the midline, and cervical nodes may be palpable. There is generally some obstruction of the nose, and inspection of the tympanic membranes may show retraction due to auditory-tube obstruction.

If a mirror view of the post-nasal space has not been obtained (although it is usually possible in children who will tolerate a tongue spatula) a soft-tissue lateral x-ray of the post-nasal space will give a good radiographic shadow of the adenoid mass, and its size in relation to the space.

Complications

Recurrent acute otitis media

Proximity of the infected adenoids to the auditory-tube openings constitutes a ready pathway of infection to the middle ear. Children are frequently seen with acute otitis media which relapses as soon as antibiotic is discontinued. While this may be due to some otological cause such as retained middle-ear effusion, the adenoids should also come under suspicion. Where there are confirmatory symptoms and signs of adenoid infection, especially with enlargement, adenoidectomy may well be the one measure required to terminate the attacks.

Chronic maxillary sinusitis

This has already received mention above. Where radiographic investigation suggests the possibility of antral infection, the adenoids should receive consideration of treatment *before* the sinus. It is almost impossible to cure chronic antral infection in children whose adenoids are also infected and enlarged until the adenoids have been removed. Removal of adenoids in itself may be curative of the sinus infection. It is usual, however, to take advantage of the anaesthetic required for removal of the adenoids to treat the sinus by a single lavage or by temporary in-dwelling polythene tube for daily lavage post-operatively.

Retention cysts of the adenoids

Chronic infection may result, as in the case of the tonsils, in the formation of retention cysts. These retention cysts occasionally reach quite a large size being usually seen in adults in whom involution of the adenoid tissue itself leaves the cyst more easily visible. Similar cysts described by Tornwaldt may form in the pharyngeal bursa (pouch of Luschka) and secrete sticky mucus but distinction is difficult on clinical examination. Cysts of the adenoids or Luschka's pouch may be treated by uncapping and thorough aspiration under general anaesthetic. Simple incision or needle aspiration will almost certainly be followed by recurrence. In the case of the adenoid cyst curettage may be required. If the cysts are symptomless (not associated with post-nasal catarrh) they may be left untreated.

Mental lethargy

While the adenoids should not be blamed for backwardness when the cause may lie in hereditary, developmental, or environmental factors, there is no doubt that, other things being equal, a child with infected and enlarged adenoids shows reduced mental alertness and less physical energy. This is not surprising in view of the universal adult experience of mental dullness when the nose is blocked, for example, during a cold.

Impaired speech

Nasal obstruction due to adenoids results in rhinolalia clausa or closed-nose voice. While this is likely to cure itself in time, it is unpleasing and productive of bad speech habits.

High arch palate

Constant mouth-breathing may be associated with impaired development of the nasal airways so that the floor of the nose (roof of palate) fails to descend. This in turn results in orthodontic disturbance and the so-called 'adenoid facies'; a pinched nose, open mouth, and narrow maxillary alveolar arch with crowded and protruding teeth.

Treatment

When adenoids are so enlarged as seriously to interfere with nasal respiration and/or middle-ear ventilation and are thought to be chronically infected there is no better treatment than adenoidectomy. While enlargement and chronic infection are more often found to be present at the same time, there are some cases where symptoms suggest chronic infection but inspection or x-ray study does not reveal significant enlargement. In these cases a regimen of medical treatment is advisable before undertaking surgery.

Medical treatment will aim at:

(1) Reducing the adenoid size still further by the use of decongestant nasal drops (ephedrine 0.5 per cent in normal saline is appropriate).
(2) Reducing infection by systemic antibiotics based on laboratory culture of nasal swabs. Swabs often will fail to grow pathogenic organisms, and then a course of broad-spectrum antibiotic must perforce be tried.
(3) Reducing volume of mucus secretion by antihistamine therapy (e.g. chlorpheniramine malleate 2–4 mg twice daily). There is no point in prolonging treatment if no improvement has been obtained after three weeks, but some patients respond and relapse, and for these repeated courses may be helpful. Others may benefit from prolonged daily oral antibiotic therapy if response has been good. But the advisability of prolonged antibiotic therapy, which carries a risk of induced organism-resistance or patient allergy, must be questioned when a probability exists of cure by surgery.

The operation of adenoidectomy

The operation is indicated, as previously discussed,

(1) When the size of the adenoids is interfering with nasal or auditory-tube ventilation, speech or feeding.
(2) When chronic infection is considered to be the cause of repeated upper respiratory infection, repeated otitis media, chronic catarrh, headache, nocturnal cough or lethargy.
(3) Especially when obstructive and infective symptoms coexist.

Removal of adenoids may be required independently of removal of the tonsils, but in practice the indications are more often present for removal of both. Whether the tonsils alone, adenoids alone, or both, are being removed the overall considerations set out under 'The operation of tonsillectomy' (on p. 142 *et seq.*) are of equal relevance. Safety, depending on appreciation of the risks involved, selection of cases, contra-indications, preparation of patient, surgical technique and post-operative care, is the overriding factor of importance. *These pages should be read before the technicalities of the operation of adenoidectomy (below) are studied.*

In order that removal of adenoids may be as complete as possible the anaesthetic should provide a relaxed palate and superior constrictor muscle, and time for adequate exploration and clearance of the retrotubal fossae of Rosenmüller. Oral intubation is desirable with the use of a Doughty split tongue piece and Davis gag. If the tonsils are being removed at the same operation the adenoids are most conveniently removed first. The post-nasal space may then be packed with ribbon gauze while the tonsils are being dissected, and in the majority of cases all bleeding will have ceased from the adenoid bed when the pack is removed at the end of the procedure.

As with the tonsil operation there are several methods of adenoid removal, using different types of curettes which may be equally successful in expert hands. The importance lies in learning one good method well. The method to be described has given satisfactory results over many years.

Technique

Stage I – engagement of curette

(1) The patient lies on his back. The surgeon stands at head of table, which is tilted 20 degrees head-down below the horizontal. The mouth is held open with the Davis gag, with the head and neck in a straight line. Head is slightly flexed to abolish convexity of upper cervical vertebrae (electric-powered suction *must* be available).
(2) The nasopharynx is palpated and adenoids identified together with auditory-tube cushions. With the examining finger, adenoid tissue lying in the fossae of Rosenmüller is displaced towards the midline. This should be no more than a gentle scraping action with the glove-protected finger-nail.
(3) A St. Clair Thomson's adenoid curette of suitable size, fitted with a cage to 'catch' the adenoids as they are scraped off, is passed strictly in the midline behind the soft palate until brought into contact with the posterior edge of the nasal septum.

Stage II – curettage

(1) The curette, in contact with the nasal septum, is pressed against the hard roof of the nasopharynx. This action pushes the adenoids through the fenestration of the curette and engages the cutting edge correctly (*Figure 6.8a*).
(2) The curette is firmly kept in contact with the roof and posterior wall of the pharynx as it is swept downwards to a level just short of the curved lower edge of the soft palate, when it is moved sharply away from the posterior pharyngeal wall to break the adenoid mass free from the mucosa (*Figure 6.8b*). If the last movement is not brisk the mucosa may not be torn through cleanly but stripped off the pharynx in unsightly ribbons. If the actions have been correctly performed

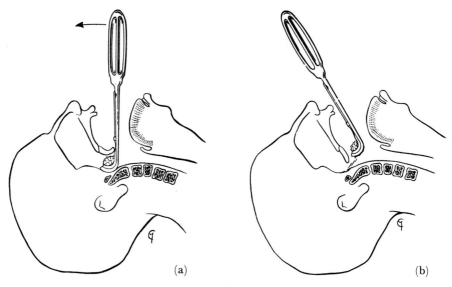

Figure 6.8   Adenoidectomy. (a) Employment of the curette; (b) curettage completed

the curette can be removed easily from the mouth with the main mass of adenoids caught in the cage. If the mass has not been cleanly removed a second stroke of the curette in the midline may succeed. If the mass still remains attached to mucosa it must be grasped in Luc's forceps and the attachment cut with scissors. Care should be taken not to injure the uvula in the process.

Stage III – removal of remnants

The examining finger is again inserted and the area searched for remnants. These will generally be found in the fossae of Rosenmüller or where the nasal septum joins the roof of the nasopharynx. The finger may again be used to scrape these areas clean. It is safer than exploring the lateral recesses with a curette which may either injure the superior constrictor muscle and cause unnecessary bleeding or scarring, or else damage the auditory-tube entrance with the possibility of post-operative disturbance of function. The use of adenoid tag forceps or punch forceps to remove remnants can be the cause of excessive and possibly dangerous bleeding.

After-care

Protection of airways

This is the same as in tonsillectomy (p. 154).

Control of haemorrhage

Primary haemorrhage (during operation)
To control bleeding occurring at the time of operation a length of folded gauze with a tape attached is packed into the nasopharynx and left in position for ten minutes. In many cases this coincides with the time taken for removal of the tonsils and the adenoid bed is dry when the pack is removed (it is always wise to attach a tape to the pack and lead it out of the mouth so that the pack cannot possibly go out of mind during the tonsillectomy).

If removal of the pack is followed by brisk haemorrhage the cause may lie with a remnant preventing proper contracture of vessels. A second curettage and packing often succeed in arresting bleeding. If removal of the pack is repeatedly followed by bleeding a pack may be left in for 12–24 hours (attached to two tapes led one through each nostril and tied in front of the nose to hold it in position, and a third tape led through the mouth and strapped to cheek to facilitate removal when the nasal tapes are untied). If the pack is not held in position by nasal tapes it may subsequently displace downwards, impact on the larynx and cause asphyxia. If left in too long a pack will lead to local sepsis which in turn may provoke further bleeding or give rise to acute otitis media. Any patient in whom it is deemed necessary to leave a pack for over 12 hours should be given antibiotic.

Reactionary haemorrhage (see also *p. 154*)
If bleeding occurs in the post-operative period turn patient on his side, raise the head slightly and attempt to control:

(1) Place ice-cold packs across bridge of nose and on back and sides of neck for reflex vasoconstriction. If the child is very restless and provided that the airway is clear and the patient is conscious, give sedation (i.m. injection pethidine 1 mg/kg body weight).
(2) If bleeding persists an inflatable post-nasal tampon may be inserted (Mawson, 1956). This is a rubber balloon attached to a fine rubber catheter which is introduced through a nostril and inflated with 20 ml of air in the post-nasal space. It is then pulled against the posterior choana and the tension maintained by strapping the catheter to the cheek, a roll of wool or gauze protecting the corner of the nostril from pressure.
(3) If bleeding still persists a post-nasal pack must be inserted. This can sometimes be done in a cooperative child without anaesthetic, but usually it is necessary to return the patient to the theatre and re-anaesthetize. *It must be emphasized that at this stage the child may be in a position of imminent danger.* It is not always easy to decide whether to wait expectantly for bleeding to stop spontaneously, especially if it appears to be diminishing, or whether to re-anaesthetize with the risks that attend re-intubation through a field obscured by blood, and of anoxia in a patient with depleted red cells. But the risks of re-anaesthetizing increase greatly with waiting, and if the child's compensatory mechanism is showing signs of failure with approaching shock there will be need not only for a hurried second anaesthetic and insertion of a post-nasal pack to arrest the haemorrhage, but also for blood transfusion. *The object of treatment will be to prevent the child ever entering this*

dangerous stage and an early decision to re-anaesthetize and repack is *always* safer than delaying.

When the child is anaesthetized intravenous infusion of dextran BP may be set up. This assists in restoration of blood volume and allows rapid substitution with blood transfusion if required. The second anaesthetic demands greater skill than the first and it is essential for it to be given by an experienced anaesthetist. The surgeon will palpate the post-nasal space with a finger. If any tags or remnants are apparent they may be reduced by morcellement with the finger or a midline recurettage may be performed. Curettage of the lateral recesses is more likely to increase bleeding. A post-nasal pack will be inserted and held in position with tapes as described above (*see* 'Primary haemorrhage'). Post-nasal packs should normally be removed not later than 24 hours after insertion. The presence of the pack promotes sepsis which in turn may promote further bleeding tendency or otitis media. Children with packs in should be given systemic penicillin.

Secondary haemorrhage
Infection of the adenoid bed may lead to secondary haemorrhage between the fifth and tenth post-operative days. Such bleeding usually stops with nasal ice packs, sedatives and penicillin injections. It is extremely rare for post-nasal packing to be required.

General care
It is very rare for reactionary bleeding to occur later than 12 hours after operation, and most small children are ready for discharge from hospital the day following. Analgesics are not required and a normal diet may be taken as soon as the child feels like it. Antibiotics are not given routinely, but a rise in temperature may indicate secondary infection when administration will be indicated.

Other complications of adenoidectomy

Unusual haemorrhage

As in the case of tonsillectomy alarming haemorrhage may very rarely occur through accidental injury of aberrant vessels. The internal carotid artery has been encountered in a dangerous looped position in relation to the nasopharynx as a congenital anomaly (McKenzie and Woolf, 1959).

Pulmonary complications (*see* p. 156)

Surgical trauma

A badly performed adenoidectomy may result in:

(1) Damage to the auditory-tube cushions with subsequent scarring. Such scarring may interfere with tubal function with liability to otitis media and deafness.

(2) *Subluxation of atlanto-axial joint.* A traumatic operation followed by infection may lead to decalcification of the vertebrae and laxity of the anterior ligament between the atlas and the axis. Muscle spasm then results in stiff neck and torticollis. The spinal cord is at risk of compression. The deformity must be reduced by traction (after radiographic confirmation of the displacement) and an immobilizing collar worn for at least ten weeks after the adenoid bed is healed (Gibb, 1969).

(3) Damage to the palate. This occurs less rarely than with tonsillectomy.

(4) Cicatricial stenosis of the nasopharyngeal aperture has been reported (Guggenheim, 1963).

Hyper-nasality (rhinolalia aperta)

The gradual involution of the adenoids that occurs in later childhood or early adolescence is not accompanied by hyper-nasality. But the sudden operative removal of a large adenoid mass may result in incompetence of the velopharyngeal isthmus with escape of air from the nose during speech. The adenoids because of their size facilitate nasopharyngeal closure. The palate becomes habituated to moving only a short distance. The tonsils may also push the posterior pillar of the fauces backwards and aid closure. If palatal movement is also subsequently hindered by post-operative scarring a serious problem of hyper-nasality may arise.

Some assessment of speech and palatal function should be made before operation, and parents should be warned that removal of the adenoids may result in hyper-nasality, but also that the effects are usually temporary. The writer has only seen one serious case of hyper-nasality in 27 years of practice. Gibb (1969) considers it probably occurs in a serious form once in every 2000 operations.

Treatment consists of remedial exercises to increase palatal movement under a speech therapist. In serious cases some form of plastic surgery to narrow the isthmus may be required.

The anginas

Angina is an ancient term (Greek *anchein*; Latin *angere*, throttle) used by Hippocrates to signify sore throat. Under it are traditionally grouped some diseases of the tonsils which, while having sore throat in common, differ in aetiology. These are Vincent's angina, monocytic angina, aphthous angina, agranulocytic angina and leukaemic angina.

Vincent's angina

This is a subacute ulcerative, usually unilateral, tonsillitis of insidious onset liable to appear, as in the trenches in the First World War, in overcrowded, insanitary and unhealthy conditions. Vincent's angina as originally described was confined to the tonsils, but in so-called 'trench mouth' the ulcerating lesions more often affect the gums, and oral mucous membrane. The disease is attributed to the symbiotic action of two organisms, *Bacillus fusiformis* and *Spirochaeta denticolata*, always present in the lesions.

Clinical features

Following a short incubation period the patient begins to feel generally unwell with headache and loss of appetite and energy, soon to be aggravated by discomfort in the throat and tender enlargement of the jugulodigastric lymph nodes (frequently unilateral).

On examination the breath is characteristically foetid, glandular enlargement is confirmed, the temperature is slightly raised and the tonsil shows a typical appearance according to the stage of the disease reached when examined.

At first the affected surface is partly covered with an exudate or an easily removable membrane. Soon the membrane thickens into a slough derived from an underlying excavating ulcer, with irregular edges. If the membrane or slough is removed in the early stages it will quickly reform. But after a week or two, the slough tends to separate permanently and the ulcer to heal.

In some cases the ulcerating process may involve the whole tonsil and extend to adjoining tissues, with subsequent scarring and loss of part of fauces or uvula. Although complications are very rare the disease has been known to spread to the larynx and bronchial tree.

Treatment

At the time of writing the standard treatment for Vincent's angina is administration of penicillin (e.g. penicillin V elixir or tablets 250 mg six-hourly) to which the responsible organisms are normally sensitive. Should the patient be debarred from receiving penicillin because of allergy, an alternative antibiotic must be selected on laboratory findings. Mouth-washes or gargles (phenol gargle BPC or sodium perborate 5 g in 250 ml of warm water), isolation and bed rest until the ulcer heals are advisable. Feeding utensils should be sterilized during the disease and toothbrushes discarded after recovery.

Monocytic angina (infectious mononucleosis, glandular fever, anginose glandular fever)

The term 'glandular fever' came into use in 1889, 'infectious mononucleosis' in 1920, 'anginose glandular fever' (from which 'monocytic angina' was coined) in 1934. Today, 'infectious mononucleosis' is widely considered the term of choice to describe the not very common, usually benign, self-limiting disease in which there is a high incidence of sore throat and, sometimes alarming, tonsillitis. Virological investigations show that the herpes-like Epstein–Barr virus is the causative agent but diagnosis still depends on the clinical, haematological and serological characteristics of the condition (Carter and Penman, 1969).

Infectious mononucleosis principally affects young patients between the ages of 15 and 30 years. The method of transmission is still not known for certain, although oral contagion through kissing or sharing of drinks is suspect.

Clinical features

Early symptoms include general malaise, fatigue, feverishness, anorexia, nausea and headache and a curious sudden distaste for cigarettes but the most consistent complaint is the sore throat (angina). Sore throat develops at some stage of the disease in 80–85 per cent of patients and, although in the majority mild, it can be severe, reminiscent of quinsy, with inability even to swallow saliva.

Signs of infectious mononucleosis are, commonly, slight pyrexia (occasionally peaking to 40°C [104°F]), bradycardia, posterior cervical adenopathy, spleno-megaly, pharyngitis and tonsillitis. Less commonly patients develop a palatal enanthem in the form of small petechiae, peri-orbital oedema, and a skin rash resembling rubella. The liver may be damaged and tests of liver function should be carried out.

The appearance of the pharynx varies from a mild hyperaemia and congestion to gross oedema with ulceration and membrane formation. When the tonsils are involved the otolaryngologist is often called in consultation because a diagnosis has been made of acute tonsillitis, and the medical practitioner is disturbed because of failure to respond to antibiotics with alarming persistence of red swollen tonsils covered with patches of dirty grey membrane (*see Plate 2, facing page 112*).

Convalescence is frequently very protracted.

Haematological and serological findings

There is a total lymphocytosis of at least 4500/mm^3 in the peripheral blood with at least 51 per cent lymphocytes in the differential leucocyte count, of which a significant number are atypical.

Serum heterophile antibody (sheep's cell agglutinin) titres rise during the first 2–3 weeks in nearly all adult patients. Demonstration of the presence of these antibodies by the Paul Bunnell–Davidson or ox-cell haemolysis tests is diagnostically specific for infectious mononucleosis.

Treatment

There is no cure for this disease, from which patients generally recover spontaneously albeit sometimes very slowly, taking several weeks. Antibiotics are useful only to prevent or treat secondary infection with bacteria (e.g. beta-haemolytic strepto-coccus), but ampicillin and amoxycillin should be avoided. Treatment is sympto-matic. For the relief of sore throat sodium perborate gargle (5 g in 250 ml of warm water) and lozenges containing chlorhexidine dihydrochloride and benzocaine (hibitane lozenges ICI) are useful.

Complete airway obstruction is extremely rare but can occur and may require temporary tracheostomy. Tonsillectomy may be indicated if the tonsils remain uncomfortable or enlarged after the infection, or if, as not infrequently occurs, the patient subsequently becomes susceptible to recurrent attacks of tonsillitis.

Aphthous angina

This is probably the same condition as the angina ulcerosa benigna of older textbooks. Aphthous ulcers may appear anywhere in the oral cavity or oropharynx. They are common on the anterior pillar of the fauces and occur on the tonsil. The ulcer is usually small, solitary and quite superficial. The aetiology is uncertain but the lesions are self-curing. Healing and relief of pain may be assisted by allowing a beta-methazone lozenge BPC (containing beta-methazone sodium phosphate equivalent to 0.1 mg beta-methazone) to dissolve slowly in the mouth near the lesion four times a day.

Giant aphthous ulcers, usually solitary, also occur on the tonsil or other parts of the oropharyngeal cavity. These are indolent, extremely painful, slow to heal and liable to relapse. Response to local medicaments is poor, but prednisolone 10 mg three times daily on a reducing dosage may be prescribed with good effect in problem cases. Relapse while on prednisolone calls for the addition of oxyphenbutazone 200 mg twice daily for 2–3 weeks.

Agranulocytic angina

In agranulocytosis the total white cell count is low and the polymorphonuclear cells may be reduced to five per cent or less. As a result of this the patients have diminished resistance to infection and frequently suffer from severe ulcerative and necrotic lesions in the mouth, on the pillars of the fauces and on the tonsils. The sore throat or mouth is an incidental symptom in a rapidly prostrating febrile illness of obvious severity that prompts further urgent investigation. The blood count is diagnostic and serves to differentiate from acute leukaemia or monocytic angina with which it may be initially confused. Treatment is the province of a physician.

Leukaemic angina

Ulcerating lesions similar to those seen in agranulocytosis and glandular fever may be seen on the tonsils of patients suffering from acute leukaemia. In the commoner myelogenous type nearly all the circulating white cells are myeloblasts and there is a severe and progressive anaemia usually of a microcytic type. A leukaemic angina may simulate agranulocytic angina with a total white-cell count below 1000. But the high proportion of immature forms on differential count serves to distinguish from the latter.

Keratosis pharyngis

This is a curious disease where the epithelium overlying aggregations of lymphoid tissue in the pharynx undergoes hypertrophy and keratinization with the production of discrete greyish-white horny spicules. These horny growths are found on the lingual tonsils, adenoids and on the lymphoid nodules that frequently become apparent on the posterior pharyngeal wall, as well as on the tonsils.

The tonsil crypts are the most frequent site of origin. In an advanced case the tonsil appears dotted with miniature cow-horns. Where the excrescences are small the condition may be confused with the caseous debris of chronic follicular (lacunar) tonsillitis but the keratotic spicules are more adherent and there is no surrounding inflammation.

The condition was formerly considered to be a mycosis because of the presence of numerous leptothrix filaments among the cornified epithelial cells. But the cause has still to be positively determined.

The excrescences cause little in the way of symptoms. But a patient looking for a source of discomfort or irritation in the throat may be alarmed at the appearance of the tonsils or pharynx. In fact the disease is benign and usually disappears spontaneously in time.

Treatment is symptomatic. There is no known specific cure. Excrescences recur if removed but it may increase comfort to scrape off all excess from the tonsil surfaces and treat with iodine (Mandl's) paint. An improvement in general health achieved by diet, holiday and exercise may have a beneficial influence.

Foreign body in tonsil

Apart from tonsillolith (p. 139) the only foreign bodies found in the tonsil with any degree of frequency are fish bones. Bones, or rather the fine cartilaginous filaments, from a herring or similar fish are especially liable to enter a crypt during swallowing and become impacted. If a patient complains of a bone stuck in the throat after eating such a fish the surgeon should pay particular attention to the tonsil area and inspect meticulously with a good headlight and mirror. It is an easy matter to extract a bone once located.

Elongated styloid process

In some cases ossification in the stylohyoid ligament prolongs the length of the styloid process until it comes into relation with the palatopharyngeus muscle. Occasionally it may penetrate the muscle and the tonsil. Such elongations are not infrequent but are of no importance unless giving rise to symptoms.

If a patient complains consistently of pain in the tonsil area, unilateral or bilateral, on swallowing, referred to the ear, and if the tonsils appear perfectly healthy without enlargement of regional lymph nodes and if nothing can be found on palpation of the neck or inspection of the pharynx to account for the dysphagia, an x-ray should be taken to exclude this condition. If the x-ray confirms the presence of elongated styloid process or processes and if finger pressure on the tonsil in a backward and downward direction reproduces the pain, a diagnosis of styloid neuralgia may be made.

Treatment

The necessity for treatment depends on the severity of pain. The only effective cure is to perform tonsillectomy, locate the tip of the elongated process and amputate a sufficient length to remove it from contact with the pharynx.

Technique

(1) Tonsillectomy.
(2) Finger papation of the posterior half of the posterior wall of the tonsil fossa to locate the tip of the process.
(3) Delivery of the process through the palatopharyngeus muscle by blunt separation of muscle fibres with non-toothed dissection forceps.
(4) Incision of periosteum over tip of process and careful stripping of periosteum from tip towards base of skull. As long as the plane of dissection is subperiosteal there is no risk of damage to adjacent structures.
(5) Amputation of exposed bony tip with bone forceps.

In unilateral cases it is advisable to remove the other tonsil in the interest of oropharyngeal symmetry.

References

Carter, R. L. and Penman, H. G. (1969). *Infectious Mononucleosis*; Blackwell, Oxford

Dudgeon, J. A. (1969). *Proceedings of the Royal Society of Medicine*, **62,** 1

Gibb, A. G. (1969). *Journal of Laryngology*, **83,** 1159

Guggenheim, P. (1963). *Archives of Otolaryngology*, **77,** 13

Morag, A. and Ogra, L. (1975). *Annals of Otology, Rhinology and Laryngology*, Suppl. 19, **84,** ii, 37

Mawson, S. R. (1956). *Lancet*, **1,** 486

Mawson, S. R., Adlington, P. and Evans, M. (1967). *Journal of Laryngology*, **81,** 777

McKee, W. J. (1963). *British Journal of preventative and social Medicine*, **17,** 49

McKenzie, W. and Woolf, C. I. (1959) *Journal of Laryngology*, **73,** 596

Roydhouse, N. (1969). *Lancet*, **2,** 931

7 Tumours of the pharynx
Douglas Ranger

Introduction

The pharynx extends from the posterior choanae to the oesophagus at the lower border of the cricoid cartilage. In accordance with its anterior openings it is conveniently subdivided into three sections – the nasopharynx, the oropharynx and the laryngopharynx (hypopharynx). For oncological purposes the Union Internationale Contre le Cancer (UICC) includes that portion of the tongue behind the line of the circumvallate papillae as part of the oropharynx.

Although Wood-Jones (1940) pointed out that morphologically and functionally the nasopharynx is a posterior extension of the nasal cavities and not truly part of the pharynx, no other name for this region has found general acceptance. However, from the functional point of view it must not be overlooked that 'nasal obstruction' is a common symptom of lesions in the nasopharynx, or 'post-nasal space' as it is sometimes called.

The pharynx contains tissues derived from all germinal layers and almost any type of neoplasm may occur there. In addition non-neoplastic cysts and tumours of developmental origin may be found in the pharynx.

Tumours arising from adjacent structures may present as swellings in the pharynx and particular examples are tumours arising from the deep lobe of the parotid gland and also from nerves such as the vagus and sympathetic. In order to present in the pharynx such tumours must be large, and if they are covered by intact mucosa and there are no other symptoms or signs they are almost certainly benign. However, as is stressed in Chapter 3, benign pleomorphic adenomas of the parotid gland are apt to recur if the capsule is ruptured and therefore it is important that tumours presenting in this way should not be subjected to any biopsy procedure through the pharyngeal mucosa. Such tumours need to be removed through an external approach and any preliminary biopsy through the pharyngeal wall makes the operation more difficult and introduces a risk of recurrence which can easily be avoided by an appreciation of the possibilities before any procedure is undertaken.

Most tumours arising in the pharynx may occur in any part of it but some, such as juvenile angiofibromas, may be found only in the nasopharynx while others may develop much more frequently in one area than another. Treatment of pharyngeal tumours will be determined by the anatomical site of origin as well as by the pathological features and therefore cannot be considered under any general heading. However, in all portions of the pharynx there are important structures lying in close proximity to the walls and unfortunately these are often involved at a relatively early stage in malignant disease.

Tumours of the nasopharynx

Anatomy

The nasopharynx or post-nasal space is a cavity, the roof of which is formed by the basisphenoid and basiocciput which slope downwards and backwards to merge with the posterior wall formed by the arch of the atlas and upper part of the body of the second cervical vertebra. The lateral part of the roof, over the pharyngeal recess, consists of the foramen lacerum and tip of the petrous temporal bone.

Laterally the space is bounded by the superior constrictor muscle and between the upper border of this muscle and the base of the skull (the sinus of Morgagni) pass the eustachian tube and levator palati muscle. Behind the opening of the eustachian tube is a lateral recess known as the pharyngeal recess or fossa of Rosenmüller. Anteriorly the space opens into the posterior choanae of the nose and inferiorly into the oropharynx. Its mucous membrane lining is of ciliated columnar epithelium above and squamous below. The exact proportion between the two types is very variable.

There is an extensive submucosal plexus of lymph vessels. Rouvière (1932) described lateral and medial retropharyngeal lymph nodes into which this plexus drains. The medial retro-pharyngeal lymph nodes lie on either side of the midline posteriorly but are inconstant and often disappear in adult life. The main lymph node station is the lateral retro-pharyngeal nodes which lie high up in the para-pharyngeal or lateral pharyngeal space near the base of the skull in front of the lateral mass of the atlas (*Figure 7.1*). They are in relation postero-laterally with the internal carotid artery,

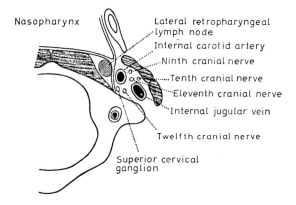

Nasopharynx
Lateral retropharyngeal lymph node
Internal carotid artery
Ninth cranial nerve
Tenth cranial nerve
Eleventh cranial nerve
Internal jugular vein
Twelfth cranial nerve
Superior cervical ganglion

Figure 7.1 Section through the nasopharynx showing its relationship to the para-pharyngeal space and its contents. Note the lateral retro-pharyngeal lymph node. (Adapted from Rouvière, 1932)

jugular vein and the ninth, tenth, twelfth cranial nerves and the superior sympathetic ganglion. The nodes drain into the upper deep cervical nodes which also receive vessels direct from the post-nasal space.

Pathology

Benign neoplasms

Although inflammatory enlargement of the lymphoid tissue of the nasopharynx is extremely common, benign tumours are rare. Cysts of developmental origin may arise from the second branchial cleft laterally or from Rathke's pouch in the midline and these are sometimes found for the first time in adult life. Craniopharyngiomas may also arise from Rathke's pouch.

Hamartomas and dermoids are also occasionally found in the nasopharynx and, although they are not true neoplasms, they are most conveniently included under this heading.

Benign tumours of mesodermal origin, such as lipomas, fibromas, neurofibromas, neurilemmomas, chondromas, and osteomas may occur rarely in the nasopharyngeal region.

Juvenile angiofibromas are possibly not true tumours. They predominantly occur in males in the adolescent period but persist into adult life and, although the sex and age incidence has led to speculation about an hormonal aetiology, biochemical assays have not substantiated this hypothesis; the patients have no consistent abnormality of pubertal development, and treatment with androgens or with oestrogens have not been effective. They arise from the roof or posterior wall of the nasopharynx from which they obtain their primary blood supply but as they extend forwards into the nasal cavities, sinuses and possibly into the pterygopalatine fossa, orbit and even the cranial cavity they acquire new blood vessels which may become more important than the original ones.

Juvenile angiofibromas are generally regarded as arising from the fibrous tissue in the basisphenoid and consist of fibroblasts and collagen in which there are large thin-walled vessels. They do not invade surrounding structures but may produce extensive erosion of bone by pressure.

Projection of a benign pleomorphic adenoma of the deep lobe of the parotid into the pharynx has been mentioned already but the primary neoplasms arising from the mucous glands of the nasopharyngeal mucosa are almost invariably malignant (*see* Chapter 3).

Malignant neoplasms

These are more common than benign tumours and in some parts of the world they account for a high proportion of all malignant neoplasms. They are of particular importance because their presence may not be suspected until they are well advanced, diagnosis may present problems and curative surgical excision is not possible.

Squamous cell carcinoma, in its varying degrees of differentiation, is by far the most common; next come lymphosarcoma and reticulum cell sarcoma. Adenocarcinoma, chondrosarcoma and chordoma are rare. Stout and Kenney (1949) collected from the literature 24 cases of plasmacytoma arising in the nasopharynx but more have been added since. Other malignancies have been reported. Differentiation of these lesions depends upon microscopic examination and so the following description will be based almost entirely on the carcinomas and lymphomas.

A special variety of epithelioma, to which the name 'lympho-epithelioma' has been given, occurs in the nasopharynx and oropharynx where there are collections of subepithelial lymphoid tissue. Clinically it is characterized by its more frequent occurrence in young subjects, its tendency to early and widespread metastasis and its sensitivity to irradiation. Histologically there are masses of lymphocytes interspersed with which are columns and sheets, often syncitial, of epithelial cells with large pale vacuolated nuclei. This growth has caused confusion because some authors have classified it among the sarcomas and hence reports of the relative frequency of carcinoma and sarcoma in the pharynx are often not comparable.

Yeh (1962) extensively reviewed a series of 1000 cases of carcinoma of the post-nasal space seen on the island of Formosa (Taiwan). He concluded that the lympho-epithelioma was not a separate entity but was an anaplastic carcinoma modified in appearance by arising in intimate association with subepithelial lymph tissues. This opinion is being generally endorsed by other pathologists. Its clinical characteristics, however, make it a useful subgroup to retain. The transitional cell carcinoma is another variety of epithelioma.

Aetiology

Squamous cell carcinoma of the nasopharynx has an interesting racial distribution. Sturton, Wen and Sturton (1966) report that it is common in the Cantonese population of the Kwantung province of China, Hong Kong and Macao. In Hong Kong it accounts for 13 per cent of all deaths from cancer as compared with about 0.5 per cent in most other countries. They say that as far as they know this high incidence does not occur in the rest of China. However, it is also prevalent in the Chinese of Singapore and Taiwan (Formosa). California has a large Chinese population, mainly derived from the Kwantung province. According to Buell and Dunn (1965) the incidence of post-nasal carcinoma in the Chinese who have emigrated to California is as high as that in Kwantung, and a male native born Chinaman in California is 40 times more likely than a white Californian to develop this neoplasm. In the first generation of Californian-born Chinamen this ratio drops to 20:1. At first sight this would seem to indicate that environment plays a large part in causing this growth but Buell and Dunn think that a genetic tendency is the more important factor and point out that immigration to California could create a genetic selectivity which would account for the drop in frequency seen in the first-generation Chinese. There may also be a genetic–environmental interaction. Sturton, Wen and Sturton suggest that environment is the more important factor and from statistics compiled from Hong Kong bring some evidence to show that exposure to the smoke of incense burning may play a part.

Other races, such as the Malays and Kenya Africans, also have a high incidence of post-nasal cancer.

Males are more commonly affected than females and the growth is more common after the age of 40. Lympho-epitheliomas, however, arise in younger patients and it is not uncommon to find them in patients under the age of 20.

The role of the Epstein–Barr virus in the aetiology of carcinoma of the nasopharynx is still not clear. Many workers including Henle *et al.* (1970) have demonstrated high antibody titres to the E–B virus in virtually all patients with extensive nasopharyngeal carcinomas and about half of those with localized disease, while the levels have been shown to fall in patients who have been treated and who have no evidence of residual tumour. Immunological similarities exist in patients with Burkett's lymphoma, nasopharyngeal carcinoma and infectious mononucleosis but the precise significance of this in relation to the aetiology of nasopharyngeal neoplasia has still to be determined.

Spread

Spread postero-laterally takes place through the sinus of Morgagni to the para-pharyngeal space (*Figure 7.1*) where lie the great vessels, the last four cranial nerves and the sympathetic chain. Paralysis of the nerves may follow but involvement of the vessels is rare. More direct lateral spread will involve the mandibular nerve as it emerges from the foramen ovale. More commonly, however, the fifth and sixth nerves are involved intracranially by spread of the growth through the foramen lacerum, which forms part of the roof of the fossa of Rosenmüller. This spread accounts for the many cases of intracranial nerve involvement in which there is no radiological evidence of bone destruction.

The carcinomas, but not the malignant lymphomas, may involve bone, and erosion of the tip of the petrous part of the temporal bone and of the basisphenoid and basiocciput occurs (*Figure 7.2a*). The sphenoid sinus may also be invaded and lateral spread will destroy the pterygoid plates and the foramina ovale et spinosum (*Figure 7.2b*).

The eustachian tube is of course very vulnerable to the spread of post-nasal growths.

Invasion of the orbit with proptosis and involvement of the optic nerve is rare and is more suggestive of a growth arising from the posterior ethmoid region.

Downward extension to the oropharynx and forwards into the nasal cavities is seen in very large growths.

Lymphatic spread
It is a characteristic of post-nasal carcinomas that they give rise to early and widespread lymph node metastases and the great majority of cases have palpable nodes when first seen. Bilateral invasion is more frequent than unilateral. These nodes are usually the upper deep cervical nodes but the middle and lower deep cervical and the accessory and supraclavicular nodes are also often enlarged. The submaxillary and sublingual nodes are frequently involved and the high lateral retro-pharyngeal nodes, which may well be the first affected in the majority of cases, are beyond the reach of the examining fingers. More than one group of nodes are commonly enlarged.

Distant spread to the lungs, bones and other viscera eventually occurs.

The spread of adenoid cystic carcinoma through Haversian canal systems and in perineural and perivascular lymphatics may lead to fatal intracranial extension of the tumour without there being any detectable evidence of recurrence of the tumour below the skull base.

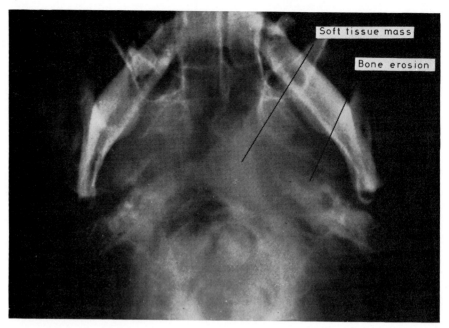

(a)

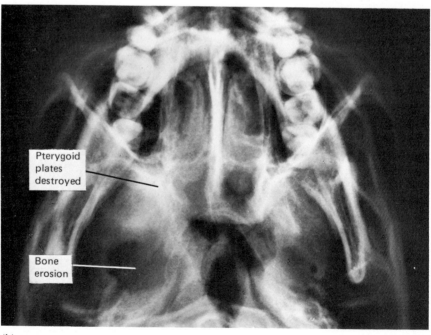

(b)

Figure 7.2 (a) Radiograph of base of skull showing soft-tissue mass and erosion of bone on the left side in a case of carcinoma of the nasopharynx. (b) A similar case, with a large skull-base defect and destruction of pterygoid plates (right side)

Symptoms

The presenting symptoms of malignant tumours may be diverse and will be considered in greater detail later. However, any mass in the nasopharynx, whether it be inflammatory or caused by a benign or malignant tumour tends to produce obstruction to the nasal airway with some associated nasal discharge, and there may also be obstruction of the eustachian tube with conductive deafness and secretory otitis media. Even in the presence of a clear nasal airway a tumour of the nasopharynx may give rise to secretory otitis.

Bleeding from nasopharyngeal tumours is uncommon even when they are malignant but this possibility should be considered in patients who present with epistaxes, especially if most of the blood runs down into the throat in the upright position. Any substantial bleeding in boys or young male adults must immediately raise a suspicion of juvenile angiofibroma, especially if there is a previous history of increasing nasal obstruction.

Malignant tumours of the nasopharynx may present with symptoms caused by their effects on the nasal airway or on the patency of the eustachian tube or because of symptoms produced by invasion of adjacent structures or because of distant spread to lymph nodes or more rarely to other organs, such as the lungs or skeleton. In some patients almost all of these features may be present when the patient is first seen in hospital and they may occur in any combination but for convenience the symptoms may be grouped under the following separate headings:

(1) Nasal.
(2) Otological.
(3) Neurological (including ophthalmological).
(4) Nodal.

The nasal and otological symptoms have already been discussed in the preceding paragraph.

Of the nerves adjacent to the nasopharynx Flatman (1954) has pointed out that the nerve of the pterygoid canal is most at risk but few patients mention any changes in watering of the eye, and any changes in nasal secretions are more commonly attributable to direct local effects. However, tests of lachrymal function may show diminution of secretion at an early stage. The most common symptom of neurological involvement is pain in the face or temporal region attributable to spread to the trigeminal nerve, the maxillary division being the one most likely to be affected. The pain is not necessarily continuous or constant and for this reason diagnoses such as 'atypical facial neuralgia' should not be made without the possibility of a nasopharyngeal tumour being considered. The next most common symptom indicating neurological involvement is diplopia resulting from involvement of the abducens nerve or, less commonly, the oculomotor and trochlear nerves. The last four cranial nerves may also be involved with dysphonia and dysphagia and weakness of the shoulder and, in more advanced disease, the facial and auditory nerves may be invaded and ocular movements and vision may be impaired by extension of the tumour into the orbit. In fact, patients have been seen in whom, with the exception of the olfactory nerve, all the cranial nerves on one side have been affected.

Lymphatic spread of carcinoma of the nasopharynx to cervical lymph nodes is common and may occur even when the primary growth is still small and not giving rise to any other symptoms. The upper deep cervical nodes are the ones most commonly noticed first but high lateral retro-pharyngeal nodes are probably invaded earlier and in lympho-epitheliomas and other undifferentiated tumours virtually all the nodes on both sides of the neck may be involved and the condition might be regarded as a lymphoma unless the possibility of a nasopharyngeal tumour is suspected and sought for.

The detection of any swelling of the neck which is considered to be an enlarged lymph node calls for a detailed examination of the structures which drain into the cervical nodes and, of course, the nasopharynx is a site which requires careful inspection, for carcinoma there may occur at almost any age and there may be no other symptoms or signs even with a large node. No biopsy of an enlarged cervical node should ever be taken until after an adequate examination has been made of all the epithelial surfaces of the head and neck, if necessary under general anaesthesia.

Diagnosis

As in many other sites, the first essential in diagnosis is to suspect the possible presence of a tumour and then to carry out the requisite examinations. As was mentioned previously, some tumours will be suspected readily because of nasal obstruction or bleeding but the same thorough examination of the nasopharynx is required in patients who have pain in the face or head for which there is no obvious cause or who have an enlarged cervical lymph node.

Examination of the nasopharynx has been dealt with in Chapter 1 and in most adults and in some children it will be possible to detect a mass in the post-nasal space without resort to general anaesthesia, by inspection with a nasopharyngeal mirror or nasopharyngoscope passed via the nose or through the mouth with retraction of the soft palate if necessary as described by Buiter (1976). In addition, radiographic examination by plain lateral soft-tissue x-rays, by xeroradiography or by tomography can demonstrate the site and size of tumours. In a few patients the instillation of a contrast solution into the nasopharynx through the nose can give valuable information and the extent of the tumour can be demonstrated most comprehensively by computerized axial tomography.

Once a lesion in the nasopharynx has been detected it is necessary to determine its nature and this is best achieved by biopsy. In some cases the tumour is so large that a biopsy specimen can be obtained readily under local anaesthesia through the nose or below the soft palate, but in a number of instances the procedure is most adequately carried out under general anaesthesia, retracting the palate and taking a biopsy with forceps passed through the nose, guided by a mirror in the pharynx or by a nasopharyngoscope.

It is important to point out that, in a number of instances of patients having neurological signs suggesting nasopharyngeal carcinoma, no abnormality can be detected even on the most careful inspection and palpation, and biopsies taken in the manner described above may reveal no sign of tumour. However, if the palate is divided transversely just in front of the soft palate attachment which is then retracted backwards to expose the nasopharynx, a wedge biopsy down to basisphenoid can be taken and this may well reveal carcinoma on histological examination.

One form of tumour can sometimes be diagnosed with precision even before a biopsy is taken. Sometimes patients are seen on account of nasal obstruction and a large smooth mass is found in the nasopharynx associated with x-ray evidence of extensive destruction of the bones of the base of the skull but without any signs of neurological involvement. A carcinoma would not produce such a picture and in those patients a plasmacytoma should be suspected; this may well be confirmed by biochemical tests including plasma protein analysis. Small localized plasmacytomas do not display these specific diagnostic features, however.

Management

Once the diagnosis has been established the decisions on management will be governed both by the pathological nature of the tumour and by its anatomical extent. While every patient requires individual assessment, in general benign tumours will usually be treated by surgical excision and malignant tumours will generally be treated by radiotherapy or by chemotherapy or by a combination of the two regimens. Although a number of patients with carcinoma will require a radical neck dissection.

Trans-palatal operations for simple benign tumours

Some benign cysts and a few pedunculated tumours can be removed satisfactorily by an operation through the mouth after retracting the palate, but in most patients a trans-palatal approach will be required. This is best carried out under general anaesthesia using an armoured oral endotracheal tube and with the mouth kept open by a suitable gag, such as a modified Doyen gag or a Boyle–Davis gag fitted either with a standard or a Doughty split blade. A pharyngeal pack should be inserted and this can be used conveniently to prevent any pressure of the tip of the tongue blade on the posterior pharyngeal wall where it could otherwise produce pressure ulceration. Tracheostomy will be required only in exceptional circumstances. While the operation can be carried out in the tonsil position with the surgeon sitting at the head of the table it is usually much more convenient to operate with the patient in a semi-sitting-up position and with the surgeon standing by the side of the patient. There also tends to be less bleeding in this position.

Before starting the operation it is helpful to infiltrate the mucosa of the floor of the nose with 1:200 000 adrenaline solution to reduce the amount of bleeding and also to facilitate removal of the palatal bone while leaving the nasal mucosa intact so that it can subsequently be divided at the most advantageous site. The mucosa of the palate is then infiltrated over the posterior portion of the hard palate and adjacent portion of the soft palate, and further forwards if a more extensive operation is planned. The injecting needle will also serve to locate the posterior edge of the hard palate with precision.

If access is required only to the nasopharynx itself then a gently curved incision extending at the midline 2 cm in front of the posterior edge of the hard palate will provide adequate exposure. If there is the need to gain access to the nose also for tumours which have extended forwards into the nasal cavities a much more curved incision can be used, even almost to the line of the gums. Alternatively a midline incision can be made forwards from the centre of the curved incision so that two triangular flaps can then be raised, one on each side. If a single curved incision is employed the mucosa of the anterior flap should be elevated from the palate for about 5–10 mm before any bone is removed in order to make it easier to insert sutures subsequently. This is a simple procedure at that stage but if it is not done and bone is resected right up to the line of the incision then subsequent elevation of the flap is more difficult and time-consuming.

The posterior flap is then stripped off the hard palate to its posterior edge and the dissection carried around the free edge on to the upper surface with a right-angled dissector. The nasal mucosa can then be separated from the upper surface of the palate and opened at a convenient point determined by the site and size of the tumour. If it is necessary to remove some of the bone of the hard palate this is best accomplished with right-angled punch forceps such as Hajek's sphenoidal punch forceps. The blades are inserted just to one side of the midline and the bone removed as far forward as required in a series of small bites and then the opening can be extended laterally as necessary. If a bilateral anterior extension is required the process is repeated on the opposite side, a transverse bite made with forward-cutting forceps at the anterior end and then the septum is readily broken across just by moving the mass slightly laterally. The edge of the septum is then trimmed with forward-cutting forceps.

After exposure the attachments of the tumour are identified and divided and any bleeding points coagulated with diathermy. The palatal incision is then closed using absorbable sutures through the full thickness of the mucosa and periosteum.

Nasopharyngeal angiofibroma

The management of a patient having a nasopharyngeal angiofibroma must start with an accurate assessment of the extent of the lesion and, particularly, whether there has been extension into any of the sinuses or the pterygomaxillary fossa and orbit or even inside the cranium. This can usually be determined by plain radiography including tomography of either the standard or computerized axial variety, but can also be demonstrated by carotid angiography which is an essential investigation in order to delineate the sources of blood supply of the tumour. Commonly this is mainly from the internal maxillary artery but there are nearly always other significant vessels arising from the middle meningeal artery and from branches of the internal carotid artery and in a proportion of patients these are the largest and most important.

As has been mentioned previously, hormonal treatment has not proved effective in controlling these tumours and, although at one time irradiation was employed extensively, it has not proved to be as effective as was hoped and there are serious disadvantages in exposing young patients to the large doses of irradiation which are required, especially so in a region where there are so many important structures which must inevitably be included in the field. Small doses of irradiation are not effective in reducing the blood supply or size of the tumour and for these reasons surgical excision of the tumour is considered to be the treatment of choice except, perhaps, for some tumours in which there is intracranial or intra-orbital extension.

Before any operation is undertaken, large quantities of blood for transfusion must be available and the blood supply of the tumour must have been delineated precisely by selective bilateral internal and external carotid angiography. This examination should not be performed until a few days before the operation has been arranged so that at the same procedure embolization of the vessels supplying the tumour can be carried out. This is not a therapeutic measure in the sense that it could ever cure the condition but when carried out a few days prior to operation the procedure does greatly reduce the blood loss during surgery and for that reason is a valuable preliminary to excision. Robertson *et al.* (1972) have reported favourably on this development and that is also the writer's experience, but the more vessels which can be embolized the more effective is the method and the procedure should not be restricted just to the internal maxillary supply.

For tumours which are confined to the nasopharynx and nasal cavities a trans-palatal approach on the lines already described will provide adequate access but there must be no hesitation in extending the removal of palatal bone as far forward as necessary and particular care should be taken to avoid damaging the surface of the tumour until an adequate exposure has been obtained. Incision of the nasal mucosa should take place away from the tumour so that it can be reflected without risk of starting troublesome haemorrhage.

When there is extension very far forward into the nasal cavities the trans-palatal approach requires to be supplemented by a lateral rhinotomy and when there is involvement of the sinuses they will need to be opened as well. In many instances extension into the infratemporal fossa can be dealt with satisfactorily by enlarging the trans-palatal incision into the sulcus posterior and lateral to the tuberosity of the maxilla, but when there is considerable lateral spread it may well prove necessary to remove the lateral and posterior walls of the maxillary sinus to gain adequate access.

Cryosurgical procedures have not proved helpful in this condition and they can introduce additional hazards by hampering access to the base of the tumour at a critical stage of the operation. Preliminary ligation of the external carotid artery is not particularly helpful and ligation of an enlarged internal maxillary artery through the posterior maxillary wall introduces an additional risk.

Chordoma

Chordomas invade tissues locally as well as eroding them by pressure and for this reason the cranial nerves tend to be involved in the spread of the disease. The tumours exhibit some degree of radio-sensitivity and the decision whether treatment should be by radiotherapy or surgical excision, or a combination of both, is governed by the extent of the tumour and the general condition of the patient. Any surgical approach is along similar lines to that described above.

Plasmacytoma

Plasmacytomas are radio-sensitive and in general this is the treatment of choice. Small localized tumours may be excised completely in the process of taking a biopsy but larger tumours, and especially those associated with extensive destruction of the base of the skull, can only be treated by irradiation.

Lymphoma

The management of patients with a lymphoma in the nasopharynx has been improved dramatically by the better understanding of the varieties of localized and generalized disease, and by the development of a wide variety of chemotherapeutic drugs. Extensive investigation of the whole patient is essential before any treatment is undertaken and the patient should be referred to one of the Oncological Units specializing in these conditions.

Carcinoma and sarcoma

Sarcoma is uncommon in the nasopharynx and essentially the treatment is almost identical to that of the very much commoner carcinomas, except that some of the tumours may be less radio-sensitive and chemotherapy may be ineffective and has obviously been less well evaluated.

As in other situations, the management of a patient with a carcinoma of the nasopharynx must start with histological evaluation of the type of tumour and by a detailed assessment of the extent of the disease. The latter has been greatly improved by the introduction of computerized axial tomography and in some instances emission tomography.

There is no possibility of effective surgical excision of nasopharyngeal carcinomas except in extremely small localized tumours discovered by chance, and those would be better treated by irradiation in any case. Accordingly, the only uncertainties with regard to treatment concern whether radiotherapy should be combined with chemotherapy in any way, and whether any involved cervical lymph nodes should be treated by radiotherapy or by radical neck dissection.

Opinions vary on the place of chemotherapy but on theoretical grounds at least there are merits in combining it with radiotherapy. There is no place at present for considering it as a substitute for irradiation but it has a place in patients who may have residual or recurrent disease after a full therapeutic course of irradiation. Supervoltage radiotherapy is the treatment of choice. In undifferentiated tumours the irradiation must be given over wide fields including both sides of the neck whether or not there are palpable lymph nodes. In well-differentiated tumours high doses locally may be necessary to eradicate the primary tumour in the nasopharynx and this may limit the amount of irradiation which can be applied over wide areas.

The presence of clinically invaded nodes in the neck will not alter the principles of treatment, which will still be primarily by irradiation, but the details of dosage will be affected. If there are residual nodes some six weeks after the completion of radiotherapy then radical neck dissection is indicated except for anaplastic tumours where chemotherapy would be regarded as a better alternative. If the persistent nodes are present on both sides of the neck it is not possible to carry out simultaneous bilateral radical neck dissection with the sacrifice of both internal jugular veins and it is necessary to defer the operation on one side for three weeks after resection of the more affected side.

Careful follow-up of patients after treatment is required. In some patients a very satisfactory examination of the nasopharynx can be obtained using the methods described previously for diagnosis. However, in a proportion of patients it is not possible by simple means to obtain a view of the nasopharynx which enables the surgeon to be confident that there is no residual or recurrent tumour. As it is important that this should be achieved repeatedly the choice lies between examination under anaesthetic at frequent intervals or else the creation of an artificial opening in the palate which will enable direct inspection of the nasopharynx from the mouth after taking out the obturator which is used to cover the opening and which is little more inconvenient than an ordinary upper denture.

This operation of fenestration of the palate is started in the same way as the transpalatal operation already described, but after sufficient bone has been removed to provide an adequate opening the mucosa of the palate is sutured to the mucosa of the floor of the nose over the bony edges around the opening. A temporary light plate is fitted as a denture at the time of operation to enable the patient to swallow soon afterwards, and a nasogastric tube is not required. A stronger prosthesis with any dentures which are also required can be fitted later when healing has occurred.

As with carcinomas elsewhere the prognosis is greatly influenced by the extent of the disease at the time treatment is instituted. Approximately 30–35 per cent of all patients survive for five years but Smith *et al.* (1963) have reported figures as high as 76 per cent for localized Stage I lesions; but for advanced tumours involving surrounding tissues the chances of five-year survival may be as low as 10 per cent.

Tumours of the oropharynx

Anatomy

The oropharynx extends from the line of the circumvallate papillae, the anterior pillars of the fauces and the free edge of the soft palate downwards to the free border of the epiglottis, and includes the tonsil and vallecula as well as that portion of the tongue lying posterior to the circumvallate papillae. The oropharynx is lined by non-keratinizing squamous epithelium containing seromucinous glands and subepithelial collections of lymphoid tissue of which the faucial and lingual tonsils are especially large masses.

Pathology

Of the benign tumours the commonest is the squamous cell papilloma which is frequently found as a sessile or pedunculated warty mass arising from the edge of the soft palate or tonsil or anywhere on the pharyngeal wall. As in the nasopharynx almost any benign tumour can occur but they are all uncommon. Also, as mentioned previously benign adenomas of the deep lobe of the parotid gland and neurilemmomas or neurofibromas arising from adjacent nerves may indent the wall of the oropharynx and present as symptomless swellings.

The most common malignant neoplasm is the squamous cell carcinoma. It may occur in any degree of differentiation, the more highly differentiated ones appearing as a rule on the soft palate and fauces. Carcinomas of the tonsil and base of the tongue are nearly always anaplastic.

Lympho-epithelioma is uncommon and even more rare are the various types of adenocarcinoma and the malignant pleomorphic tumour. Lymphosarcoma and reticulum cell sarcoma arise in the faucial and lingual tonsils.

Malignant mesodermal tumours are so rare as hardly to deserve more than passing mention.

Aetiology

Squamous cell cancer is uncommon before the age of 50 but increases in frequency thereafter. Men are about five times more commonly affected than women. Keratosis with dysplasia is well recognized as a pre-cancerous condition in the mouth but it seldom occurs in the orophranx except on the palatine arch. As with oral cancer, there is strong evidence that tobacco smoking and chewing are important causal factors: Wynder, Bross and Feldman (1957) incriminate cigars and pipes more than cigarettes. Alcohol usually in the form of spirits may also be a predisposing cause, but nearly all heavy drinkers are heavy smokers and it is difficult therefore to determine its true importance. The mucosal atrophy associated with iron-deficiency anaemia seems often to be the precursor of oropharyngeal cancer in women. Syphilis and dental sepsis are no longer important factors in this country. Another primary growth in the upper alimentary tract or lung is found in about 10 per cent of cases of squamous cell carcinoma of the mouth and oropharynx.

Lymph node involvement

According to MacComb and Fletcher (1967) and Terz and Farr (1967) about 70 per cent of carcinomas of the base of tongue and tonsil present with nodal involvement. The growths arising from the palatine arch are less aggressive and enlarged nodes are present in about 50 per cent of cases when first seen. Bilateral involvement is common from base of tongue and central soft palate lesions.

The jugulodigastric node is the one most frequently involved but deposits may occur in any node of the cervical field. This possibility, together with the fact that the metastasis may skip intervening nodes (Toker, 1963) makes anything less than a complete neck dissection an inadequate method of eradicating the disease. Distant metastases may be more common than has been suspected in the past and an incidence of up to 57 per cent of distant metastases has been reported by Gowen and de Suto-Nagy (1963) in patients dying of head and neck cancer. Arons and Smith (1961) put the incidence lower, at 23 per cent. In most of these cases local disease was still present.

Staging

It is difficult to devise satisfactory staging in the TNM notation for these lesions. Since the size of the primary growth has been shown to correlate well with the prognosis the following scheme has been suggested:

T_1 – Tumours less than 2 cm in diameter.
T_2 – Tumours between 2 and 4 cm in diameter.
T_3 – Tumours more than 4 cm in diameter.
T_4 – Massive tumours.

Symptoms

A growth in the oropharynx may become quite large before attracting attention. The first symptom is usually a disturbance of swallowing variously described as a soreness or pain or a pricking sensation as the food is passing down. Occasionally blood is spat up or the growth may be seen by a dental surgeon or the patient himself. Not uncommonly the appearance of a lump in the neck is the only abnormality noticed by the patient. Pain referred to the ear, via the tympanic branch of the glossopharyngeal nerve. Excessive salivation and foetor are late symptoms.

Examination

Two main clinical types of squamous cell carcinoma may be recognized: the exophytic (*Figure 7.3*) and the ulcerative (*Figure 7.4*). The exophytic type tends to spread superficially and the ulcerative type infiltrates deeply, but exceptions occur. An adenocarcinoma presents as a smooth non-ulcerated swelling and the malignant lymphomas as enlargement in the tonsillar fossae or base of the tongue. Ulceration supervenes eventually.

Provided good lighting is used the growths can be easily seen, though for those originating in the base of the tongue a laryngeal mirror is needed. Note should be made of any fixation of the palate or tongue and palpation with the forefinger will help in estimating the extent of infiltration. A post-nasal mirror should be used to detect extension into the nasopharynx or onto the upper surface of the soft palate.

Sometimes a carcinoma may occur deep in the base of the tongue which may not be associated with any abnormality of the surface mucosa. The presenting symptoms may be pain, possibly of the glossopharyngeal neuralgic type, or a node in the neck. It is important to remember that a carcinoma of the base of the tongue cannot be excluded merely by inspection with a spatula or a laryngeal mirror – it is essential to palpate the tongue as well if growths of this type are not to be missed.

The neck must also be examined carefully for lymph nodes both from in front of the patient and most particularly from behind the patient using the tips of the fingers.

Diagnosis

This is usually not difficult since most chronic ulcerative or proliferative lesions in the oropharynx turn out to be malignant. A biopsy, however, is necessary to confirm the diagnosis and to establish the histology of the growth, since this is of importance in

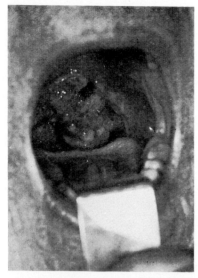

Figure 7.3 Carcinoma of the soft palate and uvula; exophytic type

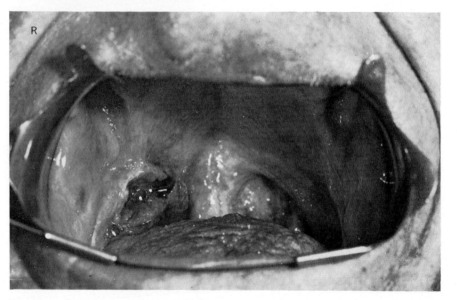

Figure 7.4 Carcinoma of the right tonsil; ulcerative type

planning treatment. In most cases the biopsy can be done under topical analgesia but a general anaesthetic may be needed in base of the tongue lesions. The anaesthetic will also help in determining the extent of the growth by allowing deep palpation in this region. Small smooth non-ulcerated lesions should be dealt with by wide excisional biopsy. In larger lesions of this kind a piece should be taken for section after reflecting healthy mucosa which is then sewn up again. Since these swellings often turn out to belong to one of the radio-insensitive adenocarcinoma groups needing wide surgical excision it is advisable to have this information beforehand, so that the patient can be prepared both mentally and physically for an extensive and possibly mutilating operation.

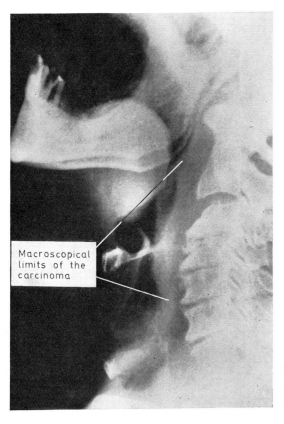

Macroscopical
limits of the
carcinoma

Figure 7.5 A lateral soft-tissue
radiograph helps to show the extent
of a carcinoma of the posterior wall
of the oropharynx

Lateral soft-tissue radiographs or xeroradiographs are often useful for demonstrating the precise location and extent of hypertrophic carcinomas in the oropharynx (*Figure 7.5*).

On the soft palate, keratosis and nicotine stomatitis raise problems as to whether malignant change has supervened. Cytological examination of scrapings from suspected areas may be helpful in these cases. Similarly, if the lesion is cleaned, dried and painted with toluidine blue two per cent aqueous solution and examined after the area has been washed with water, any malignant change will be shown up as a deeply staining area. The writer has not found this a very reliable test but it may occasionally be helpful.

Chest radiographs and blood examinations, including serological tests for syphilis, should be routine and will eliminate tuberculosis, syphilis and the blood dyscrasias from the diagnosis. A double pathology is of course always possible. A gumma before breaking down may resemble an adenocarcinoma or sarcoma and very occasionally an indolent quinsy may look like a lymphosarcoma of the tonsil. In more acute ulcers a throat swab may demonstrate Vincent's organism.

Neurilemmomas of the vagus nerve or sympathetic chain, mixed tumours of the deep portion of the parotid gland and glomus tumours sometimes form a smooth bulge in the lateral pharyngeal wall behind the tonsil pushing it forwards and medially. Secondary deposits in the tonsils have been described from bronchial carcinoma and testicular seminoma. Tonsilloliths may be deceptive and bilateral lymphosarcomas of the tonsils sometimes occur.

If biopsies are consistently non-specific the possibility of Wegener's type granuloma must be considered.

Every attempt must be made to get an immediate diagnosis; it is never justifiable to wait and see.

Management

Simple benign papillomas arising from the soft palate or tonsil can be removed easily, if it is necessary to do anything, under a local anaesthetic. Other benign tumours arising elsewhere in the oropharynx can also be excised readily enough under local or general anaesthesia depending on the site and on the patient's tolerance to stimulation of the pharynx.

It has been stressed already in the section dealing with the nasopharynx, but is repeated here because of its importance, that no attempt should be made to take a biopsy from or to excise through the pharyngeal wall any tumours which are bulging into the pharynx and which may be arising from the deep lobe of the parotid gland.

Lymphomas should be treated in special Oncological Centres as indicated for similar tumours occurring in the nasopharynx.

For carcinomas, once the diagnosis has been confirmed by histological exam-ination, the choice of treatment lies between surgical excision and radiotherapy, with or without chemotherapy in either case. Although some localized tumours might be suitable for limited excision not many lesions fall into this category and when they do they are the tumours which are likely to respond most readily to radiotherapy. With advanced disease neither form of treatment can offer a good prognosis. However, the problems associated with radical surgical excision are such that in most patients it generally seems preferable to regard radiotherapy, possibly combined with chemo-therapy, as the treatment of choice and reserve surgical excision for those patients in whom there is residual or recurrent disease following radiotherapy. One exception to this generality is carcinoma on the lateral wall of the oropharynx which is already invading the mandible in a patient who is otherwise fit. Bone involvement by the carcinoma reduces very considerably the chances of cure by radiotherapy, pain is already likely to be a very troublesome symptom and irradiation of the mandible when it is invaded by tumour is very likely to lead to bone necrosis and sequestration. Accordingly, in such patients primary excision would seem to be the treatment of choice, as being the method which is most likely to effect a cure and which will alleviate the pain and restore good swallowing function as soon as possible without troublesome sequelae.

As has been mentioned already, involvement of lymph nodes is common with carcinoma of the oropharynx and in many patients these will require treatment at the same time as the primary neoplasm. In those patients being treated by radiotherapy who have evidence of invaded nodes these should be irradiated at the same time, and radical neck dissection carried out later if the nodes persist or recur and the primary lesion has been eradicated or is being excised. In patients who are being treated initially by surgery and in whom there is nodal involvement a radical neck dissection should be performed at the same time as the primary resection.

Surgical excision and repair

No attempt will be made to discuss a number of operations which used to be performed for pharyngeal neoplasms in the days before radiotherapy had reached its present stage of development and before the use of skin flaps for repair had been established. If they are ever required under exceptional circumstances for a particular patient with an unusual problem, descriptions of them can be found in a number of older textbooks.

Nowadays there are really only two groups of operations used for radical excision of oropharyngeal carcinomas. The first is for resection of tumours involving the lateral wall and the other for tumours of the base of the tongue.

For lateral tumours in the tonsillar region it will be necessary to remove the ascending ramus of the mandible and also a variable amount of the body forwards from the angle together with the internal pterygoid muscle on the inside and the masseter muscle on the outside. This composite resection is often referred to as a 'Commando operation' and quite extensive growths can be removed in this way with a good margin of tissue externally. As repair will be effected by means of a pedicled skin flap, mucosa can also be removed over a wide area. Parts of the soft palate and side of the tongue can be included in the resection if necessary. Of the various skin flaps which can be employed to repair the pharyngeal defect the simplest and most readily accessible in most patients is the forehead flap. This can be raised immediately at the time of operation and it has a good blood supply from the anterior branch of the superficial temporal artery and, as a result, a broad forehead flap can be based on a narrow pedicle which will enable it to be folded down either deep or superficial to the zygomatic arch. With a good split skin graft applied to the donor area the cosmetic defect is not great. Nape flaps can also be used but are not so satisfactory in that they usually need to be delayed before use. Delto-pectoral flaps (Bakamjian, 1965) can also provide very satisfactory primary cover over a wide area and some surgeons prefer them to the forehead flap even though a subsequent operation is necessary in order to return the unused carrier pedicle to its original site. In a few patients it is necessary to provide skin cover externally and in those patients a deltopectoral flap is well suited for that purpose with a forehead flap being used internally, provided the integrity of the external carotid artery has been maintained.

For tumours of the base of the tongue surgical excision involves laryngectomy as well as glossectomy, for after resection of the base of the tongue alone swallowing is extremely difficult and laryngeal spill-over with consequent pneumonia is a common sequel.

Tumours of the laryngopharynx

Anatomy

The laryngopharynx or hypopharynx extends from the lower limit of the oropharynx down to the opening of the oesophagus at the lower border of the cricoid cartilage. At rest this is usually opposite the sixth cervical vertebra but during swallowing the

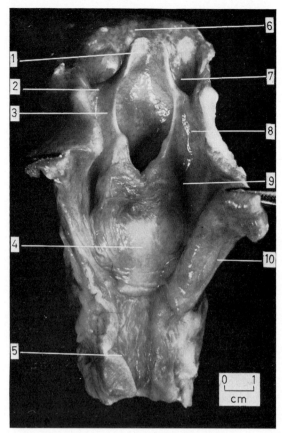

Figure 7.6 The normal pharynx and larynx opened up from behind. The contrast between the shallow upper and deep lower parts of the pyriform fossa is well shown.

1 Epiglottis
2 Pharyngo-epiglottic fold
3 Aryepiglottic fold
4 Post-cricoid region
5 Cervical oesophagus
6 Base of tongue
7 Vallecula
8 Upper pyriform fossa
9 Lower pyriform fossa
10 Postero-lateral pharyngeal wall

whole larynx is drawn upwards so that the cricoid cartilage then comes to lie opposite the fourth or fifth cervical vertebra. This point is relevant to the interpretation of barium-swallow radiographs on which lesions which are opposite the fifth or sixth cervical vertebra are often erroneously described as 'post-cricoid' when in reality they are in the cervical oesophagus 2 or 3 cm below the cricoid cartilage. This is readily demonstrated in films in which the penetration is such that the laryngeal cartilages are delineated.

The larynx projects into the laryngopharynx from the front (*Figure 7.6*) so that grooves are formed on either side of it which are known as the pyriform fossae or the pyriform sinuses or recesses. These are shallow above and are separated from the valleculae by the pharyngo-epiglottic folds. Lower down, the pyriform fossae become deeper and more cleft-like. The upper shallow part of the pyriform fossa is bounded laterally by the thyrohyoid membrane and medially by the aryepiglottic fold. The lower deeper part of the fossa is in relation laterally to the thyroid cartilage and medially to the cricoid cartilage. The post-cricoid portion of the laryngopharynx is, as its name implies, that segment on the anterior wall which lies directly behind the cricoid cartilage and for that reason the mucosa there usually appears slightly paler than elsewhere. The laryngopharynx is completed by its lateral and posterior muscular walls.

Although, anatomically, the laryngopharynx ends at the oesophageal opening at the lower border of the cricoid cartilage there is no change in the mucosa at that level and growths spread readily across the junction. A large proportion of carcinomas in this part of the alimentary canal are pharyngo-oesophageal and there would be merit in tumour classifications incorporating the cervical oesophagus into the 'pharyngo-oesophageal region' in the same way that UICC incorporates the posterior third of the anatomical tongue into the 'oropharynx' for oncological classification. It is certainly much more common for carcinoma to spread from the cervical oesophagus into the laryngopharynx than into the thoracic oesophagus.

Benign tumours

Papillomas and adenomas are very rare indeed; mesodermal neoplasms are a little more common and lipomas, fibromas and leiomyomas are occasionally reported.

These benign tumours grow very slowly and form smooth, well-defined, mobile (sometimes pedunculated) masses. They can seldom be confused with malignant tumours though their true nature can be shown only by microscopic examination. Small ones may be removed by endoscopy but larger ones need excision through the lateral pharyngotomy approach.

Cysts of the anterior surface of the epiglottis are more frequent. They are yellow in appearance and seldom grow large enough to cause symptoms. It is usually sufficient to remove most of the cyst wall endoscopically and recurrence is rare. The lining membrane consists of squamous epithelium.

Malignant neoplasms

Pathology

Malignant growths of the laryngopharynx are nearly all squamous cell carcinomas. Adenocarcinomas, malignant lymphomas, mesodermal tumours and metastatic deposits from elsewhere in the body are very rare and need only be mentioned. Their structure will be shown by the biopsy which should always be taken.

One rare tumour of very low-grade malignancy which occurs in the laryngopharynx is characterized by pain of a neuralgic type which often extends to the ear, mediated via the vagus nerve. The pain may be triggered off by eating or drinking sharp or bitter substances. Most of these very uncommon tumours have occurred in the arytenoid region although some have developed on the epiglottis. Macroscopically they usually appear as small reddish or purplish swellings which may be almost pedunculated. Histologically they appear to be *glomus tumours* and there is nothing in their histological appearance to differentiate them from the very much larger non-painful glomus tumours which are sometimes found in the larynx.

However, clinically these painful glomus tumours form a distinct group. The striking feature is the pain and in small tumours this can be relieved dramatically by biopsy excision. These tumours also tend to metastasize, possibly after several years, to regional lymph nodes and also in a very unusual manner to subcutaneous tissues and subserous layers such as under the peritoneum and pleura. These metastases are also painful and sometimes exquisitely so. They tend to be multiple and one of the writer's patients had 120 metastases removed at one operating session from subcutaneous sites scattered throughout the body. He obtained great relief from the procedure. The tumours are not radio-sensitive and local excision, possibly by partial laryngectomy, appears to be the treatment of choice. On the basis of electron-microscopic and other studies Ranger and Thackray (1979) regard these tumours as chemodectomas of an unusual clinical type. This opinion is shared by Vetter and Toner (1970) although Hyams (1975) regards them as 'oddball' poorly differentiated adenocarcinomas.

The squamous cell carcinomas are most often moderately well differentiated and macroscopically present as either exophytic or ulcerative growths. The exophytic form occurs most commonly in the upper pyriform fossa and aryepiglottic fold regions and the ulcerative in the remaining areas of the laryngopharynx. Atrophic mucosal changes elsewhere in the pharynx and oral cavity may be seen, especially in women with post-cricoid cancer, and a second primary growth is not uncommon. Carcinomas in this region are usually classified under the anatomical site in which they are considered to have originated as follows:

(1) Marginal (sometimes referred to as epilaryngeal).
(2) Pyriform fossa.
(3) Postero-lateral walls.
(4) Post-cricoid.
(5) Cervical oesophagus.

Some systems of classification place the marginal zone carcinomas with the laryngeal growths but their behaviour, symptomatology and mode of spread is such that the writer prefers to include them with the pharyngeal tumours. Upper oesophageal carcinomas are difficult to separate from the post-cricoid ones and are often grouped with them. This combined group is sometimes termed 'epi-oesophageal' (Lederman, 1962).

Frequently the growth is so advanced when first seen that it is difficult to determine its site of origin, and placing it in one of the above categories is rather a matter of guesswork. This may account in part for the reported variations in frequency with which each area is involved, but there is undoubtedly a wide geographic variation. In the United Kingdom most series of patients show that approximately half are considered to arise in the pyriform fossa and the other half from the remaining sites with the post-cricoid region being affected nearly as commonly as the pyriform fossa. On the other hand, in Canada and the United States of America the reported incidence of pyriform fossa neoplasms is considerably higher.

Relative figures are well illustrated in the following comparison of four series of patients of which the first two are from London, England, the third from Toronto, Canada and the last from Houston, USA (*Table 7.1*).

In most sites the incidence of carcinoma is much higher in men than in women but in the post-cricoid region the reverse is true.

Table 7.1

	1	2	3	4
Number of patients	848	246	230	245
Pyriform fossae	39%	50%	61%	75%
Post-cricoid	24%	41%	24%	2%
Other	37%	9%	15%	23%

1 – Royal Marsden Hospital, Dalley (1968).
2 – The Middlesex Hospital and Mount Vernon Hospital,
     MacKinnon, D.M. (personal communication).
3 – Toronto General Hospital, Bryce (1967).
4 – MD Anderson Hospital, Houston, Texas, USA,
     MacComb and Fletcher (1967).

Spread

Both the exophytic and ulcerative forms spread submucosally well beyond the macroscopic limits of the growth, especially in the poorly differentiated lesions, but the ulcerative form has a greater tendency to infiltrate deeply. Deep spread forwards and laterally leads to invasion of the thyroid cartilage and gland; medially the aryepiglottic fold and ventricular band become infiltrated and swelling and fixation of one half of the larynx develops. Paralysis of a vocal cord may also arise from direct involvement of the recurrent laryngeal nerve behind the cricothyroid joint. Post-cricoid growths tend to spread circumferentially, as well as vertically, thus producing stenosis.

The collecting vessels from the lymphatics of the mucous membrane of the laryngopharynx converge on the thyrohyoid membrane and pass through it alongside the superior laryngeal artery. Some empty into the jugulodigastric node but others spread up and down so that almost any node in the deep cervical chain may be the first to be enlarged and when one node has been involved the distribution may be even more eccentric.

Lymphatic vessels from the lower part of the laryngopharynx pass directly to the lower nodes of the deep cervical chain and to the para-tracheal nodes.

Since the lymphatic network freely crosses the midline, bilateral lymph node metastasis occurs; this is particularly common of course when the growth itself crosses the midline as in post-cricoid carcinomas.

Lymph node involvement is early and there may be a large lymph node in the neck while the primary growth in the laryngopharynx is still minute. The majority of patients already have palpable cervical lymph node involvement when they are first seen and Dalley (1968) puts the incidence of this as follows:

Marginal (epilaryngeal)	57 per cent
Pyriform fossa	66 per cent
Postero-lateral walls	55 per cent
Post-cricoid	42 per cent
Cervical oesophagus	31 per cent

Other writers have reported a similar incidence. Of more importance to the surgeon, however, would be the ability to estimate the likelihood of occult metastases in a case in which there are no palpable nodes, but there are not many figures available. Ogura and Mallen (1965) showed that of 39 cases of carcinoma of the superior and inferior hypopharynx (corresponding to our marginal and pyriform fossa divisions) 15, or 38 per cent, had microscopic involvement although clinically no nodes were palpable. The numbers are small but they conclude that this figure is high enough to justify an elective neck dissection.

Distant metastases to bones and viscera occur and are becoming increasingly recognized, possibly because patients are surviving their primary lesion for longer (Arons and Smith, 1961).

Aetiology of carcinoma

One of the problems associated with any discussion of aetiological factors is the uncertain specificity of the data on which they are based. Although there may be little doubt about the fact that the figures refer to patients having carcinoma it is often difficult to identify the precise anatomical site of the growth in the large series which are necessary for epidemiological studies. There is considerable evidence that tobacco and alcohol are factors in the development of carcinoma of the larynx/pharynx/oesophagus in general and Wynder, Bross and Feldman (1957) consider that pipes and cigars have a greater role than cigarettes in the development of carcinoma of the pharynx.

There is detailed statistical evidence of the association of one particular condition in the aetiology of carcinoma of the largyngopharynx and more particularly the post-cricoid region, although there is evidence that these patients have some increased liability to the development of carcinoma anywhere in the squamous-lined upper alimentary tract from the lips to the cardia. Nowadays, the condition is most commonly called 'sideropenic dysphagia' but it is also known as the 'Paterson–Kelly syndrome' after the two workers who described the condition separately in 1919. In some parts of the world it also used to be referred to as the 'Plummer–Vinson syndrome'.

Sideropenic dysphagia is characterized by thinning of the mucosa of the upper alimentary tract with disappearance of the rete pegs and a reduction or absence of glycogen in the cells. Clinically, this tends to be most obvious on the tongue and lips and patients commonly demonstrate the conditions referred to as superficial glossitis and angular stomatitis with cracking of the mucosa at the corners of the mouth. In the pharyngo-oesophageal region the same histological features are evident and in some patients a mucosal fold develops from the anterior wall of the upper oesophagus referred to as an oesophageal web. Erroneously these are sometimes called 'post-cricoid webs' for the reasons explained earlier in the section on anatomy. In a few patients with long-standing sideropenic dysphagia a dense fibrous stricture may form in the upper oesophagus (*Figure 7.7*) and histologically there may be necrosis of the muscle as well as fibrosis. Sometimes two strictures may be present (*Figure 7.8*).

The word sideropenia in connection with this condition serves to illustrate the commonest, most striking and most readily demonstrable deficiency (iron) but many patients have a number of other identifiable metabolic abnormalities. In association with the iron deficiency most patients have a reduced level of haemoglobin and the

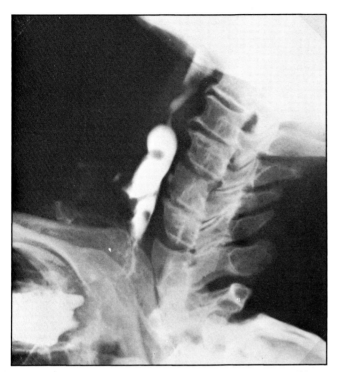

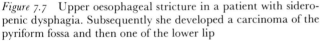

Figure 7.7 Upper oesophageal stricture in a patient with sidero-penic dysphagia. Subsequently she developed a carcinoma of the pyriform fossa and then one of the lower lip

mean corpuscular haemoglobin is low. The serum iron level is below normal limits and the iron-binding capacity is raised in approximately half the patients. In some the serum iron may be reduced even though the haemoglobin may be within normal limits. In about 20 per cent of the patients, vitamin B_{12} absorption is reduced to within the pernicious anaemia range and in about five per cent the level of serum B_{12} is pathologically low, indicating that the patient has pernicious anaemia in addition to sideropenic anaemia. In approximately half the patients there is evidence of pyridoxine deficiency as indicated by estimations of pyridoxine-dependent trans-aminases, and in some patients there is also evidence of some disturbance of tryptophane metabolism as shown by the excretion of excessive amounts of abnormal metabolites in the urine after oral administration of tryptophane. There does not appear to be any change in riboflavine metabolism in these patients.

These biochemical abnormalities found in patients with sideropenic dysphagia do not occur in patients with other strictures of the oesophagus, such as those resulting from ingestion of caustics, and for this reason they appear to be primary and causative of the condition and not secondary to the dysphagia as was originally thought by some workers such as Vinson (1922). In addition, patients undergoing gastrectomy tend to develop multiple deficiencies and Jacobs and Kilpatrick (1964) have shown that women in this category develop webs in the upper oesophagus eight times more

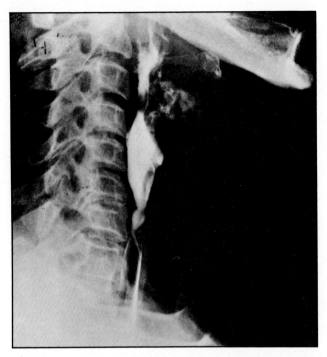

Figure 7.8 Two fibrous strictures of the upper oesophagus in a
woman with sideropenic dysphagia

commonly than a matched group of the population who have not undergone
gastrectomy.

The precise explanation of the dysphagia in those patients who do not have a
fibrous stricture is not quite clear. Most of the patients do not have a demonstrable
web on barium-swallow examination and in them it is considered that the dysphagia
results from incoordination of muscular contraction consequent upon the interference with the sensory side of the reflex arc. The same explanation probably
applies also in those patients who have a definite web. The web in itself does not
explain the dysphagia because it may be just as prominent for a time after the
dysphagia has been completely relieved by the administration of iron together with
vitamin B complex if indicated.

The association between sideropenic dysphagia and carcinoma has been amply
demonstrated by Richards (1970) who found that of 266 patients with post-cricoid
carcinoma, 35 per cent had had dysphagia for more than five years at the time of
diagnosis and a benign stricture of the upper oesophagus had been demonstrated in
9 per cent before the carcinoma developed.

Symptoms of carcinoma

A carcinoma in the laryngopharynx will first affect swallowing, except for the
marginal growths which may first produce a thickening or muffling of the voice. Since

the laryngopharynx is a fairly capacious structure and since carcinoma is at first painless, symptoms may not arise until the growth is well advanced. The symptoms at the start may be indefinite but discomfort or pain on swallowing develop, at first with solid foods only. The discomfort begins simply as a soreness or slight pricking sensation as solid food is going down, but it gradually progresses to pain, which may be referred to the ear via Arnold's nerve, and to obstruction with all acts of swallowing.

Carcinomas of the post-cricoid region and below cause obstructive symptoms earlier than those at a higher level but discomfort and pain are not so evident. In early cases the patient may say that she feels as though the food is passing over a ledge or ridge while fluids go down without difficulty. In most cases, however, obstructive symptoms are quite severe by the time the patient first seeks advice and loss of weight is usually more marked than in carcinomas arising in the other sites.

As has already been pointed out, an enlarged lymph node may appear in the neck while the primary growth is still small, before it has given rise to any throat symptoms.

In males the growth is usually seen in the sixth and seventh decades but in females post-cricoid lesions often appear earlier and cases are not uncommonly met with in the late twenties and the thirties.

The feeling of a 'lump in the throat' or the sensation of a foreign body being present, like a hair or a small pip, causing the patient to swallow constantly is not suggestive of an organic lesion. In these cases food and drink go down without difficulty and the symptoms are intermittent as against the gradually increasing severity of those caused by carcinoma.

Diagnosis of carcinoma

Most patients have had symptoms for some time when they are first seen and in them it is usually not difficult to suspect the presence of a carcinoma in the laryngopharynx or upper oesophagus, to detect it on indirect examination with a mirror or else demonstrate an irregular filling defect on barium-swallow examination, and then to confirm the diagnosis by direct examination and by taking a biopsy of the lesion for histological examination. However, the situation is much more difficult in the patients who present with symptoms other than dysphagia or an enlarged node in the neck and in those who have had treatment and who are being followed-up to ensure that there is no residual or recurrent disease. In addition, in all patients diagnosis requires not only a determination of the nature of the lesion which is present but also an assessment of its extent and this poses a number of problems. These three particular diagnostic difficulties will now be considered in more detail.

Early diagnosis
Like dysphagia, pain localized to the throat should direct attention to the pharynx, but it may be attributed erroneously to other causes without adequate examination and investigation. Vaguer symptoms such as a mild discomfort or a 'catch' in the throat on swallowing are usually attributed to anxiety, but unless there are other positive indications of the psychological nature of the disturbance and unless the symptoms subside in a short time further investigation is required.

Diagnosis after treatment

As will be discussed later, both radiotherapy and surgery are used in the treatment of carcinoma of the laryngopharynx and upper oesophagus and they are not mutually exclusive. Accordingly, after either form of treatment it is necessary to try and detect the presence of any residual or recurrent disease at the earliest possible moment while alternative treatment is still possible. Unfortunately there are difficulties in detecting further growth before it has reached an advanced stage and this is well illustrated by the very large number of patients reported in numerous series who succumb to their disease after being treated by only one modality. Although there may be differences of opinion about the relative merits of each form of treatment used as a primary measure or as a salvage procedure, there is ample evidence to support the use of a second form of treatment if the first fails and if this is not employed it is usually because recurrent disease has advanced to the stage of being untreatable before being positively identified.

Treatment of any type produces alteration of the tissues and subsequent examination is a matter of determining whether the abnormalities which are present are those which would be expected or whether they indicate that there is active tumour still present. While positive biopsies confirm the presence of growth (unless taken within a few weeks of the completion of a course of radiotherapy) negative biopsy findings in no way exclude the possibility. After both radiotherapy and surgical excision there may well be healing of the surface mucosa while there is still active growth extending in the deeper tissues (*Figure 7.9*).

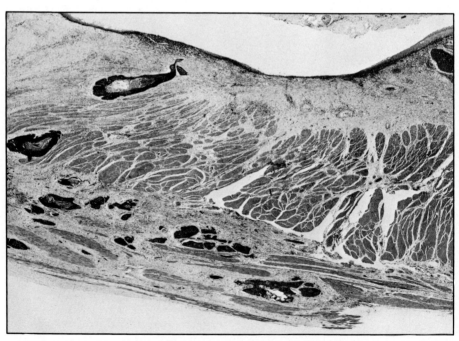

Figure 7.9   Histological section of pharyngo-oesophageal area after radiotherapy. The mucosa is thin but intact and a biopsy would have been negative in most areas unless it had penetrated the muscular wall. (Reproduced by courtesy of the Director, Bland Sutton Institute of Pathology)

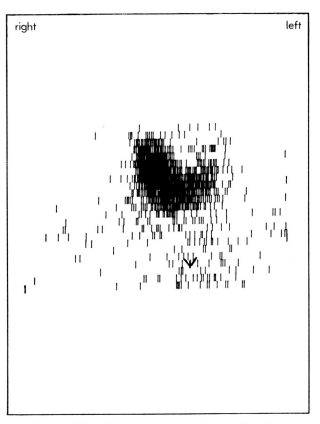

right   left

Figure 7.10 Thyroid scan in a patient with pharyngo-
oesophageal carcinoma showing invasion of the left lobe of the
thyroid gland. (Reproduced by courtesy of the Director,
Department of Nuclear Medicine, The Middlesex Hospital
Medical School)

Diagnosis of the extent of the tumour

As has been mentioned already in the section on pathology, carcinoma of the
laryngopharynx tends to spread in submucous tissues well beyond the surface limits of
the growth and the extent of this can be difficult to judge. It is never easy to assess
possible involvement of deep strictures in the neck with any accuracy although this
will be clear if there is a paralysis of the recurrent laryngeal nerve. While involvement
of the thyroid gland may be revealed on a thyroid scan (*Figure 7.10*) there may still be
spread into the gland even when the scan is normal.

Detection of lymph node involvement is also impossible in the early stages and the
common criterion of palpability is dependent on so many factors that it can usually be
regarded as merely the detection of advanced disease in the nodes. As was mentioned
previously, Ogura and Mallen (1965) demonstrated histological involvement in 38
per cent of patients who had no palpable nodes and this has also been the writer's
experience. In 37 patients operated on in the absence of detectable nodes no less than
13 (35 per cent) had histologically invaded nodes and in 8 (22 per cent) there was
bilateral involvement.

For these reasons even the most careful examinations and investigations of patients with carcinoma of the laryngopharynx tend to underestimate the true extent of the disease to a significant degree, and Harrison (1970) has shown that this occurs in about 40 per cent of patients as judged by examination of resected specimens by serial section. This is of great importance in considering the management of patients with this condition.

Management of patients with carcinoma

Unfortunately a number of patients have such advanced disease when they are first seen that curative treatment is not possible or it may be excluded by other medical conditions. In them palliative treatment must be governed by the predominant symptom for which relief is necessary and in many of these patients there is little that can be done. A gastrostomy which enables the patient to obtain nourishment but which does nothing to allow the swallowing of saliva or to avoid inhalation pneumonia cannot be regarded as palliation.

In patients who are otherwise reasonably fit and whose growth is not so advanced that the possibility of cure is excluded, the methods of treatment available are radiotherapy and surgery with or without cytotoxic chemotherapy. Although considerable advances have been and are still being made in the field of cytotoxic agents the position at present can be summed up by saying that the stage has not been reached when chemotherapy could be advocated as more than an adjuvant method of treatment for carcinoma of the laryngopharynx, but that its use in conjunction with radiotherapy or surgery offers the possibility of controlling blood-borne metastases and residual pockets of tumour in a way that is not possible otherwise. The precise details of chemotherapeutic regimens and their relationships to the timing, fractionation and dosage of irradiation are too complex to be considered here but are referred to in Volume 1.

As has been mentioned above, the use of either radiotherapy or surgical excision does not preclude the possibility of also employing the other form of treatment subsequently and there are thus four possibilities open to the clinician responsible for advising the patient:

(1) Radiotherapy followed by surgical excision if required for recurrence (salvage surgery).
(2) Radiotherapy followed routinely by surgical excision (elective surgery).
(3) Surgical excision followed by radiotherapy if required for recurrence (salvage radiotherapy).
(4) Surgical excision followed routinely by post-operative radiotherapy (elective radiotherapy).

Although those are the theoretical possibilities, it has been explained already in the section on diagnosis that the vast majority of patients placed in treatment groups (1) and (3) never have salvage treatment because of the difficulty in diagnosing recurrent disease at a time when curative treatment could still be considered. For this reason it is important that the particular risks inherent in that course of action should be recognized by the clinician concerned so that they can be weighed against the risks and disability resulting from a course of radiotherapy post-operatively, or a surgical excision after a radical course of radiotherapy. To appreciate those risks and to regard them as acceptable under the circumstances can easily be justified, but a number of people experienced in dealing with these patients consider that the risks of delay in diagnosis outweigh the hazards of elective treatment.

In considering this problem some statistics are of value. In an extensive series of 568 patients with pharyngo-oesophageal carcinoma treated by radiotherapy, Lederman (1962) reported an overall five-year survival figure of 59 (10.4 per cent). Of the 244 patients with epi-oesophageal growth (post-cricoid and upper oesophageal) only 19 survived for five years (7.8 per cent), and for the 416 patients in all sites who had lymph node involvement at the time of treatment the five-year survival figure was only 25 (6 per cent). Even for the most localized Stage I tumours with no lymph node involvement there were only 12 out of 36 patients who survived for five years (33 per cent). Similar figures have been reported by others such as Dalby (1964) and it follows from this that if radiotherapy is used as the primary treatment there will be at least 60 per cent of the patients who require further treatment in the form of surgical excision and, overall, 90 per cent will need operation. The question which requires consideration is whether the diagnosis of residual disease in those 60–90 per cent of patients will be achieved in time to allow further curative treatment. The reports based on series treated by radiotherapy alone suggest that in practice large numbers of patients have become inoperable before a diagnosis of radiotherapy failure is established.

In considering surgical excision it is necessary to refer to treatment of the lymph nodes as well as the primary site, but in view of the very high incidence of nodal involvement with carcinoma of the hypopharynx it is more convenient to consider the problems as combined rather than separate.

Surgical procedures

In theory it might be possible to treat some very localized carcinomas in the laryngopharynx by limited excision through a lateral pharyngotomy approach, but such tumours are rarely seen and if a small tumour of this type is not eradicated by radiotherapy there are probably sound reasons why subsequent surgery should excise more tissue than appeared to be involved initially. Accordingly, in practice, there is virtually no place for local surgical excision for carcinoma of the laryngopharynx. Because of the anatomical features of the region all curative resections must involve the larynx as well as the pharynx. Although partial laryngectomy (with partial pharyngectomy) has been advocated for the treatment of some growths in the pyriform fossae the results have been disappointing and total laryngectomy is regarded as a necessity by most workers in this field.

In association with total laryngectomy, if the growth is restricted to the upper part of the laryngopharynx there may well be enough mucosa which can be retained to effect closure of the pharynx by direct suture of the cut edges. In contrast to this, if the growth is in the lower part of the laryngopharynx there will be no possibility of excising the lesion adequately and preserving sufficient mucosa to effect reconstruction, and in that case the whole pharynx and larynx need to be removed and continuity restored by other means. These two types of operation will now be discussed.

Laryngectomy and partial pharyngectomy

A number of growths in the upper part of one pyriform fossa are suitable for a procedure of this type. Because lymph nodes are involved in approximately 70 per cent of patients with carcinoma of the pyriform fossa it is usual to combine the resection with a block dissection of the neck on the affected side. The lobe of the thyroid gland on that side should also be included in the resected specimen.

The writer prefers to use a large U-shaped skin flap which can be extended if necessary by an additional incision from a point low on the vertical limb of the incision obliquely downwards to the point of the shoulder. However, this is required only exceptionally if the U incision is made broad enough.

The pharynx is opened at the tip of the epiglottis after reflecting the mucosa of the vallecula off the anterior surface and the growth can then be visualized and resection carried out together with an ample margin of apparently healthy tissue. It must be remembered that there is considerable mucosa available in the upper part of the laryngopharynx and there is no virtue in preserving more than is required to provide a lumen the same size as the oesophagus. Even if it is necessary to reduce the lumen to even smaller dimensions it will be adequate provided the diameter after suture is no less than 7–8 mm.

The cut edges of the pharyngeal mucosa are sutured after insertion of a nasogastric tube and the skin closed in the usual way with suction drainage of the wound.

Laryngopharyngectomy (total laryngectomy and pharyngectomy)

For growths in the lower part of the pyriform fossa, in the post-cricoid region and in the upper oesophagus, it is necessary to resect the whole of the larynx and laryngopharynx and, because of the incidence of lymph node involvement, a bilateral block dissection may also be required. Even in the absence of palpable nodes pre-operatively it is the writer's experience that all these patients have enlarged nodes at operation and in 35 per cent of such patients active growth is demonstrated in the nodes. It is not possible, because of the mortality and severe morbidity, to include both internal jugular veins in the resection at the same operation, and therefore it is necessary to preserve the internal jugular vein on the side which appears to be less affected on palpation after dividing the sternomastoid muscles and the strap muscles to give better access to the fingers.

For this operation also the writer prefers a wide U-shaped incision. After the decision mentioned above has been made, the block dissection is carried out on the less affected side and after the jugular vein on that side has been dissected clear and preserved, the block dissection is carried out on the opposite side including the internal jugular vein.

The pharynx is then separated from the pre-vertebral tissues after the inferior thyroid arteries have been ligated and the whole laryngopharynx and larynx are ready for removal together with the whole thyroid gland and the blocks of tissue from each side of the neck.

Apart from being somewhat more extensive than a total laryngectomy or a total laryngectomy combined with a partial pharyngectomy, the excision involved in a laryngopharyngectomy is not much more complex or difficult. The real problem lies in the restoration of continuity of the alimentary canal after the resection. This will, of course, have been planned before any decision is made about operation and will be undertaken as part of the procedure, but for descriptive purposes it is convenient to discuss it as a separate problem as it is a major decision which has to be made but one which does not affect the excision of the growth up to the point described above.

Restoration of continuity of the alimentary tract after laryngopharyngectomy

The oesophagus has a segmental blood supply and, despite a few reported successes, it is not usually possible to effect a mobilization of the oesophagus which will enable it to be brought up for anastomosis to the pharynx after resection. The methods which are currently in use to restore continuity can be classified as follows:

(1) Repair with a plastic tube.
(2) Repair using skin.
(3) Visceral repair.

These will now be considered in more detail.

Repair with a plastic tube
Silicone rubber tubes are advocated by Stuart (1966) and they have the advantage of simplicity and the fact that the lower end can be inserted into the oesophageal lumen without sutures being required and so a considerable length of oesophagus can be resected without opening the chest. Difficulties arise in obtaining a water-tight seal between the pharynx and the upper end of the tube.

Repair using skin
While split skin grafts wrapped around a moulded tube have been used, they are very liable to give rise to fistulae and to stenosis and cannot be used after radiotherapy.
    The most suitable skin flaps are the delto-pectoral flaps and Stell (1973) and others regard them as providing the most satisfactory form of repair in the majority of patients. They have the advantage that an abdominal operation is not required but the method has the disadvantage that only a limited length of oesophagus can be resected and reconstituted without opening the chest. Also, fistulae and stenosis may occur and a longer average stay in hospital is required.

Visceral repair
Although it is possible in some cases to effect continuity between the pharynx and oesophagus by the use of revascularized segments of intestine, the method is fraught with difficulty and the anastomosis of small veins in particular is liable to be unsure. For this reason the procedure has no wide application and the visceral repairs which are used are in effect limited to transposition into the neck of either the stomach or the colon. Both procedures have had considerable success and many surgeons regard them as providing the most satisfactory method of restoring swallowing and speech after laryngopharyngectomy.
    Visceral transposition has the great advantage that it effects an immediate repair of

the pharynx and oesophagus and the whole length of the gullet can be removed so that there is no lower limit to the level of resection. Swallowing is restored within a few days and most patients are eating almost a normal diet within a week or two. Also, the repair can be regarded as durable in the sense that swallowing tends to be maintained even when recurrent growth develops in the neck.

Fistulae are uncommon and stenosis is unknown when stomach is used and is seldom seen when colon is transposed.

However, the procedure does impose a more major operation on the patient and it requires the cooperation of an experienced surgeon who is well versed in the techniques of handling abdominal viscera.

Both stomach and colon have their own advantages and disadvantages which may determine the choice in a particular patient but in many the decision may merely reflect the particular experience and preference of the surgeon concerned.

Two particular advantages of transposing the stomach are that it has an excellent blood supply and when it is used only one anastomosis is required and that is in the neck. On the other hand, mobilization of the stomach requires extensive and meticulous dissection and in a few patients there is some tendency to reflux and to dumping. On balance, stomach is the viscus of choice of Le Quesne and Ranger (1966), Harrison, Thompson and Buchanan (1978) and others. Although colon was originally chosen by some surgeons more now seem to prefer stomach.

Colon has the advantage that mobilization is more straightforward even though it also needs to be performed meticulously and no large raw area is left subsequently. It also preserves the normal gastric reservoir but three anastomoses are required of which two are in the abdomen. Although anastomoses should not give rise to any difficulty complications can occur. In general, colon has a much more fickle blood supply than stomach and although Slaney and Dalton (1973, 1979) have had considerable success with this method in a series of 74 patients, other workers have experienced a number of vascular failures.

Repair procedures of this type should not be undertaken by the 'occasional' surgeon in the field of laryngopharyngectomy and it is necessary to discuss only the general principles of the operations rather than the minute details which are, nevertheless, critical to the success of the procedure.

The blood loss during the operations is in the range of 200–1000 ml and an adequate supply of blood must be available. The patients must be assessed carefully before operation to ensure that they are physically fit, and adequate time must be taken to ensure that they are well adjusted to the effects of the resection and the repair. An experienced anaesthetist is required and after operation the patients are best nursed in an Intensive Care Unit for 24–48 hours. Pre-operative assessment must include studies of thyroid and para-thyroid function.

At operation the two surgical teams should start their procedures synchronously, but if a bilateral block dissection of the neck is included the abdominal surgeon will complete the mobilization before the neck dissection is finished. This has advantages in that the viscus can remain in its natural environment for a while after mobilization before being moved to the neck. Best swallowing is obtained if the stomach or colon is transposed via the posterior mediastinum after complete removal of the oesophagus which can be freed in its whole length by finger dissection from above and below without opening the chest.

At the end of the operation and before the patient leaves the theatre a radiograph of the chest must be taken and, if there is a pneumothorax present, this must be dealt with appropriately by aspiration or insertion of an intercostal drain attached to a water seal unless the pneumothorax is very small. In any event the radiograph must be repeated after a few hours.

Post-operatively regular checks must be made of blood calcium levels and appropriate steps taken as required. In spite of the extent of the resection there are a few patients in whom there does not appear to be any disturbance of calcium metabolism and who need no calcium replacements. There can be no routine treatment in this respect and every patient's requirements must be assessed individually.

Prognosis after laryngopharyngectomy

Figures are not easy to compare because of the types of patient treated. In series where there is a wide difference between the numbers of patients treated by radiotherapy and those treated by surgery it is reasonable to assume that there has been considerable selectivity in the choice of patients for laryngopharyngectomy and better results might be expected. Again, more advanced tumours can be treated when visceral repair is employed because a greater length of oesophagus is removable.

Although the writer has not seen any recurrent tumour become manifest for the first time more than three years after laryngopharyngectomy, the five-year survival figures are not the same as those for three years because some patients succumb during the interval either due to recurrence which was present at three years or else they die of inter-current disease and this is not surprising in view of the age of the patients.

In their large series of 74 patients, Slaney and Dalton (1979) had a five-year survival figure of 29 per cent. Le Quesne and Ranger (1966) in a series of 54 patients had 24 per cent five-year survivors and Harrison, Thompson and Buchanan (1978) report a 29 per cent three-year survival in a series of 56 patients. The operative mortality has been defined somewhat differently in the various series but about 10 per cent of the patients have died in hospital following operation.

These survival figures for patients treated in a number of instances by radiotherapy as well as surgery and having, in the main, very advanced disease, must be compared with the figures quoted earlier for radiotherapy. The figures are, in fact, not much below the very best figures for radiotherapy alone reported by Lederman (1962) and by Dalby (1964) in respect of selected groups of small localized lesions without any evidence of nodal metastasis.

At present it is not possible to compare the effects of elective surgery after radiotherapy with salvage surgery.

References

Arons, M. S. and Smith, R. R. (1961). 'Distant metastases and local recurrence in head and neck cancer', *Annals of Surgery*, **154**, 235–240
Bakamjian, V. (1965). 'A two-stage method for pharyngoesophageal reconstruction with a primary pectoral skin flap', *Plastic Reconstructive Surgery*, **36**, 173–184
Bryce, D. P. (1967). 'Pharyngectomy in the treatment of carcinoma of the hypopharynx', In: *Cancer of the Head and Neck*, pp. 341–356;

Butterworths, London and Boston

Buell, P. and Dunn, J. E. Jnr. (1965). 'Cancer mortality among Japanese Issei and Nisei of California', *Cancer*, **18**, 656–664

Buiter, C. T. (1976). *Endoscopy of the Upper Airways*; Excerpta Medica, Amsterdam

Dalby, V. M. (1964). 'Treatment of post-cricoid carcinoma by combined intracavitary and external radiation', *Clinical Radiology*, **15**, 251–255

Dalley, V. M. (1968). 'Cancer of the laryngopharynx', *Journal of Laryngology*, **82**, 407–419

Flatman, G. E. (1954). 'Discussion on treatment of carcinoma of nasopharynx', *Proceedings of the Royal Society of Medicine*, **47**, 547–560

Gowen, G. F. and DeSuto-Nagy, G. (1963). 'The incidence and sites of distant metastases in head and neck carcinoma', *Surgery, Gynecology and Obstetrics*, **116**, 603–607

Harrison, D. F. N. (1970). 'Pathology of hypopharyngeal cancer in relation to surgical management', *Journal of Laryngology*, **84**, 349–367

Harrison, D. F. N., Thompson, A. E. and Buchanan, G. (1978). 'Radical resection for cancer of the hypopharynx, and cervical oesophagus with repair by stomach transposition', *British Journal of Surgery*, in press

Henle, W., Henle, G., Hung-Chiu Ho., Cachin, Y., Clifford, P., De Schryver, A., De-The, G., Diehl, V. and Klein, M. (1970). 'Elevated titers to Epstein–Barr virus in nasopharyngeal carcinoma, other head and neck neoplasms and control groups', *Journal of the National Cancer Institute*, **44**, 225–231

Hyams, Vincent, J. (1975). 'Unusual tumours of the larynx', *Canadian Journal of Otolaryngology*, **4**, 332

Jacobs, A. and Kilpatrick, G. S. (1964). 'The Paterson–Kelly syndrome', *British Medical Journal*, **2**, 79–80

Kelly, A. Brown (1919). 'Spasm at the entrance of the oesophagus', *Journal of Laryngology*, **24**, 285–289

Lederman, M. (1962). 'Carcinoma of the laryngopharynx', *Journal of Laryngology*, **76**, 317–334

Le Quesne, L. P. and Ranger, D. (1966). 'Pharyngolaryngectomy, with immediate pharyngogastric anastomosis', *British Journal of Surgery*, **53**, 105–109

MacComb, W. S. and Fletcher, G. H. (1967). *Cancer of the Head and Neck*, Williams and Williams, Baltimore

Ogura, J. H. and Mallen, R. W. (1965). 'Surgery of cancer of the laryngopharynx', In: *Proceedings of the Eighth International Congress of Oto-Rhino-Laryngology*, pp. 167–171; Excerpta Medical, Amsterdam

Paterson, D. R. (1919). 'A clinical type of dysphagia', *Journal of Laryngology*, **24**, 289–291

Ranger, D. and Thackray, A. C. (1979). *Painful Glomus Tumours of the Larynx*, in press

Richards, S. H. (1970). 'Postcricoid carinoma and the Paterson–Kelly syndrome', *Journal of Laryngology*, **85**, 141–152

Robertson, G. H., Biller, H., Sessions, D. G. and Ogura, J. H. (1972). 'Presurgical internal maxillary embolisation in juvenile angiofibroma', *Laryngoscope*, **82**, 1524–1532

Rouvière, H. (1932). *Anatomie des Lymphatiques de l'Homme*; Masson et Cie, Paris

Slaney, G. and Dalton, G. A. (1973). 'Problems of viscus replacement following pharyngo-laryngectomy', *Journal of Laryngology*, **87**, 539–546

Slaney, G. and Dalton, G. A. (1979). 'Carcinoma of the hypopharynx and its surgical treatment', *Journal of the Royal Society of Medicine*, in press

Smith, R. R., Frazell, E. L., Caulk, R., Holinger, P. H. and Russell, W. O. (1963). 'The American Joint Committee's proposed method of stage classification and end results reporting applied to 1320 pharynx cases', *Cancer*, **16**, 1505–1520

Stell, P. (1973). 'Cancer of the hypopharynx', *Journal of the Royal College of Surgeons, Edinburgh*, **18**, 20–30

Stout, A. P. and Kenney, F. R. (1949). 'Primary plasma-cell tumours of upper air passages and oral cavity', *Cancer*, **2**, 261–396

Stuart, D. W. (1966). 'Surgery in cancer of the cervical oesophagus. Plastic tube replacement', *Journal of Laryngology*, **80**, 382–396

Sturton, S. D., Wen, H. L. and Sturton, O. G. (1966). 'Etiology of cancer of the nasopharynx', *Cancer*, **19**, 1666–1669

Terz, J. J. and Farr, H. W. (1967). 'Carcinoma of the tonsillar fossa', *Surgery, Gynecology and Obstetrics*, **125**, 581–590

Toker, C. (1963). 'Some observations on the distribution of metastatic squamous carcinoma within cervical lymph nodes', *Annals of Surgery*, **157**, 419–426

Vetter, J. M. and Toner, P. G. (1970). 'Chemodectoma of the larynx', *Journal of Pathology*, **101**, 259–265

Vinson, P. (1922). 'Hysterical dysphagia', *Minnesota Medicine*, **5**, 107–108

Wood-Jones, F. (1940). 'The nature of the soft palate', *Journal of Anatomy, London*, **74**, 147–170

Wynder, E. L., Bross, J. J. and Feldman, R. M. A. (1957). 'A study of the etiological factors in cancer of the mouth', *Cancer*, **10**, 1300–1323

Yeh, S. (1962). 'Histological classification of carcinomas of the nasopharynx with a critical review as to the existence of lympho-epitheliomas', *Cancer*, **15**, 895–920

8 Hypopharyngeal diverticulum (pharyngeal pouch)

R F McNab Jones

The relatively common type of pharyngeal pouch, correctly known as a hypopharyngeal diverticulum, is a posterior pulsion pouch which occurs between the upper thyropharyngeal fibres and the lower cricopharyngeal fibres of the inferior constrictor muscle.

The inferior constrictor muscle arises from the oblique line on the lamina of the thyroid cartilage, and from the side of the arch of the cricoid cartilage (*Figure 8.1*). It has two parts: an upper oblique part, the thyropharyngeus; and a lower circular part, the cricopharyngeus.

The fibres of the thyropharyngeus are inserted into the median raphe of the pharynx. Its upper fibres are supported by the overlapping fibres of the middle and superior constrictors, but its lower fibres lack this support below the level of the vocal cords and are, furthermore, thinned out. This leaves a potentially weak area above the cricopharyngeus (*Killian's dehiscence*).

The cricopharyngeus is thicker than the other pharyngeal muscles and it extends

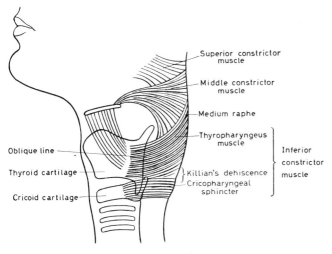

Figure 8.1 Anatomy of the lower pharynx

around the pharynx, without interruption, from one side of the cricoid arch to the other. There is no raphe here. The muscle acts as a sphincter at the lower extremity of the pharynx and it is continuous with the circular muscle coat of the oesophagus. It is normally closed, except for momentary relaxation during the act of deglutition, and it has a different nerve supply from the other constrictors.

All the nerve fibres to the constrictor muscles, except those destined for the cricopharyngeal sphincter, leave the brain stem in the cranial root of the accessory nerve, and pass thence to the vagus. Most of these fibres pass in its pharyngeal branch to the pharyngeal plexus, whence the constrictor muscles are innervated. However, the sphincter derives its nerve supply from the recurrent laryngeal nerve and the external laryngeal branch of the superior laryngeal nerve.

The rare congenital pouches arising in the sites of the branchial clefts were discussed by Wilson (1962) in his Semon Lecture.

Aetiology

There is still much controversy about the cause of hypopharyngeal diverticula.

Negus (1950) believed that tonic spasm of the cricopharyngeus muscle prevented the downward passage of the bolus and that the relatively weak area of the posterior pharyngeal wall (Killian's dehiscence) gave way to the long-continued pressure within the pharynx above the sphincter, with eventual herniation.

A more commonly held theory is that of a neuromuscular incoordination. This postulates that there is a delay or failure of relaxation of the cricopharyngeal sphincter at the end of the second stage of swallowing, that is, that the diverticulum results from an achalasia rather than a spasm.

Kodicek and Creamer (1961) were unable to find any evidence to support a theory of faulty relaxation or achalasia of the cricopharyngeal sphincter as a cause of pharyngeal pouch. They measured the intraluminal pressures of the pharynx and the sphincter in five patients with pouches, through fine water-filled polythene tubes attached to manometers; the resting tone of the sphincter was normal and, on swallowing, normal relaxation was recorded.

As Korkis pointed out in 1958, neither of these theories explains the absence of diverticulosis in this area in cases of long-standing stenosis of the upper oesophagus; nor do they explain how it is that the condition appears to be permanently cured by adequate excision of the pouch, even though the alleged cause remains.

Wilson (1962) agrees with this view and goes further by saying there is no dehiscence above the cricopharyngeal sphincter; indeed, in many dissections of the pharynx, he has found that the lower fibres of the thyropharyngeus are transverse and usually overlap the cricopharyngeus. 'To produce a pouch', he adds, 'there must certainly be increased hypopharyngeal pressure, and this can only be produced by a descending peristaltic contraction of the inferior constrictor when the upper sphincter of the gullet is closed.'

He further states that, in examining the barium radiographs of patients with these pharyngeal pouches, there are two constant features: in the first place, there is always some residual barium after the act of swallowing has been completed; and secondly, the pharynx is usually larger than normal (megapharynx). In some patients with a megapharynx, according to Wilson, there is a 'primary swallow' which is initiated by the tongue, with elevation of the pharynx, peristaltic contraction of the constrictors and relaxation of the upper sphincter of the gullet; but these patients take large mouthfuls and leave a residue of food, and also of air, in the pharynx after the sphincter has closed. Then, in these patients a 'secondary swallow' takes place – a voluntary act – not initiated by the tongue at all, but a consciously initiated contraction of the constrictor muscles immediately after the primary swallow, while the sphincter is closed; that is to say, increased pressure is produced between the contracting portion of the inferior constrictor above and the closed gullet below. This, so Wilson believes, gives rise to the herniation which subsequently becomes a pouch.

Ardran, Kemp and Lund (1964), in a cine-radiographic study, have emphasized that all the above theories are based on studies of established pouches and not on pouches in the process of formation. The swallowing abnormalities noted by those authors may therefore be the result rather than the cause of a pouch. Their cine-radiographs were taken on 35 mm film at 25 frames per second.

In normal subjects, the films showed a wave of peristalsis in the pharynx produced by the contracting pharyngeal constrictors. This wave, which includes the sphincter, sweeps down the upper digestive tube in a progressive fashion, squeezing the bolus from top to bottom 'like squeezing the toothpaste out of a tube'.

The common factor in all patients with pouches, from very small to very large, was the early closure of the cricopharyngeal sphincter, usually but not invariably in association with weakness or incoordination of the pharyngeal peristaltic wave.

Continuing their analogy, these authors show that, if one starts to squeeze a tube of toothpaste from the bottom, and then suddenly (with the other hand) squeezes it near the top, a bulge will occur in the tube between the two flattened parts. The squeeze near the top produces the same effect as the sudden early contracture of the sphincter; the bulge represents the pouch. Thus the pouch is formed when the sphincter is contracting and not when it is relaxing. In fact, relaxation is usually adequate.

It is difficult to say whether these diverticula are caused by the early contraction of the cricopharyngeal sphincter or by the later arrival of the peristaltic wave in the pharynx, but Ardran, Kemp and Lund believe it is most likely that the fundamental upset is the early contraction of the cricopharyngeus muscle ahead of the expressor action.

In contra-distinction to Wilson's view that a 'secondary swallow' against a closed sphincter is responsible for the formation of a pouch, Ardran, Kemp and Lund have emphasized that, except in one case in their series, the pouch (in the earliest stage of development) was always visualized during the first swallow, never as the result of an obstructed second swallow.

Another aetiological factor may be spasm of the cricopharyngeus caused by reflux oesophagitis. Hunt, Connell and Smiley (1970) and Delahunty *et al.* (1971) both reported evidence of increased cricopharyngeal tone in patients with reflux oesophagitis. Stanciu and Bennett (1974), using different techniques for recording intraluminal pressures, found no increase in the resting tone of the upper oesophageal sphincter in patients with proven reflux oesophagitis. Todd (1974) studied 121 cases of hypopharyngeal diverticula, six of whom were known to have a hiatus hernia.

A few families show a high incidence of the condition. The author (1959) recorded five cases in two generations of one family and others have noted this familial tendency.

Pathology

The pouch is composed usually of mucosa and fibrous tissue only. As it enlarges, the pouch sags downwards behind the oesophagus and may reach the mediastinum. The opening of the pouch becomes more and more a direct continuation of the pharynx and the oesophageal opening becomes concealed in front of the mouth of the pouch. As more food enters the pouch, pressure is exerted on the oesophagus from behind to cause oesophageal obstruction.

Originating posteriorly, the pouch usually passes down to the left of the oesophagus, much less commonly to the right.

A hypopharyngeal diverticulum may be complicated by carcinoma within the pouch, usually in its lower two-thirds. A carcinoma confined to the neck of the pouch is very rare but has been reported.

The recurrent laryngeal nerve may be implicated by a large pouch, especially when it is complicated by neoplasia.

Clinical features

Pharyngeal pouches occur most commonly in late middle age, and they are three or four times more common in men than in women.

Their cardinal symptoms are dysphagia, often of long standing, and regurgitation of undigested food, often foetid; this causes bad breath.

Discomfort may be caused by the excessive collection of saliva in the pouch, and as the sac grows the patient takes longer and longer to complete a meal. This is a source of growing social embarrassment.

A swelling in the neck may be present, usually on the left side. It may gurgle and empty on external pressure.

Cough may be caused by overflow of fluids from the diverticulum into the larynx, or rarely by compression of the recurrent laryngeal nerve, the latter also causing occasional hoarseness, especially when the pouch contains a carcinoma.

Emaciation will eventually result from oesophageal obstruction or from neoplastic changes, the latter diagnosis being always suggested when there is blood in the regurgitated material. Small pouches are not uncommonly asymptomatic.

Diagnosis

In most cases, radiography with a barium-swallow will show a characteristic retort-shaped swelling, which may extend into the mediastinum. It will also demonstrate the septum between the gullet and pouch (*Figure 8.2*).

Cine-radiography may demonstrate the earliest tendency to herniation and is useful in demonstrating the results of treatment.

Turner (1963), reporting the radiographic findings in two cases of hypopharyngeal diverticulum with carcinoma, emphasized that when an interruption is found in the normally smooth outline of a barium-filled pouch, and when this is continuous with a

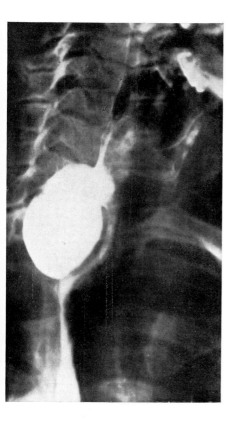

Figure 8.2 Barium-swallow: pharynx and upper oesophagus. The radiograph demonstrates a pharyngeal pouch of moderate size. The septum between the pouch and the oesophagus is well demonstrated

filling defect in the interior of the pouch, the diagnosis is very likely to be that of carcinoma. If such an appearance is quite constant after an interval of one or more days, the diagnosis is practically certain.

Treatment

No treatment is necessary for very small pouches, but if symptoms persist dilatation of the cricopharyngeal sphincter may give relief of varying duration. More lasting results may be effected by the use of a hydrostatic bag (Negus, 1950). However, such methods rarely give permanent relief.

If it can be accepted – and it probably can be accepted – that the site of obstruction in cases of hypopharyngeal diverticula lies at the cricopharyngeal sphincter, then it would seem rational, at least in early cases, to divide the circular muscle fibres of the cricopharyngeal sphincter by an external route. This may be compared with Heller's operation for achalasia of the cardia or Ramstedt's operation for infantile pyloric stenosis, and such a procedure has been supported by Spencer Harrison, who advises that this should be followed by inversion of the sac by means of a purse-string suture, bringing together neighbouring tissues over the gap in the posterior pharyngeal wall.

Myotomy of the cricopharyngeus muscle would seem to be a simple, safe and successful alternative to excision or endoscopic diathermy in small pouches, especially when a prominent cricopharyngeus muscle is shown in the x-ray. After the myotomy, the cricopharyngeal and oesophageal muscles should be dissected from the underlying mucosa for about half the circumference of the mucosal tube, to allow the mucosa to protrude freely through the incision. Ellis *et al.* (1969) have reported 18 cases in which a myotomy was performed; in four it was combined with excision, in another four with suspension, of the pouch. Fourteen patients became symptom-free; three had only occasional symptoms of dysphagia; and only one, who had a large pouch, had no relief at all.

More radical surgical procedures are difficult and unsatisfactory at this stage, but they offer the only hope of permanent relief in more advanced cases.

Excision of the pouch

The pre-operative preparation is important. The patient should be admitted three days before operation so that his general condition may be assessed. These patients are often elderly, with chronic chest infection. The bacteriology of the sputum is investigated and suitable antibiotic therapy instituted before the operation. Physiotherapy can help the chest condition. The pouch is washed out twice daily for 48 hours pre-operatively, using a wide-bore stomach tube. Twenty-four hours pre-operatively, the patient is asked to swallow a coloured thread half-a-metre in length, the proximal end of which is taped to the cheek. When the operation commences this thread will always be seen to have entered the oesophagus.

The operation commences with a direct pharyngoscopy when the operator must:

(1) Follow the thread to identify the oesophageal opening in the anterior wall of the pouch.
(2) Dilate the cricopharyngeus.
(3) Pass a size 18 French gauge nasogastric tube into the stomach.
(4) Pack the sac gently with paraffin flavine ribbon gauze, leaving the proximal end protruding from the mouth.

The neck incision is best made as a collar incision centred to the left of the midline, 1.5 cm below the level of the cricoid cartilage. Alternatively, the incision may be made along the anterior border of the left sternomastoid muscle from the hyoid to the sternum. Appropriate skin flaps, including the platysma, are raised, and the anterior border of sternomastoid identified. Dissection between this and the midline structures, with division of the omohyoid muscle (*Figure 8.3a*) and ligation of the middle thyroid veins, allows separation of the sternomastoid and carotid sheath laterally from the larynx, trachea, thyroid, pharynx, and oesophagus medially. Gentle dissection with gauze-tipped forceps should reveal the sac, made bulkier by the flavine paraffin gauze. In order to dissect this free it is usually necessary to identify and ligate the inferior thyroid artery. Even large diverticula well down in the mediastinum dissect out easily. They should be handled gently and grasped with a Babcock or similar tissue forceps.

The larynx is now rotated to the right by a retractor under the lateral edge of the thyroid ala (*Figure 8.3b*). This allows better access to the area of the neck of the diverticulum. The thin muscle layer on the diverticulum is carefully dissected from

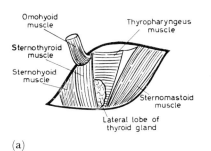

(a)

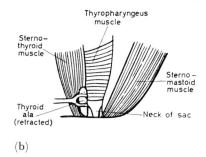

(b)

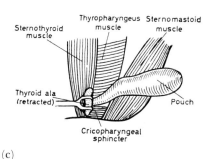

(c)

Figure 8.3   Excision of a pharyngeal pouch. (a) Omohyoid muscle divided; (b) neck of sac exposed; (c) pouch mobilized

the fundus down towards the neck where it forms a small collar (*Figure 8.3c*). Identification of the neck is facilitated by palpation of the nasogastric tube. Marker forceps are now placed at each end of the neck and the anaesthetist removes the gauze pack from the sac.

The mucosa of the sac is severed at the neck between the forceps and the anaesthetist temporarily removes the nasogastric tube. The small finger of the operator's left hand is gently inserted into the oesophagus through the opening in the pharynx. This facilitates accurate division of the fibres of the cricopharyngeus down to the mucosa. The site of division should be postero-lateral and well away from the recurrent laryngeal nerve where it enters the larynx close to the articulation between the inferior horn of the thyroid and the cricoid cartilage. The nasogastric tube is now re-inserted into the oesophagus under vision.

The pharyngeal opening is closed in layers with oo chromic catgut on an atraumatic needle. An inverting stitch is used for the mucosa, and muscle is stitched together over this in such a way as to form an adequate covering without narrowing the pharynx and risking a post-operative stricture.

Haemostasis is secured and the wound drained down to the pharyngeal repair via a separate inferior stab incision. Suction should not be applied to the drain for fear of promoting a salivary fistula.

In uncomplicated cases the drain is removed on the third post-operative day and the feeding tube after 5–7 days. Antibiotic therapy is continued for at least one week post-operatively.

In good hands serious complications are rare. The commonest is salivary fistula. Todd (1974) and McKay (1976) both found the incidence was 20 per cent but they healed rapidly. Recurrent nerve paralysis and surgical emphysema may occur but the older surgeons' fear of fatal mediastinitis is not relevant today.

A difficult problem is post-operative stenosis at the site of the neck closure. This is due to over-enthusiastic removal of mucosa and is made more likely if the pharynx is sutured without an oesophageal tube *in situ*. It may require repeated dilatation. McKay found that only one of his 30 cases suffered from this complication, while in Todd's series of 48 cases, three developed stenosis.

Carcinoma may develop in the diverticula probably as a result of mucosal irritation from food stasis. Dohlman, who popularized endoscopic division of the party wall between oesophagus and pouch, reported that, following this treatment the mucosa in the fundus of the sac returned to a healthy state (Dohlman and Mattson, 1960). However, Juby (1969) and McKay (1976) both report one case each where carcinoma developed in a pouch after Dohlman's operation. They both use this as an argument that diverticulectomy is the treatment of choice. If carcinoma occurs within a pouch, wide local excision is recommended by Garlock and Richter (1961). Where the growth has spread outside the pouch, radical excision of the pouch and adjacent oesophagus is required with a stomach pull-up replacement.

Endoscopic diathermy

Under certain circumstances, especially when the barium-swallow suggests that the sac is adherent to the adjacent oesophageal wall, division of the septum between the gullet and the pouch, after the method originally described by Dohlman, has gained favour with many laryngologists. It may be particularly useful in patients who have become emaciated by prolonged dysphagia or are unfit (by reason of some general disease of poor or uncertain prognosis) for major surgery, but it is also applicable to many large or medium-sized pouches. It is not to be recommended for a small sac, nor for a very large one extending well down into the thorax, nor when it is very difficult to find the opening into the oesophagus.

Dohlman and Mattson (1960) reported the results of treatment by the endoscopic operation in nearly 100 cases, without mortality or serious complications; and more recently White (1968) has reported a small series of nine cases treated satisfactorily by this method, emphasizing that excision can be carried out subsequently without undue difficulty if the diathermy operation fails to relieve symptoms or is followed by recurrence.

Dohlman uses a bivalved oesophageal speculum (*Figure 8.4a*). After dilatation of the oesophageal opening the anterior blade is inserted into the oesophagus, the posterior blade entering the pouch. As the instrument is advanced, the 'septum' between gullet and pouch forms a bulky horizontal mass which contains the cricopharyngeal sphincter (*Figure 8.4a*). This is grasped with the jaws of the diathermy forceps (*Figure 8.4b*) and a coagulating current is applied until the tissues held by the forceps become blanched. The forceps are withdrawn, and an insulated spatula (*Figure 8.4c*) introduced into the pouch. Finally, the coagulated tissues are divided by a cutting current applied through the insulated knife (*Figure 8.4d*).

Simpson (1964) has devised an improved modification of Dohlman's diathermy forceps (*Figure 8.5*) which can be introduced through the ordinary oesophageal speculum of Negus. The spatulate end enters the pouch as the cutting part is introduced carefully into the oesophagus. The jaws are opposed only when the

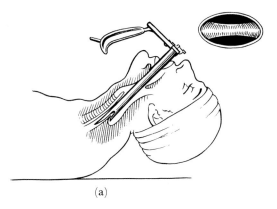

(a)

Figure 8.4 Dohlman's operation. (a) The Dohlman bivalved speculum in position (inset shows the horizontal 'septum'); (b) diathermy forceps;
(c) spatula; (d) diathermy knife

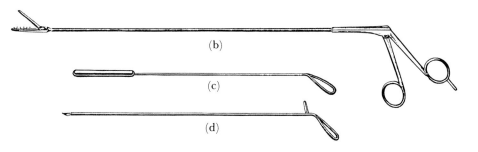

(b)

(c)

(d)

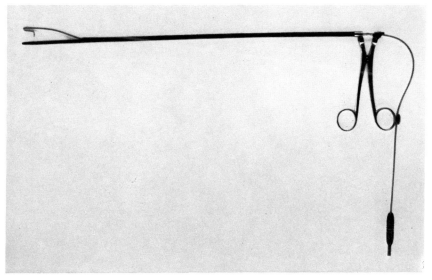

Figure 8.5 Simpson's diathermy forceps. (Reproduced by courtesy of Mr. J. F. Simpson
and the Photographic Department, St. Mary's Hospital, London)

cutting 'knife' has passed beyond the sphincter. The instrument is withdrawn in the closed position, while a cutting current is applied.

An oesophageal feeding tube should be left in position for four or five days, and systemic antibiotic cover is given for the same period.

A barium-swallow after diathermy division of the septum will, of course, show that the pouch is still present; but it also shows in successful cases that the barium is no longer held up and there is no regurgitation.

Despite reports of isolated instances of carcinoma following a Dohlmann operation, it is known that such a lesion may develop spontaneously in one of these diverticula; and the procedure, or one of its modifications, has given very satisfactory symptomatic relief in many cases, including some in which the lesion has been present for so long that the patient's general condition precluded radical excision.

Division of the septum may have to be repeated several times, an average of three in Juby's series, and mediastinitis has been known to occur.

Diverticulo-oesophagostomy

Jackson, Slack and Williams (1960) have recorded a case of a very large pouch occurring in a man 57 years of age, who had had a history of regurgitation of food for five years. The pouch was so large and descended so far into the thorax that they regarded the case as unsuitable for excision through the neck or diathermy division through the endoscope.

The pouch was therefore exposed in the chest and the lower end of the pouch was anastomosed to the oesophagus, by an end-to-side anastomosis.

Two weeks later, the patient was swallowing well and had gained 4.5 kg in weight and the barium-swallow demonstrated a good stoma; ten weeks after the operation, he was still swallowing well and had gained 12.5 kg.

References

Ardran, G. M., Kemp, F. H. and Lund, W. S. (1964). 'The aetiology of the posterior pharyngeal diverticulum; A cineradiographic study', *Journal of Laryngology*, **78,** 333

Delahunty, J. E., Margulies, S. I., Alonso, W. A. and Knudson, D. H. (1971). *Laryngoscope*, **81,** 570

Dohlmann, G. and Mattson, O. (1960). 'The endoscopic operation for hypopharyngeal diverticulum', *Archives of Otolaryngology*, **71,** 744

Ellis, F. H., Schlegel, J. F., Lynch, V. P. and Payne, W. S. (1969). 'Crico-pharyngeal myotomy for pharyngo-oesophageal diverticulum', *Annals of Surgery*, **170,** 340

Garlock, J. H. and Richter, R. (1961). 'Carcinoma in a pharyngo-oesophageal diverticulum: A case report', *Annals of Surgery*, **154,** 259

Hunt, P. S., Connell, A. M. and Smiley, T. B. (1970). *Gut*, **11,** 303

Jackson, J. W., Slack, W. and Williams, R. A. (1960). 'Pharyngeal pouch treated by diverticulo-oesophagostomy', *Lancet*, **1,** 470

Jones, R. F. McNab (1959). *Lancet*, **ii,** 350

Juby, H. B. (1969). 'The treatment of pharyngeal pouch', *Journal of Laryngology*, **83,** 1067

Kodicek, J. and Creamer, B. (1961). 'A study of pharyngeal pouches', *Journal of Laryngology*, **75,** 406

Korkis, F. Boyes (1958). 'The aetiology, diagnosis and surgical treatment of pharyngeal diverticula', *Journal of Laryngology*, **72,** 509

McKay, I. S. (1976). 'The treatment of pharyngeal pouch', *Journal of Laryngology*, **90,** 183

Negus, Sir Victor (1950). 'Pharyngeal diverticula. Observations on their aetiology and treatment', *British Journal of Surgery*, **38,** 9

Stanciu, C. and Bennett, J. R. (1974). 'Upper oesophageal sphincter yield pressure in normal

subjects and in patients with gastro-
oesophageal reflux', *Thorax*, **29,** 459

Todd, G. B. (1974). *Journal of Laryngology*, **88,** 307

Turner, M. J. (1963). 'Carcinoma as a
complication of pharyngeal pouch', *British
Journal of Radiology*, **36,** 206

White, I. L. (1968). 'Endoscopic treatment of
hypopharyngeal diverticula'. *Californian
Medicine*, **109,** 374

Wilson, C. P. (1962). 'Pharyngeal diverticula,
their cause and treatment' (Semon Lecture),
Journal of Laryngology, **76,** 151

9 Oesophageal conditions in the practice of ear, nose and throat surgery
R F McNab Jones

General considerations

Symptoms of disease of the oesophagus

Dysphagia

Difficulty in swallowing will usually lead the patient quickly to his doctor. Few discomforts are as alarming or distressing. In the presence of this symptom clinical examination, radiography and endoscopy will be promptly undertaken. In the absence of dysphagia, however, the possible oesophageal significance of the other symptoms discussed below is all too easily overlooked. Investigation and diagnosis then will be unnecessarily late.

Since dysphagia can be caused by virtually any abnormality or disease affecting the tongue, pharynx or oesophagus, there is little point in compiling or memorizing a 'list of causes'. It is helpful, however, to consider some categories of causes, particularly in that they may cause characteristic patterns of difficulty in swallowing.

Inflammations of the throat give rise to painful difficulties at the beginning of the act of swallowing. In the upper oesophagus they cause a feeling of obstruction with pain which may necessitate a second voluntary act of deglutition to get the bolus down. At the lower end of the oesophagus they cause discomfort for a few seconds, subsiding spontaneously as the bolus is first checked by muscular spasm and then slowly moved through into the stomach.

Organic stricture (fibrous or neoplastic) causes obstruction (but seldom pain), whose severity depends upon the 'tightness' of the stricture. If it is high in the oesophagus or in the hypopharynx a sensation of choking is felt during swallowing, a double effort may be necessary, and coughing and choking result from spill-over into the laryngeal inlet. The patient quickly learns to restrict each swallow to the small amount that can be contained above the stricture without rising above the watershed of the arytenoid eminences. Strictures in the middle or lower oesophagus do not usually cause bronchial tree spill-over unless associated with recurrent laryngeal nerve paralysis or tracheo-oesophageal fistula.

Localization of the site of obstruction is notoriously unreliable. Stimulation of the afferent receptors anywhere in the oesophagus tends to be referred to one place in a particular patient. This site may be anywhere from the epigastrium to the hyoid bone (Edwards, 1976).

Neuromuscular disorders of deglutition as a rule cause greater difficulty with liquids, either because of regurgitation into the nose (past a paralysed palate) or by laryngeal spill-over if the laryngeal sphincters are paralysed. Often such patients can manage better with soft solid food, in contrast to those with an organic stricture, who swallow liquids more easily than solids.

When the oesophagus is compressed or distorted by a lesion outside its wall dysphagia is usually not very severe, and localization by the patient of the level of the hold-up is often rather vague. Liquids may be swallowed quite freely, while solids will go down if well chewed and given sufficient time to pass.

If dysphagia develops only slowly or is of long standing (for example, in some cases of Paterson–Brown Kelly syndrome) it may come to be accepted and tolerated so that the patient only mentions it when specifically questioned on the point. Conversely, the rapid onset of a similar degree of narrowing (e.g. due to a neoplasm) causes great distress and rapid loss of weight due to insufficient food intake.

The normal act of swallowing allows a bolus to pass from mouth to stomach in 8–10 seconds. The sensation of true dysphagia, due to an organic lesion, is therefore felt within 15 seconds of the initiation of the act of swallowing. Pseudo-dysphagia is a sensation which comes on 15 seconds or more after swallowing. Two common examples of this are the 'lump in the throat', relieved by swallowing; and a sensation of food being stuck in the neck, or retrosternally, which comes on an hour or more after eating.

Regurgitation

Painless regurgitation of undigested food is indicative of a dilated viscus above an obstruction. In its most marked form, due to achalasia of the cardia, regurgitation occurs when the patient lies down. In contrast, the regurgitation due to lesions of the upper oesophagus happens during a meal. When it is due to the emptying of a pharyngeal diverticulum the act of regurgitation relieves temporarily the dysphagia caused by the distension of the pouch with food.

Acid regurgitation from the stomach into the throat is associated with a bitter taste, or a burning sensation in the precordium and back, and is caused not by obstructive lesions but by failure of the cardiac sphincteric mechanism (as in hiatus hernia).

The quantity of regurgitated contents can help in diagnosis. In achalasia this may be between 50 and 200 ml while, in cases of carcinoma or other strictures, the amount is usually less than 25 ml.

Pain

When caused by oesophageal disease pain may be felt in the epigastrium, in the substernal region, in the back (particularly in the left scapular region) or in the root of the neck. Referral of pain to the vagus nerve territory of the ear is rare, and may originate even from the lowest part of the oesophagus, as in reflux oesophagitis.

If the pain is associated with, or aggravated by, swallowing its significance is readily appreciated. If dysphagia is slight or absent, however, oesophageal pain may be erroneously attributed to diseases of the heart, lungs or stomach.

Bleeding

Gross haemorrhage from the oesophagus is rather uncommon and is usually due to varices. A few patients with neoplasms or inflammatory disease may vomit or regurgitate blood-stained fluid. Fresh blood appearing in quantity in the throat without effort may arise from lesions near the upper end of the oesophagus.

Respiratory symptoms

Recurring attacks of bronchitis or bronchopneumonia complicate the progress of any disease of the oesophagus associated with laryngeal spill-over, or tracheo-oesophageal fistula. Progressive deterioration of pulmonary function may be so severe that it dominates the clinical picture. The underlying oesophageal cause may even be missed altogether. *Hoarseness*, whether due to an obvious cord paralysis, or to laryngitis, or to the simple weakness of cachexia, should always arouse suspicion of an oesophageal lesion.

General symptoms

Loss of weight is the most important of these, and occurs rapidly in the presence of oesophageal obstruction. General malaise and the symptoms of anaemia are frequently observed and justify suspicion of oesophageal disease if their cause is not readily apparent on clinical examination.

Physical examination

When symptoms suggest the possibility of an oesophageal lesion a routine physical examination of the patient's chest, abdomen and cardiovascular and nervous systems must be followed by attention to the following special points:

(1) Evidence of wasting and dehydration must be noted.
(2) Inspection and palpation of the neck (for thyroid enlargement, palpable lymph nodes and inflammatory or neoplastic masses arising from the pharynx or oesophagus). Absence of laryngeal crepitus against the vertebral column is noted in some cases of carcinoma of the post-cricoid or upper oesophageal region.
(3) Mirror examination of the pharynx and larynx (for palatal or vocal cord paralysis, ulceration or tumour). Even though all of these visible regions may be normal, pooling of saliva in the pyriform fossa of one or both sides is strongly suggestive of a lesion at a lower level.
(4) In completing his special examination the laryngologist will inspect the mouth

and tongue for clinical evidence of anaemia, in the form of glossitis, atrophy of lingual papillae, and cracks or healed fissures at the corners of the mouth.

The patient should then be given something to drink, and his performance of deglutition is observed. This simple test should never be omitted. Coughing, choking, pain, 'double-effort', and regurgitation are much easier to assess in the clinic than by hearsay. If swallowing is repeated while the examiner palpates the root of the neck a typical gurgling sensation will be felt under the hand in cases of pharyngeal pouch.

Laboratory investigations

(1) Blood examination is always indicated to determine the presence of anaemia associated with Paterson–Brown Kelly syndrome, carcinoma, or oesophageal bleeding. Occasionally, serological tests for syphilis will be necessary.
(2) Bacteriological investigations are seldom helpful, but in rare conditions such as diphtheria, fungus infections or tuberculous disease of the oesophagus, examination of a throat swab, specimens of sputum, or oesophageal washings may assist diagnosis.
(3) Exfoliative cytology has been shown to be of value in carcinoma of the oesophagus (Klayman, 1955). A Ryle's tube is passed to the level of the lesion and through it saline lavage and suction are performed. The aspirated fluid is centrifuged and the residue is suitably fixed, stained and examined microscopically.
(4) Examination of the stools for occult blood will usually give positive findings in the presence of malignant or other bleeding disease of the oesophagus, but the test has only slight diagnostic value.

Radiographic examination

Routine plain films

Routine plain films must include:

(1) Postero-anterior views of the chest and mediastinum, to show pulmonary fibrosis or tumour, enlargement or displacement of the mediastinum, aortic aneurysm, and the size and shape of the heart.
(2) Lateral soft-tissue views of the neck to show the outlines of the larynx, trachea, vertebral column, and the vertical band of soft tissues representing the post-cricoid area and cervical portion of the oesophagus (*Figure 9.1a*). Pathological widening of this band may indicate a tumour or cellulitis. Surgical emphysema, a fluid level within an abscess cavity or a persistent gas bubble in the upper oesophageal lumen are all significant abnormalities detectable in this projection.

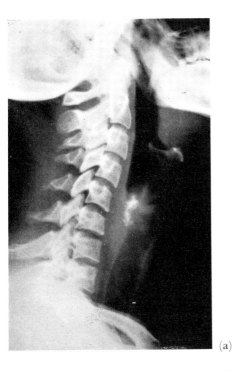
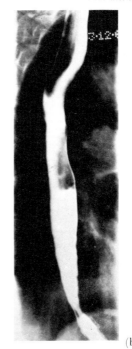

(a)   (b)

Figure 9.1   (a) Lateral radiograph of the neck. Note the normal soft-tissue shadow between the trachea and vertebral column; (b) normal barium-swallow appearances of the thoracic part of the oesophagus

Fluoroscopic screening and contrast studies

These are normally done together and permanent records of the radiologist's observations are made by means of 'still' exposures and cine-photography. The latter technique is finding an increasing usefulness, especially in cases where slow-motion study of abnormal deglutition can contribute to the analysis of neuromuscular disorders.

The technique of conducting these examinations is not described here. The clinician must always try to indicate to the radiologist the likely level of the lesion, so that the examination can be as brief and informative as possible. This is particularly important in patients who are weak and ill. It is also very important to warn the radiologist of the possibility of inundation of the bronchial tree in cases with laryngeal 'spill-over' or suspected broncho-oesophageal fistula. In these cases the examination should begin with the swallowing of a small amount of iodized oil which would do no harm if it were to 'go the wrong way'.

In screening these cases the radiologist will follow the passage of a mouthful of barium and use it to indicate the outlines of the oesophageal lumen, its mucosal folds, the form and position of physiological and pathological constrictions, and the rate and smoothness of the peristaltic waves. The lower end of the oesophagus, the cardia and the stomach are all observed. When sufficient barium has collected in the stomach the patient is placed in Trendelenburg's position and manual pressure is applied to the stomach. This manoeuvre demonstrates the presence of hiatus hernia, and the competency or otherwise of the cardiac sphincteric mechanisms. The normal barium-swallow appearances are shown in *Figure 9.1b*, and are described in more detail in Volume 1.

Figure 9.2 (*below* and *opposite*) illustrates some typical deformations of the normal

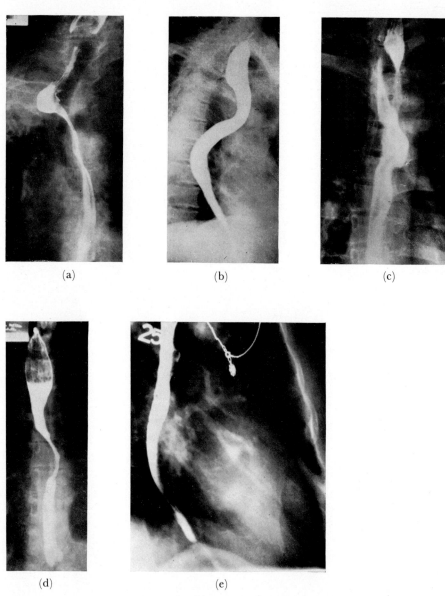

(a)   (b)   (c)

(d)   (e)

Figure 9.2   Deformations of the oesophagus by lesions outside its wall, as seen in barium-swallow radiographs. (a) Extreme displacement and kinking caused by the traction of fibrosis in the right upper lobe of the lung (healed pulmonary tuberculosis); (b) distortion due to a large aortic arch aneurysm; (c) spiral filling defect due to aberrant right subclavian artery passing behind the oesophagus (dysphagia lusoria); (d) compression of the middle third of the oesophagus by mediastinal lymph node metastases (carcinoma of the breast); (e) cardiac enlargement. The gullet is compressed by the dilated left atrium

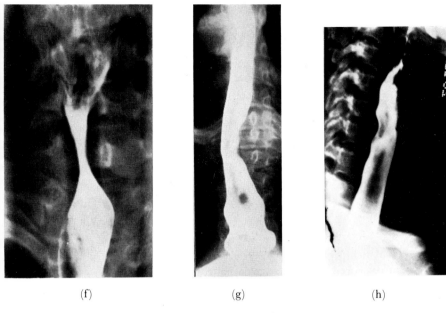

(f)   (g)   (h)

Figure 9.2 (contd)   (f) Symmetrical indentation of cervical oesophagus by pressure of a diffuse goitre; (g) sideways displacement of cervical oesophagus by neoplasm of right lobe of thyroid; (h) scalloping of posterior outline of oesophagus due to cervical osteophytes

oesophagus by extrinsic lesions. These deformations are best shown radiographically, are important in the differential diagnosis of dysphagia, and some of them may be contra-indications to oesophagoscopy. Their importance to the oesophagoscopist is therefore very great.

Oesophagoscopy

Direct endoscopic inspection of the oesophagus by means of a straight rigid tube was reported in 1868 by Kusmaul, who used professional sword-swallowers as subjects. Really satisfactory instruments and techniques were only developed, however, with the invention of electrical lighting systems. In more recent times the Jacksons and many other oesophagologists have established the clinical applications of the method. During the last 30 years oesophagoscopy has come to be taken for granted as a simple diagnostic routine, practised more or less regularly and uneventfully by non-specialists, such as thoracic surgeons and physicians, as well as by laryngologists. This facilitation has been accelerated by modern anaesthetic techniques which have reduced the difficulties and hazards. Oesophagoscopy nevertheless is still potentially one of the most dangerous of all procedures, and the laryngologist bears a great responsibility to maintain the highest possible standards both in the performance and in the teaching of the technique. Oesophagoscopy should only be done when definite indications are present, and these must always be assessed in terms of likely benefit to the patient. Mere confirmation of diagnosis is no justification if no advantage can accrue to the patient by it.

Flexible fibre-optic oesophagoscopes are currently being developed for use under topical anaesthesia, permitting safer inspection, biopsy and photography. Without doubt, when these tools are adopted in general use many advantages will be gained, but at the time of writing the standard techniques about to be described are not superseded, nor are they likely to be in the foreseeable future in any cases requiring intra-oesophageal manipulations.

Common sense should dictate who should perform a given oesophagoscopy. Clearly, the thoracic surgeon should inspect lesions of the middle or lower oesophagus, such as carcinoma or hiatus hernia, when trans-thoracic surgical treatment may be envisaged. Lesions of the hypopharynx and upper oesophagus are primarily the laryngologist's concern. An impacted foreign body should be removed by the most competent endoscopist available at the time – almost invariably this person is a laryngologist. Specific indications for oesophagoscopy emerge later in this chapter. Some contra-indications must now be considered.

Contra-indications to oesophagoscopy

(1) Aneurysm of the aorta.
(2) Severe spinal deformities, such as kyphosis or advanced osteophytosis of the bodies of the cervical vertebrae.
(3) Advanced 'general' disorders such as heart, kidney or liver failure.

Other factors may make oesophagoscopy difficult. These are prominent upper teeth, a narrow mandibular arch, a stiff, short and thick neck, and moderate degrees of kyphosis. Such difficulties can usually be overcome with patience and skill, but they may occasionally dictate the abandonment of the investigation.

Instruments

The oesophagoscope is basically a rigid metal tube. Lighting may be distal (as in the Jackson type), proximal through obliquely-placed side tubes (Negus), or proximal in the form of an external light source directed down the tube by a mirror or prism (Bruning, Killian, Haslinger). The most effective lighting is undoubtedly the remote source applied by a flexible fibre-optic cable, and the Negus type of instrument lends itself particularly well to this improvement.

The different types vary considerably in the design of their distal ends. These differences are seen in the obliquity of the mouth of the tube, and in the thickened 'rolled' leading edge of some patterns. In cross-section types range from a very flat oval to a virtually circular shape. Several lengths are available in each of the various patterns, so that the endoscopist can operate at the shortest practicable working distance whatever the level of the lesion. An extremely useful short tube is the so-called 'oesophageal speculum', which allows inspection of the upper 10–12 cm of the oesophagus as well as the hypopharynx.

Other essential equipment includes: (a) metal suction tubes in various lengths to suit the oesophagoscopes to be used; (b) various grasping and biopsy forceps; (c) bougies in a series of graduated sizes.

In addition, special devices will be needed for particular cases. These may include foreign-body forceps, hydrostatic dilators, equipment for the introduction of metal or plastic tubes, snares, or special syringes.

The operating table must be versatile in its tilting arrangements, and the section supporting the head must be easily raised and lowered, ideally by the operator himself. Some surgeons favour the special Negus head-rest, which facilitates movement from side to side as well as up and down.

Anaesthesia

Preparation of the patient includes examination of the teeth. Any which are decayed or loose must be noted. Elaborate and fragile dental works such as 'jacket crowns' are easily overlooked and may be damaged if the patient is not questioned on this point. Mirror laryngoscopy is required to detect any oedema which might be aggravated by endoscopic manoeuvres. Retained food, as in diverticula or achalasia should be cleared away as well as possible by lavage through an oesophageal tube.

A general anaesthetic is almost invariably preferred nowadays. The fasting patient receives suitable pre-anaesthetic medication. The surgeon requires complete relaxation of the jaws, neck and pharyngeal muscles, easily attained with modern anaesthetic drugs. A cuffed orotracheal tube guarantees the airway and permits assisted respiration when necessary. Passed through the mouth, the tube obtrudes less upon the oesophagoscopist's field than does a nasotracheal tube.

It is difficult to imagine circumstances in which a local anaesthetic would be unavoidable for oesophagoscopy today. The skilful anaesthetist required to give a 'general' is far more ubiquitous than the well-equipped oesophagoscopist. The patient himself is probably safer under a modern general anaesthetic than under a 'local'.

Technique

The patient is placed on the operating table, and his head is supported either by an assistant or by a special head-rest. The head must be lifted so that the cervical spine is flexed and the occipito-atlantoid joint is extended. A piece of gauze is placed so as to protect the upper lip and teeth, and the lubricated oesophagoscope is passed through the mouth and backwards over the tongue. From this stage onwards all landmarks must be plainly seen through the oesophagoscope and the instrument may only be advanced when the lumen of the gullet is clearly in view, and in line. Utmost gentleness is essential, otherwise the pharynx or oesophagus will be perforated. The epiglottis is first seen and behind it the anaesthetist's tube. About 4 cm lower and more posteriorly the arytenoids are next defined. The beak of the oesophagoscope is then passed behind the larynx and lifted so as to open the hypopharynx. Very gentle progress strictly in the midline for a further 2 cm or so will bring into view the cricopharyngeal sphincter which opens to receive the oesophagoscope if the patient is completely relaxed. This is the most dangerous and difficult step, and the surgeon must take time to be absolutely sure of the entrance to the oesophagus. Often the sphincter will open after a short wait, or additional relaxant may be needed before progress can safely be made. Some surgeons advocate the insinuation of a fine bougie which defines the lumen and can then be followed through the 'narrows' of the pharyngo-oesophageal junction.

Beyond this point progress is usually easier, but the oesophageal lumen must always be directly in view, and in line, each time the instrument is advanced. Some opening and closing of the lumen in concert with respiratory movements will be apparent. Below the aortic arch the oesophagus swings forwards and the head of the patient must be progressively lowered. When the cardia is reached the head will be lower than the shoulders, and the oesophagoscope will be pointing towards the left anterior superior iliac spine.

Every part of the oesophageal wall is closely examined. Small areas can be magnified with a suitable lens attached to the proximal end of the oesophagoscope. The cardia is recognized by the appearance of a redder mucous membrane and by the cessation of the respiratory movements.

Removal of the instrument is done slowly and the walls of the oesophagus are re-examined. 'On the way out' the unfolding mucosal pattern may reveal small abnormalities or a foreign body overlooked during introduction of the oesophago-scope. The head must again be positioned throughout so that the oesophagoscope is properly aligned at all stages during its withdrawal.

Hazards

Apart from damage to the lips and teeth due to rough technique, the chief danger in oesophagoscopy is perforation of the oesophagus. Strict observance of the rules outlined above will prevent this accident in most cases. The danger arises chiefly when force is used to overcome difficulties. Awkward jaws and teeth, a short stiff neck, and vertebral osteophytosis multiply the dangers.

In children there is some danger of compression of the trachea by the oesophago-scope. This can cause anoxia, despite the endotracheal anaesthetic technique. Adequate theatre lighting is essential so that the onset of cyanosis can be noted immediately if this complication arises. It cannot be emphasized too strongly that if the patient becomes 'blue' and there is no apparent reason for it, the oesophagoscope must be completely withdrawn and the anaesthetist must be given sole access to the mouth.

Surgical exposure of the oesophagus

Throughout its length the oesophagus is very deeply placed, and surrounded by vital structures. Its blood supply is segmental, not longitudinal, and is jeopardized if more than about 5 cm of the viscus is mobilized. An outline is given below of the usual routes by which the oesophagus may be approached at operation.

In the neck

An incision is made along the anterior border of the sternomastoid muscle from the level of the clavicle to the level of the hyoid bone. The deep cervical fascia is opened in the same line, and the carotid sheath is displaced laterally. The thyroid gland is displaced anteromedially by blunt dissection and the middle thyroid vein is ligated and divided. The thyroid gland is then further displaced forwards and the vertebral column is palpated. The pre-vertebral fascia is then identifiable and immediately anterior to it the visceral compartment of the neck enclosed in the parapharyngeal fascia. The latter must be opened to expose the oesophagus, and the inferior, thyroid artery may first require division if it impedes access. In this region the recurrent laryngeal nerve must be carefully preserved.

By means of this approach localized strictures and tumours of the cervical oesophagus can be removed. Oesophagotomy for removal of a foreign body (when endoscopic removal has failed), the repair of an oesophageal perforation, or the drainage of a para-oesophageal abscess are carried out by the same route. By blunt (finger) dissection downwards alongside the oesophagus an upper mediastinal abscess may be opened and drained.

In the chest

Trans-pleural thoracotomy on the right side gives access to the entire thoracic oesophagus, after division of the azygos vein. Left thoracotomy exposes the oesophagus from the aortic arch downwards, and provides in addition wide access to the abdominal contents through the left half of the diaphragm.

Extrapleural access can be gained by posterior mediastinotomy. This is the preferred route for drainage of a para-oesophageal abscess, but it does not give sufficiently wide exposure for surgical attack upon the oesophagus itself.

In the abdomen

Left upper laparotomy exposes the lowest 3 or 4 cm of the oesophagus and the gastro-oesophageal junction.

In the operation of total oesophagectomy blunt finger dissection from the abdomen and from the neck can mobilize the entire viscus prior to its withdrawal through the neck wound, without the necessity for a trans-thoracic exposure.

Pathology and treatment of diseases of the oesophagus

Congenital abnormality of the oesophagus

In order to understand the congenital anomalies of the oesophagus it is necessary to recall its development. It is formed from that part of the primitive foregut immediately caudal to the pharynx, and three salient features should be noted:

(1) At about the fourth week of intra-uterine life, the median laryngotracheal groove appears in the ventral aspect of the foregut. As the groove deepens, its lips

approximate and fuse, forming the laryngotracheobronchial tree ventrally, and the oesophagus dorsally (*Figure 9.3*). Incomplete fusion explains the presence of a fistula between the oesophagus and trachea, which usually occurs at the level of the bifurcation of the latter.

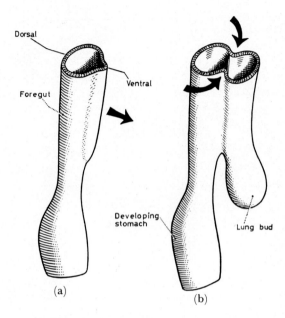

Figure 9.3   The development of the oesophagus and trachea. (a) The laryngotracheal groove is appearing in the ventral aspect of the foregut; (b) the lips of the groove are closing in and separating the developing lower respiratory tract from the alimentary canal

(2) In the early stages of the developing oesophagus there is such proliferation of its lining membrane that the lumen is almost obliterated, but later the wall becomes thinner and the normal lumen is restored. Interference with this latter stage may result in atresia.

(3) Again, early in its development, the oesophagus is exceedingly short, but later it has to undergo rapid lengthening, for the developing lungs push the stomach caudally. This may explain some cases of short oesophagus, although it is probable that reflux oesophagitis is more often responsible for this condition.

Types of abnormality

(1) Atresia (*see* Vogt's classification *opposite.*)
(2) Tracheo-oesophageal fistula without atresia.
(3) Congenital oesophageal stenosis.
(4) Short oesophagus.

Atresia

Vogt (1929) classified congenital atresia of the oesophagus as follows:

Type I. Absence of the oesophagus.

Type II. Cases in which both upper and lower segments of the oesophagus end in blind pouches.

Type III. Atresia of the oesophagus with tracheo-oesophageal fistula: (a) fistula is between upper oesophageal segment and trachea; (b) fistula is between lower oesophageal segment and trachea; (c) fistulae are between both oesophageal segments and trachea.

According to Belsey and Donnison (1950) the incidence of oesophageal atresia is distinctly greater than 1 in 800, and much the most common type of malformation is atresia, in association with a fistula between the trachea or left main bronchus and the lower segment of the oesophagus (*Figure 9.4*). The upper segment of the oesophagus

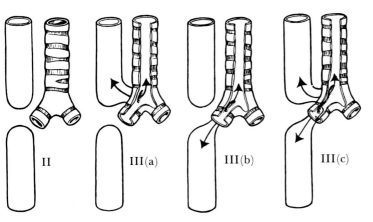

Figure 9.4   The types of congenital oesophageal atresia according to Vogt's classification (*see text*). Type III (b) is the most common

ends blindly. This type – Vogt Type III (b) – accounts for approximately 80 per cent of all congenital oesophageal abnormalities, a fact of supreme importance to all medical personnel associated with the newly born. All the other types of congenital abnormality are much less common.

Diagnosis of congenital oesophageal atresia
Excessive salivation, cyanosis and inability to swallow fluid soon after birth constitute the triad, which should suggest the possibility of congenital oesophageal atresia to the medical or nursing attendant, and the infant should be immediately transferred to a unit fully equipped to deal with this emergency. A lubricated rubber catheter passed through the nose or mouth will be held up in the upper oesophageal segment, and the diagnosis is often confirmed by introducing 1–2 ml of iodized oil into the catheter and taking x-ray films (*Figure 9.5*). The blind end of the upper oesophagus is seen to be

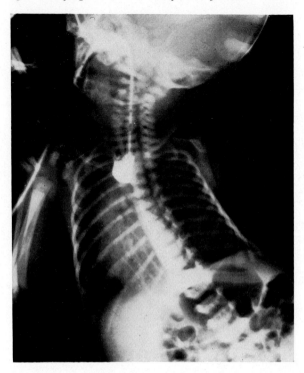

Figure 9.5   Radiograph showing oesophageal atresia. (Mr. David Levi's case)

pear-shaped and regular in outline. A pencil-line airway may be demonstrable leading from the bifurcation of the trachea to the stomach and is said to represent air in the lower oesophagus. Barium must not be used under any circumstances, as its entry into the lungs would be disastrous – in fact, Nixon and Wilkinson (1963) decry the use of any opaque medium, for there is likely to be some spillage into the lungs, predisposing to bronchopneumonia. If the x-ray films suggest the presence of gas in the stomach and the passage of a catheter has been arrested in the upper oesophageal segment, the diagnosis of atresia of the oesophagus, with tracheo-oesophageal fistula, may be made with confidence.

Management

Once the diagnosis has been established it is essential to commence supportive therapy, including intravenous fluids and oesophageal suction, although these measures do not obviate the infant's chief hazard – the passage of gastric juice up the lower oesophageal segment and through the fistula into the tracheobronchial tree.

Operation is usually by the right trans-pleural route, although in some circumstances the approach may be extrapleurally or from the left side. Ideally, the two oesophageal segments are defined, the fistula is closed and anastomosis between the two segments is completed, but many cases are fraught with difficulty. Other anomalies, such as imperforate anus, may be present, further handicapping the infant, and it is necessary to search for these. There is not infrequently some degree of prematurity. It may be possible only to perform cervical oesophagostomy and gastrostomy, and to delay reconstitution of the oesophagus until a later date. Intensive post-operative care is necessary and involves special positioning of the infant, oxygen therapy, pharyngeal aspiration, antibiotics and meticulous attention to fluid balance (Benson *et al.*, 1962). Yet, in spite of the hazards attending these procedures, results have continued to improve and impressive series of anastomosing operations have been placed on record, as for example that of Ty, Brunet and Beardmore (1967) in which no less than 15 cases of repair are quoted with 'zero operative mortality'.

The entire subject of oesophageal atresia and tracheo-oesophageal fistula is covered in very great detail by Freeman (1969) who gives an exhaustive bibliography.

Tracheo-oesophageal fistula without atresia

This is a condition of exceeding rarity, but the case histories described are of great interest: Franklin (1958); Helmsworth and Pryles (1951); Imperatori (1939); Mullard (1954); Negus (1929); and Robb (1952–53).

It is important to remember that it is by no means necessarily inconsistent with life as, for example, is the Vogt Type III (b) deformity and, consequently, diagnosis is sometimes delayed for a very long time. The condition must be considered if feeding the infant causes choking and cyanotic attacks, and these symptoms may be more pronounced when fluids are administered and the infant is placed in certain positions. Recurrent pulmonary infections are likely to occur.

The diagnosis is confirmed by radiography using contrast media, and by bronchoscopy and oesophagoscopy.

The approach used by the thoracic surgeon in order to effect closure of the fistula varies according to the site of the latter, and the surgery is fraught with difficulty. However, gratifying cases of cure have been reported.

Congenital oesophageal stenosis

Congenital strictures and cases of stenosis of the oesophagus are very rare. In the past the term has, without doubt, often been applied where the stenosis has been the result of reflux peptic oesophagitis. This error is less likely to be made if it is recalled that, in the acquired type of stricture, dysphagia gradually increases in severity, particularly after the infant commences to take solids, whereas in true congenital stenosis dysphagia is present from birth. If, on oesophagoscopy, as a result of finding normal mucosa below the site of the stricture, a diagnosis of true congenital stricture is made, the treatment consists of dilatation with gum-elastic bougies over a long period.

Short oesophagus

There has been much confusion on this subject in the past, but it is now considered that cases of true congenital short oesophagus are extremely rare, and Barrett (1954), who has made a detailed study, considers that the term 'congenital short oesophagus' should be reserved for those cases which are true anomalies. The confusion has arisen from the fact that cases of short oesophagus, although dubbed 'congenital', have in fact been produced after birth by reflux of gastric juice. The oesophagitis caused by this reflux leads to fibrosis and, eventually, shortening of the viscus.

Olsen and Harrington (1948), in a review of 220 cases of short oesophagus, considered that of these only four per cent were really congenital, and Allison, Johnstone and Royce (1943), Sweet (1954) and many others, have found a similar state of affairs.

Injuries of the oesophagus

External wounds

External wounds may involve the cervical oesophagus as a result of suicidal 'cut-throat', gunshot wounds, or very rarely as a surgical accident in the course of a tracheostomy operation. If the patient survives the immediate wounding the oesophagus must be exposed surgically and repaired over an in-dwelling oesophageal feeding tube. The neck wound may require debridement and free drainage to forestall the dangers of mediastinitis. Systemic broad-spectrum antibiotics must be given in large doses. Associated injuries to the larynx, recurrent laryngeal nerves, or trachea will necessitate tracheostomy in most cases.

Spontaneous rupture

Spontaneous rupture of the oesophagus is rare. It occurs in the lowermost part of the thoracic oesophagus and is caused by sudden localized distension during vomiting. Mediastinitis always results, and often empyema as well. The condition is rapidly fatal if not recognized and treated. Diagnosis depends upon the history of vomiting, severe pain in the chest or epigastrium, and the radiographic evidence of mediastinal emphysema and pleural effusion. Perforation of a gastric or duodenal ulcer requires consideration in differential diagnosis, while in some cases coronary thrombosis, pulmonary embolus, or dissecting aneurysm of the aorta may need to be excluded.

Immediate treatment consists of intravenous fluids and systemic antibiotics. Nothing is allowed by mouth. As soon as possible thoracic surgical treatment must be given. Early drainage of the infection and repair of the oesophageal wall offer the best hope of recovery.

Accidental perforation

Accidental perforation of the oesophagus from within its lumen results from penetration by metallic pointed foreign bodies such as an open 'safety' pin, or by spicular fish or meat bones.

Perforation is also a complication of oesophagoscopy and the danger is greater when the oesophagus is abnormal. The risk is especially great during the removal of foreign bodies, dilatation of strictures, and when biopsy material is being taken.

Symptoms and signs develop quickly, but at first the patient is not as desperately ill as would be the case with the massive contamination of the mediastinum caused by spontaneous perforation during vomiting (*see earlier*). If the perforation is in the upper oesophagus, crepitus due to surgical emphysema in the neck may be detectable within an hour or so of the accident. *After every per-oral endoscopy the neck should be routinely palpated one to two hours later for this reason.* A plain radiograph (*Figure 9.6a*) confirms the diagnosis. If the oesophagus is perforated near its lower end clinical signs of surgical emphysema in the neck and over the chest wall are slower to appear, and the first indication of disaster will then be severe substernal or epigastric pain, which the patient notices as soon as he recovers from the anaesthetic.

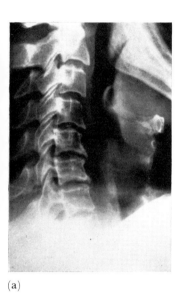

(a)

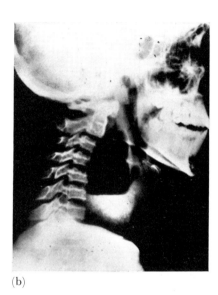

(b)

Figure 9.6   (a) Surgical emphysema in the soft tissues of the neck, following perforation of the cervical oesophagus; (b) retro-oesophageal and retro-pharyngeal abscess, with fluid level and gas above, due to infection after an upper oesophageal perforation

As soon as the diagnosis is clear, the patient is forbidden to take anything whatsoever by mouth. A small dose of morphine may be necessary for relief of pain. Intravenous fluids and systemic antibiotics are given. Operative treatment may be deferred for a few hours, since in many cases a gradual improvement in the local and general condition is seen.

Indications for operation are:

(1) Increasing surgical emphysema.
(2) Abscess formation (*Figure 9.6b*).
(3) Evidence of pleural effusion.
(4) Progressive worsening of the general condition.

If the site of perforation is likely to be at a level above the arch of the aorta a cervical approach is made (p. 228). The oedematous tissues of the visceral compartment of the neck are explored and drained. In early cases a gush of saliva may be released but, later, pus will be found. Goligher (1948) advocates the earliest possible intervention and immediate repair of the torn viscus. However, this is only possible if the tear can be found, and if the tissues are as yet not oedematous and friable. In most cases only drainage can be achieved. If necessary, saliva or pus must be sought in the mediastinum by finger dissection downwards along the oesophageal wall. At the end of the operation a small oesophageal tube is passed gently from the nose into the stomach.

If the perforation is known to be below the level of the aortic arch, or the early development of pleural effusion makes this seem likely, the aid of a thoracic surgeon is essential since posterior mediastinotomy or possibly a trans-thoracic repair of the torn oesophagus is urgently required.

The management of any case of perforation of the oesophagus presents very great difficulties. If the site and cause of the perforation are known it becomes much easier to decide what to do, but these patients quickly become very ill and a second oesophagoscopy to locate the tear is not likely to give positive findings and may be very dangerous. Massive dosage of broad-spectrum antibiotics, and shrewd decision as to the timing and route of surgical drainage are the two essentials in treatment. The mortality of this complication is less than in the pre-antibiotic era, but it is still formidable.

Corrosive injury of the oesophagus

The swallowing of corrosive poisons is usually accidental in children and suicidal in adults. Strong solutions of caustic alkali are a rare household commodity in England, while the strong acids, such as sulphuric, nitric and hydrochloric, are only found in industry. The greatest damage when these poisons are swallowed is seen in the mouth and in the lower third of the oesophagus. While the mouth burns contribute largely to the patient's agony it is the injury to the oesophagus which determines the long-term outlook. The immediate question of survival hinges upon the acute disturbance of acid–base equilibrium and renal function, and upon the incidence of laryngeal oedema and bronchopneumonia. The last-named respiratory complications are more serious in cases due to ingestion of corrosives which give off injurious fumes such as strong ammonia, hydrochloric acid and fuming nitric acid.

Immediate treatment is directed towards the relief of shock and pain, and the neutralization of the corrosive by an appropriate weak acid or alkali given by mouth. Intravenous fluids and systemic (parenteral) antibiotics are commenced as soon as possible. Careful watch is kept for signs of laryngeal oedema which may call for tracheostomy. In close collaboration with the chemical pathologist the acid–base equilibrium and renal function must be studied and controlled by suitable regulation of the intravenous fluid–electrolyte input.

Prevention of stricture formation
An impassable stricture, usually of the lower oesophagus is extremely likely to occur if burning penetrates the muscular wall of the viscus. Modern therapy is aimed at preventing this by means of the insertion of an in-dwelling nasogastric tube within the first day or two of the illness. This, if done gently, is not as dangerous as it was once thought to be. Some authorities recommend oesophagoscopy at the earliest possible moment, although there seems to be little therapeutic advantage in this. The main thing is to get a tube down and keep it there until two or three weeks later when the

patient is ready for solid food. (A good bolus of well-chewed solid food is the best dilator of all if there is a lumen for it to pass through, and some muscle to drive it down.)

Systemic steroid therapy, if begun in the first two or three days of the illness, is considered to be effective in keeping fibrosis (and therefore stenosis) to a minimum.

In recent years cervical oesophagostomy has been found useful, especially in children, in permitting early and well-tolerated oesophageal intubation. Rubber is preferred to plastic for the tube in these cases because its physical properties are said to be more effective in preventing stricture formation. It has also the advantage later that if stenosis threatens, frequent passage of bougies is possible without the necessity for either training the patient to swallow them, or frequent general anaesthetics.

Delayed stenosis may develop after two or three months or even longer. It is less likely if the patient perseveres with a normal diet, but in all cases regular surveillance and repeated barium-swallow examinations should be maintained for at least six months. The treatment of an established stricture is discussed in more detail on p. 251 *et seq.*

Foreign bodies in the oesophagus

A complete study of foreign bodies in the oesophagus and upper respiratory tract was made by Jackson and Jackson (1936), who published records of over 3000 patients who had ingested foreign bodies. This is by far the largest series of cases. Each case history is described in detail with endoscopic findings, description of the foreign body and the type of forceps used for removal. Alpin (1934), Diggle (1932), Flett (1945), Mosher (1935), Phillips (1938), and Schlemmer (1920) reported on similar but smaller series.

Aetiology

Statistics show that coins and bones are the most common foreign bodies to lodge in the oesophagus. Open safety-pins and lumps of meat are the next in order of frequency. Jackson says that poor children who are not given individual attention and who are left to feed themselves at an early age are more liable to swallow a foreign body (Jackson and Jackson, 1936). The incidence of foreign bodies rises in old people who get lumps of meat impacted in the oesophagus; this may be due to the lack of propulsion efficiency or to the fact that the patient is often edentulous and therefore unable to masticate his food properly.

Dental factor
A patient who has an artificial denture is unable to detect a fish or meat bone in the mouth as easily as a person with a normal palate, and is therefore more likely to swallow a foreign body. Tough meat, if improperly chewed, may become impacted. If the denture or plate is ill-fitting or broken it may itself be swallowed and this occasionally occurs while the patient is drunk or asleep.

Oesophageal factor

Local conditions of the oesophagus may determine the impaction of a foreign body. A stricture of the oesophagus is more likely to occlude the passage of a small foreign body which would normally pass through. In a carcinomatous stricture the first sign of this disease may be the lodging of a foreign body, with the sudden onset of dysphagia or even aphagia.

Type of food

Carelessness in the preparation of food is a factor in the lodging of a foreign body. Certain types of food are eaten very rapidly because the patient does not suspect the presence of bones. Stews and soups may contain meat with splinters of bone attached if the meat has been prepared with a chopper. Fish cakes may also contain bones which may become impacted in the alimentary tract.

Voluntary swallowing

Foreign bodies are swallowed voluntarily by patients who attempt suicide, by prisoners and by mentally ill patients.

Types of foreign body

Foreign bodies may lodge in the oesophagus by reason of the nature of the foreign body. Coins and disc-shaped objects which pass through the mouth and pharynx of a child may then lodge in the upper part of the oesophagus. Open safety-pins stay in the oesophagus because of the resilience of the pin when the point is uppermost or by penetration of the oesophageal wall when the point is downwards.

Site

Coins lodge usually in the upper end of the oesophagus. Meat and soft foreign bodies may lodge above a stricture, and sharp foreign bodies, such as meat bones, may lodge anywhere, but most commonly in the upper end of the oesophagus.

Pathological changes caused by the foreign body

Coins may stay in the oesophagus for many months and cause only a slow ulceration of the oesophageal wall, but meat- and fish-bones will very soon give rise to ulceration, peri-oesophagitis and other complications.

History

The patient, if an adult, may be able to give a very accurate account of the type and shape of the foreign body swallowed. He is very often able to point to the exact site of the obstruction, particularly if the foreign body is lodging in the upper part of the oesophagus. When the foreign body is in the middle or lower third of the oesophagus localization is not so accurate and the pain is referred to the back or behind the sternum. The pain is of a sharp, 'cutting' nature, is worse with attempts to swallow, and occurs at the same place every time the patient swallows. A smooth foreign body may give rise to only a vague sensation of discomfort and not to actual pain. In children who cannot give a history, the presence of a foreign body may be unsuspected for several months. Dysphagia is nearly always present and is due to the size of the foreign body or inflammatory reaction and spasm caused by its presence.

At first there is only slight difficulty in swallowing but later the difficulty becomes more pronounced. There is also regurgitation of food and later regurgitation of blood-stained saliva and mucus. In the later stages when the obstruction is complete there may be pulmonary symptoms produced by the overflow of the oesophageal contents, which suggests the presence of a foreign body in the child's respiratory tract.

Examination

The patient must be observed during the act of swallowing. When a sharp foreign body is lodging in the upper part of the oesophagus, in the larynx or in the post-cricoid region, swallowing gives a definite expression of pain. Examination of the neck may show a tender swelling in the lower part of the neck medial to the sternomastoid muscle; this swelling is usually caused by the inflammatory reaction around the foreign body, by actual abscess or by surgical emphysema which is recognized by the accompanying crepitus. Tucker (1925) and Wright (1934) stressed the importance of tenderness on pressure on the trachea, and the former observer considers it pathognomonic of the presence of a foreign body in the cervical oesophagus if, on movement of the trachea and larynx towards the point of maximum tenderness, there is marked exacerbation of pain.

The mouth, pharynx, tonsillar region and base of the tongue must be examined with the use of a headlight and spatula. A small sharp foreign body, such as a fish bone, may lodge in the base of the tongue or tonsillar crypt, although the patient may be convinced that the foreign body has actually been swallowed. The area around the foreign body is bruised and inflamed.

Indirect pharyngoscopy and laryngoscopy must be extremely thoroughly carried out. Each part of the pharyngeal wall must be minutely studied in the mirror, otherwise the tip of a small fish bone almost completely buried in the tissues will be overlooked. If the patient can localize his pain to one side or the other, then the foreign body, or the laceration caused by its passage, must be above the cricoid level and should be visible in the mirror. Most foreign bodies which can be seen with the mirror can be removed without recourse to general anaesthesia. After receiving careful explanation of what is to be done, the patient cooperates by holding his own tongue in a piece of gauze, leaving the surgeon free to hold his mirror in his left hand and a pair of suitably angled grasping forceps in his right. The forceps are guided down the throat until the foreign body can be grasped and withdrawn. There must of course be no blind 'grab' – every step must be clearly observed in the mirror. There is no greater reward in all laryngology than to see the relief and gratitude of a patient who, in a matter of moments, is relieved of a fish bone in the pharynx. The technique, which requires a little practice, is well worth cultivating.

If no foreign body can be seen in the laryngeal mirror further investigations are necessary.

Radiological examination (*Figure 9.7*)

Plain films of the neck and chest are taken. If the foreign body is not revealed the neck, thorax and abdomen are screened. If an opaque shadow is still not seen a little barium sulphate is given and its passage down the gullet observed. The opaque

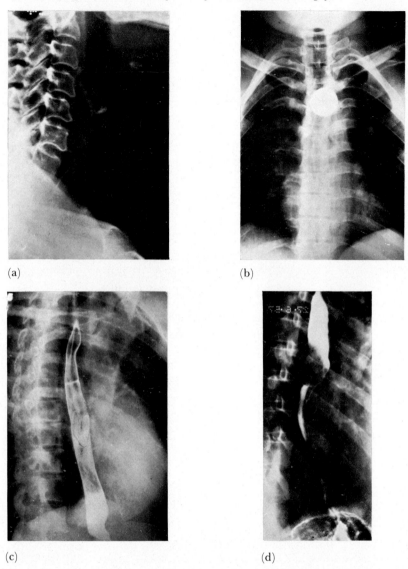

(a)   (b)

(c)   (d)

Figure 9.7   Foreign bodies in the oesophagus. (a) Chicken bone at thoracic inlet; (b) coin in the oesophagus of a child; (c) plastic denture faintly outlined by barium in the mid-thoracic oesophagus; (d) meat bolus, impacted at level of aortic arch

medium may be held up at one point and may actually outline the foreign body, or the flow of barium may be split. If the barium cannot be easily dislodged by further swallowing or washed down with water the presence of a foreign body is to be strongly suspected. An air bubble in the oesophagus in the region of the hold-up is very often indicative of a foreign body. In a difficult case a pledget of cotton-wool soaked in barium paste, or a gelatin capsule filled with barium may impact upon the foreign body, thus revealing its presence and position.

Management of a patient

The diagnosis is sometimes difficult if the foreign body is small and not opaque and if the radiological examination is inconclusive. If there is any doubt about the presence of a foreign body an oesophagoscopy is imperative. Even if the symptoms improve rapidly the patient must be kept under observation until he is completely symptom-free. Abrasion of the oesophageal mucosa will give some pain and cause dysphagia but usually these symptoms disappear rapidly. Increase of pain and dysphagia indicates the presence of a foreign body or some more serious damage to the oesophageal wall and warrants more active treatment, such as endoscopic examination.

Treatment

Although oesophagoscopy for the removal of a foreign body may be an emergency operation, the surgeon must have knowledge of the nature, size and site of the foreign body, and if possible a replica should be examined.

Coin in the oesophagus of a child
The radiological examination must be repeated immediately before the endoscopy is done because the coin may have passed into the stomach if there has been a delay between first seeing the patient and endoscopic examination. The oesophagoscope used is a small Negus type (35 cm in length), but an oesophageal speculum or even an anterior commissure laryngoscope may be the only instrument necessary in a small child if the coin is impacted in the upper end of the oesophagus. The instrument should be passed slowly because it is very easy to override the foreign body, especially if it has been in the oesophagus for some time, in which case it is coated with mucus. Any food debris is removed by suction. The operator must pass the oesophagoscope as near to the foreign body as possible, making sure he does not push the foreign body ahead. The coin must be maintained in the centre of the field. Alligator forceps are then passed and the coin is seized firmly and brought out until it impinges on the end of the oesophagoscope. The forceps are fixed by the surgeon at the proximal end of the oesophagoscope so that the foreign body, forceps and oesophagoscope can be pulled out of the oesophagus together. Care must be taken, when the foreign body is passing the cricopharyngeus, that the coin is turned so that it lies in the coronal plane. Often, despite this, it slips off when being pulled over the sphincter and may be found lying in the hypopharynx; for its removal a laryngoscope is then necessary.

A sharp foreign body in the oesophagus
A sharp foreign body such as a meat bone or fish bone may lodge anywhere in the oesophagus and, unless the position is verified by a radiograph, a full-length oesophagoscope must be used.

The anaesthetist must take care not to pass the intratracheal tube blindly because it may accidentally go into the oesophagus and cause the foreign body to perforate the oesophageal wall. The oesophagoscope is passed until the foreign body is seen and the surgeon must resist any temptation to extract the foreign body quickly without noting the position of its sharp edge. The problem is not simply to remove the foreign body but to remove it with little or no risk to the patient. Mucus, food debris, and any barium which has been left after an x-ray examination, are removed by suction. If the end of the foreign body is free the forceps are passed and the end is gripped. If any bleeding occurs a swab soaked in adrenaline is introduced. If the ends of the foreign body are buried in the oesophageal wall, manipulation is necessary to try to release one end and to get a point of the foreign body into the tube, so that its long axis is parallel with the oesophagoscope.

A small bone may be extracted through the oesophagoscope, but a large one should be treated as for a coin and removed with the oesophagoscope and forceps. The patient should be kept under close observation because this type of foreign body is likely to cause complications.

Meat and soft foreign bodies

Meat and soft foreign bodies are extracted piecemeal. Cancer of the oesophagus may present as a case of an impacted food bolus. Therefore, after endoscopic removal of the impacted meat or other food it is important to pass the oesophagoscope again and to check that there is no underlying intrinsic oesophageal lesion. If the patient refuses to undergo oesophagoscopy or if there is some contra-indication to endoscopy, the method advised by Richardson (1945) should be tried. In this method papain, which contains enzymes similar to pepsin, is given by mouth. This solution acts in an acid medium and is said to digest 30 times its weight of lean meat. A five per cent solution dissolved in ten per cent alcohol is used and 1 ml is given by mouth every 15 minutes. The obstruction is said to be relieved in 2–3 hours without any reaction or complications. If no treatment at all is given the meat will be digested in time but this may take 7–14 days.

Safety-pin in the oesophagus

An open safety-pin presents no difficulty if the sharp point is distal. If the point is proximal there is often great difficulty, and several methods have been devised to overcome it. If it is not too large it may be possible to turn the pin in the oesophagus, or alternatively to manipulate the point of the pin into the lumen of the oesophagoscope. Some endoscopists prefer to cut the pin *in situ* using endoscopic shears, or to close it with Clerf's or similar forceps. If all else fails, the pin may be grasped with rotation forceps at the ring, pushed into the stomach and allowed to rotate and then be extracted through the oesophagus with the point trailing.

Denture in the oesophagus

A denture in the oesophagus presents many hazards. The radiograph should be studied carefully with special regard to the hooks and points on the denture. During oesophagoscopy the hook should, if possible, be manipulated into the lumen of the oesophagoscope before extraction. The denture may be impacted and may have to be divided *in situ*. If there is any gross trauma of the oesophagus by the foreign body or if any previous manipulation has been performed endoscopic removal should be delayed, and it is better to wait until the inflammatory reaction has subsided and do the oesophagoscopy some days later. In the meantime the patient should be treated as for a peri-oesophagitis or perforation of the oesophagus with systemic antibiotics.

External operation for removal of foreign body

The majority of foreign bodies which lodge in the oesophagus can be removed endoscopically. Guisez, in a series of 530 foreign bodies, had only to remove three, or 0.6 per cent, by the external route. There are instances, however, in which an external operation is preferable.

The majority of foreign bodies are situated in the upper or cervical part of the oesophagus. Large and irregular foreign bodies, such as dentures, may present great difficulty in removal. Oesophagoscopy may so injure the oesophagus as to cause great damage and complications.

The following types of foreign bodies may require removal by the external route:

(1) An impacted foreign body.
(2) A foreign body producing peri-oesophagitis after unsuccessful attempts at removal through the oesophagoscope.
(3) A peri-oesophageal abscess with a foreign body lodging in the abscess itself.

Inflammation of the oesophagus

Aetiology

Apart from the inflammatory changes which result from corrosives and foreign bodies, inflammation can occur from a number of other causes.

Diphtheritic, tuberculous, and *syphilitic oesophagitis* are all rare today. Each occurs as a complication of its 'parent' disease, and will be recognized by its characteristic type of ulceration at oesophagoscopy, presence of membranous exudate, bacteriological investigations and, where appropriate, biopsy findings. Treatment is that of the causative disease.

Fungal infection occasionally causes oesophagitis with marked dysphagia. It may complicate a thrush (monilial) infection of the mouth and pharynx in infants and young children. It can also occur in elderly or debilitated patients, causing the acute onset of severe dysphagia with considerable pain. Very occasionally fungal oeso-phagitis is a complication of broad-spectrum antibiotic therapy. Treatment consists of correction of dehydration, parenteral administration of vitamins, and a suspension of nystatin given by mouth every 2–3 hours. In very severe cases a nasogastric feeding tube may be needed for a few days.

Non-specific types of oesophagitis

Gastric and duodenal juices in the oesophagus set up chronic inflammatory changes, with ulceration, pain, dysphagia and sometimes bleeding. Acid, pepsin and bile salts are probably the most important factors in this process (Gillison *et al.*, 1972). The condition may occur as a result of protracted vomiting, or very rarely may be due to secretion of gastric acid and enzymes by islets of gastric mucosa in the walls of the oesophagus. As a congenital condition these islets are considered to be a rare curiosity. The most common cause of lower oesophagitis is hiatus hernia (*see later*), in which derangement of the cardiac sphincteric mechanism allows frequent re-gurgitation. Gastric contents are especially likely to rise in the oesophagus when the patient lies down. In late cases chronic inflammation is followed by fibrosis and stricture formation.

Localized inflammation of the wall of the oesophagus may be caused by the pressure of an oesophageal feeding tube if it is retained for long periods. Oesophagitis is invariably present above strictures, and in achalasia of the cardia, due to stagnation of undigested food particles. Inflammatory changes, with superficial erosions, are commonly observed in relation to large varices of the lower oesophagus in cases of portal hypertension. Reflux oesophagitis is a frequent complication of oesophagogastric anastomosis when this technique is used to restore continuity after partial oesophagectomy. At its upper end the oesophagus is sometimes involved in the inflammatory changes of Paterson–Brown Kelly disease (*see* Chapters 1 and 2).

Leucoplakia

Long-continued irritation of the oesophageal lining can result in the formation of areas of leucoplakia and the risk of carcinoma. Localized patches of hyperkeratosis and pre-malignant change are seen in chronic oesophagitis due to almost any of the above-mentioned causes.

Diagnosis

The diagnosis of oesophagitis is usually evident from the history, barium-swallow and oesophagoscopic findings.

Treatment

The cause is removed whenever possible. The gullet is rested by restriction of diet to soft foods and fluids. Gastric acidity is reduced by appropriate alkalis taken by mouth. The most effective remedy is Gaviscon, an antacid/alginate compound. Bennett (1976) attributes its efficacy to the formation of a non-irritant gel which floats on the gastric contents and is therefore the main component of any reflux into the oesophagus. It may be re-inforced in the early stages of treatment with any standard antacid, excepting ones containing polymethyl siloxane.

If these drugs are not effective by themselves metoclopramide, which increases the tone of the lower oesophageal sphincter and improves oesophageal motility, may be added to the regimen.

The H_2-receptor blocker, cimetidine, is effective in reducing gastric secretion. It gives good symptomatic relief but patients experience immediate return of symptoms when administration ceases. Gastric reflux is prevented as far as possible by the avoidance of bending and stooping, avoidance of 'indigestible' foods, and over-eating, and by persuading the patient to sleep propped up in a sitting position. It is important to persuade the patient to abandon any smoking habit. In cases due to hiatus hernia successful weight reduction helps a great deal, while the failure of medical treatment indicates surgical repair of the diaphragmatic hiatus (*see below*).

Hiatus hernia

Hiatus hernia may be defined as a displacement of the stomach into the lower mediastinum through the oesophageal opening of the diaphragm. Two main types are recognized (*Figure 9.8*).

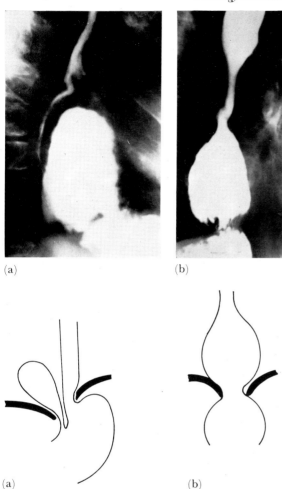

(a)   (b)

(a)   (b)

Figure 9.8 Hiatus hernia. (a) Para-oesophageal type; (b) 'sliding' type with associated stricture formation at and above the displaced cardia

Para-oesophageal hernia

A peritoneal sac leads from the abdominal cavity upwards alongside the oesophagus. Within the sac a varying amount of the stomach is found, but the cardia lies at or below the level of the diaphragm. Flavell (1963) states that this type of hiatus hernia is always congenital, although the more usual view has been that in most cases it is an acquired condition.

Sliding hernia

Laxity of the hiatal orifice permits the entry of the gastro-oesophageal junction into the thorax whenever intra-abdominal pressure is raised. This process is almost literally the 'thin end of the wedge', and once it has begun to occur, the hiatus becomes more and more widely stretched, and more and more of the stomach follows the cardia into the chest. The angulation between the oesophagus and stomach is lost, and with it muscular control of the gastro-oesophageal junction. Reflux oesophagitis is then inevitable, and may lead to fibrous stenosis and shortening of the oesophagus.

Although this kind of hernia occurs in infants and children, it is common in middle-aged and elderly patients. It is probably due to the well-known causes of raised abdominal pressure – obesity, flatulence, constipation, pregnancy and corsets. Most of these factors beset humanity when the muscles, including the diaphragm, are somewhat past their prime. Flavell points out that crush injuries of the abdominal region may cause hiatus hernia, even in young patients with good muscles.

Management

In the *para-oesophageal* cases oesophagitis is absent, and diagnosis may therefore be long delayed. Breathlessness on exertion if the herniation is large, or anaemia secondary to ulceration and bleeding in the thoracic portion of the stomach, may be overlooked or attributed to other causes, unless a barium-swallow is done. Treatment is surgical. The stomach is replaced in the abdomen and the hiatus is repaired.

Sliding hiatus hernia is characterized by the symptoms of reflux oesophagitis, in addition to breathlessness if the hernia is large. Complications such as bleeding and stricture formation are common, and are pressing indications for surgical repair of the diaphragm. Thoracic surgeons, naturally enough, advocate surgical treatment as the principal line of attack in hiatus hernia. The hardships and hazards endured by the elderly patient, in whom many years of conservative treatment have merely served to postpone operation until he is no longer fit to undergo it, are a grim warning. Each individual case will be assessed carefully on its merits. In very early cases, in the very old and in infants, it will usually be best to adopt medical treatment (*see* p. 244). Severe cases, those with complications, and those becoming worse despite conservative treatment, should be advised operation. The newer techniques of gastroplication (Belsey, 1966; Logan, 1967; Nissen, Rossetti and Markman, 1965) in which effective valvular action is restored at the lower end of the oesophagus, are reported to give satisfactory results and a very low recurrence rate.

Achalasia of the cardia or cardiospasm

In considering the various causes of dysphagia, achalasia of the cardia or 'cardiospasm', although not commonplace, is by no means rare, and is therefore of importance to the laryngologist.

In this condition there is degeneration of the ganglion cells in Auerbach's plexus. No coordinated peristalsis occurs in the oesophagus and the lower oesophageal sphincter fails to relax in response to each swallow. As a result, there is retention of food in the oesophagus and distension of the lumen which gradually increases to produce the gross mega-oesophagus seen in museum specimens. In the early stages the muscles of the oesophageal wall are healthy but gradually they become atrophic and the wall thins down while the mucosa becomes ulcerated through food stasis. There is an increased incidence of carcinoma developing as a result of these changes. Joske and Benedict (1959) estimated the chances as seven times the normal, while Ellis (1960) in his series, found a 20 per cent incidence of carcinoma.

Aetiology

This has aroused much interest and controversy, and the cause remains unknown. The essential pathological change is probably in the ganglion cells of Auerbach's plexus. There is round-cell infiltration and sclerosis in the plexus and in the smooth muscle fibres of the oesophageal wall. Similar changes also occur in the striated muscle of the upper third of the oesophagus, in the lower oesophageal sphincter and sometimes in the muscles of the upper part of the cardia of the stomach. Cosella *et al.* (1964) have also found degenerative changes in the neurones of both vagal trunks and in the cells of their central nuclei. It has been postulated that these occur secondarily to the loss of the Auerbach ganglion cells by trans-synaptic retrograde degeneration.

Earlam (1972) proposes the theory that the original degeneration occurs *in utero* and is due to temporary ischaemia of this area during rotation of the gut while there is still a large umbilical hernia. Because of the especial sensitivity of nerve tissue to oxygen lack this could damage the ganglion cells but leave the other tissues unaffected.

Chagas' disease is an infection with *Trypanosoma cruzi*, and occurs mainly in South America and especially in Brazil. The course is prolonged but over a period of up to 30 years the trypanosomes infiltrate the intermuscular lymphatics of the gut wall and gradually destroy the ganglion cells. Changes in the colon are six times as common as in the oesophagus. When the latter is affected the changes exactly mimic achalasia. This is important evidence that the oesophageal changes in achalasia do start in the ganglion cells.

Clinical picture

The condition is of more frequent occurrence in men than in women. It may occur at any age, but is most often seen between the ages of 30 and 60, a common early symptom being epigastric discomfort, or a feeling of fullness in the upper abdomen.

Later dysphagia occurs, but unlike the unrelenting and slowly progressive dysphagia of malignant disease of the oesophagus, it may be marked by temporary remissions. After these early symptoms have been present for many months or even years regurgitation is noticed. The volume regurgitated is at first slight, but after a time becomes more bulky, until eventually enormous quantities of frothy mucus mixed with swallowed food and fluids may be brought back. Loss of weight is moderate and, as a rule, by no means so pronounced as in oesophageal malignancy.

In advanced cases pulmonary complications, due to inhalation, are common, and pulmonary osteo-arthropathy is described in association with the condition.

Diagnosis

Radiological examination and oesophagoscopy confirm the diagnosis (*Figure 9.9a*). In the earliest stages the lower oesophagus is spindle-shaped, and the meal passes in a narrow ribbon-like stream into the stomach. Later, the obstruction and dilatation become more marked and no barium enters the stomach. A fluid level may be

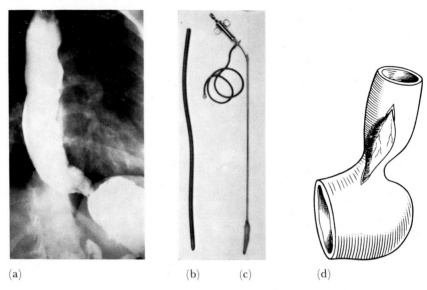

(a)   (b)   (c)   (d)

Figure 9.9   Achalasia of the cardia. (a) Typical radiographic appearances; (b) Hurst's mercury-filled bougie; (c) hydrostatic dilator (Negus); (d) Heller's operation showing the incision of the muscle coats

demonstrated, and in advanced cases the oesophagus will hold as much as 500 ml of fluid.

The oesophagus may be fusiform, spindle-shaped, pear-shaped or S-shaped; fusiform dilatation is most common. At first there is spasm involving the cardia and cardiac ampulla; Allison (1943) has demonstrated that the mucosal junction lies above the constricted portion. In the earliest stages there is only moderate dilatation in the plain muscle segment above the constriction, up to the level of the aorta, and above this the dilatation is much greater. Later, the lower segment becomes more dilated, but the upper segment still remains the wider portion.

No normal peristalsis occurs, and if waves are seen they are irregular in the lower segment or plain muscle portion. In the late stages of the disease the oesophagus shows no peristalsis, the muscular tissue becomes atrophic and the mucosa is thickened. This thickening is responsible for the visibility of the organ without barium. It is important to note that the outline of the lower end of the oesophagus is smooth and regular as distinct from the irregular outline often (but not invariably) seen in cases of malignant disease.

Oesophagoscopy is mandatory. Not only has the diagnosis to be confirmed, but a coexisting carcinoma must be carefully excluded. Oesophageal carcinoma complicating achalasia constitutes a well-known diagnostic trap, and Groves (1956), who reviewed the literature, himself adding two cases, drew attention to the difficulty of diagnosis. He emphasized that oesophagoscopy, with careful study of the entire length of the oesophagus, is called for, pointing out that even direct endoscopy may fail to demonstrate a large tumour if the oesophageal wall is dilated and obscured by retained food and secretion. There are many parallel instances where the finding of a relatively benign condition may obscure and delay the diagnosis of a coexisting sinister lesion.

The patient should be admitted two days before oesophagoscopy. The oesophagus should be washed out twice daily with a wide-bore stomach tube and the diet must be liquid. After anaesthesia is induced, but before passage of the oesophagoscope, the viscus should be aspirated through a wide-bore catheter. These measures will avoid wasting much time clearing the oesophagus of retained food before proper inspection can begin. The mucosa lining the dilated oesophagus is generally found to be unhealthy and may be ulcerated and bleed readily. Longitudinal folds can often be seen. The oesophagoscopist may have the feeling that he is groping in a strange and almost boundless territory, and it is not always a matter of simplicity to find the cardia. Once found, however, a large bougie should pass with ease; in fact, any difficulty encountered in instrumentation calls for careful exclusion of malignant stricture.

Treatment

Conservative treatment by drugs such as octyl nitrite has, on the whole, been disappointing, but one form of conservative treatment which has been used for many years and is undoubtedly of value is regular dilatation by means of a Hurst mercury bougie (*Figure 9.9b*). This method has the advantage that it can be used by the patient himself, the bougie either being swallowed before each main meal, or less frequently in less severe cases. It is of importance that on the first occasion of bouginage an x-ray should be taken in order to confirm the presence of the bougie in the cardiac sphincter.

In other cases dilatation with a Negus hydrostatic bag (*Figure 9.9c*) is carried out under direct vision through a wide-bore oesophagoscope. The empty bag is introduced through the sphincter, then slowly filled with water, stretching the muscle. This method of dilatation may have to be repeated several times but often affords lasting relief.

Dilatation with Starck's expanding metal dilator is hardly mentioned in any article or textbook which considers the treatment of this condition. The methods and the results of treatment are recorded by Starck (1934, 1936) and by Schindler (1956) in a total of 500–600 cases without a fatality and minor complications in less than two per cent.

The method is used by a few surgeons in this country, but Scott-Brown (personal communication) reports 30 years' experience with this dilator with no fatality, no complications in any case, and excellent results in 80 per cent of cases after one dilatation. It is important to carry out a sudden dilatation without an anaesthetic and when the cardia is in spasm. It is only in those cases where the spasm yields before rupture of the fibres takes place that a further 1–3 dilatations are necessary.

This method of treatment has also been used in a few cases of failed cardio-myotomies without any complications and with good permanent results (Scott-Brown, 1964).

Bennett and Hendrix (1970) report their experience of the Hurst–Tucker dilator. This has an inflatable cuff near the distal end of a Hurst mercury bougie. The cuff is radio-opaque and has a maximum diameter of 3 cm. It can be passed under radiological control and the cuff pressure is measured by a manometer. Most patients were dilated up to a pressure of 618 mmHg (12 psi). Treating 61 patients they had good results in 70 per cent of cases. However, in three cases they could not pass the bougie at the initial attempt and in three cases the oesophagus was torn.

Operative treatment is by Heller's operation of cardiomyotomy, first described in 1914 and again in detail by Barlow (1942).

The approach is via the abdomen or a left-sided thoracotomy, and after exposure an anterior longitudinal incision is made through the muscular wall at the cardio-oesophageal junction down to, but not through, the mucous membrane (*Figure 9.9d*). Ellis (1962) has drawn attention to the remarkable propensity of the muscle to heal, with possible recurrence of symptoms, and the importance of making a long incision (at least 12 cm) and carrying out submucous dissection. However, despite recurrence of symptoms and reflux oesophagitis in a few cases, extremely good results are claimed (Acheson and Hadley, 1958; Douglas and Nicholson, 1959; le Roux and Wright, 1960). In some cases, however, operations of the Wangensteen-type (1951) in which portions of redundant oesophagus and stomach are excised are considered more appropriate.

Diverticula of the oesophagus

The following section refers to pouches or diverticula of the oesophagus proper and has no bearing on diverticula of the hypopharynx, which are more common and more familiar to the ear, nose and throat surgeon. Unfortunately, the term 'oesophageal pouch' is still sometimes inaccurately used to include both the oesophageal and the hypopharyngeal variety.

It is usual to classify diverticula of the oesophagus as of the 'pulsion' type or the 'traction' type, and Barrett, in a classical paper on this subject in 1933, added a third variety: the 'traction–pulsion' diverticulum.

Pulsion diverticula

These are due to herniation of the mucous membrane through the muscular walls of the oesophagus. The underlying cause may be a congenital weakness or defect in the muscle, and increasing pressure from retained food leads to an increase in the size of the pouch.

Most of these pulsion diverticula occur in the lower two-thirds of the oesophagus and cause, at first, dyspepsia and a sensation of fullness in the chest and, later, dysphagia due to pressure on the oesophagus below. The diagnosis is established by barium-swallow and oesophagoscopy, and treatment, if called for, consists of removal of the pouch by thoracotomy. If a pouch is not causing symptoms and is discovered accidentally no active treatment is advised.

Traction diverticula

Traction diverticula occur most commonly in the middle third of the oesophagus (*Figure 9.10a*) and are caused by adhesions between the latter and adjacent structures. This region contains numerous lymph nodes, and the most common cause of a

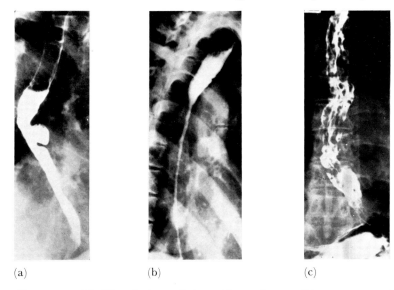

(a)   (b)   (c)

Figure 9.10   (a) Diverticulum of the mid-oesophagus; (b) severe corrosive stricture; (c) oesophageal varices

traction diverticulum of the mid-oesophagus is fibrosis following tuberculous disease of these nodes.

In contrast to the smooth downward convexity of the pulsion diverticulum, the traction pouches, which may be multiple, tend to have an irregular outline and to be directed upwards; thus, food is unlikely to collect in them, although fatal mediastinitis has been recorded as a result of perforation (Smith, 1928).

Non-malignant strictures of the oesophagus

Aetiology and pathology

Most oesophageal strictures, apart from the congenital type which is uncommon, are a complication of acute or chronic oesophagitis which has encroached on the muscular layer of the oesophageal wall. Serious damage results from the swallowing of corrosive poisons and very young children may develop a stricture after swallowing hot fluids. Damage to the muscular layers of the oesophagus by hasty removal of a foreign body or from prolonged impaction of a foreign body, causing peri-oesophagitis and abscess formation, may give rise to stenosis. Reflux oesophagitis due to hiatus hernia, or prolonged vomiting, may cause ulceration in the lower end of the oesophagus and this ulceration may give rise to a simple stricture.

At the upper end of the gullet, stricture and web formation occur in association with the Paterson–Brown Kelly syndrome. In the middle third of the oesophagus there may be a congenital narrowing and Brown Kelly (1936) considers that during adult life a superimposed infection may cause further narrowing of the oesophagus. Simple strictures may also follow external injury to the oesophagus and occur very occasionally in typhoid fever and in scarlet fever. The most common post-operative complication of operations which entail oesophageal anastomosis is a fibrous stricture at the suture line. Fibrotic stenosis of the oesophagus also occurs as a late development in scleroderma, a rare form of collagen disease.

Complications
If an untreated stricture becomes impermeable or so narrow that it is easily blocked by food and debris, malnutrition, dehydration and starvation may result. Chronic infection of the lungs from regurgitation and aspiration of oesophageal contents can occur, especially in children; occasionally there is malignant change in the scar.

Symptoms

After the ingestion of a caustic, the patient has difficulty in swallowing caused by acute ulcerative pharyngitis, and when initial reaction has subsided there is usually a period during which the patient swallows without any apparent difficulty. The medical attendant may hope that the return of normal swallowing will indicate that no permanent damage to the oesophagus has occurred, but only too soon dysphagia re-appears with the formation of a stricture. At first the dysphagia may be only slight and intermittent owing to temporary obstruction of the lumen of the stricture caused by an irritative spasm and inflammatory reaction. In untreated patients fluids and even saliva are eventually regurgitated. The sudden onset of complete oesophageal obstruction in a patient who had previously only slight difficulty in swallowing indicates a 'corking' of the lumen of the stricture by a hard foreign body such as a bolus of food.

Examination

On general examination no clinical abnormality, apart from malnutrition, may be found. Radiography with barium-swallow will show the site of the narrowing.

Some observers have noted that strictures after the swallowing of corrosives are more common at the sites of normal narrowing of the oesophagus, at the crossing of the left bronchus, at the upper end of the oesophagus and at the diaphragmatic narrowing. The oesophagus is only moderately dilated above the stricture and never to the degree shown in achalasia of the cardia.

In a stricture which is caused by instrumental trauma or by a congenital defect the lumen is regular and the length of the stenosis short, but in a stricture due to corrosive poisoning the lumen of the oesophagus is irregular and the stricture is long and multiple (*Figure 9.10b*). The differential diagnosis between simple and malignant strictures of the oesophagus by radiological methods is often difficult, especially if there is no definite history of trauma to the oesophageal wall. Above a carcinomatous stricture there is little or no dilatation of the oesophagus and the stricture itself has a more tortuous and irregular channel than the simple type.

Oesophagoscopy

Above a simple stricture the oesophageal mucosa may be normal, but if the stricture has been present for some time evidence of chronic oesophagitis will be apparent. The oesophageal lumen may be central or eccentric and if the stricture is very narrow the oesophagus above will be dilated and will contain debris and food particles. Near the stricture the mucosa is dull and thickened, and granulation tissue may be present. The stricture is recognizable by the pallor of the mucosa and by the lack of elasticity of the oesophagus. When an attempt is made to pass the oesophagoscope further along the lumen the rosette appearance of the normal oesophageal mucosa changes to a dull white inelastic membrane.

Treatment

The stricture must be examined through the oesophagoscope and preliminary dilatation performed under direct vision. The wide Negus oesophagoscope is ideal for this method of treatment because it allows an unobstructed view of the end of the bougie. The contents of the oesophagus must be aspirated until an accurate view of the lumen of the stricture can be obtained. The stricture is dilated by the use of tapering soft fine gum-elastic bougies. These are passed in increasing sizes until difficulty is experienced. There are many types of bougie in use: the flexible gum-elastic bougie of Jackson, the olive-headed bougies of Vinson and the dilatable bougies of Tucker and Negus. There may be a small amount of bleeding after the passage of the dilator in the early stages of treatment. Care has to be taken because there is a tendency for the bougie to pass into a pocket next to the lumen of the stricture and to cause a false passage. Dilatation by bougie under direct vision is the first and principal method of treatment. Dilatation may have to be done very frequently and even when the stricture is fully dilated the patient should be kept under observation, and any return of dysphagia will necessitate further treatment. The patient should be advised to take care with food and should always masticate properly and avoid swallowing large lumps of food which may lodge in the oesophagus.

In a case requiring frequent dilatation the patient may be taught to swallow the bougie himself. No force is used. Many endoscopists maintain that blind bouginage is dangerous and quote Truman, the French clinician, who said that 'a patient using a bougie would sooner or later die of the instrument'. The practice of blind bouginage is not often done now but some laryngologists advise the use of a Hurst mercury tube which can be used by the patient himself.

Impermeable stricture
An impermeable stricture is rare. If a gastrostomy has been performed and dye, taken through the mouth, cannot be found in the gastric contents, then the obstruction is said to be complete. Usually there is a pin-point opening through the stricture and, with practice, a twisted silk thread can be swallowed or a very small bougie coaxed through the lumen. Closure of the stricture occurs slowly except when it is 'corked' by a foreign body. It is usually in neglected cases that an impermeable stricture occurs.

Oesophagoscopy must be done as a preliminary measure in an attempt to dilate the stricture. If no passage is found a gastrostomy should be performed. Such an operation is also necessary if an adequate and permanent dilatation cannot be maintained or if the mechanical obstruction is causing starvation. A gastrostomy gives physiological rest to the oesophagus, allows any inflammation to subside and very often enables bouginage to be restarted.

Treatment of the impermeable stricture is difficult. Among many methods which have been advised are:

(1) Establishment of the lumen by oesophagoscope: the oesophagus is ballooned from above, and forceps or a small metal bougie is pushed through the occluding membrane.
(2) Combined oesophagoscopy from above and bouginage from below.

Retrograde bouginage

A stricture which cannot be dilated from above may still be permeable from below where the lumen narrows like a funnel towards the lesion, and the entrance to the stricture is concentrically placed. A small oesophagoscope is inserted through the gastrostomy into the lower oesophagus and bougies are then passed up through it. It is a help if the patient can swallow a thread which finds its way through the stricture and is recovered from the gastrostomy opening. The bougie can then be attached to the thread and guided up through the stomach to the stricture by gentle traction upon the upper end through the mouth. Alternatively, the ends of the thread may be joined to form an endless loop, by which olive-shaped dilators, graduated in size, can be drawn up through the stricture.

By whatever method it is achieved bouginage must be continued, daily at first, and later at longer intervals. Neglect of follow-up care all too often results in the return of severe obstruction or aphagia. Bouginage is more often successful with short annular strictures than with long tubular ones.

Surgical treatment

If bouginage fails to establish or maintain a satisfactory lumen external operation is required. The type of operation depends on the upper level at which the oesophagus is diseased. Strictures of the lower half may be dealt with by oesophagectomy, mobilization of the stomach and an oesophagogastric anastomosis above the level of the aortic arch. If the upper oesophagus is also involved the anastomosis may be made in the neck. In some cases a jejunal or colonic transplant may be preferable to bringing up the stomach. The thoracic surgeon today has a wide choice of techniques for dealing with these problems, thanks to the progress of the last 20 years in oesophageal surgery for cancer.

In frail elderly patients unfit for major thoracic surgery, the failure of bouginage to give lasting benefit justifies insertion of a Souttar, Celestin or Mousseau Barbin tube (*see* pp.258–259).

Oesophageal varices

Cirrhosis of the liver due to any cause gives rise to portal hypertension, and this raised pressure results in varicosity wherever the portal and systemic venous systems converge. At the lower end of the oesophagus such varicosities form an irregular, tortuous mesh in the submucosa. They are subject to repeated trauma by swallowed food, and often the overlying mucosa is affected by reflux oesophagitis. Sooner or later haematemesis occurs, with grave danger to life.

The condition may be diagnosed by barium-swallow (*Figure 9.10c*) and oesophagoscopy which reveals varicosities reaching high into the oesophagus and, at the lower end, projecting into its lumen.

Treatment

When life is immediately in danger from profuse bleeding the most effective treatment is by means of a Sengstaken tube. This is passed into the stomach, the lower balloon is inflated and traction is applied so that the veins of the cardia are compressed from below. The upper balloon is then used to compress the veins in the lowest part of the oesophagus.

Some workers, notably Macbeth (1955), advocated strongly the use of sclerosing injections for the control of bleeding. A special syringe designed for use through the oesophagoscope is necessary. The method has not found much favour, despite the obvious advantages as compared with the Sengstaken tube, or external operative measures.

Definitive treatment consists of porto-caval anastomosis, which can relieve the causative portal hypertension. Partial oesophagogastrectomy destroys the faulty collateral venous circulation and, by diminishing gastric secretions, lessens the risk of oesophagitis. This procedure is indicated in cases in which porto-caval anastomosis is not feasible.

Neoplasms of the oesophagus

Benign neoplasms

Benign tumours are very rare. Leiomyoma, occurring as a tumour of smooth muscle, arises usually in the lower one-third of the oesophagus. It may reach a large size as an encircling submucosal mass which can be completely shelled out at thoracotomy without resection.

Other benign tumours, such as fibroma, papilloma, haemangioma and cysts, can occur at any level, and rarely are pedunculated so that they can be regurgitated into the mouth. Such tumours may be suspected from the history and the barium-swallow findings. Oesophagoscopy permits their diagnosis and endoscopic removal.

Malignant growths

Fibrosarcoma, leiomyosarcoma, lymphosarcoma, melanosarcoma and rhabdo-myosarcoma are exceedingly rare.

Carcinoma

Squamous-celled carcinoma is the most common tumour at any level in the oesophagus. At the lower end a fair proportion of adenocarcinomas are found. These arise from mucous glands in the oesophageal wall, or by extension of gastric carcinoma upwards, beyond the cardia.

Oesophageal carcinoma occurs most frequently after the age of 50, and is many times more common in men than in women. The cause is unknown, but predisposing factors are recognized, such as long-standing chronic oesophagitis, fibrous stricture, achalasia of the cardia, and Paterson–Brown Kelly syndrome.

The tumour, usually ulcerative in form with surrounding submucosal extensions, soon encircles the oesophagus. Obstruction follows, partly from stenosis and partly from the intraluminal mass of the tumour. Less often a fungating tumour distends the lumen from within, although it fails to encircle the gut, and obstruction is then less marked.

Direct spread of the growth occurs in submucosal lymphatics and this may result in 'satellite' ulcers at a distance, with apparently normal tissue intervening. Extrinsic spread involves the mediastinal contents, especially the trachea and bronchi leading to fistula formation, the recurrent laryngeal nerves causing vocal cord paralysis, and the great vessels. Metastases occur in the lymph nodes of the mediastinum, root of neck, and coeliac area. Secondary (blood-borne) deposits are common in the lungs and the liver.

Symptoms
It must be emphasized that obstruction sufficiently marked to cause symptoms occurs late in the course of the disease. Once established, dysphagia is rapidly progressive and in a matter of weeks loss of weight and dehydration are severe. Total obstruction may occur at any time due to the impaction of a fragment of food. Dysphagia of long standing is more likely to be due to a non-malignant cause than a cancer, but it must be remembered that benign disease of the oesophagus may conceal the later onset of a carcinoma. Pain due to oesophageal carcinoma is not common, and usually is a sign of spread in the mediastinum.

Diagnosis is made as a result of the systematic investigations described at the beginning of this chapter. Some comments regarding the radiographic and endoscopic findings are now made.

Radiography (Figure 9.11)
Soft tissue films are taken to show whether there is any enlargement of the visceral tissues at the root of the neck or in the mediastinum. Barium-swallow is then carried out. This immediately outlines the upper end of the lesion, and if it is permeable, a trickle passes on through the stricture. An irregular filling defect, an everted upper edge to the mass, and the familiar 'rat-tailed' attenuation of the barium stream are all

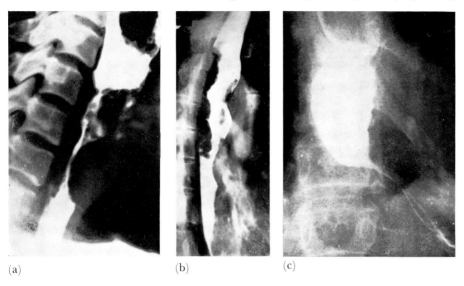

(a)   (b)   (c)

Figure 9.11   Carcinoma of the oesophagus. (a) Growth at and below the cricopharyngeus level; (b) growth at mid-thoracic level – a long ragged filling defect; (c) carcinoma of the lower end. Differential diagnosis from benign stricture due to reflux oesophagitis may be difficult

suggestive of malignant disease. The lower limit of the tumour can sometimes be roughly indicated by the use of Trendelenburg's position, which allows barium to flow back again to the lesion. The examination must be abandoned if opaque medium enters the bronchial tree through a broncho-oesophageal fistula. Radiography can be relied upon always to show the level of the lesion (unless the latter is so small that a normal picture is produced), but differential diagnosis between benign and malignant strictures can be difficult.

Oesophagoscopy is essential in any case of suspected malignancy of the oesophagus, and in all cases in which abnormal radiographic appearances are noted in the gullet. The site of the ulcer or stricture is inspected and the distance of the lesion from the line of the upper teeth or alveolar margin is measured.

The type of ulceration is noted. A rough hard knobbly surface indicates the probable presence of malignancy, whereas a softer stricture with surface ulceration is more likely to result from reflux oesophagitis.

Inspection of the upper surface of a stricture will give no clue as to the length of gullet involved in the stricture, but by passing a Jackson type of bougie through the stricture and then withdrawing it until the shoulder of the upper part of the bougie is felt to be caught by the lower surface of the stricture, the surgeon may gain some idea of its length.

Whenever an oesophagoscopy is carried out an examination of the main bronchial tree should be made at the same time if malignant disease is suspected. In many cases the gullet becomes involved by direct extension from an undiagnosed bronchial growth. In other cases a primary oesophageal cancer spreads into the tracheo-bronchial tree. If either of these complications is present it indicates that the lesion has progressed beyond all help of any treatment other than alleviation of symptoms.

Biopsy

In all cases, a piece of tissue should be removed through the oesophagoscope for microscopic examination. Special forceps are made for this purpose and care must be taken to avoid injuring the wall of the oesophagus to such an extent that a perforation is produced.

Before advising radiotherapy or operative treatment, it may be necessary to carry out more than one biopsy. It is not possible to be certain of obtaining a positive report of malignancy from one small piece of tissue, and in suspected cases a negative microscopic report calls for a further oesophagoscopy and removal of another specimen for examination.

Palliative treatment consists of maintaining the nourishment of the patient by keeping the oesophagus permeable.

The stricture of the gullet can be prevented from becoming complete by dilatation followed by the introduction of a rigid tube (*Figure 9.12*).

Dilatation with bougies alone produces such a short period of freedom from obstruction that it is hardly worth considering.

If the site of obstruction lies below the thoracic inlet a Souttar's tube may be inserted through the oesophagoscope. The technique is illustrated in *Figure 9.12*.

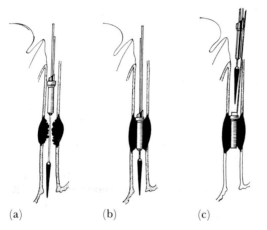

(a)   (b)   (c)

Figure 9.12 Technique of inserting Souttar's tube through the oesophagoscope. (a) After gentle dilatation of the lumen the Souttar's tube is passed down along the metal guide; (b) the flange of the tube is seated firmly onto the upper rim of the growth; (c) the guide is withdrawn while the tube is held in position with the ring-shaped introducer. The latter is then removed and the position of the tube finally scrutinized before withdrawal of the oesophagoscope

Owen's plastic tubes are usually more satisfactory. They are easier to insert and more comfortable for the patient. Radiotherapy can be given with the tube *in situ* and extra irradiation dosage can be given by temporary insertion of a caesium-loaded bougie through the Owen's tube without increasing the danger of pulmonary fibrosis. Because of their flexible nature and small weight they are tolerated in the cervical oesophagus and occasionally even in the post-cricoid region. These tubes are inserted by sliding them over a fine bougie passed through the stricture (*see Figure 9.13*). The oesophagoscope is removed, the bougie remaining in position to guide the tube. The latter is passed behind the larynx with a finger and then gently pushed on by the oesophagoscope which is re-inserted around the bougie. When the tube is snugly seated on the growth the bougie, and then the oesophagoscope, are finally removed. If these measures fail the standard Mousseau–Barbin technique must be used (*Figure 9.14*). A laparotomy is done and the stomach is opened. The stricture is then dilated from above, through an oesophagoscope, and a medium-sized bougie is passed through and retrieved from the stomach. The tail of the tube is fixed to the upper end

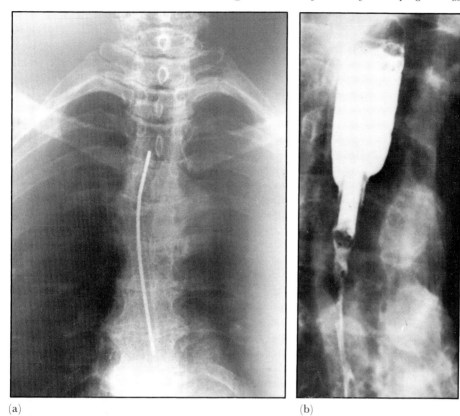

(a)   (b)

Figure 9.13   Owen's tube used in carcinoma of oesophagus showing (a) caesium bougie within the tube; (b) blockage of tube by food

of the bougie, which is then pulled through from below. The tube slides down through the mouth until its flange is seated upon the stricture. Finally, the tube is cut across just below the cardia, and the stomach is closed. This technique is best done by two teams of surgeons, and is greatly improved by the use of Crossling's bougies (Crossling, 1961) (*Figure 9.14*). Better functional results have recently been claimed for Celestin's nylon and latex tube which is more flexible, and less liable to cause pressure necrosis around the rim of the funnelled upper end.

Intubation may not be well tolerated in the cervical part of the oesophagus. Here, and in the post-cricoid region, severe obstruction can be managed by the insertion of a nasogastric feeding tube, pending the outcome of radiotherapy or the decision to undertake radical excision. Gastrostomy merely for the prolongation of hopeless misery should be avoided, although there may be cases in which it may be necessary to improve the general condition in preparation for an attempt at curative operation.

In cases where radiotherapy is likely to be used, plastic, and not metal, tubes should be insisted upon for all these manoeuvres.

All patients with in-dwelling oesophageal tubes must be instructed to eat a liquidized diet washed down with copious draughts of fluid.

Treatment by radiotherapy
The majority of cancers of the oesophagus are inoperable. A small proportion of them

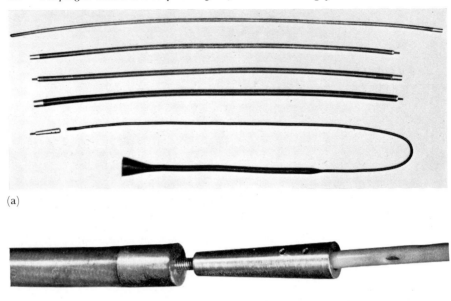

(a)

(b)

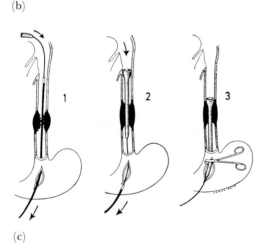

(c)

Figure 9.14 Technique for inserting Mousseau–Barbin tube. (a) Crossling's graduated screw-ended bougies (there are six in the complete set), with metal adaptor, and a Mousseau–Barbin plastic tube. The bougies are assembled as a continuous rod, passed through the mouth and drawn out at the gastrostomy wound; (b) method of attaching the tail of the Mousseau–Barbin tube to the threaded bougie; (c) three stages in pulling down the tube onto the growth (*see text*)

can be improved by radiotherapy, and an even smaller number may be apparently cured. Endoscopic application of radium, and interstitial radon or gold seeds, have been virtually abandoned in favour of external irradiation. The ability to deliver effective tumour doses has increased with the availability of tele-cobalt beam therapy and, in some centres, mega-voltage x-ray or computerized tracking equipment.

Significant damage to the lungs is now largely avoided and even if treatment fails the patient's plight is not worsened by it. In cases of satisfactory tumour regression a fibrous stricture remains, requiring dilatation at intervals.

Cytotoxic drugs
In malignant disease of the oesophagus regional infusion is not possible, and the use of these drugs has been restricted to general systemic administration. Up to this time

there is no convincing evidence of worthwhile palliation of symptoms, but their use is justified if no other treatment is possible.

Oesophagectomy
Thoracic surgery offers the best chance of cure, and a fair chance of palliation if cure should fail, in carcinoma of the lower and middle thirds of the oesophagus. The decisions as to operability and choice of technique are extremely complex, and outside the endoscopist's province.

Inoperability is beyond dispute in cases having involvement of the bronchial tree, or recurrent laryngeal nerve, or distant metastases.

At the present time it is considered that growths above the aortic arch should be treated only by radiotherapy, but modern techniques of total oesophagectomy, with colon, jejunal or stomach transplantation may in the future provide a better line of attack.

Carcinomas of the cervical oesophagus are rarely operable, but if an adequate margin of healthy oesophagus is present between the tumour and the thoracic inlet, it is the laryngologist who must decide whether to proceed or rely upon radiotherapy. Such tumours can be excised by means of slightly modified techniques, as described for the hypopharynx in Chapter 8. In practice, simple oesophagectomy is rarely indicated here, and involvement of the trachea, larynx or recurrent laryngeal nerves will dictate oesophagopharyngolaryngectomy. The addition of total thyroidectomy increases the chances of total clearance of local spread of the disease, but inability to remove the mediastinal lymph nodes adequately is responsible for the very high failure rate for this type of operation.

General diseases affecting the oesophagus

Scleroderma

This is a rare collagen disease in which there is atrophy and fibrosis of smooth muscles. There are marked changes in the hands and feet due to vascular impairment. The oesophagus may be affected. The ganglion cells are normal but there is slowly progressive impairment of oesophageal motility, dilatation of the lower oesophagus and laxity of the lower oesophageal sphincter. As a result, reflux oesophagitis is common and over 30 per cent of cases develop a hiatus hernia. Dysphagia is mild and the usual medical anti-reflux regimen should be instituted. Poor oesophageal motility has also been noted in many cases of systemic lupus erythematosus.

Motor neurone disease

This causes poor oesophageal motility but the upper oesophageal sphincter is normal. In this condition and other neurological conditions affecting the upper alimentary tract – such as Parkinson's disease, polyneuritis and poliomyelitis – the oesophageal abnormalities are always over-shadowed by the pharyngeal difficulties of initiating swallowing and laryngeal spill-over.

Diabetic neuropathy

Diabetics who show evidence of autonomic neuropathy complain of diarrhoea, vomiting, impotence and bladder dysfunction. Radiology shows that a majority of them also have poor oesophageal motility, a weak lower oesophageal sphincter and marked reflux. However, they rarely have severe oesophageal symptoms and this may be due to the commonly associated gastric atrophy and achlorhydria.

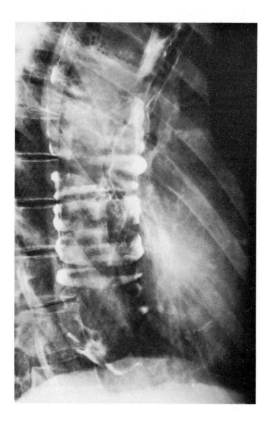

Figure 9.15   A dilated oesophagus with tertiary contractions in senility

Senility

Along with other muscles the oesophageal walls may become very weak and atrophic in the aged. This is demonstrated in dramatic form by barium studies which show a dilated oesophagus with small tertiary contractions (*Figure 9.15*). Fortunately, these changes seem to cause few symptoms although similar pharyngeal weakness may be very troublesome.

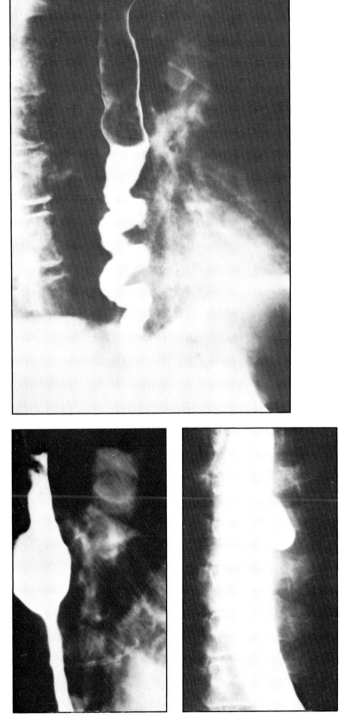

Figure 9.16   The bizarre radiological changes seen in chronic diffuse
oesophageal spasm

Chronic diffuse oesophageal spasm

This is really a radiological diagnosis. A variety of changes are seen on barium-swallow studies which appear to be due to irregular and incoordinated muscular contractions. These can produce most interesting and bizarre x-ray appearances and a collection of these is shown in *Figure 9.16*. The patients are usually elderly and symptoms few. Some patients have intermittent chest pain and dysphagia. If the latter is persistent, endoscopy is indicated to exclude a neoplasm and allow dilatation as required.

References and bibliography

Acheson, E. D. and Hadley, G. D. (1958). *British Medical Journal*, **1**, 549

Allison, P. R. (1943). *Journal of Thoracic Surgery*, **12**, 432

Allison, P. R. (1946). *Journal of Thoracic Surgery*, **15**, 308

Allison, P. R., Johnstone, A. S. and Royce, G. B. (1943). *Journal of Thoracic Surgery*, **12**, 342

Alpin, M. (1934). *Monatsschrift für Ohrenheilkunde u. Laryngo-Rhinologie*, **68**, 1172

Barlow, D. (1942). *British Journal of Surgery*, **29**, 415

Barrett, N. R. (1933). *Lancet*, **1**, 1009

Barrett, N. R. (1954). *British Journal of Surgery*, **42**, 231

Belsey, R. H. R. (1966). *Proceedings of the Royal Society of Medicine*, **59**, 927

Belsey, R. H. R. and Donnison, C. P. (1950). *British Medical Journal*, **2**, 324

Bennett, J. R. (1976). 'Medical management of gastro-oesophageal reflux', *Clinics in Gastro-enterology*, Vol. 5, No. 1, ch. 13, pp. 175–185

Bennett, R. B. and Hendrix, T. R. (1970). 'Treatment of achasia with pneumatic dilatation', *Modern Treatment*, Vol. 7, No. 6, pp. 1217–1228

Benson, C. D., Mustard, W. T., Ravitch, M., Snyder, W. and Welch, K. J. (1962). *Pediatric Surgery*, Vol. 1, p. 266; Year Book Publishers, Chicago

Chesterman, J. T. (1965). *British Journal of Surgery*, **52**, 601

Cosella, R. R., Brown, A. L., Sayre, G. P. and Ellis, F. H. (1964). 'Achalasia of the oesophagus; pathologic and etiologic considerations', *Annals of Surgery*, **160**, 474–486

Crossling, F. T. (1961). *British Medical Journal*, **1**, 1032

Diggle, F. H. (1932). *British Medical Journal*, **1**, 277

Douglas, K., and Nicholson, F. (1959). *British Journal of Surgery*, **47**, 250

Earlam, R. J. (1972). 'Hypothesis: a vascular cause for aganglionic bowel', *American Journal of Digestive Diseases*, **17**, 255–261

Edwards, D. A. W. (1976). 'Evaluation of

dysphagia', *Clinics in Gastro-enterology*, Vol. 5, No. 1, ch. 4

Ellis, F. G. (1960). 'The natural history of achalasia of the cardia', *Proceedings of the Royal Society of Medicine*, **53**, 663–666

Ellis, F. G. (1962). *Annals of the Royal College of Surgeons of England*, **47**, 466

Ellis, F. G., Kauntze, R., and Trounce, J. R. (1960). *British Journal of Surgery*, **47**, 466

Ellis, F. G., Kauntze, R., Nightingale, A., and Trounce, J. R. (1960). *Quarterly Journal of Medicine*, **29**, 305

Etzel, E. (1942). *American Journal of Medical Science*, **203**, 87

Flavell, G. (1963). *The Oesophagus*; Butterworths, London and Boston

Flett, R. L. (1945). *Journal of Laryngology*, **60**, 1

Franklin, R. H. (1958). *Proceedings of the Royal Society of Medicine*, **51**, 595

Freeman, N. V. (1969). In *Neonatal Surgery* (Eds P. P. Rickham and J. H. Johnston); Butterworths, London and Boston

Gillison, E. W., de Castro, V. A. M., Nybus, L. M., Kusakari, K. and Bombeck, G. T. (1972). 'The significance of bile in reflux oesophagitis', *Surgery, Gynecology and Obstetrics*, **134**, 419–424

Goligher, J. C. (1948). *Lancet*, **1**, 985

Groves, J. (1956). *British Journal of Surgery*, **43**, 413

Heller, E. (1914). *Mitteilungen aus den Grenzgebieten der Medizin und Chirurgie*, **57**, 141

Helmsworth, J. A. and Pryles, C. V. (1951). *Journal of Pediatrics*, **38**, 610

Hurst, A. (1943). *Journal of Laryngology*, **58**, 60

Imperatori, C. J. (1939). *Archives of Otolaryngology, Chicago*, **30**, 352

Jackson, C. (1922). *Laryngoscope*, **32**, 139

Jackson, C. and Jackson, C. L. (1915). *Peroral Endoscopy and Laryngeal Surgery*, The Laryngoscope Co., St. Louis

Jackson, C. and Jackson, C. L. (1933). *Archives of Otolaryngology*, **18**, 731

Jackson, C. and Jackson, C. L. (1936). *Diseases of the Air and Food Passages of Foreign Body Origin*; Saunders, Philadelphia

Joske, R. A. and Benedict, E. B. (1959). 'The role of benign oesophageal obstruction in the development of carcinoma of the oesophagus', *Gastro-enterology*, **36,** 749–755

Kelly, A. Brown (1936). *Journal of Laryngology*, **51,** 78

Klayman, M. I. (1955). *Annals of International Medicine*, **43,** 33

Logan. Quoted in *Current Problems in Surgery* (1967). Eds M. M. Ravitch, E. H. Ellison, O. C. Julian, A. P. Thal and O. H. Wangensteen); Year Book Medical Publishers, Chicago

Macbeth, R. G. (1955). *British Medical Journal*, **2,** 877

Mosher, H. P. (1935). *Surgery, Gynecology and Obstetrics*, **60,** 403

Mullard, K. S. (1954). *Journal of Thoracic Surgery*, **28,** 39

Negus, V. E. (1929). *Proceedings of the Royal Society of Medicine*, **22,** 527

Negus, V. E. (1955). In: *Diseases of the Nose and Throat* (6th edn); Cassell, London

Nissen, R., Rossetti, M. and Markman, I. (1965). *Prensa médica Argentina*, **52,** 2510

Nixon, H. H. and Wilkinson, A. W. (1963). In: *Congenital Abnormalities in Infancy* (Ed. A. P. Norman); Blackwell, Oxford

Olsen, A. M. and Harrington, S. W. (1948). *Journal of Thoracic Surgery*, **17,** 189

Phillips, C. E. (1938). *Journal of the American Medical Association*, **111,** 998

Richardson, J. R. (1945). *Annals of Otology*, **54,** 328

Robb, D. (1952–53). *Australia and New Zealand Journal of Surgery*, **22,** 120

Roux, B. T. le, and Wright, J. T. (1960). *British Journal of Surgery*, **48,** 619

Schindler, R. (1956). *Annals of International Medicine*, **45,** 207

Schlemmer, F. (1920). *Archiv Klinische Chirurgie*, **114,** 37

Smith, M. K. (1928). *Annals of Surgery*, **88,** 1022

Starck, H. (1934). *München-medizinische Wochenschrift*, **81,** 1794, 1805

Starck, H. (1936). *Sonderdruck aus 'Knolls' Mitteilungen für Ärtze*. Jubiläuausgabe

Sweet, R. H. (1954). *Thoracic Surgery* (2nd edn); Saunders, Philadelphia

Terracol, J. and Sweet, R. H. (1958). *Diseases of the Oesophagus*; Saunders, Philadelphia

Trounce, J. R., Deuchar, D. C., Kauntze, R. and Thomas, G. A. (1957). *Quarterly Journal of Medicine*, **26,** 433

Tucker, G. J. (1925). *Journal of the American Medical Association*, **84,** 511

Ty, T. C., Brunet, C. and Beardmore, H. E. (1967). *Journal of Pediatric Surgery*, **2,** 118

Vogt, E. C. (1929). *American Journal of Roentgenology*, **22,** 463

Wangensteen, O. H. (1951). *Annals of Surgery*, **134,** 301

Wright, A. J. (1934). *Journal of Laryngology*, **49,** 175

Methods of examining the larynx and tracheobronchial tree
John Groves and Stewart W Clarke

The larynx

The complete investigation of laryngeal disease may necessitate examination by external palpation, indirect laryngoscopy, direct laryngoscopy, stroboscopy and radiography, and biopsies and swabs may be taken. It is hardly possible to list all the indications for the various procedures; the experience and judgment of the examiner must determine which of the investigations are necessary.

Palpation of the larynx

Palpation of the larynx may yield useful information and constant practice is necessary to acquire the skill to detect minor deviations from the normal.

Before palpating the neck sufficient clothing must be removed to give a free and unrestricted approach and the neck is first inspected in a good light.

To obtain the necessary muscular relaxation the patient should sit with his head slightly flexed; the examiner stands behind and palpates the neck and larynx with the finger tips of both hands. It is rarely necessary for the patient to lie down, and palpation from in front is unsatisfactory.

The prominence of the pomum Adami is first identified and the wings of the thyroid cartilage are carefully examined for any thickening, tenderness, or alteration of shape or position. The thyroid notch is easily found and just above this can be felt the hyoid bone; the greater cornua of the hyoid can be grasped between the fingers and thumb of one hand as they run upwards and backwards below the mandible. Below the thyroid cartilage the anterior surface of the cricoid cartilage forms an important surgical landmark. In adults it lies at the level of the sixth cervical vertebra but in children it may be as high as the lower border of the fourth cervical vertebra. Although about seven rings of the trachea are present in the neck they cannot be palpated even when the neck is fully extended. The isthmus of the thyroid gland lies over the second, third and fourth tracheal rings.

The movements of the larynx should be noted: the larynx is stationary during quiet respiration but on deep breathing and in laryngeal stenosis respiratory excursions occur, the larynx descending on inspiration and ascending on expiration. The larynx also moves upwards on swallowing and during the production of high notes. It can be moved from side to side on the vertebral column, with which it is in contact, and a peculiar grating sensation is often felt; this must not be mistaken for pathological crepitus.

Attention should also be paid to the other structures of the neck, particularly the regional lymph nodes. It should be remembered that paralysis of the sternomastoid and trapezius muscles may occur in association with laryngeal palsies.

Indirect laryngoscopy

In many cases indirect laryngoscopy, considered with the history, will be sufficient to establish a diagnosis. It is a straightforward procedure which should be within the capabilities of every practitioner; and it ought to be more frequently employed than it is. Cases would then be diagnosed earlier with consequent improvement in the results of treatment.

In order to obtain a satisfactory view of the larynx, the examiner must be accustomed to using frontal illumination. A good headlamp is as satisfactory as light reflected from a forehead mirror and is easier for the beginner. Several laryngeal mirrors of different sizes are needed, also a spirit lamp and a gauze square for holding the tongue. If a spirit lamp is not available the mirror can be warmed in a bowl of hot water. The examiner may wear a mask or shield to protect his face in infected cases.

The cooperation and relaxation of the patient are essential to the success of an examination, and before he begins the examiner should explain what he is going to do and how he would like the patient to help. The patient's position is important: he should sit with his body upright and his head held level; the examiner sits facing him and draws the head a little forward from the shoulders. Any dentures the patient may be wearing are removed, and the largest mirror which will conveniently fit at the back of the patient's throat is selected; a small mirror gives a less complete view of the larynx and pharynx, and may slip behind the soft palate when the mirror is raised to elevate it. The mirror is warmed by holding it, face downwards, in the flame of a spirit lamp and, before it is introduced into the patient's mouth, its temperature is tested on the examiner's hand or cheek. The patient is asked to put out his tongue and, covering it with the gauze square, the examiner takes hold of it with the thumb and middle finger of his left hand; the forefinger lifts the upper lip out of the way, and rests on the incisor teeth for steadiness (*Figure 10.1*). At this point the patient is asked to breathe steadily in and out through his mouth in order to separate the tongue and soft palate, otherwise the mirror cannot be placed in position. The warmed mirror, held in the right hand like a pen, is passed face-downwards over the tongue (with care not to touch the tongue and smear the surface with saliva) and placed firmly against the base of the uvula, lifting it upwards and backwards; the shaft rests against the angle of the mouth for support. The examiner focuses his light on the mirror and, by tilting the mirror in different directions, the reflected images of the various structures of the larynx and laryngopharynx may be seen (*Figure 10.2*).

The ease with which the larynx may be seen varies from patient to patient, but by going about it in the right way the number of difficult cases may be reduced to a minimum. Success depends to a great extent on the patient's relaxation, and gentleness in handling is therefore most important. The tongue should be held firmly

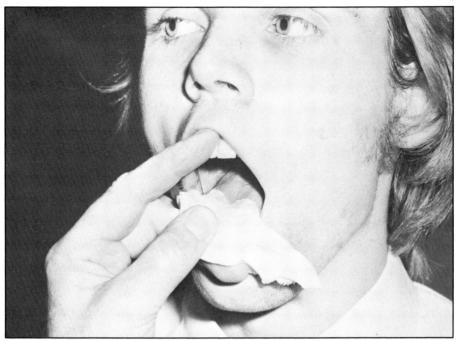

(a)

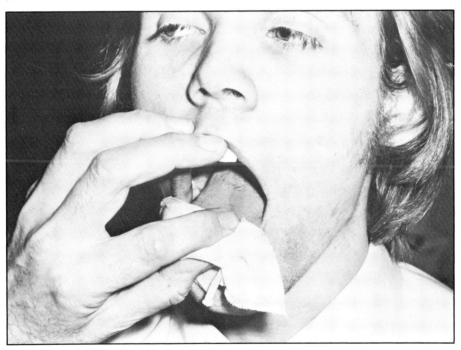

(b)

Figure 10.1 (a) Holding the patient's tongue for indirect laryngoscopy; (b) alternative technique sometimes preferable if the tip of the tongue is short. The ring finger can be passed backwards and used as a tongue depressor if necessary

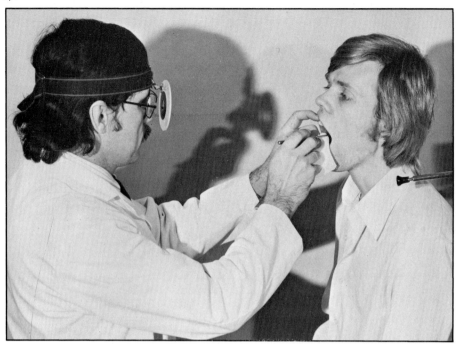

(a)

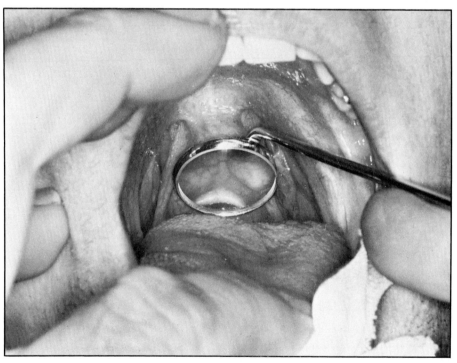

(b)

Figure 10.2 (a) Indirect laryngoscopy. Note the 'forward' position of the patient's neck, and his well-relaxed posture; (b) the mirror lifts the uvula and reveals the epiglottis and valleculae

in position, but not dragged upon or pinched. Too much downward pull will press the lower surface of the tongue against the lower incisor teeth, causing pain, or even laceration of the frenum. A mirror which is placed firmly against the soft palate and deliberately tilted as required is much better tolerated than one which only just touches it and which slides about when moved to bring the laryngeal structures into view. Even so, there are many patients who retch or gag when the mirror is put into position and in these cases the soft palate must be anaesthetized by spraying with a four per cent lignocaine aerosol, or by the patient sucking an amethocaine or lignocaine lozenge.

It is possible to see the base of the tongue, the larynx, and the upper portions of the hypopharynx and pyriform fossae by indirect laryngoscopy, but all these structures will not appear at one time in the laryngeal mirror, and the examiner has to piece together the various images into a complete picture. Each structure should be inspected in turn, and it is advisable to keep to the same order of inspection in every case. It is only by adhering to a regular routine of inspection that one may be certain of not missing any detail. Before the examination is completed the mirror may have to be taken out and re-inserted several times to give the patient a rest.

Structures visible on indirect laryngoscopy

The first structures seen are the anterior surface of the epiglottis, the base of the tongue and the valleculae. Raising the mirror and tilting it downwards brings into sight the entrance to the larynx. It is bounded in front by the upper edge of the epiglottis, behind by the mucous membrane between the arytenoid cartilages, and on each side by the aryepiglottic folds. The epiglottis is a flattened, leaf-like structure, covered with pale mucous membrane, across which a few blood vessels arborize. Its shape varies a good deal, and it is more folded upon itself in infants and young children than in adults. It may overhang the larynx, making it almost impossible to get a good view of the interior (*Figure 10.3*). The posterior surface of the epiglottis forms a slight elevation, known as the tubercle, just above the anterior commissure of the vocal cords. Running postero-medially from the lateral margins of the epiglottis to the arytenoid cartilages on each side is a free fold of mucous membrane. This is the aryepiglottic fold. It is thin in front, but thickens behind, where it contains the cartilages of Wrisberg and Santorini. Beneath these are the eminences formed by the arytenoid cartilages, and in between is the interarytenoid space.

The ventricular bands lie immediately above the vocal cords and appear to be in contact with them; the ventricles of the larynx cannot usually be seen by indirect laryngoscopy. The vocal cords run backwards from the angle of the thyroid cartilage to the vocal processes of the arytenoids, forming the triangular aperture of the rima glottidis. In the mirror-image the vocal cords appear as flat, ribbon-like structures with sharp, free margins. They are glistening white in colour, and there should not be any vessels visible on their surface. The motility of the cords should be observed during quiet respiration and by making the patient phonate, saying 'e-e-e-e'. If there is no paresis or fixation, the cords and arytenoids will approximate and the interarytenoid space will be obliterated (*Figures 10.3 and 10.4*).

Below the vocal cords is the subglottic space, the walls of which are hidden from view but, further down, the first two or three rings of the trachea may be seen anteriorly.

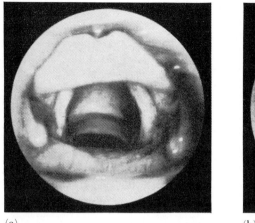
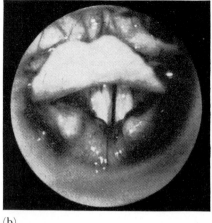

(a)   (b)

Figure 10.3   Indirect laryngoscopy. (a) During inspiration; (b) during phonation. Note how clearly the cartilages of Wrisberg stand out in the aryepiglottic folds. (Reproduced by courtesy of Dr. Paul H. Holinger and the Editor of *Annals of Otology, Rhinology and Laryngology*)

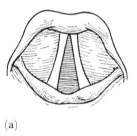
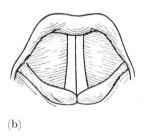

(a)   (b)

Figure 10.4   Indirect laryngoscopy. Diagrams of larynx: (a) during quiet respiration; (b) during phonation

The larynx lies in contact with the posterior wall of the pharynx, and moves away from it only on deglutition; thus the lower half of the hypopharynx cannot be seen. The entrances to the pyriform fossae can be seen in the mirror and a little more of the fossae becomes visible on phonation, but complete inspection is not possible by the indirect method of examination.

The image of the larynx seen in the mirror is reversed antero-posteriorly but not from side to side. That is to say, the anterior commissure will appear to point away from the examiner and the right-hand structures will be seen on his left.

The most difficult part to bring into view is the anterior commissure, and the larynx cannot be passed as normal until this has been inspected. It is often invisible during quiet respiration, but if the patient is asked to say 'e-e-e-e' the larynx elevates and the epiglottis tilts forwards, uncovering the anterior commissure. In some cases the overhang of the epiglottis may be so marked that this manoeuvre fails. Occasionally this is simply due to the nervousness and tenseness of the patient and re-examination a day or two later when he is less apprehensive may succeed. If not, the examiner will have to hook the epiglottis forward with a curved probe or special epiglottis retractor, the patient holding his own tongue to free the examiner's hand. Another obstacle to satisfactory examination is the fact that the tongue may elevate on phonation and hide the mirror, just when a view is most wanted; this can be overcome by using a tongue depressor, or by drawing the tongue well across to one side of the mouth while viewing the mirror in a line between the lateral border of the tongue and the anterior faucial pillar.

Children are difficult to examine by indirect laryngoscopy and direct inspection is usually required if it is necessary to see the larynx. Sometimes, however, a sufficiently good view can be obtained if the mirror is placed almost horizontally against the hard palate, instead of the uvula, so that the cough reflex is not elicited.

Observations during examination

During examination the observer must look for, and assess the significance of, any abnormal appearances. There may be injection, swelling, oedema, proliferation or ulceration; and the movements of the vocal cords may be impaired. In those parts of the larynx and pharynx which cannot be seen in the mirror, a lesion may produce visible indications that will lead to correct diagnosis. For example, impairment of movement of a vocal cord may be due to a hidden subglottic growth, and frothy saliva in the pyriform fossae may be traced to a low laryngopharyngeal or upper oesophageal carcinoma.

Observation of the cartilage of Wrisberg in the aryepiglottic fold may be of assistance in the diagnosis of laryngeal paralysis, especially in differentiating paralysis from fixation of the crico-arytenoid joint. In the latter case, the cartilage retains its normal upright position, braced by the action of the posterior crico-arytenoid muscle. In recurrent laryngeal nerve paralysis this action fails, and the cartilage droops forward over the posterior end of the vocal cord, making it appear shorter than its fellow.

Indirect laryngoscopy is used mainly for diagnosis. In the past, various manipulations such as laryngeal biopsy, removal of innocent growths and cauterization of tuberculous ulcers, were done under indirect laryngoscopic control. They demand considerable skill and, since more accurate work can be done by direct laryngoscopy, the modern operator seldom troubles to acquire it. However, it is still sometimes convenient to take a biopsy of a large malignant growth by this method and

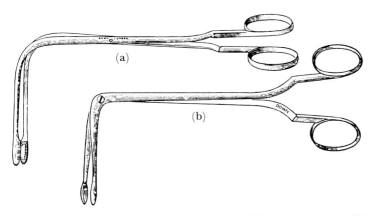

Figure 10.5 Mackenzie's laryngeal forceps. (a) With serrated jaws; (b) with scoop jaws. (Reproduced by courtesy of Down Bros. and Mayer & Phelps Ltd)

Mackenzie's spoon-bladed forceps are recommended (*Figure 10.5*) (Thomson and Negus, 1955).

The laryngeal mirror is also useful in guiding the manipulations for anaesthetizing the larynx and trachea for direct laryngoscopy and bronchoscopy, and when bronchograms are required iodized oil may be introduced into the trachea via the larynx.

The operator requires both hands free to carry out these procedures under indirect vision, and the tongue has to be held by an assistant or by the patient himself. The operator usually holds the laryngeal mirror in his left hand and the instrument in his right hand.

Fibre-optic laryngoscopy

Inspection of the respiratory tract has been revolutionized by the development of flexible fibre-optic equipment in recent years. Fibre-glass bundles within a sealed plastic sheath, with appropriate lenses at either end (and only a few millimetres in diameter) can transmit a good-quality image of the endoscopic view, as well as bright illumination to the field from an external light source. Internal control cables allow tilting of the tip as much as 90 degrees to scan the field of view while an internal channel permits introduction of miniature biopsy forceps. Fibre-optic bronchoscopy is discussed fully later in this chapter (p. 303). For laryngoscopy the fibrescope is chiefly useful in adults where, because of anatomical difficulties or intolerance of the mirror, indirect laryngoscopy proves impossible. The method is quick and simple and can be done without detention of the patient or disruption of a busy clinic. A detachable camera allows permanent photographic records to be made.

Technique

Lignocaine four per cent aerosol is applied with a few metered doses to the (wider) nasal cavity, to the oropharynx and back of the tongue, and to the laryngeal inlet with an angled jet. Adequate topical anaesthesia results within five minutes. The fibrescope is lubricated with lignocaine jelly, the illumination is tested and the focus adjusted. Its tip is then passed gently along the floor of the nose. The downward curvature in the nasopharynx is negotiated by a remotely controlled tilting of the tip, after which a further insertion of 5–7 cm gives a view of the epiglottis. Slipping downwards behind this structure the instrument then reveals the glottis, albeit from a distance of about 5 cm. The image, though small, is sharp because of the very great depth of focus inherent in the optical design. By a combination of rotating the instrument and tilting its tip, the cords are kept in the centre of the field of view while insertion continues to give a closer (and larger) 'picture'. The laryngeal interior is scanned minutely at all stages; biopsy forceps will yield a useful specimen if a lesion is revealed, and photographs can be taken if a permanent record is needed.

Fibre-optic laryngoscopy is of potentially very great value in diagnosis and follow-up work. In economic terms alone the technique justifies the capital costs of the equipment, by the avoidance of hospitalization for these essential purposes. It does not, however, permit curative excision of endolaryngeal lesions, for which micro-laryngoscopy under general anaesthetic is essential.

Direct laryngoscopy

By this method the larynx is looked at directly through a rigid endoscope. Except for injuries and diseases of the cervical spine, there are very few contra-indications to its use. When there is marked laryngeal obstruction, preliminary tracheostomy may be necessary. The examination may not be possible when severe trismus exists.

The design of laryngoscopes has evolved from Chevalier Jackson's, through Negus' and Kleinsasser's, with many variations and modifications. Modern instruments employ the proximal lighting of Negus, vastly improved since his time by fibre-optic technology with remote light source (*Figure 10.6*). Use of the binocular operating microscope has in the last decade become routine for most laryngoscopies. For this reason tubes with cylindrical cross-section have been largely superseded by wider, but tapering tubes which at the wider, proximal end are transversely oval in section. This

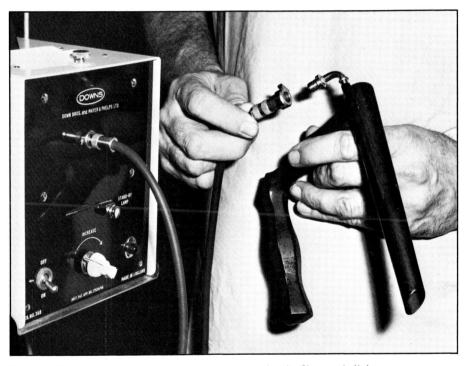

Figure 10.6 A modern laryngoscope being connected to its fibre-optic light source

allows binocular vision under the microscope, and gives more space for passage of instruments (*Figure 10.7*).

The Mackintosh laryngoscope (*Figure 10.8*) is used by most anaesthetists for routine endotracheal intubation, and is often ideal for the removal of foreign bodies

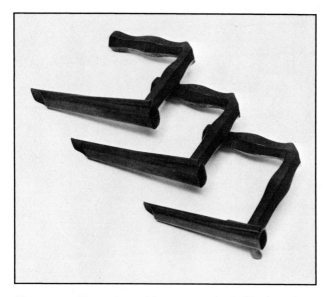

Figure 10.7   Three sizes of laryngoscope suitable for micro-laryngoscopy. Note the oval cross-section at the proximal (viewing) end of this pattern

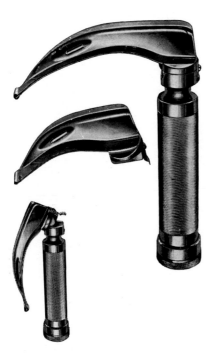

Figure 10.8   Mackintosh laryngoscope. (Reproduced by courtesy of The British Oxygen Company)

arrested in the vallecula and the region of the laryngeal aditus. The tip is placed in the vallecula, in front of the epiglottis which is lifted forwards with, and by, the tongue.

Anaesthesia

Even if the airway is compromised general anaesthesia is nowadays preferred to rigid endoscopy under local anaesthetic. Fibre-optic laryngoscopy under topical anaesthesia will often solve the immediate diagnostic problem, without added risk and with minimal discomfort for the patient. In infants and young children Chevalier Jackson used to teach that no anaesthetic at all should be used, but it is now considered wiser and safer to give a general anaesthetic. The relaxation and control given by well-administered general anaesthesia enables the surgeon to make a more thorough examination and perform his manipulations with greater accuracy than when he has to contend with a conscious patient.

General anaesthesia

For children from two to seven years old trimeprazine tartrate is an excellent pre-medication. It is given by mouth $1\frac{1}{2}$ hours before operation at a dose rate of 3–4 mg/kg. An intramuscular injection of 0.4–0.6 mg of atropine is also given half-an-hour before the operation is due to begin.

Above the age of seven years pethidine and atropine are probably preferable to Omnopon and scopolamine because they do not depress the cough reflex so much. Pethidine 10 mg/6.35 kg (1 stone) for children and a full dose of 100 mg for adults is given with 0.6 mg of atropine 45 min pre-operatively by intramuscular injection.

The introduction of the muscle relaxant drugs has been of great help in per-oral endoscopy and nowadays most laryngoscopies and many bronchoscopies are performed under their influence. Adults are induced with intravenous thiopentone followed by intravenous suxamethonium and when relaxation has been obtained a small-bore (7 mm) endotracheal tube is passed through the nose or the mouth. Anaesthesia is maintained through the tube with nitrous oxide, oxygen and halothane. The tube lies in the posterior commissure and most of the larynx can be thoroughly inspected while it is in position. It is removed or displaced by the laryngoscope to allow inspection of the posterior commissure and adjacent regions. The recent introduction of Carden's endotracheal tube with Venturi-assisted respiration gives much improved access to the larynx.

For the average adult, the dose of thiopentone is usually 300 mg and that of suxamethonium 50 mg. (Further details of anaesthesiology are given in Volume 3.)

Instruments

'Wide-mouthed' laryngoscopes (modified Kleinsasser type) in a range of sizes are ideal for micro-laryngoscopy and must always be at hand as first choice. In cases of difficulty due to anatomical problems of prominent teeth, large tongue, short, narrow-angled mandible, or stiff cervical spine, the Negus tubes with their smaller diameter are necessary to allow insertion through the easier angle offered laterally between the molar teeth. In addition to this choice of endoscopes, one should be equipped to proceed without delay to oesophagoscopy, bronchoscopy or even tracheostomy as the case proceeds. A great range of biopsy forceps, suction tubes and

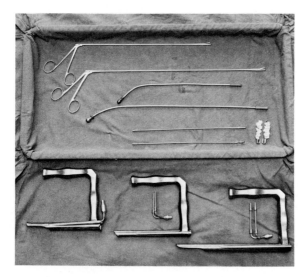

Figure 10.9 Negus standard and anterior commissure laryngoscopes, with oesophageal speculum, and grasping forceps, suction tubes and swab-carriers. Note the fibre-optic light carriers

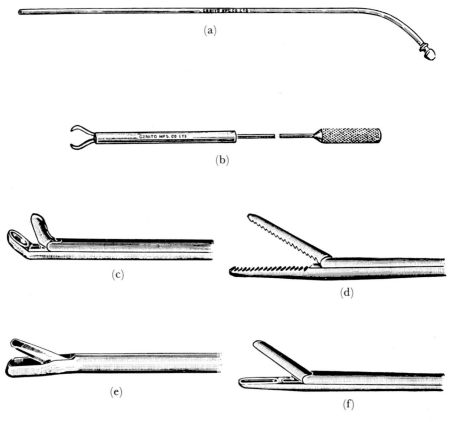

(a)

(b)

(c)

(d)

(e)

(f)

Figure 10.10 Instruments used in direct laryngoscopy. (a) Aspirating tube, Chevalier Jackson, open end; (b) swab holder, Coolidge; (c) nodule forceps, Chevalier Jackson; (d) grasping forceps, Chevalier Jackson; (e) biopsy forceps, Taylor; (f) cutting forceps, Patterson. (Reproduced by courtesy of The Genito–Urinary Manufacturing Company Ltd)

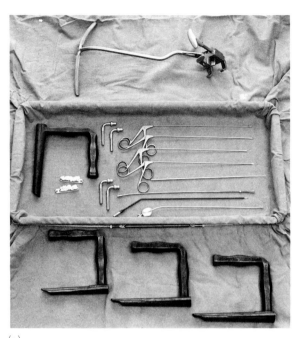

Figure 10.11   (a) Basic instruments for micro-laryngoscopy; (b) magnified view of micro-laryngeal instruments.

1 Diathermy electrode
2 Angled cupped forceps
3 Straight cupped forceps
4 Fine serrated grasping forceps
5 Scissors
6 Sickle knife

(a)

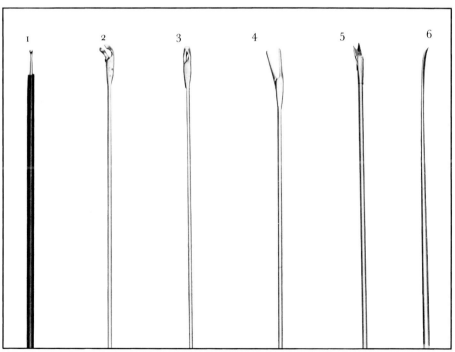

(b)

micro-surgical instruments need to be available, though few will be used in any one case (*Figures 10.9, 10.10* and *10.11*).

Modern theatre sterilizing practice based on pre-set trays prepared in a sterilizing centre ('TSSU') creates organizational problems for frequently performed operations in which such a truly vast variety of instruments needs to be *instantly* to hand. The problem is soluble but only by very expensive re-duplication of equipment. The alternative of the traditional formalin sterilizing cabinet (*Figure 10.12*) still deserves consideration, especially in hospitals otherwise dependent on remote 'central' sterilizing services, perhaps many miles away.

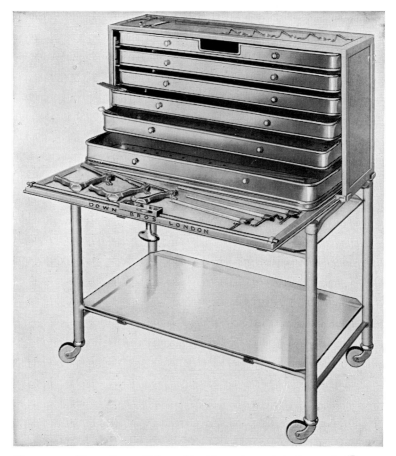

Figure 10.12   Formalin sterilizing cabinet for endoscopic instruments. (Reproduced by courtesy of Down Bros. and Mayer & Phelps Ltd)

Non-sterile equipment must include a fibre-optic light source, powerful suction pump, and binocular operating microscope fitted with a long-focus (400 mm) objective lens.

Position of the patient

The anaesthetized relaxed patient lies supine with an ordinary pillow under the occiput. The head-flap of the table is included in the sterile head-drape so that the surgeon can himself adjust its elevation without becoming unsterile and with complete precision. An assistant (to hold the head extended on the neck and the neck flexed forward from the thorax) is seldom needed but is a great help in anatomically difficult cases. The special Negus head-rest (*Figure 10.13*) is favoured by some, but not considered essential. A strong metal bridge is positioned (*Figure 10.14*) for the Loewy support before draping is completed.

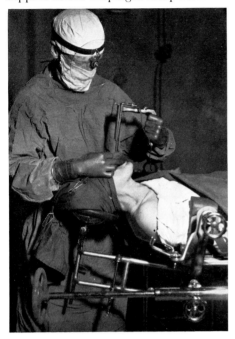

Figure 10.13 Use of the Negus head support, a technique still favoured by some workers (*see text*). Under the drapes, the surgeon has personal control of the various adjustments of head position. Note also the transparent plastic disc to protect the surgeon's eyes; a sensible precaution for those who do not wear spectacles

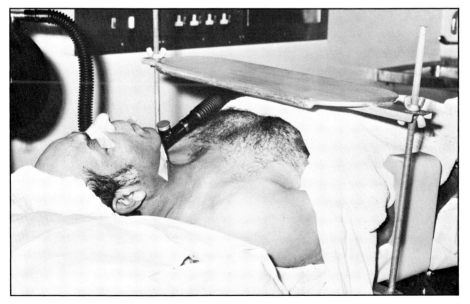

Figure 10.14 Adjustable metal bridge supported from table-rails. This takes full pressure of the Loewy support (as in *Figures 10.18, 10.21* and *10.22*) without interfering with anaesthetic tubes, and avoids pressure upon the patient's chest wall

Examination

The examination should be conducted with full aseptic precautions to prevent the carrying of infection from one patient to another.

The method of holding and introducing the laryngoscope is shown in *Figures 10.15, 10.16, 10.17* and *10.18.* Care must be taken to protect the teeth, lips, and tongue from

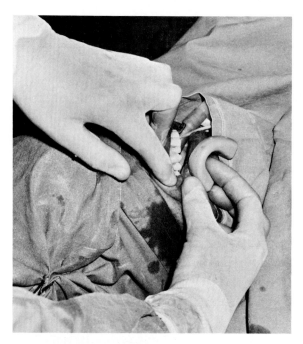

Figure 10.15 Insertion of a plastic guard to protect the upper teeth

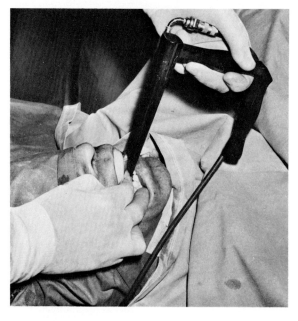

Figure 10.16 Fingers of right hand protecting lips while beak of laryngoscope slips backwards a little to the right side of the midline of the tongue

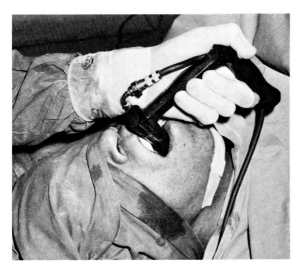

Figure 10.17   The laryngoscope is now behind the epiglottis which is being lifted forwards to establish the final definitive view required

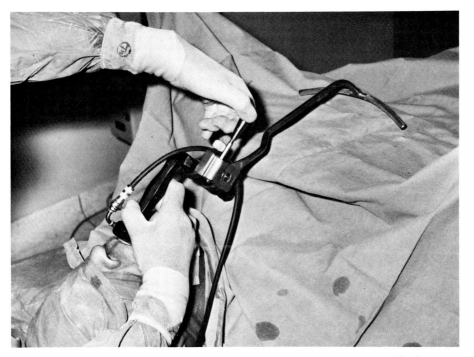

Figure 10.18   The Loewy support, clamped to the laryngoscope, being extended by its worm-and-rack to stabilize the exposure. Its counter-pressure is against the (draped) metal bridge above the chest

pressure and laceration at every stage. Generous lubrication and unhurried, gentle work are required. *Figure 10.15* illustrates an excellent dental guard. When the posterior one-third of the tongue is reached, the laryngoscope is directed to the midline and elevated slightly, bringing the epiglottis into view (*Figure 10.19*). Its tip is then guided behind the epiglottis, advanced about 1 cm and elevated. This is effected by *lifting* upwards and forwards with the left hand. There must be no *levering* of the laryngoscope on the upper teeth or gums. Only the posterior part of the larynx (*Figure 10.20*) is usually seen at first, and further elevation may be necessary to bring the anterior commissure into view. At this stage the Loewy support (*Figure 10.18*) can be fitted and judicious use of the extension screw will give a better view of the anterior half of the larynx. If it still remains out of sight, it may be helpful to alter the position

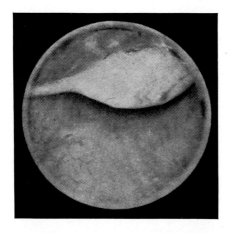

Figure 10.19 Direct laryngoscopy. Epiglottis and posterior pharyngeal wall. (Reproduced by courtesy of Dr. Paul H. Holinger and the Editor of *Annals of Otology, Rhinology and Laryngology*)

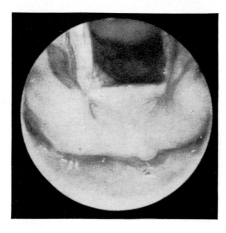

Figure 10.20 Direct laryngoscopy. Posterior part of larynx. (Reproduced by courtesy of Dr. Paul H. Holinger and the Editor of *Annals of Otology, Rhinology and Laryngology*)

of the head by raising or lowering it a little; sometimes it is useful to get an assistant to press the thyroid cartilage back from the outside. Although it is rightly taught that pressure on the upper teeth must be avoided or minimized, every experienced laryngologist knows that in some cases it is inevitable. Patients should be warned of the possibility, albeit a slight one, of chipping of an incisor, or even dislodgment of a loose tooth. The surgeon has to use all his judgment and skill in difficult cases to ensure that no cancers are overlooked even if this means that some dental risks must be taken from time to time. If a lesion is in the posterior part of the larynx the laryngoscope must be placed behind the anaesthetic tube, lifting it forwards.

When the required exposure of the larynx is finally achieved and stabilized the operating microscope is brought into position (*Figures 10.22* and *10.23*).

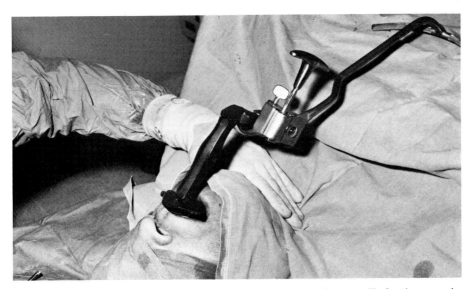

Figure 10.21 Backward displacement by external pressure on the larynx will often improve the view of the anterior commissure. This can equally well be done by an unsterile assistant's hand, underneath the drapes

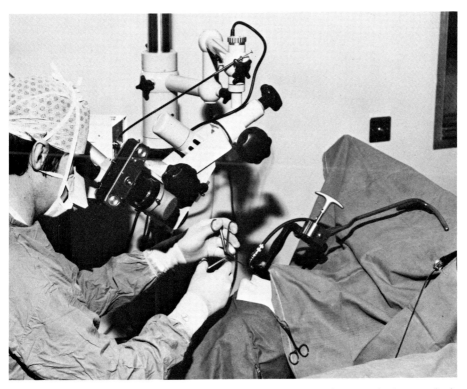

Figure 10.22 Micro-laryngoscopy. Although not depicted here, the anaesthetist must be in overall control and must be given the airway without a moment's delay if problems arise demanding it

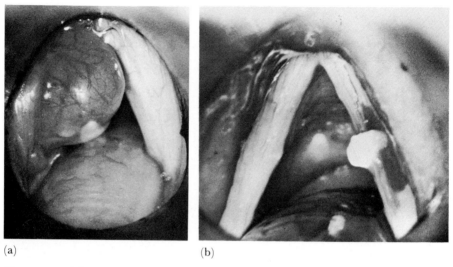

(a)   (b)

Figure 10.23   Micro-laryngoscopy. (a) Ventricular cyst; (b) carcinoma of vocal cord

The standard laryngoscope gives a general view of the larynx, but the anterior commissure laryngoscope is more useful for a detailed examination and for exposing the anterior commissure of the larynx. The tip of the anterior commissure laryngoscope can be used to lift up the ventricular bands, so that the interior of the ventricle is exposed and it can be passed between the vocal cords to inspect the subglottic region.

Comparison of direct and indirect laryngoscopic appearances

Direct laryngoscopy gives the more accurate picture of the larynx, and the student should understand the reasons why the larynx looks different in the reflected mirror image. In indirect laryngoscopy, the angle at which the mirror has to be held causes some foreshortening in the antero-posterior diameter, so that the apparent length of the vocal cords and aryepiglottic folds is reduced, and a lesion of the vocal cord will appear to be nearer the arytenoid cartilage than it really is. The line of vision also is different in the two methods. The mirror, placed posteriorly in the pharynx, reflects the light downwards and forwards into the laryngeal aperture, and thus, in effect, the examiner is looking at the larynx from above and behind. From this viewpoint it is impossible to see much of the anterior surface of the interarytenoid space (*see Figure 10.3*). With the direct laryngoscope, however, the whole of the area is exposed (*see Figure 10.20*). In the mirror-image a false impression of the depth of the larynx is given and it looks much shallower than it really is. The ventricular bands appear to be in contact with the upper surface of the vocal cords, which look flat and white with sharp free margins. Direct laryngoscopy reveals the true depth of the larynx, the presence of the ventricle between the true and false cords, and the fact that the cords are actually slightly rounded and faintly pink in colour.

Stroboscopy

The vibrations of the vocal cords during phonation are much too rapid to be followed by indirect laryngoscopy, but with the stroboscope an effect of slowing down can be achieved, enabling them to be followed and analysed by the naked eye. This apparent slowing down is brought about by the use, during indirect laryngoscopy, of an interrupted source of light. The original means of producing the interruptions was by a disc with holes in it, set before the light and rotated at varied speeds by an electric motor.

If, when the patient phonates, the frequency of the note uttered corresponds exactly with the frequency of the flashes of interrupted light, the same phase of the vocal cord movement will be illuminated by each flash and the cords will appear to be motionless. If, however, the speed of the disc be so altered that there is a difference of 1 cycle/second between the frequency of the note and the light flashes, a slightly different phase of the vocal cord vibration will be illuminated by each flash, with the original phase re-appearing at the end of one second. It will appear, therefore, as though only one excursion of the vocal cords is taking place each second. This obviously greatly facilitates the study of the physiology of speech and analysis of faults of voice production.

Instruments are now commercially available which automatically adjust the frequency of the light interruptions to the note produced by the larynx. This makes the examiner's task much easier than formerly when he had to control the frequency of the light interruptions himself.

Radiography of the larynx

Radiographs of the larynx are useful in conditions other than malignant disease. Foreign bodies are rare in the larynx, but those that become impacted are usually metallic and so can be easily shown. Fractures of the laryngeal cartilages may be demonstrated, and also oedema, with narrowing of the airway and surgical emphysema. The degree and extent of laryngeal and tracheal stenosis may be shown by x-ray examination, and after tracheostomy and in the treatment of stenosis a radiograph is useful to check the position of the tracheostomy tube and any intralaryngeal mould that may have been used. A retropharyngeal abscess appears as a considerable thickening of the pre-vertebral soft tissues.

Tomography

Tomograms of the larynx are often more useful than lateral skiagrams in the demonstration of growths and stenosis. The vocal cords, ventricular bands and the ventricle of the larynx can be defined, and thickening of the cords and obliteration of the ventricle are readily seen when they are involved by growths. As in ordinary radiographs, the most important point to be learnt from tomography in carcinoma of the larynx is the amount of subglottic spread that has taken place.

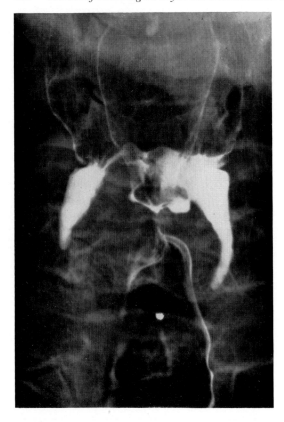

Figure 10.24 Laryngogram showing a right subglottic neoplasm

Laryngograms

Study of laryngograms may give additional information as to the site, size and spread
of a laryngeal neoplasm (*Figure 10.24*) and so help in deciding upon the right
treatment. The accuracy of assessment of a growth by this method is higher than by
ordinary methods but the interpretation of the films needs much study and practice.

The tracheobronchial tree

Indirect methods of examining the tracheobronchial tree

Much information can be gained from clinical examination of the chest, accompanied by suitable x-rays including tomography where indicated and backed up by
tests of pulmonary function.

Clinical examination of the chest

Finger clubbing, cyanosis and tachypnoea should be looked for and the chest then examined in the classical manner by inspection, palpation (of the apex beat, trachea and movement), percussion and auscultation.

Inspection
The normal chest may be slightly asymmetrical, but usually moves equally on both sides. Exaggeration of this asymmetry may be seen with pigeon chest and pectus excavatum. With underlying pleural effusions or fibrosis the chest may appear flattened and less mobile (e.g. frozen chest).

Percussion
The chest should be percussed from top to bottom, front and back, areas of dullness due to collapse or consolidation determined, and the stony dullness of a pleural effusion sought.

Auscultation
This should be carried out over all lung areas, comparing the two sides, and the normal vesicular breath sounds appreciated. Underlying consolidation leads to bronchial breath sounds (similar to those usually heard over the trachea) and these are occasionally heard through a pleural effusion. More often the pleural effusion leads to obliteration of breath sounds. Added sounds include crackles (synonym, crepitations or *râles*) due to opening of small airways, and wheezes (synonym, rhonchi) due to critical narrowing of small airways. The third type is the leathery noise of a pleural friction rub. Crackles indicate pneumonic consolidation, heart failure if basal, or fibrosing alveolitis for instance; transient crackles which clear on deep breathing or coughing may be heard at the lung bases in normal individuals. Wheezing may be of variable pitch and is heard in patients with airways obstruction from chronic bronchitis or asthma. Stridor is usually inspiratory and indicates upper (laryngeal or tracheal) airways obstruction, either intrinsic (e.g. tumour) or extrinsic (e.g. goitre) in type.

Radiography

A chest x-ray is vital for any patient with suspected lung or intrathoracic disease. The usual posterior–anterior (PA) 2 m standard film suffices, if necessary supported by a lateral view. If abnormalities are shown on these, then further views including tomography may be indicated. This is particularly important for lesions at the apex or at the hilar regions where differentiation from the pulmonary vessels may be difficult.

Pulmonary function tests (Clarke, 1976)

As their name suggests, these test pulmonary function, changes in which may support a particular diagnosis. Unlike lung histology, for example, they rarely give a definitive diagnosis. However, they may provide key evidence in disorders such as asthma, characterized by variable airways obstruction and monitored by wide swings in peak expiratory flow rate (PEFR).

The standard pulmonary function tests are summarized in *Figure 10.25*. They can be grouped under dynamic lung volumes which include FEV_1, FVC, FEV_1/FVC, and PEFR; static lung volumes including VC, RV and TLC; and gas transfer, where carbon monoxide is used as a test gas. Space is left for other tests such as skin-prick allergy tests, important when dealing with hay fever and asthma.

With airways obstruction, whether due to asthma, chronic bronchitis or emphysema, the dynamic volumes and flows are much reduced and may be reversed with an inhaled bronchodilator (e.g. salbutamol), an integral part of the testing. The degree of reversibility gives a clue as to which of these three entities is present, asthma usually being largely reversible (> 20 per cent). At the same time airways obstruction leads to compensatory hyperinflation of the lungs with a high residual volume and RV/TLC ratio.

With the static lung volumes, significant reduction (< 80 per cent) indicates a restrictive defect, whether caused by changes in the chest wall, pleura or lung proper. In this case a fall in gas transfer usually suggests parenchymal lung disease such as fibrosing alveolitis or sarcoidosis. Naturally, these findings will be correlated with the appropriate chest x-ray. If the patient is cyanosed or dyspnoeic, then arterial blood gases may be done, though this is essentially an invasive procedure while the foregoing are not.

In conclusion, much can be gained from careful evaluation of the patient and the chest with chest x-rays and pulmonary function tests. This can lead to a more precise indication for or diagnosis at endoscopy.

Bronchoscopy

Although bronchoscopy was brought to its present state of perfection by the skill and enthusiasm of laryngologists, notably Killian in Germany, Chevalier Jackson in the United States of America and Negus in Great Britain, its practice has now passed into the hands of the chest surgeons and physicians who naturally want to see the lesions they are to treat. However, the laryngologist still has occasion to examine the respiratory passages below the larynx and he should therefore have a knowledge of the anatomy of the bronchial tree, of pulmonary diseases and of the technique of bronchoscopy.

Instruments and equipment

It is impossible to describe more than a few of the instruments that have been devised for use in bronchoscopy. Some, though rarely needed, may be essential in an emergency and it should be realized that it will not be possible to improvise or find substitutes while the operation is in progress. Each clinic must therefore carry a number of instruments which will be used very rarely or should be prepared to hand on to a larger unit all but the simplest and most routine cases. The following is a list of instruments which will meet most requirements.

Royal Free Hospital - Department of Thoracic Medicine
PULMONARY FUNCTION REPORT

M/F
M/S/W

Diagnosis

Hospital No.
Surname
First Names

D. of B.

Branch

Ward/Dept.
Consultant
Doctor's Signature   Date

Ht.   cm. Wt.   Kg. Smoking:

LUNG VOLUMES			Predicted	Observed	% Predicted	After Broncho-Dilators
Vital capacity	VC	L				
Forced vital capacity	FVC	L				
☐ Forced expiratory volume. 1 sec.	FEV₁	L				
FEV₁/FVC		%				
Peak flow rate	PFR	L/min				
Expiratory reserve volume	ERV	L				
Residual volume	RV	L				
☐ Functional residual capacity	FRC	L				
Total lung capacity	TLC	L				
RV/TLC		%				

GAS TRANSFER		Predicted	Observed
Lung transfer			
T₁CO ml/min/mmHg			
Rebreathing PⱴCO₂	mmHg		
☐ Arterial PO2	mmHg		
″ PCO2	mmHg		
″ pH	units		
″ Base	mEq/L		
OTHER TESTS:			

COMMENTS:

RF 230 I

PULMONARY FUNCTION REPORT

Figure 10.25   A form for recording pulmonary function tests

Bronchoscopes; rigid, Negus – adult and child ranges (i.e. 4.8–11 mm outside diameter; 27.5–40 cm length), with direct vision (46 cm length), retrograde (48 cm length) and 90° telescopes. Flexible fibre-optic bronchoscope. Snares, forceps (*see Figures 10.31 and 10.33*), aspirating tubes, sputum traps, sponge holders, etc. Negus 'split' laryngoscope (*Figure 10.36*), optional.

Rigid bronchoscopes. Fundamentally, a bronchoscope consists of a hollow brass tube, which is slanted at its distal end and which has a small handle at the proximal end. Accurately placed breathing-holes are situated in the side walls of the distal part of the tube, to allow respiration to take place through the bronchi which are not occupied by the bronchoscope. Various small auxiliary tubes are incorporated into the main bronchoscopic tube for the purposes of lighting and aspiration, and for insufflation of oxygen and of anaesthetic vapours.

Bronchoscopes have been designed to fit the bronchi at various developmental ages and at various depths in the bronchial tree. The bronchi will not tolerate dilatation, and bronchoscopes of greater diameter than the air passages to be explored should never be used as the results of the over-distension of a bronchus may be very serious and rupture is generally fatal.

The diameters of the bronchoscopes are limited also by the size of the glottis and of the laryngeal cavity. In an adult the glottis is a triangle measuring approximately 12 × 22 × 22 mm, which permits the passage of a tube not exceeding 12 mm in diameter without risk of injury. Subglottic oedema may occur as a result of the passage of an instrument too large to be tolerated by this region, or by too prolonged or too frequently repeated bronchoscopic examinations in a previously normal larynx. The duration of a bronchoscopic examination in a small child should never exceed 20 min, and it should be repeated only at reasonable intervals. Other causes of subglottic oedema are trauma caused by undue force or improper direction during the insertion of the bronchoscope, rough manipulation of instruments and injury inflicted by a foreign body during its extraction.

Subglottic oedema is a serious lesion which may necessitate early tracheostomy and which sometimes may prove fatal.

The Negus bronchoscope illustrated in *Figure 10.26* is to be preferred to the original Jackson ones. The proximal third of the Negus bronchoscope, which remains

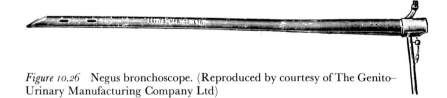

Figure 10.26   Negus bronchoscope. (Reproduced by courtesy of The Genito–Urinary Manufacturing Company Ltd)

in the mouth and pharynx, is expanded and this affords more room for inspection and the introduction of instruments. It is also more economical of space, having a finer light carrier which is held in a groove, not a tube, so increasing the effective lumen of the bronchoscope.

Bronchoscopic telescopes. Bronchoscopic telescopes (*Figure 10.27*) are of great value in the examination of the subglottic region, the trachea and the bronchi since they give a wide-angle magnified view of the area under inspection. Direct vision, 90° and retrograde telescopes are available. When in use they are kept standing in a vessel containing hot water (covered at the bottom with cotton wool to prevent damage to the lens) to prevent fogging when they are passed down the bronchoscope.

Aspiration tubes. Jackson's open-ended aspirating tubes and Negus' tubes with detachable gum-elastic ends are most generally useful (*Figure 10.28*). The original Luken's specimen collector (*Figure 10.29*), or sputum trap, has been superseded by plastic disposable traps which are used routinely. An efficient suction apparatus is necessary and is usefully incorporated in an endoscopic table. They must in every case be spark-proof to avoid explosion of anaesthetic vapours.

In addition to suction tubes, sponges are needed to dry the field and to clean the light of the bronchoscope. They are made from selvedge ribbon gauze in several sizes and are held in Coolidge's sponge holders.

Forceps. Almost all bronchoscopic forceps are of a tubular type and they are so constructed that a slender tube works over a stilette which carries spring-spread jaws. The forceps are made in lengths which vary from 40 cm to 60 cm, as required for use through the different bronchoscopes; and a very delicate or 'mosquito' size is available for the infant and suckling bronchoscopes.

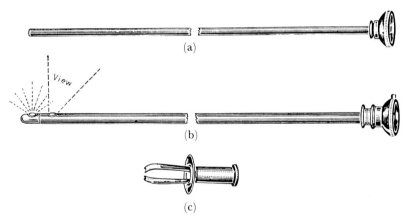

Figure 10.27 (a) Direct-vision bronchoscopic telescope; (b) retrograde broncho-scopic telescope; (c) spring clip adapter with shield for holding telescope in position in laryngoscope. (Reproduced by courtesy of the Editor of *Lancet*)

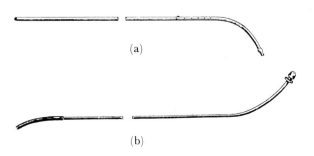

Figure 10.28 Aspiration tubes. (a) Jackson's open end aspirating tube. (Reproduced by courtesy of W. B. Saunders, Philadelphia); (b) Negus' aspirating tube with flexible gum-elastic end. (Reproduced by courtesy of The Genito–Urinary Manufacturing Company Ltd)

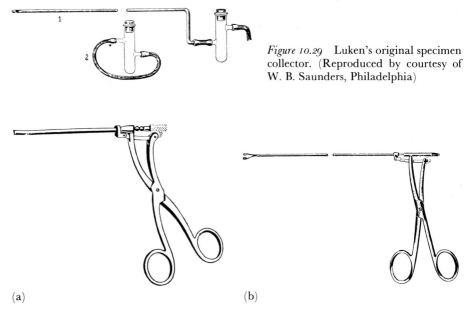

Figure 10.29 Luken's original specimen collector. (Reproduced by courtesy of W. B. Saunders, Philadelphia)

(a)   (b)

Figure 10.30 (a) Chevalier Jackson's bronchoscopic forceps handle. (Reproduced by courtesy of W. B. Saunders, Philadelphia); (b) Negus' modification of Chevalier Jackson's bronchoscopic forceps handle. (Reproduced by courtesy of The Genito–Urinary Manufacturing Company Ltd)

The stilette and tube are fixed in the handle mechanism. The Chevalier Jackson handle is illustrated in *Figure 10.30*; the Negus modification of this, which gives more steadiness to the tip of the forceps, is also shown. A ratchet handle may be substituted for the above if it is desired to lock the forceps on to a foreign body or tumour. The forceps jaws are screwed on to the stilette and the degree of their closure and the extent of their opening are adjusted by the thumb-nut on the proximal end of the stilette.

To close the forceps the handle must be used so that the cannula is forced down on the jaws, causing them to approximate. The handle must not be manipulated so that the jaws are pulled into the cannula as this causes their tips to recede from the target. *Figure 10.31a* illustrates the correct method of closure of the forceps by pushing the cannula on to the jaws. It also illustrates the correct fingering of the handle and the method of making traction for the withdrawal of the forceps with the grasped object. *Figure 10.31b* shows the incorrect method of these manoeuvres by which the object is grasped insecurely and the shaft of the forceps is dragged out of the line of the bronchoscope.

Most of the jaws were designed by Chevalier Jackson for the removal of foreign bodies or for obtaining specimens of tissue, and the more frequently used types are illustrated in *Figure 10.32*. They have either straight ends or side-curved ends; the latter are of more general use. Each forceps should have its own handle and the set-screws should be on the right side in order to be out of sight.

Brock's biopsy forceps (*Figure 10.33*) have the advantages of simplicity and a more rigid shaft.

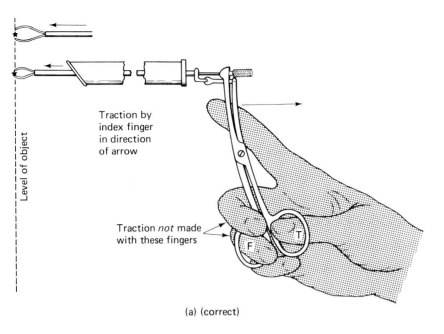

Traction by
index finger
in direction
of arrow

Level of object

Traction *not* made
with these fingers

F   T

(a) (correct)

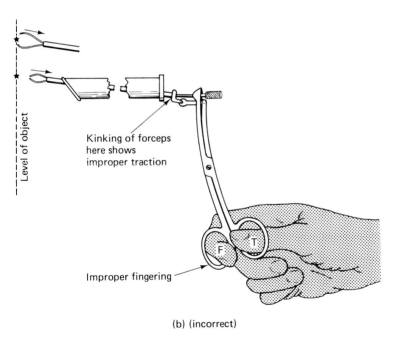

Level of object

Kinking of forceps
here shows
improper traction

F   T

Improper fingering

(b) (incorrect)

Figure 10.31 (a) Diagram of correct fingering of forceps, manner of closing forceps on object and method of making traction. The thumb and ring finger are inserted into the handle rings. These fingers are used for opening and closing forceps only. All traction is made with index finger, which is placed high on the handle. (b) Diagram showing incorrect method of fingering, closure of forceps and traction whereby object may be missed and forceps kinked

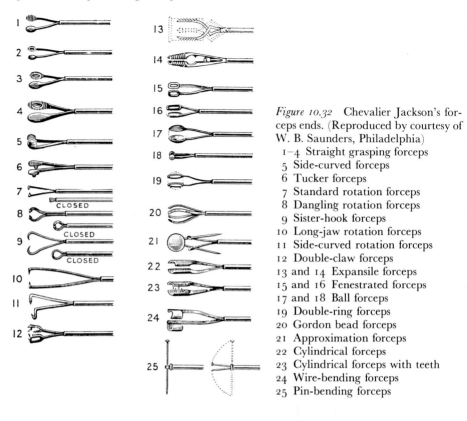

Figure 10.32   Chevalier Jackson's forceps ends. (Reproduced by courtesy of W. B. Saunders, Philadelphia)

1–4 Straight grasping forceps
5 Side-curved forceps
6 Tucker forceps
7 Standard rotation forceps
8 Dangling rotation forceps
9 Sister-hook forceps
10 Long-jaw rotation forceps
11 Side-curved rotation forceps
12 Double-claw forceps
13 and 14 Expansile forceps
15 and 16 Fenestrated forceps
17 and 18 Ball forceps
19 Double-ring forceps
20 Gordon bead forceps
21 Approximation forceps
22 Cylindrical forceps
23 Cylindrical forceps with teeth
24 Wire-bending forceps
25 Pin-bending forceps

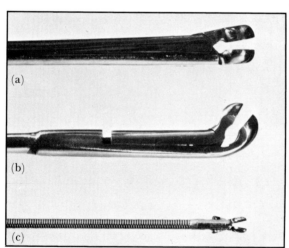

Figure 10.33   (a) and (b) Brock's straight and angled bronchial biopsy forceps; (c) flexible biopsy forceps for use in the fibre-optic bronchoscope

Anaesthesia

In rigid bronchoscopy, as in direct laryngoscopy, general anaesthesia is replacing local analgesia.

Local analgesia

This is carried out in the same way as for direct laryngoscopy with the addition that, besides dropping the lignocaine into the interior of the larynx, a further 2 ml are dropped between the cords into the trachea. This is better than injecting the solution through the cricothyroid membrane.

General anaesthesia

This is also carried out initially as described under direct laryngoscopy. Since a bronchoscope has to be passed, however, an endotracheal anaesthetic tube cannot be used. The anaesthetist, therefore, after inducing with thiopentone and suxamethonium, fully inflates the patient's lungs with oxygen. Alternatively, anaesthesia may be maintained through a small-bore catheter. The bronchoscope is then passed and the examination started. Ventilation is continued by means of the Sanders technique, described in Volume 1.

A biopsy should not be taken nor the bronchoscope removed until spontaneous respiration is returning.

In young children, deep inhalation anaesthesia with nitrous oxide, oxygen and halothane is sufficient for a short examination and spontaneous respiration is not abolished.

Technique of rigid bronchoscopy

It is unnecessary to state that, except in cases of extreme emergency, all patients before bronchoscopy must have a thorough clinical and radiological investigation, and a routine examination of the nasal fossae, nasopharynx, pharynx and larynx, and they must be prepared in the usual manner for general anaesthesia. Aseptic precautions must be observed during bronchoscopy as in any other major surgical procedure.

Position of the patient

It is customary to carry out bronchoscopic examination while the patient is lying in the dorsally recumbent position. The patient is so placed that the head and shoulders extend beyond the table, the edge of which supports the thorax at about the midscapular region; and the head is held by an assistant or a head-rest as may be preferred.

As may be seen from *Figure 10.34*, the trachea does not pursue a horizontal course in the thorax, but is directed downwards and backwards. In order to bring the axes of the buccal cavity and pharynx into line with those of the larynx and trachea, therefore, the head and neck must be elevated so that the occiput is about 10 cm above the level of the table and the head must be extended at the atlanto-occipital joint as shown in *Figure 10.34*. This position is well maintained with the Negus head-rest.

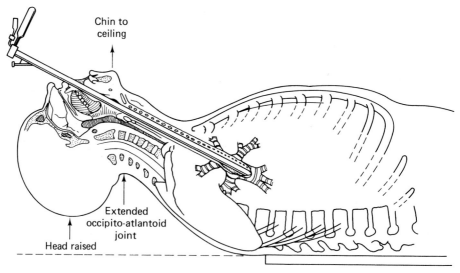

Figure 10.34   Diagram of position of patient's head and neck for bronchoscopy

Introduction of the bronchoscope

If bronchoscopy is carried out under surface analgesia, it is essential that the procedure and the sensations to be endured shall be explained fully to the patient, so that he may be freed from apprehension and in order that his cooperation may be obtained.

Some laryngologists expose the glottis with a laryngoscope and pass the bronchoscope through this into the trachea; others pass the bronchoscope directly through the glottis into the trachea without the aid of a laryngoscope.

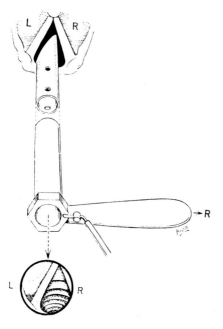

Figure 10.35   Diagram showing method of insertion of bronchoscope through glottis

In young children and infants it is always advisable to expose the glottis with a laryngoscope before passing the bronchoscope.

If the bronchoscope is inserted through the laryngoscope after exposure of the glottis, its handle is rotated to the right so that a full view of the left vocal cord is obtained through the bronchoscope (*Figure 10.35*). In this position the tip of the bronchoscope is situated in the long axis of the glottis and it can be inserted gently and easily into the trachea.

When the bronchoscope has been advanced a short distance into the trachea, the handle of the laryngoscope is rotated to the left, its slide is removed (*Figure 10.36*), and the laryngoscope is then withdrawn.

If the bronchoscope is to be passed directly, without the aid of a laryngoscope, it should be held in the right hand by the shaft – not by the handle – in a pen-like manner, and the patient's upper lip should be retracted by the surgeon's left index finger.

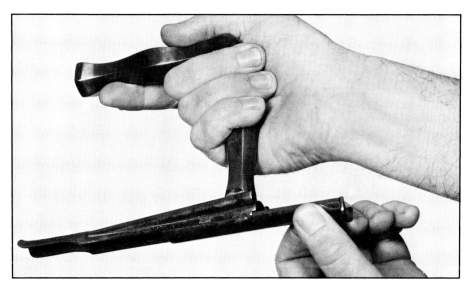

Figure 10.36   The Negus laryngoscope, which is in two separable halves, for removal after introduction of a rigid bronchoscope through it into the upper trachea

The bronchoscope is inserted to the right of the anterior two-thirds of the tongue and its tip is directed towards the midline when the posterior third is reached. The epiglottis is the first landmark and when this has been identified it is lifted forward on the tip of the bronchoscope to expose the glottis. The bronchoscope is then rotated to the right and so directed that a good view of the left cord is obtained, when the bronchoscope can be inserted gently into the trachea.

When the trachea is entered it is recognized as an open tube with whitish cartilaginous rings, while the expiratory blast is felt and tubular breathing is heard through the bronchoscope.

If a direction-vision bronchoscopic telescope is to be used, it is taken from the vessel of hot water, the lens is dried and it is passed down the bronchoscope until the walls of the trachea are in focus. It is then clipped to the bronchoscope when it can be used with – or as part of – the bronchoscope. It will be necessary to remove the telescope periodically in order to clean the lens, which must be warmed each time in hot water before re-insertion into the bronchoscope.

The axis of the bronchoscope should be made to correspond as nearly as possible with that of the trachea; any secretion must be removed by aspiration and the walls of the trachea inspected by 'weaving' the bronchoscope from side to side or by use of a 90° telescope which is self-illuminated.

The carina is recognized as a sharp vertical spur separating the orifices of the two main bronchi. As the carina is situated to the left of the midline the lumen view of the left main bronchus is very incomplete, and in order to view this adequately the tip of the bronchoscope is turned to the left while the patient's head and neck are flexed slightly to the right.

After identification and examination of the carina and of the main bronchial orifices, the main bronchi should be entered in turn, the tip of the bronchoscope being rotated in the direction of the bronchus to be examined and the head and neck flexed and rotated to the opposite side.

The bronchial orifices then must be identified seriatim as in *Figure 10.37*.

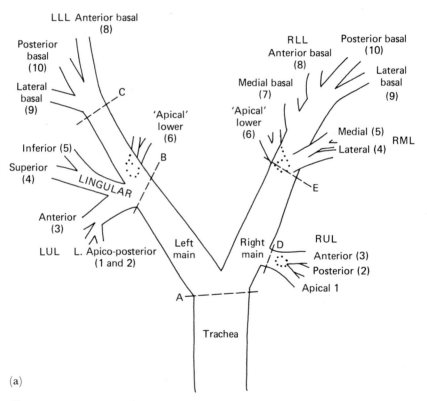

(a)

Figure 10.37   (a) Diagram of the bronchial tree. (b) Subdivisions of bronchial tree as seen at bronchoscopy. (A) Carina and main bronchi (from lower end of trachea); (B) left upper and lower lobe bronchi (from left main bronchus); (C) left lower lobe segmental bronchi; (D) right upper lobe segmental bronchi (through 90° telescope); (E) right middle and lower lobe bronchi (from right main bronchus)

As a rule, it is impossible to visualize more than a short length of the lumen of any tertiary bronchus through the bronchoscope; and there may be considerable variation of the origins of the tertiary bronchi within 'normal' limits.

The right upper lobe bronchus joins the lateral aspect of the main stem 1 or 2 cm below the level of the carina at an angle of 90°. This bronchus, though sometimes difficult to find, can always be identified by its vertical spur, and can be examined either directly or indirectly with a retrograde bronchoscopic telescope. Direct examination permits a very limited lumen view, although it is frequently possible to see the orifice of its antero-lateral branch. In order to see into the right upper lobe bronchus, the tip of the bronchoscope is directed to the right and extreme flexure of the head and neck to the left is made.

The right upper lobe bronchus can be viewed more satisfactorily through a retrograde bronchoscopic telescope, and, as a rule, it is possible to view the orifices of its three segmental branches through the telescope.

The right middle lobe bronchus is the only bronchus which joins the right stem bronchus on its anterior aspect, and its almost horizontal spur can be brought into view by directing the tip of the bronchoscope to the right, and dropping the head of the patient until the tip bears strongly on the anterior wall of the right bronchus.

The left upper bronchus, which is about 5 cm from the carina, can be examined

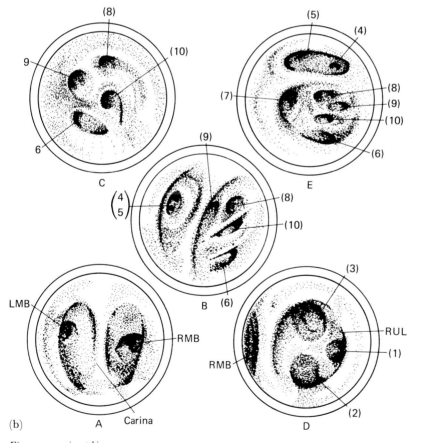

(b)

Figure 10.37 (contd.)

more easily than the right upper lobe bronchus by a similar manoeuvre. The tip of the bronchoscope is directed to the left, the head and neck are flexed strongly to the right and the head is rotated to the right. It is usually possible to visualize the division of the lingular lobe bronchus into its upper and lower segmental bronchi.

The left upper bronchus can also be viewed very satisfactorily through a retrograde bronchoscopic telescope.

Tracheoscopy

The trachea will be inspected during the course of bronchoscopy. If it is desired to inspect the trachea only, the Negus tracheoscope (*Figure 10.38*) is a most useful instrument. It is passed in the same way as a bronchoscope and its shorter length and greater diameter gives a more satisfactory field for inspection.

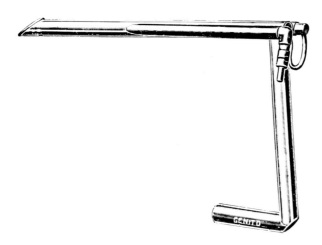

Figure 10.38   Negus tracheoscope. (Reproduced by courtesy of The Genito–Urinary Manufacturing Company Ltd)

Fibre-optic bronchoscopy

Description

Until the last decade bronchoscopy has been done solely with the rigid tube. The recent introduction of the flexible fibre-optic bronchoscope has made bronchoscopy technically simpler and more rewarding (Sackner, 1975).

The fibre-optic bronchoscope is essentially a longer version of the flexible laryngoscope, with added refinements (*Figure 10.39*). The internal guide wires enable the operator to flex the tip in two directions (from 130 degrees to 180 degrees) depending on the model used. Coupled with rotation of the instrument, this gives a wide field of

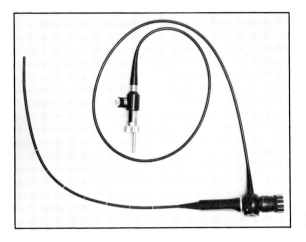

Figure 10.39   Fibre-optic bronchoscope

vision. The bronchoscope is about 700 mm in overall length with a working length of about 600 mm, a shaft diameter of about 6 mm and internal channel diameter of about 2 mm. The instruments have a suction attachment for the internal channel and are supplied with biopsy forceps and brushes. At present they are at an intermediate stage of development and are constantly being refined. The trainee fibre-optic bronchoscopist requires about three months' practice and 50 assisted bronchoscopies before being considered fully trained.

Technique of flexible fibre-optic bronchoscopy

Most fibre-optic bronchoscopies are performed by the direct trans-nasal route under local anaesthesia, similar to that described on p. 274 for fibre-optic laryngoscopy. Failing this, the trans-oral route may be used though this is slightly more difficult. Occasionally, in particularly anxious patients, bronchoscopy may be done under general anaesthesia. In small children, the small rigid bronchoscope may be necessary, because the diameter of the current fibre-optic bronchoscope is such as partially to occlude the airway.

The patients are fully evaluated beforehand by clinical and radiographic examination and testing of pulmonary function, which includes as least spirometry (forced expired volume in 1 second – FEV_1; forced vital capacity – FVC; peak expiratory flow rate – PEFR), with arterial blood gases if hypoxaemia is suspected. The latter can usually be corrected with nasal oxygen during the procedure. The patients have the procedure explained to them to allay anxiety and one hour beforehand pre-medication is given, either Omnopon 10–20 mg with Scopolamine 0.2–0.4 mg, pethidine 50–100 mg with atropine 0.3–0.6 mg or diazepam 5–10 mg with atropine. The patient lies comfortably, semi-recumbent on a couch with the bronchoscopist on the right side facing. Positions can be varied to suit the bronchoscopist. Lignocaine aerosol (four per cent) is sprayed into the wider nostril and sniffed back, then over the pharynx and finally over the back of the tongue with an angled jet to reach the larynx. The bronchoscope is lubricated with lignocaine gel (two per cent) and steered gently through the nose under direct vision and steadily to the larynx. The larynx is anaesthetized with a 2 ml 'bolus' of lignocaine (four per cent) injected through the central channel directly on to the vocal cords. This stage takes less than five minutes. The instrument is then passed gently through the larynx with a no-touch technique to avoid coughing. The larynx, the trachea, the carina and both bronchial trees are examined in a systematic manner, particular attention being paid to the site of any suspected lesion. At the conclusion a report is written, and the form illustrated has been found useful (*Figure 10.40*).

Biopsy – forceps and brush

Flexible cupped biopsy forceps (*see Figure 10.33*) can be introduced through the central channel and multiple biopsies taken of endobronchial lesions under direct vision, or of localized or diffuse lung lesions under fluoroscopic control.

The specimens are small, reflecting the small size of the forceps, but the diagnostic yield is high and considerably better than with the rigid bronchoscope. The specimen should be placed in a few ml of ten per cent formalin in a universal container and handled by an experienced technician.

The brush has stiff nylon bristles mounted on the tip of a flexible wire. This may be used for brushing lesions visible directly or fluoroscopically. On withdrawal the brush is smeared on to a clean, dry slide and then placed in a fixative and stained in the conventional way.

Aspiration

A suction tube is connected to the internal channel of the bronchoscope via a T-piece to allow controlled intermittent suction. A sputum trap is included routinely in the line so that samples may be sent for bacteriological and cytological examination.

Indications for bronchoscopy – rigid and fibre-optic

The indications for bronchoscopy are similar whichever instrument is used. Thus, any patient with an unexplained symptom such as cord palsy, haemoptysis, signs such as slowly resolving pneumonia, or abnormalities on chest x-ray such as lung shadows, masses or collapse, should be bronchoscoped.

The rigid bronchoscope allows adequate visualization of the bronchial tree to the origin of the lower lobe segmental bronchi. Only the orifice and 0.5–1.0 cm of the inferior aspect of the right and left upper lobe bronchi can be seen, though the sub-divisions may be inspected (but not biopsied) with a 90° telescope.

By contrast, the fibre-optic bronchoscope extends the range of vision considerably throughout the bronchial tree, enabling inspection and biopsy of all segmental and sub-segmental bronchi in each lobe. Thus, hitherto inaccessible upper lobe lesions are now readily diagnosed.

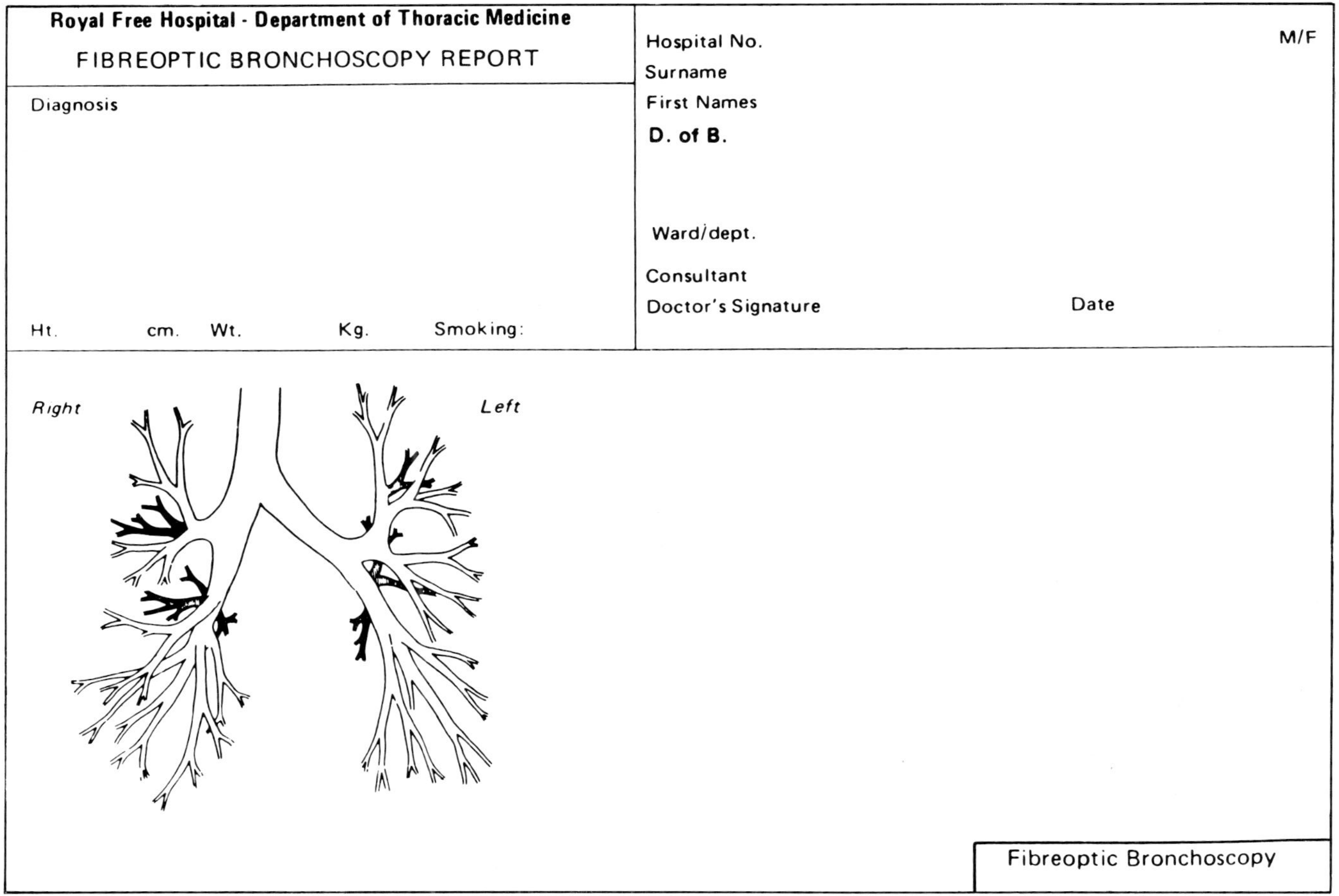

Royal Free Hospital - Department of Thoracic Medicine
FIBREOPTIC BRONCHOSCOPY REPORT

	Hospital No. M/F
Diagnosis	Surname
	First Names
	D. of B.
	Ward/dept.
Ht. cm. Wt. Kg. Smoking:	Consultant
	Doctor's Signature Date

Left

Right

Fibreoptic Bronchoscopy

Figure 10.40   A form for reporting bronchoscopic findings

While rigid bronchoscopy has been used principally for the diagnosis of bronchial carcinoma, the advent of the fibre-optic instrument has widened the diagnostic range considerably: many medical lung disorders can now be diagnosed with this added facility. These disorders include sarcoidosis, fibrosing alveolitis and other causes of diffuse pulmonary shadowing (*Figure 10.41*), unresolved pneumonia and tuberculosis. Additionally, the bronchoscope can be used for aspirating mucus plugs in post-operative patients or in those on the Intensive Care Unit. Furthermore, there are virtually no contra-indications such as cervical spondylosis, nor side effects from fibre-optic bronchoscopy. Consequently, in centres equipped for fibre-optic bronchoscopy this may be the examination of choice. Current trends support this contention. There remains one firm indication for rigid bronchoscopy, namely an impacted foreign

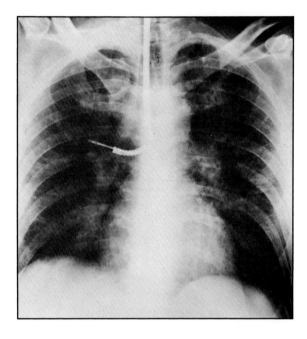

Figure 10.41 Chest x-ray of a man with diffuse pulmonary shadowing, showing fibre-optic bronchoscope *in situ*. The tip is positioned in the right upper lobe bronchus and the forceps extended distally into the posterior segmental bronchus ready for bronchial biopsy. Transbronchial lung biopsy was also done in this particular patient

body, even though special foreign body forceps are now made for use with the fibre-optic bronchoscope.

In general, the technique for fibre-optic bronchoscopy is much simpler than for rigid bronchoscopy, requiring no anaesthetist or theatre, and lending itself to out-patient bronchoscopy. Although the instrument is expensive the cost-effectiveness is high.

An up-to-date review is given by Clarke (1977).

Other diagnostic procedures

In patients with cord palsy, for instance, *mediastinoscopy* may reveal nodes compressing the left recurrent laryngeal nerve. Biopsy of these nodes should reveal the diagnosis. On occasion percutaneous *needle biopsy* of hilar or paratracheal nodes under careful fluoroscopy may likewise confirm a suspected diagnosis.

References

Baclesse, F.(1938). *Le Diagnostique Radiologique des Tumeurs Malignes du Pharynx et du Larynx*; Masson, Paris

Clarke, S. W. (1976). *British Journal of Hospital Medicine*, **15,** 137

Clarke, S. W. (1977). In: *Advanced Medicine* (Ed. G. M. Besser), Vol. 13, p. 230; Pitman Medical, London

Holtz, S., Power, S. E., McGavran, M. H. and Ogura, J. (1963). *American Journal of Roentgenology*, **89,** 10

Jackson, C. and Jackson, C. L. (1937). *The Larynx and its Diseases*; Saunders, Philadelphia and London

Kleinsasser, D. (1968). *Microlaryngology and Endolaryngeal Surgery*; Saunders, Philadelphia and London

Lewy, R. B. (1953). *Archives of Otolaryngology*, **58,** 444

Negus, V. E. (1947). *Proceedings of the Royal Society of Medicine*, **40,** 849

Sackner, M. A. (1975). *American Review of Respiratory Diseases*, **111,** 62

Thomson, St. Clair and Negus, V. E. (1955). *Diseases of the Nose and Throat*; Cassell, London

11 Congenital diseases of the larynx
R Pracy

Differences between the infant and the adult larynx

The differences between the infant and adult larynx are both structural and functional.

Structural differences

The infant's larynx is both relatively and absolutely smaller than the adult larynx. It lies higher in the neck and is tucked in under the back of the tongue. This makes examination of the larynx difficult even if it is carried out under general anaesthesia. The largest diameter of the airway at the level of the glottis in a newborn baby of 3.15 kg weight is 6 mm. The diameter of the cricoid immediately below the glottis is even smaller (4 mm). The supporting cartilages are very soft and may not provide sufficient substance to act as a rigid frame upon which the intrinsic laryngeal muscles can work. In infants 30–50 per cent of larynges show elongation and narrowing of the supraglottis with an 'omega-shaped' curling of the petiole of the epiglottis, short aryepiglottic folds and a narrow laryngeal introitus. In about ten per cent of larynges the supraglottis is covered with very lax tissue which may seem to spill over the glottis and fill the pyriform sinuses. The direction of the airway is straighter in the infant than it is in the adult. The measurements given above refer to a 3.15 kg baby and allowance must therefore be made for the size of the child in estimating the possible size of the airway.

Functional differences

As in the adult, so in the child, the larynx has a respiratory, an alimentary and a phonatory function. The respiratory function is instinctive, the alimentary function is acquired with relatively little difficulty and at least in part by instinct. Phonatory function is acquired as a result of imitation, experiment and much practice. A hearing child born of deaf parents acquires speech less rapidly than a child born to hearing parents. A newborn child normally exercises its respiratory function instinctively.

The vocal cords abduct during inspiration. The alimentary function or protection of the lower airway during swallowing is by no means as perfectly developed, and it is a commonplace experience to find a baby choking over both solid and liquid food once it attempts to take food from either a cup or a spoon. The larynx has an abundant and highly sensitive nerve supply and once a foreign body stimulates the inner surface of the laryngeal introitus a violent reflex response is initiated and the whole larynx may pass into a severe spasm and into a period of prolonged breath-holding associated with vivid colour changes in the baby's face. This is a protective response and the sensitivity of the mucosa is considerably lessened as the child grows into adult life. Since the newborn child has no phonatory ability it has to rely on its cry to attract attention when it is in distress and it is well known that the volume of this cry can be out of all proportion to the size of the baby.

Symptoms and signs of laryngeal disease in the newborn

Stridor

Stridor is a noise made by obstruction of the passage of air into or out of the lower respiratory tract. Where the obstruction lies at the entrance to the tracheobronchial tree the noise appears on inspiration and is called 'inspiratory stridor'. The actual sound may vary with the obstructing lesion but the most common form of inspiratory stridor has a musical crowing quality and is traditionally called 'croup'.

Crying and cough

Obstruction of the airway gives rise to distress and the infant tends to be restless and to cry. In cases where the lesion prevents a complete apposition of the vocal cords the cry may be weak or 'wheezy' and on occasion the cry may be absent although the child is making all the other signs of crying such as grimacing and turning his head from side to side and rotating his clenched fists.

Cough frequently accompanies the cry where there is an irritative lesion of the larynx and this cough may have a harsh metallic sound.

Dyspnoea

Many children with laryngeal stridor have no dyspnoea, but where the obstruction narrows the airway by more than 1.5 mm in a 3.15 kg baby some degree of difficulty in breathing is always present. Signs of difficult breathing may be sought:

(1) In the face, where the nostrils dilate and the lips may be cyanosed and surrounded by an area of pallor.
(2) In the neck, where violent inspiratory movements cause the whole larynx and

trachea to move downwards towards the mediastinum. This is due to high negative pressure in the pleural cavity which in effect 'sucks' the larynx and the trachea into the thorax, and if the tracheal cartilages are soft may lead to tracheal collapse. This movement of the trachea into the thorax is known as 'tracheal plunging'. When tracheal plunging is very marked it may also be possible to see movements in the muscles of the neck which are used to increase the movements of the thoracic cage.

(3) In the chest, where excessive muscular effort directed to drawing air through a narrow glottis will be accompanied by recession of the intercostal spaces. The earliest place where this is seen is in the lower and lateral part of the chest wall. When the effort becomes more violent the whole sternum may be sucked in towards the spinal column as well as moving up and down with movements of the thoracic cage.

Congenital diseases of the larynx

For many years there was no satisfactory classification of the causes of stridor in infancy. Confusion existed about nomenclature and it was not until 1952 that the first satisfactory classification was introduced by Wilson. This was a most valuable contribution in a difficult area of disease. It has certainly not been improved upon, and will therefore be used here (*Table 11.1*).

Table 11.1

Congenital anatomical abnormalities	*Tumours and cysts*	*Inflammatory conditions*	*Neurological abnormalities*	*Trauma*	*Foreign body*
Laryngomalacia (congenital laryngeal stridor)	Benign neoplasms	Acute laryngitis	Tetany (laryngismus stridulus)	Birth injury	Vegetable foreign body
Bifid epiglottis	Cysts of the larynx	Acute laryngo-tracheo-bronchitis	Neonatal tetany	Post-natal injury (e.g. caused by intubation)	Non-vegetable foreign body
Congenital stenosis of the larynx (webs of the larynx)		Diphtheric Post-diphtheritic stenosis	Recurrent nerve paralysis		
		The exanthemata (measles, whooping cough)			
		Tuberculosis			

Feeding difficulties

The young child who has not learned the adult method of feeding usually finds added difficulty if there is any kind of laryngeal lesion. Anything which interferes with the sphincteric action of the supraglottis may lead to stimulation of the sensitive mucosa on the false cords. This will cause not only choking and breath-holding but also overspill into the tracheobronchial tree.

General symptoms and signs

The child who cannot breathe easily and who has difficulty in feeding does not thrive. He will therefore tend to be weak and underweight. However, there are other general effects which are less obvious. Repeated overspill into the tracheobronchial tree leads ultimately to chest infections and absorptive toxaemia. Inadequate oxygen intake and a high pCO_2 result in alterations in the acid–base equilibrium. There will also be some measure of cerebral anoxia and to compensate for this the cardiovascular centre will be stimulated leading to a rise in pulse rate. Prolonged severe cerebral hypoxia may lead to brain damage and physical and mental retardation. It is therefore extremely important that assessment of the cause of the obstruction to the respiration should be made at the earliest possible opportunity. Before a description is given of the various lesions which may give rise to obstructed airways, the routine assessment of the patient presenting with symptoms of laryngeal obstruction will be described. This assessment may be difficult and time-consuming. It requires patience on the part of the laryngologist and the use of keen clinical observation.

Assessment

When symptoms and signs of laryngeal obstruction are manifest the baby is transferred to hospital and nursed in an incubator with humidity and oxygen supplied. If time permits, that is to say if the patient is not in need of urgent relief of the obstruction, the history may be obtained from the mother or person who first noticed the symptoms of distress. The surgeon will want to know how long the noise has been present. If there is any abnormality in the baby's cry? Has he a cough? Is there a feeding difficulty? Has there been any gain in weight since birth? Is the noise louder when the baby is asleep or awake? Does it disappear during sleep or waking periods?

An assessment must then be made of the child's general condition, and particular attention should be paid to the general nutrition. The child with a paralysed vocal cord will experience considerable feeding difficulty and will in consequence tend to be under-nourished. The overweight baby obviously does not have a feeding difficulty but may well have a feeding problem. Since oxygen requirements are related to surface area of the body the overweight baby is particularly at risk. His larynx will be of normal size for a child of his age yet his oxygen requirements will be greater. Therefore, if for any reason the laryngeal airway is further narrowed he will be plunged into respiratory distress more rapidly. This is the sort of child who at six months develops laryngismus stridulus. Once the general impression of the state of nourishment has been obtained the baby should be examined for signs of dyspnoea.

The general colour, whether there is pallor or cyanosis should be noted. Abnormal movements of the alae nasi, trachea, larynx and neck muscles or in-drawing of the intercostal spaces should be recorded. If it is at all possible it is useful to hear the noise which it is claimed the child is making, and the place in the respiratory cycle at which the noise appears is very important. The quality of the noise will help in making the diagnosis. It is often helpful to listen both at the nares and the larynx to hear if the noise is present. Much, too, can be learned by placing the examining ear on the baby's back and listening to perhaps 30 or 40 respirations. Help may also be obtained by placing a stethoscope over the child's larynx and listening to the respiration. It may be possible to determine by the use of this instrument whether the obstruction is supraglottic, glottic or subglottic. Once the position of the noise in the cycle has been fixed the baby should be placed in various positions. Sometimes a change in position may eliminate the noise altogether. Thus, in Pierre–Robin syndrome, in which the micro-gnathia associated with a relatively large tongue and a cleft palate causes pressure on the supraglottis, the distress can be relieved at once by placing the baby face-down on the surgeon's knee. In less clear-cut conditions it can be very profitable to spend perhaps half to three-quarters of an hour turning the baby from side to side and adjusting the position of the head relative to the trunk in order to find out in which position the noise is least obtrusive. However, even if the probable diagnosis can be arrived at by such manoeuvres it is imperative that every child with stridor should undergo a direct examination of the larynx in order that the cause may be determined and treatment if possible instituted.

Paediatric anaesthesia is now a specialty in its own right, and the good paediatric anaesthetist will make it possible for the surgeon to examine the larynx in a calm and methodical manner and this is absolutely essential if an accurate diagnosis is to be made.

Anaesthesia

The child is anaesthetized with thiopentone and when it is asleep it is saturated with oxygen administered through a face mask. After about ten minutes the larynx is sprayed with a measured dose of 0.5 per cent of lignocaine according to the weight of the patient. At this stage the size of the larynx should be determined by the use of a standard set of endotracheal tubes. Finally, a rubber catheter is passed through the

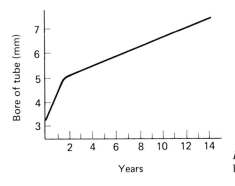

Figure 11.1 Norms for tubes accepted from birth to 14 years

nasal cavities into the larynx and is used to supply oxygen while the examination is being carried out. In this way it is possible to have a period of 10–15 minutes for laryngoscopy which is more than adequate.

Laryngoscopy

Once again a routine procedure is all-important. When a baby is to be examined to determine the cause of respiratory obstruction the surgeon must look for:

(1) Abnormalities of structure.
(2) Abnormalities of function.
(3) Pathological processes superimposed upon an otherwise normal laryngo-tracheobronchial tree.

Both hands may be required in order to carry out some endoscopic surgical procedure and it is therefore essential that the laryngoscope should be fixed in position. No endoscopic examination of a case of stridor is complete without tracheobronchoscopy.

The following instruments are required:

(1) Kleinsasser's infant laryngoscopes – blackened.
(2) Negus' infant tracheoscope.
(3) Infant and suckling bronchoscopes if possible, with Hopkin's telescopes.
(4) Loewy laryngostat and fixation (*Figure 11.3*).

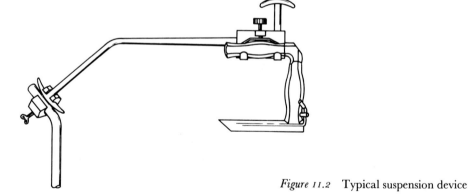

Figure 11.2   Typical suspension device

The instrument is introduced through the right-hand side of the patient's mouth, while the first finger of the operator's left hand is placed between the upper and lower alveolus (*Figure 11.3*). When the laryngoscope tip reaches the level of the uvula it is possible to see the catheter and this acts as a reliable guide to the larynx. The first stage in the examination is to pass the beak of the laryngoscope anterior to the epiglottis into the vallecula. In the infant this causes the laryngeal introitus to come into line with the optical axis of the laryngoscope. It allows a good overall view of the larynx and it ensures that in looking for paralysis or paresis of a cord a false diagnosis

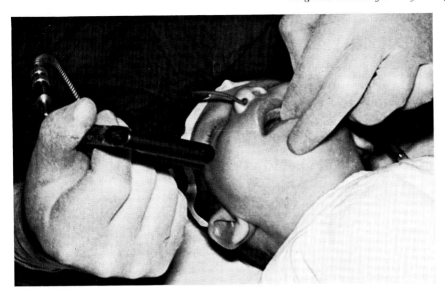

Figure 11.3 Direct laryngoscopy, first stage. (Note the nasotracheal catheter for anaesthetic gases and oxygen)

of paralysis is avoided because there is no pressure on the aryepiglottic fold. A diagnosis of vocal cord paralysis is only made when failure of the cords to move is clearly seen with the laryngoscope in this position (*Figure 11.4*). The beak should now be used to lift up the epiglottis and in this way the vocal cords, false cords and subglottic regions are inspected. If for some reason subglottic stenosis is suspected the rubber catheter can be removed.

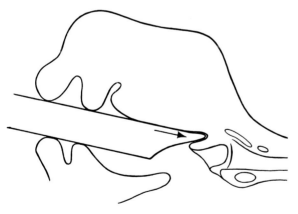

Figure 11.4 The beak of the laryngoscope in the valleculae allows an undistorted view of the vocal cords and their movements

The operating microscope has made it possible to obtain a much better view of the larynx and a standard 400 mm objective used for adult laryngoscopy is also used for examination of the infant's larynx. This enables the surgeon to gain a satisfactory view and at the same time to carry out any required operative endoscopic treatment.

When laryngoscopy has been completed the laryngoscope should be removed and the tracheobronchial tree examined for abnormal narrowing, evidence of a tracheo-oesophageal fistula and for possible abnormal pulsation due to aberrant artery formation.

Management of the newborn child with laryngeal obstruction

Two main factors have to be considered in planning the management of the patient. These are:

(1) An adequate supply of correctly humidified air.
(2) Adequate nourishment.

Many babies with stridor do not need assistance with their airway unless they develop some form of respiratory inflammation. However, about one-third of those babies will experience some feeding difficulty in the early months of life. They will be slow feeders and show a marked tendency to cough and splutter as the milk goes the wrong way. It has been found that such babies often progress more rapidly if they are introduced to a semi-solid weaning diet at an earlier age (4–5 weeks) than is usual. If some artificial assistance with the airway is necessary two possibilities are open to the surgeon; which one he chooses will depend upon how long it will have to be maintained. In the short term the most satisfactory form of airway, if it can be introduced, is the in-dwelling endotracheal tube; for all other cases the method of choice is tracheostomy (*see* Chapter 19).

A formal tracheostomy is carried out through the second, third and fourth tracheal

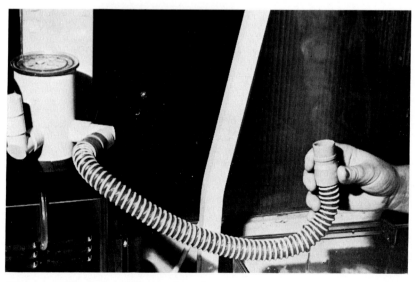

Figure 11.5   Humidifier delivers a fine mist

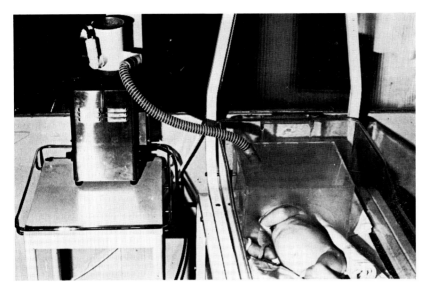

Figure 11.6 Humidifier in use

rings and a No. 14 or 16 tracheostomy tube is introduced. The tubes are of two sorts, plastic and the more traditional silver.

Where it is felt desirable that the expiratory thrust should be maintained, a valved tracheostomy tube should be fitted once the situation has stabilized. Whatever form of artificial airway is decided upon it is imperative that the air supply to the baby is properly humidifed. Adequate cold humidification greatly reduces the problems such as crusting and the cleaning of the tubes. This can be supplied by one of several forms of ultra-sonic atomizer (*Figures 11.5* and *11.6*) which deliver a fine mist of particles of less than 5 μm in diameter. If this is done and aspiration of excessive secretions using a no-touch technique with disposable sterile gloves is followed there are few difficulties in maintaining a small baby's tracheostomy in the short term.

In the long term, however, humidification in an incubator cannot be maintained because of the water-logging effect it has upon the baby's skin. Once the cause of the obstruction has been treated and de-cannulation is possible, the cannula may be removed. If it has been present for some months it may be helpful either to pass an endotracheal tube for 12 hours or to carry out such measures as are recommended in Chapter 19.

Disorders of structure

Laryngomalacia (congenital laryngeal stridor)

Wilson (1952) regarded this condition as an entity. However, experience shows that although there may be no difference to be distinguished in the history or clinical examination of the child, there are considerable differences in the possible laryngoscopic appearances.

Classically the child with congenital laryngeal stridor makes a crowing noise on inspiration because the superstructure of the larynx is driven in by the in-coming inspiratory tide of air and when the two sides of the larynx meet vibration occurs (*Figure 11.7*). The classic description of congenital laryngeal stridor attributed to Lambert Lack, Brown Kelly and Paterson is still seen.

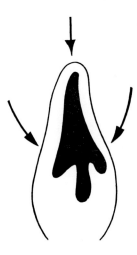

Figure 11.7   Laryngeal superstructure in congenital laryngeal stridor

The epiglottis is much elongated, folded on itself and has suspended from it thin and generally short aryepiglottic folds, which leave a very small entrance to the larynx. It may be difficult to introduce an endotracheal tube but once the tube is introduced it will be found that the glottis accepts the tube of normal size for the age of the child. It has, however, to be emphasized that not all children with this anatomical abnormality suffer from stridor; there must be an attendant abnormality for this to occur. A second category may be distinguished and to this it would seem appropriate to give the name 'laryngomalacia'. Here the entrance to the glottis can be clearly seen but the whole laryngeal superstructure is soft and appears to be oedematous. The glottis admits a normal-sized endotracheal tube for the age of the child but when the baby is relaxed the whole laryngeal superstructure vibrates producing a crowing noise. Furthermore, cinemicro-laryngoscopy shows that in some cases there is a failure of coordination of movement between the two sides of the larynx.

Clinical picture
Babies with these abnormalities are brought for advice for two reasons. First, they make a crowing noise on inspiration when they are asleep and they may also make it when they are awake. Second, babies with this abnormality experience feeding difficulties and fail to thrive. Wilson stated that the condition is essentially benign and disappears by the age of two-and-a-half years. Very few of these children ever die of their abnormality but experience shows that the noise may persist for up to five years. The child may be slow to gain weight and suffer many chest infections on the way through childhood. No treatment has been found to be effective and such empirical and radical procedures as amputation of the epiglottis have no place in modern

laryngology. As with all cases of stridor the parents should be instructed to bring the child to hospital immediately if the child's respiratory distress increases.

Bifid epiglottis

This is an extremely rare condition. From the accounts which are available it would seem that the symptoms are more acute in onset and more severe in effect than congenital laryngeal stridor. Cases have been described in which one or other half of the epiglottis becomes impacted in the glottis causing severe laryngeal obstruction. Amputation of the epiglottis after a preliminary tracheostomy is said to cure the condition, but with modern surgical techniques it would appear more logical to pare the edges and try to suture the two halves together.

Laryngeal webs and atresia

Laryngeal webs and atresia are not very uncommon. Webs are of two varieties. In the first variety the anterior end of the vocal cords are united by a transparent membrane which can easily be divided by using Kleinsassers' scissors and by keeping the vocal cords apart with a silastic sheet until re-epithelialization has taken place. The second variety of web presents a more complex problem and is associated with an abnormality of the anterior arch of the cricoid cartilage. The vocal cords are fused over perhaps two-thirds of their length and the cricothyroid ligament arises from the upper and posterior surface of the cricoid; it passes upwards and posteriorly to fuse with the web. Simple division of this web is not therefore possible.

When a laryngeal web is large enough to produce symptoms the infant will be brought for advice because of stridor or weakness of the voice. This will increase in severity during attempts at crying and coughing and it will be accompanied by a marked reduction in the volume of the voice. Dyspnoea may be extreme and may be associated with cyanosis and a high pCO_2.

Treatment of larger laryngeal webs
This is a complicated problem. The child should be left with an artificial airway until the larynx is large enough to make surgery possible. Through a median thyrotomy the web is divided along the line of one vocal cord. The submucosal tissue is then carefully dissected under the operating microscope using micro-surgical instruments and great care is taken to leave an intact epithelium (*Figure 11.8*).

The mucosa is then sutured back into the anterior commissure and the vocal cords re-aligned and the anterior commissure re-constituted. The larynx is splinted with silastic sheeting for three weeks to allow epithelialization of the raw cord.

Subglottic stenosis

Subglottic stenosis is a condition which has attracted attention in the past 20 years. This has been associated with improvements in paediatric anaesthesia and the

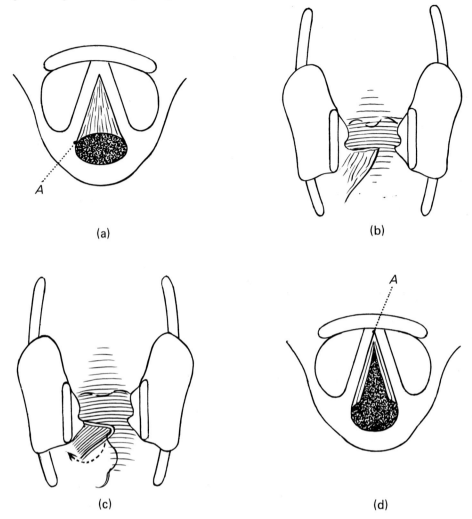

Figure 11.8 Operative correction of laryngeal web. (a) Laryngoscopic appearance of web; (b) thyrotomy with incision along the line of left vocal cord; (c) submucosal dissection of web under the microscope; (d) mucosa turned forward to provide mucosal cover for right vocal cord

introduction of routine direct laryngoscopy under general anaesthesia. The condition is not uncommon and if the degree of stenosis is severe it will give rise to a severe harsh barking kind of stridor and dyspnoea.

Mustapha discovered that one per cent of individuals have a larynx which accepts an endotracheal tube one size smaller or one size larger than normal for the age, and 1 in 1000 individuals accepts a tube which is two sizes smaller or two sizes larger than the norm for the age. It is this latter group of children who must be regarded as suffering from subglottic stenosis which is likely to produce problems.

The narrowing is due to considerable thickening of the cricoid cartilage, and is largely confined to the anterior arch and lateral parts of the ring of the cricoid. It is not uncommon for subglottic stenosis to be associated with other congenital abnormalities such as tracheo-oesophageal fistula. This increases the difficulties of treatment. The outcome in such cases may be fatal. Minor degrees of subglottic stenosis are tolerated reasonably well but constant vigilance is necessary in order to treat the increased dyspnoea which occurs when the airway is further narrowed by an infection and inflammation.

Symptoms and signs
Children with subglottic stenosis are not usually seen at birth unless the abnormality is accompanied by other conditions such as tracheo-oesophageal fistula. In this event the diagnosis is made by the anaesthetist trying to intubate the child for the repair of the fistula. More usually the child is brought for advice at two or three months when, perhaps after having gained weight and having had a respiratory infection, the characteristic brassy two-way stridor becomes more pronounced and infection is slow to clear. The diagnosis is made by the anaesthetist and laryngologist working together after the larynx has been inspected. The glottis is found to be of normal dimensions and the vocal cords mobile. Attempts are made to pass an endotracheal tube with a diameter appropriate to the size of the child. This is held up against the site of the obstruction and the cricoid.and it is then withdrawn and an attempt is made to pass a smaller tube. The size of the largest tube to pass the obstruction is taken to be the diameter of the airway at that point, and recorded (*Figure 11.9*).

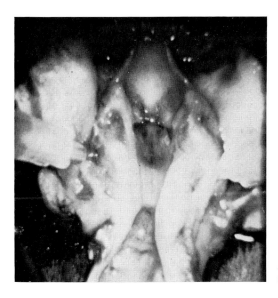

Figure 11.9 Congenital subglottic stenosis

Prognosis
The child who manages to survive the first two or three months of life with subglottic stenosis can be expected to survive into adult life unless overtaken by some overwhelming infection such as acute laryngotracheobronchitis. Extra care has to be taken when respiratory inflammation occurs and it is probably wiser to nurse the baby in hospital where oxygen and added humidity are at hand. Cases are followed up in the Out-patient Department until all symptoms have completely disappeared.

Treatment
Because the narrowing is due to cartilage rather than fibrous tissue nothing is gained

from procedures such as dilatation with bougies. Indeed, these do positive harm by damaging the delicate mucous membrane in the area of the cricoid narrowing and possibly resulting in ulceration and further stenosis. If the obstruction is severe and the airway inadequate the right treatment is the establishment of a tracheostomy well below the stenosis. The tracheostomy tube must be equipped with an expiratory valve and the development of the lower airway kept under constant review by routine direct laryngoscopy and measurement of the lumen at the site of the obstruction.

Surgical treatment

Various attempts have been made to correct subglottic stenosis by surgery, but perhaps the most satisfactory results are obtained by the use of the Evans and Todd (1974) operation. In this operation which is carried out under the operating microscope a median thyrotomy is performed, the vocal cords are visualized and the excessive narrowing of the ring is thinned by sculpting out the cartilage under direct vision. The cricoid is divided in steps (*Figures 11.10* and *11.11*) as are the upper rings of the trachea. Once the redundant cartilage has been removed the mucosa is spread to

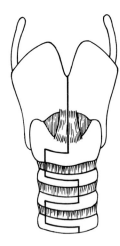

Figure 11.10   Incision in larynx and trachea

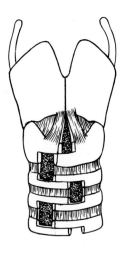

Figure 11.11   Position of cricoid and tracheal rings at closure

cover as much as possible of the increased diameter, and the cricoid and upper rings of the trachea are distracted and sewn in a new position in order to increase the lumen. In this way it is possible to increase the diameter of the obstruction by up to 2–3 mm.

Posterior laryngeal cleft

This very rare condition has in many cases been diagnosed in the *post-mortem* room. This is because (a) the extreme rarity means that the surgeon does not consider the possibility and (b) the area is difficult to visualize adequately. The cricoid lamina and a variable portion of the posterior wall of the trachea are divided by a cleft. The protective action of the supraglottic sphincter is lost and food and saliva spill through the cleft into the tracheobronchial tree. Frequent chest infection occurs, there is considerable difficulty in feeding and the child fails to gain weight. Cyanosis and apnoeic attacks are not uncommon.

Symptoms and signs
Feeding difficulties, and stridor which is usually 'two way' are present from birth. Coughing, spluttering and cyanosis may all be the cause for the initial consultation. The baby is restless and fails to gain weight. On examination, there may be obvious discolouration of the face and perhaps excess saliva around the lips. The baby may be febrile and coarse sounds may be heard in the chest.

Diagnosis
The laryngotracheobronchial tree should be examined under general anaesthesia. Particular care should be taken with the examination of the party wall between the trachea and the upper oesophagus. The cleft may not be easy to visualize even with modern endoscopes. However, it may be possible to pass a probe or bougie from the trachea to the oesophagus without withdrawing it from the larynx. If this appears to be the case then the area should be examined further by contrast-radiography.

Prognosis and treatment
Once a cleft is diagnosed the only possible line of treatment if the child's life is to be saved is surgical closure of the cleft. However, before any attempt is made to carry out the closure, an attempt should be made to obtain the most favourable chest condition. Postural drainage, tube feeding, physiotherapy and aspiration all have their part to play. Antibiotics should be given pre-operatively. The cleft is closed by paring the edges and sewing up the deficit in layers. The child must be tube-fed for 3–4 days after the operation.

Disorders of function

Paralysis of the vocal cords

Some degree of weakness of one or both vocal cords is one of the more common congenital lesions of the larynx. About 25 per cent of all cases of stridor in infancy which are examined are found to have vocal cord weakness. Unilateral vocal cord weakness is much more common than bilateral. Unilateral vocal cord weakness appears to be associated with difficult labour and birth and may perhaps be associated with the use of instruments at the time of delivery. The right and left vocal cords are affected to about the same extent. Bilateral vocal cord paresis is usually not complete and is therefore abductor in type. It is seen most commonly in cases of hydrocephalus which result from repair of a meningomyelocele. Examination of the vagus nerve in a child who died with hydrocephalus associated with bilateral abductor paresis showed that the nerve had become stretched over the anterior margin of the foramen magnum as a result of the brain stem being forced downwards through the foramen by raised intracranial pressure. This seemed to offer a reasonable explanation of how the vocal cord weakness occurred.

Symptoms and signs
The child whose stridor is due to vocal cord paresis frequently is stridulous only when making some physical effort. If the paresis is unilateral, therefore, the noise will become obvious on crying, coughing or straining at stool, and he will sleep quietly. Babies with bilateral paresis on the other hand are in more or less constant distress. All children with laryngeal paralysis have feeding difficulties. This is due to the liquid diet coming into contact with the unrelaxed crico-pharyngeus and being bounced back over the larynx, and the consequent overspill results in infection of the tracheobronchial tree. For this reason the babies tend to be weak and fail to gain weight. Feeding takes a very long time. Direct laryngoscopy will confirm the diagnosis. There are, however, pitfalls for the inexperienced laryngologist, and restriction of movement of the right hemilarynx which may be caused by the introduction of the laryngoscope through the right side of the mouth and posterior to the epiglottis. Wilson (1952) recommended that the laryngoscope beak should be introduced into the vallecula anterior to the epiglottis. Slight pressure in a caudal direction causes the axis of the glottis to straighten out at right-angles to the optical axis of the laryngoscope and this does not hinder the movement of either vocal cord. The diagnosis of paresis should therefore be made only with the laryngoscope in this position. Bilateral vocal cord paresis is confirmed by passing an endotracheal tube between the vocal cords when the symptoms will be completely relieved.

Prognosis and treatment
Unilateral vocal cord paresis seems to recover in about 50 per cent of cases. The larynx is observed at regular intervals up to 18 months. It is possible that the other 50 per cent form the hard core of the so-called idiopathic lesions seen in adult life. However, the baby has a stormy infancy with repeated respiratory infections and a very slow gain of weight. Since the swallowing of liquids presents difficulties for these children an improvement in the general condition can often be brought about by the introduction of a semi-solid weaning diet at an earlier age than usual.

Bilateral paresis has a more serious prognosis. Many cases of bilateral paresis are associated with hydrocephalus and when the intracranial pressure has risen to such a degree that stretching of the vagus occurs, the prognosis is grave indeed and the child very unlikely to survive.

When there is no associated hydrocephalus the laryngologist is faced with a most difficult decision. It may not be necessary to carry out a tracheostomy in early infancy when the infant is relatively inactive and yet the occurrence of respiratory inflammation which is to be anticipated as part of normal development may precipitate a crisis which will call for immediate relief of the obstruction. Further-more, the establishment of a permanent tracheostomy in a small baby imposes great difficulties in management on the mother, and the child may have to spend its early life in hospital which is certainly not ideal. The number of cases in this category is small and it is not possible to offer any dogmatic opinions about the course to be followed in each case. However, it has proved possible to steer such cases through the anticipated respiratory inflammations of infancy and childhood without finding it necessary to establish an artificial airway. If at any time it did become necessary to pass an in-dwelling endotracheal tube or to carry out a tracheostomy then airway relief would have to be permanent because de-cannulation would not be possible. Plastic procedures directed towards the improvement of the airway (such as arytenoidectomy) should be deferred until the age of 14–16 years when the surgeon can count upon the confidence and cooperation of his patient which are so essential to the success of the procedure.

Tumours and cysts

In the course of development of the tissues of the larynx and its surrounding structures many complicated phases of foldings are encountered and it is not surprising, therefore, that abnormalities occur when these processes are not completed with that precision normally to be expected in embryology. Three varieties of cysts may occur:

(1) Defects of lymph vessel formation may result in cystic hygroma (lymphangioma in the region of the floor of the mouth and larynx).
(2) Dermoid cysts may occur in the aryepiglottic folds.
(3) Mucous cysts are seen in the false cords and may extend laterally.

Congenital cysts of the larynx are rare. Their presence is made known in a very dramatic way in that the newly-born baby has great difficulty in breathing and intubation is called for urgently in the labour ward.

Clinical picture
The neonate makes violent efforts to breathe. These are unavailing and standard procedures of the midwife are not effective in clearing the airway. The child's colour and pulse deteriorate rapidly and the anaesthetist is called to pass a tube. On examination of the larynx the normal anatomy is completely obscured by a rounded swelling which passes over the midline obstructing any view of the vocal cords. An experienced anaesthetist usually has no difficulty in intubating the baby. After intubation the colour and the pulse improve and the child should then be transferred to the theatre for treatment by the laryngologist.

Treatment
Since the endotracheal tube cannot be removed until the cyst has been evacuated

treatment must be carried out in the first hours of the child's life. It is not necessary to make a tracheostomy and if possible, because of the difficulties of de-cannulation in small infants, tracheostomies should be avoided. Temporary improvement may be effected by removing the top of the cyst with forceps and evacuating the fluid. The disadvantage of this procedure is that the cyst rapidly fills up and it becomes necessary to repeat the procedure. The infant's larynx is so small and sensitive that repeated instrumentation is to be avoided if at all possible. A modified diathermy needle has been developed for use in these cases. A suction tube is covered with an insulated coating and fitted with a terminal for a diathermy lead. The stilette of the sucker is replaced with a sharpened trocar, the cyst is punctured by means of the trocar and the contents are aspirated by the application of suction when the trocar has been withdrawn. As the fluid is aspirated the superstructure of the cysts falls in and adheres to the mouth of the sucker. The redundant mucosa can then be destroyed by the application of a weak diathermy current. Larger laryngeal cysts may be too big to be dealt with in this way and when the cyst fills the pyriform fossa and extends over the midline of the glottis it is preferable to excise it through an external, horizontally-placed incision using the approach described by Trotter (1920) for lateral pharyngotomy. The cyst can be separated easily from the lax laryngeal submucosal tissues by blunt dissection. The airway is protected for 24 hours by an in-dwelling endotracheal tube, and remarkably little post-operative oedema follows this procedure.

Tumours

Congenital tumours of the larynx are rare. The larynx is composed of a variety of ectodermal and mesodermal derivatives and any of these can give rise to benign tumour formation, causing symptoms which are present at birth. These tumours may be divided into two categories:

(1) *Pedunculated*: including fibroma, lipoma and leiomyoma. They tend to arise from the posterior surface of the larynx and aryepiglottic folds.
(2) *Sessile*: including chondroma and haemangioma. They arise from the cartilage and blood vessels in the larynx.

Clinical picture

Tumours of the larynx present with dysphagia, dyspnoea, stridor, or with a combination of all three symptoms. Pedunculated tumours fall back into the hypopharynx and tend to give rise to serious difficulty only when the child attempts to swallow. The tumour is then squeezed upwards and comes to lie over the entrance of the larynx causing the baby to cough and choke. Once the tumour has been removed the symptoms are cured.

Chondroma and haemangioma present with stridor and dyspnoea. Chondroma of course is only diagnosed by direct laryngoscopy. Haemangioma may be suspected if the baby is seen to have multiple cavernous haemangiomata of the skin of the head and neck (*Figures 11.12* and *11.13*). Direct laryngoscopy may show that there is a single large lesion on one false cord which is interfering with the movement of the true cord and thus giving rise to symptoms. The more usual appearance is of multiple

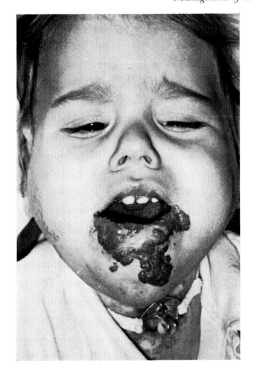

Figure 11.12 Congenital haemangioma of larynx and face

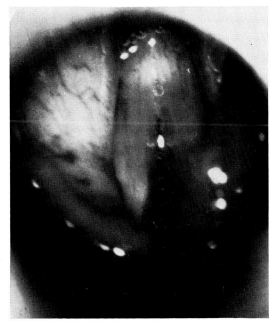

Figure 11.13 Congenital haemangioma. Direct laryngoscopy revealing large swelling of left false cord

haemangiomata arising over the whole supraglottis and also in the subglottic regions immediately below the true vocal cords. Haemangiomata of this type may be associated with abnormal lymph vessel development. Thus, a baby born with multiple congenital cavernous haemangiomata may have minimal symptoms at birth but, as development takes place, the symptoms increase and become much more severe as the lymphangiomatous element increases in size. There appears to be a tendency for isolated haemangioma to regress at about 12 months of age.

Treatment
Pedunculated tumours are removed most satisfactorily by a snare. Chondroma is best treated when the larynx has enlarged somewhat. Therefore, if the dyspnoea is considerable, a permanent tracheostomy must be made, and an expiratory valve fitted and the child left to develop for perhaps 2–3 years before any attempt is made at excision.

Treatment of haemangioma
If the haemangioma is causing respiratory distress at birth a tracheostomy must be made because the distress will certainly increase in the first months of life. Since the natural history of the condition is that regression takes place at about 12 months of age it may be possible to leave the child with a tracheostomy and expiratory valve and to observe the progress of the lesion. Recent work has suggested that steroids might be helpful in bringing about a regression of the lesion, but personal experience does not confirm this finding. Three forms of treatment are therefore available:

(1) *Radiotherapy.* Experience has not shown this to be of much help and the surgeon must bear in mind that a percentage of children so treated may have a disturbance of growth of the area irradiated and may even develop a carcinoma at that site in later life.
(2) *Sclerosing agents.* Hypertonic saline and sodium morrhuate have been used. However, the distribution of the sclerosing agent in the subcutaneous tissues is difficult to control and there may be a severe post-operative sloughing and resultant laryngeal stenosis and fibrosis.
(3) *Destruction by other agents.* Laser, diathermy and cryoprobes have all been described as being useful in this condition. These agents are applied locally to the tumours, small areas being treated at frequent sessions. This appears to offer the best hope of treatment of the supraglottic lesion and it may be possible to treat the subglottic lesions through a thyrotomy at about the age of three years.

References

Evans, J. N. G. and Todd, G. B. (1974). *Journal of Laryngology*, **88,** 589

Pracy, R. (1964). *Proceedings of the Royal Society of Medicine*, **58,** 268

Pracy, R. (1970). *Journal of Laryngology*, **84,** 37

Pracy, R. (1971). *Journal of Laryngology*, **85,** 1263

Trotter (1920). *Journal of Laryngology, Rhinology and Otology*, **25,** 289

Wilson, T. G. (1952). *Diseases of the Ear, Nose and Throat in Children* (2nd edn), p.249; Heinemann, London

12 Laryngeal trauma and stenosis
D P Bryce

The thyroid cartilages and the cricoid cartilage form the framework of the larynx. Each thyroid ala articulates with the cricoid cartilage at the cricothyroid joint. Enclosed in this box are the muscles and membranes which make up the true and false cords, aryepiglottic fold and the epiglottic and arytenoid cartilages. In youth the laryngeal cartilages are soft and elastic but later in life ossification occurs which makes them brittle and prone to fracture.

The laryngeal inlet may be closed-off from the pharynx above, but at the level of the distal end of the cricoid cartilage, the lumen opens directly into the trachea. The larynx lies anterior to the cervical spine and may be crushed against it. Anteriorly the mandible tends to protect the larynx from direct injury unless the head is extended which is usually the case when the larynx is injured as in automobile accidents.

Injury to the larynx may result from direct trauma to the thyroid cartilages with fracture and displacement of the cartilage and tearing and injury to the intra-laryngeal structures. Similar injury may result from elastic displacement of the thyroid cartilages and cricoid cartilage without fracture. The laryngeal mucosa may be injured by surgical procedures in the larynx or because of laryngeal intubation to establish an airway for anaesthesia or respiratory assistance.

Laryngeal stenosis results from the replacement of ulceration or lacerations of laryngeal mucosa by scar. Displacement of laryngeal cartilages with subsequent infection, perichondritis, and granulations will ultimately produce scarring and stenosis. Laryngeal stenosis may be the late stage of injury or laryngeal disease in which the disease process is controlled but is replaced by fibrous tissue which distorts the laryngeal lumen and may cause respiratory obstruction. Such stenosis results most commonly from the effects of extensive malignant or chronic inflammatory disease.

A variety of congenital laryngeal stenoses are seen in infancy. Most commonly these may be intracordal webs or stenosis of the subglottis because of inadequate canalization or an abnormality of the cricoid cartilage.

Open wounds

Gunshot wounds may injure the larynx. Wounds with knives and razors and other sharp weapons may open the larynx and this may sometimes occur with self-inflicted neck incisions.

Diagnosis

Open wounds of the larynx will often prove fatal before the patient can obtain any medical treatment. In those patients who survive, laryngeal involvement will usually be obvious because of bubbling of blood due to air passing in and out of the wound during respiration.

Treatment

Treatment is usually required urgently to establish a free airway and prevent more blood from entering the bronchial tree. Under these circumstances an emergency tracheostomy is required and this will be rendered more difficult if there is extensive haematoma formation. In a few patients it may be possible as an emergency measure to pass a tube into the larynx through the opening resulting from the wound.

Once a tracheostomy has been established the wound of the larynx can be dealt with on general principles; foreign bodies must be removed, devitalized tissue excised and the mucosa sutured. No raw surfaces must be left uncovered but the skin edges must never be sutured under tension. Where a large amount of skin from the neck has been destroyed it may be necessary to advance or re-arrange flaps.

An antibiotic will be required and prophylaxis against tetanus is advisable. Oedema persists for several days and the tracheostomy must be maintained until there is a clear airway through the larynx and there is no longer any risk of laryngeal swelling from tissue reaction to the trauma or from secondary infection. Difficulty in swallowing will usually necessitate the use of a nasogastric tube for feeding purposes for several days post-operatively.

Complications

The acute complications from open wounds result from haemorrhage or aspiration of blood and these require urgent and appropriate treatment as soon as an adequate airway has been established.

A further complication may result from injury to the recurrent laryngeal nerves as a result of the original injury. The resulting laryngeal paralysis cannot be corrected by suture of the nerves but must be dealt with later by injection or lateralization of the cords as indicated.

Late scarring with resulting laryngeal stenosis may occur if there has been loss of mucosa within the laryngeal lumen.

Closed injuries

Closed injuries to the larynx result from direct anterior trauma which crush the cartilaginous laryngeal box against the cervical spine. It is usually necessary for there to be a degree of extension of the head so that the mandible which otherwise protects the larynx is moved out of the way.

These injuries today are most commonly seen as the result of automobile and motorcycle injuries when the passenger is thrown forward against the windscreen or instrument panel. It may result from falls in the house or from deliberate blows to the neck in assault cases.

In cold countries such injuries are commonly seen from snow-mobile accidents or from blows from hockey sticks.

More rarely, severe laryngeal injury may result from abortive attempts at suicide from hanging.

Pathology

In moderately severe injuries because of the elasticity of the laryngeal cartilages extensive haematoma formation with arytenoid displacement, laceration of the laryngeal mucosa with subcutaneous emphysema, and pharyngeal laceration with haemoptysis may occur without cartilaginous fracture or displacement.

In more severe injuries laryngeal cartilage fracture with displacement will occur and four mechanisms can be recognized:

(1) *Lateral glottic fracture.* Force acting laterally against the thyroid alae will cause a vertical fracture through the thyroid ala at about its midpoint (*Figure 12.1*). The

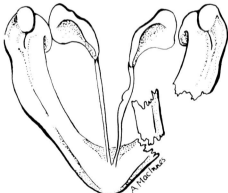

Figure 12.1 A lateral glottic fracture. The thyroid ala is fractured and displaced with damage to the vocal cord musculature. (From *Operative Surgery*, 3rd edn Eds C. Rob and R. Smith. *Nose and Throat*, Butterworths, London and Boston)

posterior segments are displaced posteriorly and medially and there may also be a displaced fracture of the superior rim of the cricoid cartilage. Such displacement results in tearing of the homolateral vocal cord with paralysis and shortening of the cord. The arytenoid cartilage may also be displaced medially and anteriorly into the laryngeal lumen.

(2) *Supraglottic laryngeal fracture.* In this condition the superior half of the thyroid alae

is fractured and displaced superiorly and posteriorly carrying with it epiglottic cartilage and tearing the supraglottic mucosa along the level of the ventricle (*Figure 12.2*). Significant denuding of the arytenoid cartilage of mucosa may result. Usually vocal cord action is not affected.

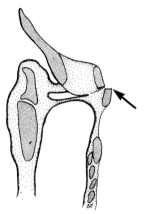

Figure 12.2   The arrow points to the fracture of the thyroid alae which is characteristic of a supraglottic fracture of the larynx. The posterior displacement of the supraglottic structure is illustrated. (From *Operative Surgery*, 3rd edn Eds C. Rob and R. Smith. *Nose and Throat*, Butterworths, London and Boston)

(3) *Separation of the larynx and trachea at the inferior border of the cricoid cartilage.* In this case the larynx is torn from the trachea and there may be several centimetres of separation between the two (*Figure 12.3*). The subglottic mucosa may be torn away from the larynx and there may be fractures of the cricoid ring. Bilateral

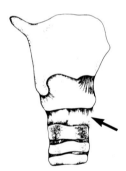

Figure 12.3   The commonest tracheal traumatic injury is crico-tracheal separation as seen in this diagram at the site of the arrow. Airway obstruction results in the acute phase and subglottic scarring and stenosis is characteristic of the chronic form. (From Bryce, D. P., 'Laryngotracheal injury and repair', *Recent Advances in Otolaryngology Series*, in press [Eds T. R. Bull, J. Ransome and H. Holden]; Reproduced by permission of Churchill-Livingstone, Edinburgh)

recurrent laryngeal nerve injury is almost always associated with this injury. In severe cases there may be an associated traumatic tracheo-oesophageal fistula.

(4) *Multiple comminuted fractures.* As a result of a severe crushing blow acting posteriorly on the larynx a multitude of cartilaginous fractures may result with gross displacement and laceration of laryngeal mucosa (*Figure 12.4*). No particular pattern can be determined in these cases as the larynx is merely a mass of mobile fractured cartilaginous fragments.

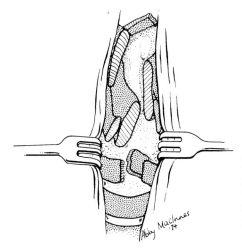

Figure 12.4 The most severe of the laryngo-tracheal injuries is seen here, illustrating multiple comminuted laryngeal cartilage fractures. If not corrected complete laryngeal stenosis will result. (From *Operative Surgery*, 3rd edn Eds C. Rob and R. Smith. *Nose and Throat*, Butterworths, London and Boston)

Symptoms and signs

In severe crush injuries of the larynx the most prominent feature is the obstruction of the airway requiring immediate alleviation by tracheostomy. If the mucosa has been torn there will be bleeding into the airway and surgical emphysema which may be extensive over the chest and face as well as the neck and may involve the mediastinum. Cough may be a troublesome feature and will add to the emphysema. There is nearly always great difficulty in swallowing.

In less severe injuries which do not immediately jeopardize the airway, pain or discomfort is usually present, especially on coughing, speaking or swallowing. Hoarseness is common but the presence of a normal or near-normal voice in the early stages does not necessarily indicate that the injury is only slight. The subsequent development of scar tissue in the damaged larynx may lead to obstruction of the airway if treatment is not undertaken early.

Injuries to other parts of the body, such as the chest and the face, may also occur at the same time and require treatment.

Diagnosis

The diagnosis of the extent and nature of the injury is of prime importance as this will determine the method of treatment. Accurate examination of the patient may be impossible as severe laryngeal injuries are usually associated with other more demanding problems. Head, chest and cervical spine injuries may complicate the laryngeal problem and in such cases, after an airway has been established, it is possible to delay adequate examination for ten days if necessary and still effect an acute repair.

The chief diagnostic point to be determined is whether or not an open reduction of the laryngeal fracture is required. Gross haemoptysis and subcutaneous emphysema may resolve completely without surgical intervention. Cartilaginous fracture with displacement is the indication for open reduction at the earliest possible moment.

Clinical evidence of laryngeal cartilaginous deformity may be obtained by palpation of the neck. In supraglottic fractures, for example, there will be loss of the normal laryngeal prominence and this is evidence of displacement which must be replaced by open reduction. The examination of the pharynx and larynx is usually impossible in severe injuries but if loose pieces of fractured cartilage are seen in the pharynx this is evidence of fracture and an indication for open reduction. These are the only two absolute indications for primary exploration of the neck (Bryce, in press).

The emergency treatment of closed laryngeal injuries is indicated by the severity of the injury and by the extent of the associated injuries of the head or chest. An airway must be established if it is compromised, haemorrhage must be controlled and other indicated supportive measures must be taken. If associated injuries take precedence to the laryngeal injury definitive repair to the larynx, if indicated, must be deferred.

A decision must be made to proceed with open reduction of the larynx or merely to observe the patient until evidence of significant injury requiring correction becomes apparent. In the absence of evidence of laryngeal displacement a policy of observation should be adopted.

If there is evidence of cartilaginous displacement, open reduction of the injury is indicated as soon as is reasonably possible. During exploration the injury can be classified as suggested previously under 'Pathology' and the appropriate repair can be carried out (Bryce, 1976).

In general, the displaced fragments of cartilage must be replaced and the mucosal laceration repaired. If necessary, skin or mucosal grafting may be used. It may also be advisable to mould the fragments about an in-dwelling laryngeal stent in order to provide stability. This is particularly necessary when a multiple comminuted fracture is being managed.

Complications

The complications of such acute injuries may result from inadequate replacement or repair in the form of scarring and late stenosis.

Recurrent laryngeal nerve injury is unavoidable in some of the injuries and later appropriate treatment will be necessary.

In severe injuries the wounds may become infected leading to perichondritis, scarring, deformity, and eventual stenosis of varying degrees. In less severe injuries, significant webs may develop anteriorly or posteriorly in the larynx. If not recognized these may result in cord fixation and airway obstruction.

Burns and scalds

The laryngeal mucosa may be damaged by the inhalation of burning gases or of very hot air from a fire, by the inhalation of steam or irritant gases, and also by the swallowing of corrosive liquids. In all these injuries there is likely to be associated damage to the mucosa of the mouth and pharynx and often to the trachea as well. The effects are erythema and oedema and also necrosis of the mucosa and, perhaps, of the underlying tissues as well.

Treatment

Thermal injuries to the larynx when severe are almost always fatal because of associated injury to the lungs. This is particularly true when associated with smoke inhalation. A most careful assessment of the patient is necessary and non-invasive supportive methods of treatment should be stressed. The place of tracheostomy in such patients is somewhat controversial because of the inevitable introduction of infection by the procedure. Early consultation is indicated in these cases and treatment should be as conservative as possible.

In severe laryngeal burns almost inevitably late stenosis will result and will have to be managed at that time.

Foreign bodies

Foreign bodies which are inhaled into the air passages seldom become impacted in the larynx but pass through it into the trachea and bronchi (*Figure 12.5*). Impaction in the larynx is more liable to occur in children than in adults. Coins and other similar objects may lodge in the larynx and care must be exercised in prescribing tablets or capsules for children. These have been known to be inhaled rather than swallowed and have, on occasion, become wedged in the larynx between the true and false cords with fatal consequences. In adults, food – particularly a piece of poorly masticated meat – may enter the larynx and be held there due to spasm of the muscles. Also bizarre foreign bodies occasionally become impacted in the larynx. The museum of one institute contains the pharynx and larynx of an edentulous man with a billiard ball stuck in the laryngeal inlet.

Acute trauma from intubation

The general acceptance of intubation anaesthesia for most surgical procedures has resulted in many relatively minor laryngeal injuries. The anaesthetist tends to intubate the larynx relatively blindly and as a result occasionally will damage the mucosa of the laryngeal inlet, usually the aryepiglottic folds or false cords, and this may result in intubation granulomas, which are characteristically present at the site of the laceration. These are often quite firm and may be large enough to cause respiratory obstruction. Initially, they have a broad base which tends to become narrowed and if merely observed may often be coughed out but would otherwise have to be removed by biting forceps. Dislocation of the arytenoid may result from traumatic emergency intubation; this is a relatively rare complication, however, and is best managed by the removal of the dislocated cartilage if it is obstructing the airway or interfering with speech. In some cases the arytenoid may be fixed back into its position, but there will never be normal cord movement following this manoeuvre. Lacerations in the anterior commissure by intubation may result in an anterior laryngeal web, which, if the mucosa is denuded bilaterally to any great extent, will extend posteriorly and may restrict the airway. This particular complication is best

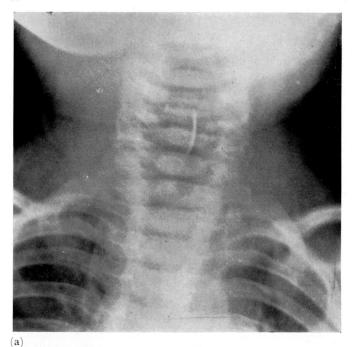

(a)

(b)

Figure 12.5   Radiographs of piece of eggshell in the larynx of a child. (a) Antero-posteral view showing eggshell seen 'end-on'; (b) lateral view – eggshell not visible. (From Douglas Ranger, *Trauma and Stenosis of the Larynx*, 3rd edn, Vol. IV, Figure 128; Butterworths, London and Boston)

managed by the insertion of a laryngeal keel which holds the denuded areas apart until they become epithelialized.

More seriously, the use of large intubation tubes may affect the mucosa of the subglottis within the cricoid ring. This causes circumferential ulceration and may produce respiratory obstruction for a period of time following the anaesthesia. It rarely proceeds to subglottic stenosis. Care by the anaesthetist to use tubes of a proper size will prevent this complication.

The intubation of patients in order to provide support for their respiratory function has in recent years been a much more common cause of acute laryngeal injury often leading to stenosis. This particular injury is frequently seen in the Respiratory Units and Special Care Units of the general hospitals and only recently has been almost completely controlled by the use of special non-irritating tubes (*Figure 12.6*) and by the recognition of the proper care of the patient who is intubated for this purpose. In

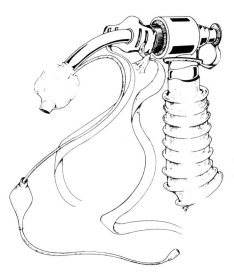

Figure 12.6 Prevention of laryngotracheal injury during assisted respiration with positive pressure is obtained by the soft flabby cuff on the tracheostomy tube illustrated here, and the mobile adjustment to the respirator which reduces movement and tugging on the tracheostomy tube. (From *Operative Surgery*, 3rd edn Eds C. Rob and R. Smith. *Nose and Throat*, Butterworths, London and Boston)

general, the injuries from intubation to provide assisted respiration have caused injury to the larynx because of pressure on the laryngeal mucosa associated with movement and the ever-present infection. The use of special adaptors which connect the tube to the respirator have reduced greatly the amount of movement, and the use of the soft inflatable cuffs and smaller tubes have prevented, to a large extent, the more serious injuries that were seen several years ago, both in the subglottis and in the trachea (Scott, personal communication).

In the Respiratory Units where excellent nursing care and the best of equipment is available, very little prolonged injury is now seen from intubation. However, acute lesions can still be recognized.

The nasotracheal tube tends to apply pressure to the larynx posteriorly and causes ulceration of the vocal cord at the arytenoid level and in the subglottis posteriorly and laterally. This is particularly true if the intubation is prolonged (*Figure 12.7*). In general, intubation that is prolonged beyond six or seven days will cause some acute laryngeal injury due to ischemic necrosis and infection at the site of tube pressure. These injuries can be observed if all of the patients intubated are routinely examined

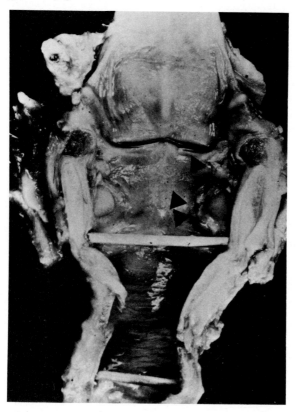

Figure 12.7 A cadaver specimen which demonstrates at the arrowheads, ulceration produced by a nasotracheal tube in the posterior commissure of the larynx, and of the mucosa of the vocal processes of the arytenoid cartilages. (From Bryce, D. P., 'Laryngotracheal injury and repair,' *Recent Advances in Otolaryngology Series*, in press [Eds T. R. Bull, J. Ransome and H. Holden]; Reproduced by permission of Churchill-Livingstone, Edinburgh)

on extubation and if this examination is persisted with for several months. Most commonly in the immediate post-intubation period a grey sloughing ulceration can be seen posteriorly in the larynx and in extreme cases may be circumferential. The amount of obstruction from this ulceration may be sufficient to cause tracheostomy but very few such injuries go on to permanent stenosis so that after observation the ulceration heals, the respiratory obstruction diminishes, and the patient may have his tracheostomy tube removed, if it was necessary to introduce one.

Treatment

The treatment of laryngeal injuries resulting from intubation or anaesthetic intubation is ideally prevention. The use of appropriate tubes for anaesthesia and the training of personnel and the use of modern non-traumatic equipment in Respiratory Units will prevent most of these injuries. When the ulcerations have occurred in the anterior commissure, in the interarytenoid area, or in the subglottis, conservative methods of observation should be adopted until it is clear that some permanent scarring and stenosis will result. This requires routine, careful examination so that the ensuing scarring and stenosis will be recognized at the earliest possible date. The use of steroids and moisturized air, although generally accepted, is debatable and should be used with caution.

Very little else can be done for treatment of the acute injury from intubation until there is evidence of scarring, at which point the appropriate surgical correction will have to be embarked upon.

Stenosis

Laryngeal stenosis is defined, for this discussion, as a narrowing of the airway at the larynx due to scarring and distortion, and not as the result of active tumour or disease.

Causes

(1) Congenital abnormalities.
    (a) Atresia.
    (b) Web.
    (c) Subglottic stenosis.
(2) Trauma.
    (a) Stenosis due to direct trauma.
    (b) Stenosis as a result of operative procedures.
    (c) Stenosis resulting from injury to the larynx secondary to intubation.
(3) Chronic infection.
(4) Laryngeal malignancy.
(5) Pathology.

Congenital abnormalities

Complete laryngeal *atresia* as a result of defective canalization of the tracheobronchial tree is seldom compatible with life. It is complete closure of the glottis at or above cord level by a firm fibrous membrane.

Laryngeal webs seen in infancy are incomplete atresias and may be quite firm and fibrous or very thin and web-like. The anterior commissure is usually involved in the web.

Subglottic stenosis may appear in the infant as a thin or thick scar in the cricoid ring. This may be congenital in nature due to imperfect formation or secondary to instrumentation or acute infection in the neonatal period. More seriously, the cricoid ring may be excessively thick resulting in an intractable narrowing of the airway.

Traumatic stenosis

Traumatic stenosis is by far the commonest form of laryngeal narrowing in the adult. Laryngeal fracture and displacement of cartilage results in scarring which, when severe, always obstructs the airway. The severe comminuted form of fracture, if not treated in the acute phase, will result in a complete stenosis and loss of the usual anatomical landmarks of the larynx. The supraglottic fracture causes an elliptical supraglottic web, which in minor degree is difficult to diagnose, but when severe is an obvious stenosis due to the posterior displacement of the epiglottis and the supraglottic structures. Characteristically laryngotracheal separation causes cricoid fracture and will produce complete stenosis if not repaired in the acute period.

Operative laryngeal procedures to remove benign and malignant tumours may result in significant stenosis. Most commonly, laryngeal polyps and papilloma, which extend into the anterior commissure when removed, may result in loss of mucosa on both vocal cords anteriorly, which causes an anterior web formation during the healing process. This might be quite a heavy scar with considerable anterior depth.

The removal of malignant tumours from the larynx by partial vertical or partial horizontal laryngectomy is a recognized, appropriate, surgical method for dealing with such tumours. In the case of the vertical hemilaryngectomy, a sufficient amount of the opposite cord may have to be sacrificed, so that significant laryngeal stenosis results. Stenosis results frequently from other, less common operations, which strive to maintain some laryngeal structure while eradicating the malignant disease.

When intubation has resulted in acute ulceration of the larynx, the resulting stenosis may occur at the anterior or posterior commissure or in the subglottis. Most commonly the laryngeal injury is posterior, because of the posterior position of the tube, which denudes the arytenoids and the posterior lateral walls of the cricoid ring of their mucosa. The resulting scar slowly forms and contracts, fixing the arytenoid movement and thus bringing the cords to the midline with greatly reduced or absent motility. At the same time the posterior interarytenoid scar slowly compromises the airway by reducing the antero-posterior diameter of the glottic chink.

The cuff of the endotracheal tube, when inflated to excessive pressures, or if positioned incorrectly, may cause circumferential ischemia of the mucosa in the cricoid ring. This may be so serious after only two or three days of intubation that irreversible necrosis of the membrane and the perichondrium results, with subsequent circumferential scarring in the subglottic region, causing serious airway obstruction. This subglottic stenosis is the most difficult to manage and the most serious of the laryngeal stenoses in the adult.

Chronic infection

The chronic infections of the larynx, such as tuberculosis, scleroma, syphilis, leprosy, and glanders, are rarely seen except in some isolated geographical areas. Their treatment may occasionally be followed by sufficient laryngeal scarring and distortion to produce significant stenosis.

More commonly, perichondritis of the laryngeal cartilages produces distortion and subsequent stenosis which may be significant. This is most often seen following injury, or surgery to the larynx, or following radiotherapy for malignant disease. When the laryngeal malignancy is ulcerated and infected, perichondritis may complicate radiotherapy and extreme laryngeal destruction may result. Excessive doses of irradiation may produce the same effect.

Management of laryngeal stenosis

The proper management of severe laryngeal stenosis is a difficult and demanding problem. The site and extent of the stenosis must be determined by clinical and radiological means and the general physical condition of the patient must be considered. The surgical management of a patient of this type may require prolonged intubation and stenting because of the dangers of infected material being in the airway and their aspiration. The patient must have a normal pulmonary function to withstand the difficulties inherent in this type of surgery.

The techniques of surgical correction of the various stenoses have been described elsewhere (Bryce, 1976). In general, dilatations, usually repeated on a multitude of occasions, have not been successful in maintaining an adequate lumen in the larynx when the scarring is severe. Whenever possible, the scarred areas must be excised and the normal structure of the larynx restored (Gerwat and Bryce, 1974). This is particularly true with severe subglottic stenosis. After such excision of scar an intraluminal stent is usually required to support the restored lumen and to allow mucous membrane to grow beneath it and to resurface the denuded areas. The use of skin and mucous membranes as grafts, for this purpose, has a limited application. The stent is ideally soft and flexible (*Figure 12.8*) and yet strong enough to resist the pressures of the post-operative scar retraction. If possible, it may have a lumen to

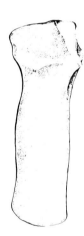

Figure 12.8 A moulded silastic stent for use to support laryngotracheal reconstructions. (From *Operative Surgery*, 3rd edn Eds C. Rob and R. Smith. *Nose and Throat*, Butterworths, London and Boston)

allow some respiratory exchange through the mouth. It should not absorb the salivary secretions so that it can be left in place for a prolonged period of time without becoming offensive. A cadaver moulded stent is ideal.

If considerable reconstruction of the airway is necessary, prosthetic materials have proven to be of no value. Infection (always present in the airway) and the movement of respiration inevitably result in their extrusion and rejection. Autogenous skin cartilage and bone may be used but this requires prolonged and repeated surgical stages and should be embarked upon only as a last resort.

During the post-operative period after excision, and during the time when a stent must be in place, a tracheostomy is of great importance. Most cases of significant stenosis will have had a previous tracheostomy. During the course of the excision of the scar, however, the tracheostomy should be replaced at some distance from the area of anastomosis. The tracheostomy should be of adequate size to allow proper respiration and great care must be taken in its placement because the in-dwelling stent will make oral respiration impossible.

In some cases of severe and extensive stenosis, surgical excision and anastomosis and all other methods of reconstitution of the airway may fail. In these cases, it is often necessary to provide prolonged stenting for a year or more to allow the walls of the scarred tracheal tube to become stable. For this purpose the most effective tube is the 'Montgomery T-tube' (*Figure 12.9*) which is so beautifully designed that it may be left in place for many years, if necessary, and it is capable of being cared for and cleaned by the patient.

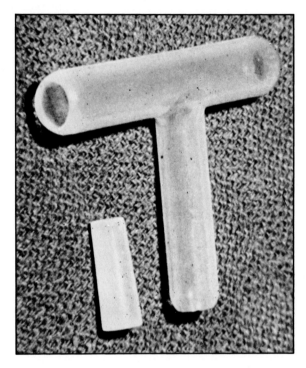

Figure 12.9   A 'Montgomery T-tube' to prevent tracheal stenosis

Not all laryngeal stenoses are of such severity that the surgical techniques of excision and direct anastomosis will be necessary for their correction. Dilatations, submucosal scar excisions, followed by stenting, widening of the airway by opening the cricoid ring anteriorly and posteriorly, have all been successfully used in some cases and should be part of the armamentarium of the surgeon who is in charge of these cases.

Conclusion

Trauma to the larynx and the stenosis which results from inadequate management of the acute problem are important and demanding clinical problems requiring considerable knowledge on the part of the surgeon for their management. These conditions have become more common recently as a result of the increased use of the motor car and other related vehicles and because of the development of special respiratory care centres in our major hospitals. The surgical techniques are complicated and require special training for the laryngeal surgeon. The rewards, however, are great. Most of the patients are young and are faced with the problem of prolonged or permanent tracheostomy, to the degree that they may lose their voice permanently and be unable to breathe through their mouths. The restoration of normal function in such patients is one of the most rewarding experiences for the surgeon.

References

Bryce, D. P. (1976). In: *Operative Surgery* (Ed. John Ballantyne); Butterworths, London and Boston

Bryce, D. P. (in press). In: *Recent Advances in Otolaryngology* (Eds T. R. Bull, J. Ransome and H. Holden); Churchill-Livingstone, Edinburgh

Gerwat, M. B. and Bryce, D. P. (1974). *Laryngoscope*, **84,** 940–957

13 Acute laryngitis
L F W Salmon

Introduction

Acute inflammatory changes in the larynx may be produced by all the classical causes of inflammation. Thus the damage inflicted by a variety of pathogenic organisms, trauma of different kinds, chemical irritation, excessive heat, ionizing radiation and the antigen–antibody reaction all occur as agents in the aetiology of acute laryngitis. Often more than one of these factors is involved. It is unusual for the irritant concerned to act only on the larynx and as a rule the respiratory tract in general is affected, though chiefly the upper respiratory passages. The clinical picture produced, therefore, will be that of the overall illness, not simply of the laryngitis. In certain cases the inflammatory changes occurring in the larynx are of secondary importance and may be overlooked or at least over-shadowed by the primary condition as in accidental injury, when a foreign body lodges in the larynx, after some lesion has been surgically removed from the vocal cord or a laryngeal neoplasm treated with radiotherapy. Certain of the inflammatory diseases which characteristically run a chronic course and which will be described in the next chapter may present as acute laryngitis or will have emerged insidiously from acute beginnings.

The most important generalization, however, concerns the serious nature of acute infective laryngitis in infants and young children in whom, in contrast with adults, it is often a grave and sometimes dangerous illness. This type of laryngitis will therefore be described separately for the two age groups.

Acute infective laryngitis in the adult

Aetiology

This disease is usually a consequence of acute infection of the nose and pharynx, generally the common cold. The infecting agent is a virus although bacterial superinfection occurs almost always. As well as the rhinoviruses and the influenza virus, adenoviruses have been identified. Among the bacteria colonizing the mucous membrane damaged by the virus are found beta-haemolytic streptococci, *Haemophilus influenzae* and, less commonly, pneumococci. *H. influenzae* may also reach the larynx by way of the blood stream as, rarely, may *Salmonella typhi*.

Laryngitis in measles, chicken-pox and other childhood infections is dealt with in the section devoted to acute laryngitis in infants and young children where an account of diphtheritic laryngitis also appears. Smallpox, regularly listed under this heading in the past, is now chiefly a matter of historical interest.

When acute laryngitis complicates the common upper respiratory infections it is popularly called 'simple' laryngitis.

Simple laryngitis

Predisposing factors

There can be few adults who have not at some time experienced this familiar minor illness. Because most cases are caused by colds, it may be argued that whatever predisposes to colds predisposes to acute laryngitis. It is certainly likely that a dry and dusty environment and exposure to the irritant tars in tobacco smoke are important in this connection.

As in the case of children, some adult patients are more than usually susceptible. They fear catching cold because experience has taught them that they are likely to develop laryngitis in the course of it. Moreover, they are not necessarily those who live in centrally heated homes with no humidification, work in noisy, dusty conditions or misuse their voices. As long ago as 1880, Morrell Mackenzie noted that 'previous attacks, especially if several times repeated, increase the susceptibility of the individual to a renewal of the affection'. However, this begs the question and the cause of this susceptibility remains uncertain.

Pathology

Simple acute laryngitis as it is encountered today does not often provide material for microscopical examination but Eggston and Wolff (1947) describe all the histological characteristics of acute infection elsewhere. At first there is vascular dilatation, diapedesis of polymorphonuclear leucocytes and marked oedema. Later, lymphocytes and fibroblasts appear (*Figure 13.1*).

Not only are the vocal cords inflamed but considerable swelling of the supraglottic tissues occurs, particularly of the vestibular folds and between the arytenoid cartilages. In severe cases the whole thickness of the mucous membrane may be involved in the inflammatory reaction and even the intrinsic muscles. Exfoliation of areas of epithelium may sometimes occur resulting in superficial ulceration.

It is rare today for the infection to attack the skeletal structures of the larynx. Apart from this complete resolution is the rule and this accords with the familiar clinical course.

Writing in the third edition of this book, Maxwell Ellis refers to paralysis of one or other vocal cord occurring occasionally in the course of acute laryngitis. He considers

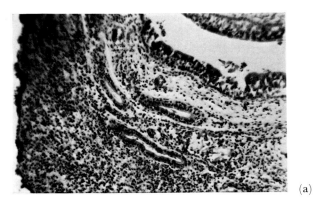

(a)

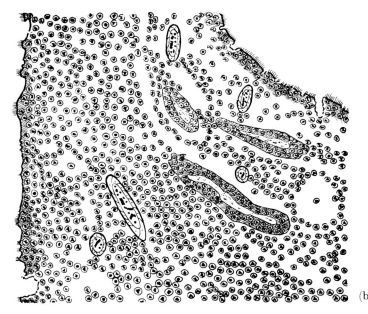

(b)

Figure 13.1 (a) Photomicrograph of a section through the mucous membrane of the larynx of a child aged five who died 12 hours after the onset of an acute respiratory tract infection. There is a heavy infiltration of neutrophils and lymphocytes together with vascular congestion and oedema. Areas of the epithelium have been destroyed and have desquamated. (b) A diagram of the photomicrograph in (a)

it to be due to peripheral neuritis and to escape diagnosis except when detected by a laryngologist. It can be expected to recover spontaneously.

The clinical features

A number of the symptoms and signs commonly ascribed to laryngitis are those of the causative illness rather than of the laryngeal involvement. The feeling of chill or even a slight rigor, the fever and malaise, the dryness and later rawness of the throat, all mentioned in classical accounts, are examples of this.

The complaints attributable to the laryngitis are those related to disturbed phonation. These may appear quite suddenly. There is a lowering of the tone of the voice with a curious unreliability of pitch. Huskiness, often worse on waking, becomes increasingly troublesome until after a few days the voice resembles a croak. Attempting to speak may be distinctly painful. Occasionally the patient becomes aphonic, sometimes because the cords are so loaded as to vibrate only with an effort greater than the patient is prepared to make, sometimes because he prefers to mouth his words than utter such a strangled sound. At first clearing the throat is difficult and ineffective and the attempt results in a croupy sound. The onset of cough suggests a spread to the lower air passages but when present it is hard, unproductive and often quite painful. Respiration is almost never embarrassed in the adult but inspiration may be a little prolonged and, rarely, accompanied by a hint of stridor.

Usually, after a further few days, secretions from the inflamed mucosa become more plentiful and less viscid. The patient derives satisfaction and some relief from clearing the throat although doing so may leave behind a slight and brief feeling of rawness. From this point recovery is not often long delayed, the illness running its course in some 7–10 days.

However, recovery may be delayed or even incomplete when the patient insists on attempting to use his voice throughout the illness or starts to use it strenuously during the productive phase. Even in the absence of this provocation, perhaps because of the damage done to the mucous membrane by a particularly virulent virus, sticky secretions continue to be produced which compel him to make often abortive attempts to clear his voice long after every other trace of the attack has disappeared.

The examination findings

The findings on general examination and of the ears, nose and throat apart from the larynx are clearly of importance but will not be described here.

The appearance of the larynx will vary with the stage of the disease. At first there is generalized hyperaemia spreading to reach the vocal cords at a time corresponding with the earliest voice changes. The cords then look glazed and somewhat injected but within a day or two may become so vascular as to match the colour and appearance of the ventricular bands. The oedema and swelling give a generally rounded contour to the cords. The mucosa, particularly of the false cords and of the interarytenoid region, assumes a dusky red velvety appearance and interarytenoid swelling may be sufficient to interfere with proper approximation of the cords. The free portion of the epiglottis does not as a rule share in the inflammation which is characteristically symmetrically distributed. The occurrence of submucosal haemorrhages is not common and is suggestive of a traumatic factor, for instance coughing, hawking or retching.

Secretions are not greatly in evidence but may be seen stringing out between the cords as they part, remaining heaped up, characteristically at the junction of the anterior and middle thirds. Muco-pus seen in the interarytenoid region has its origin in the trachea and clings to the inflamed mucosa in spite of the patient's efforts to clear it.

The patchy ulceration and epithelial desquamation described by pathologists and in older texts is rarely seen today.

Diagnosis

The diagnosis will be suggested by the characteristic onset in the course of an infection involving the upper respiratory tract. The laryngoscopic appearance will go a long way towards confirming it. Laryngitis is the usual diagnosis to suggest itself to the practitioner confronted with a hoarse patient and only the laryngologist is likely to examine the larynx before deciding how to proceed. The consequences of treating the patient without excluding diseases more serious than laryngitis, even early carcinoma or, in many parts of the world, tuberculosis of the larynx would be avoided if it were borne in mind that acute laryngitis runs a short self-limiting course and failure to recover within a week or two makes laryngoscopic assessment imperative without further delay.

Complications

Perichondritis, chondral necrosis and laryngeal abscess seem to have complicated acute laryngeal infections not infrequently in the past, particularly in such serious illnesses as smallpox and typhoid fever. They are very rare now though still reported from some parts of the developing world. An account appears later in this section (p. 368).

Some degree of oedema is a constant feature of infection in the larynx as elsewhere but it may be severe enough to dominate the picture, particularly in children and the debilitated. It may be caused by factors other than infection, however, and therefore merits separate consideration (p. 371).

Treatment

The only effective treatment is voice rest and voice rest means silence. A stage whisper can be as injurious to the inflamed cords as conversational speech. Attempts to speak are strongly inhibited during the height of the attack because phonation is likely to be difficult or even painful but during the following days it becomes easier and many patients may then struggle to talk or hurry back to work, thereby delaying recovery.

Patients susceptible to acute laryngitis are more at risk if the need to rest the voice is ignored because if recovery is incomplete when subsequent attacks occur, chronic laryngitis may become established.

Professional voice users, particularly singers, actors, entertainers and teachers may find it more difficult to follow advice about voice rest than other sorts of patient (*see also* Chapter 16. They may be tempted to undertake a performance or engagement before recovery is complete and then find themselves compelled to cancel several more.

Antibiotics are widely prescribed although their value in general is equivocal. The use of the appropriate antibiotic is advocated, however, where fever and toxaemia are conspicuous and where there is purulent expectoration. In these events, however, it is probably the lower air passages which are the therapeutic target.

Supportive treatment

The patient should be advised that he will be more comfortable, less of a menace to others and likely to get well sooner if he will confine himself to bed throughout the illness. However, such advice will often be ignored with the implied consequences. He should also be advised to avoid spirits and tobacco but may default over this too.

The value of steam inhalations medicated with tincture of benzoin co., pine, menthol or eucalyptus is not disputed and the corollary is that the air of a centrally heated room should be humidified also. The fluid intake should be greater than usual and fresh lemon juice has the reputation of helping to clear the throat. If cough is troublesome a sedative cough mixture may help. Dover's powder is indeed an excellent remedy and some patients find aspirin useful at night. Soluble aspirin should be used. The once popular astringent and vasoconstrictor applications sprayed into the larynx are ineffective and perhaps harmful; however, a case may be made out for their use where singers, speakers and other performers demand help in an emergency.

Acute supraglottic laryngitis (epiglottitis)

Described in 1900 by Thiesen, it was at first regarded as a disease ôccurring only in children and then rarely. However, since Le Mierre and his associates observed it in adults in 1936, adult cases appear to have been on the increase (Hawkins *et al.*, 1973) and Richards and Kander (1977) give an account of nine such cases occurring in South Wales over a ten-year period. Although the rapid onset of asphyxiating respiratory obstruction is not the usual course in the adult as it is in the child, nevertheless it is a dangerous illness whatever the age and deserves a full account.

Aetiology

In 1941 Sinclair recognized this variety of acute laryngitis as due to *Haemophilus influenzae*, type B. The organism produces a bacteraemia which may become localized as meningitis, pneumonia, pyarthrosis, osteomyelitis or epiglottitis. The steady reduction in incidence with increasing age was considered to occur as the result of an increasing amount of circulating antibody. It has been suggested that the universal use of antibiotics in infants and young children may be altering this process and, in support of this, increases in the number of adult cases of meningitis and respiratory infections as well as epiglottitis due to *H. influenzae* are being reported. The accounts of epiglottitis in adults include many cases where the organisms identified on culturing throat swabs have been found to be not *H. influenzae* but others including *Streptococcus viridans*, *Staphylococcus pyogenes* and *Diplococcus pneumoniae*. These cases seem generally to run a more benign course so far as respiratory obstruction is concerned.

Hawkins and his associates suggest that supraglottic laryngitis due to *H. influenzae* is a serious illness liable to rapidly progressive respiratory obstruction in adults just as it is in children, and that the less severe course and better prognosis in adults is because a proportion of the adult cases are not cases of *H. influenzae* bacteraemia with localization in the epiglottis, but supraglottic laryngitis due to other organisms. Blood culture is always positive in the cases caused by *H. influenzae* and should always be undertaken in this kind of laryngitis as a guide to prognosis and treatment.

Pathology

The acute inflammatory changes are curiously localized to the epiglottis, pharyngo-epiglottic and aryepiglottic folds, ventricular bands and arytenoids (that is to the supraglottic larynx) the vocal cords and subglottic tissues being spared. Not infrequently in the adult the aryepiglottic folds and false cords are more involved than the epiglottis so that supraglottic laryngitis is a more comprehensive description than epiglottitis.

Both the mucosa and submucosa are heavily infiltrated with neutrophils and show micro-abscesses. These may occasionally coalesce to form large abscesses requiring surgical drainage. Oedema and hyperaemia are always marked features and responsible for the progressive respiratory obstructions characteristic of the *H. influenzae* infections.

Clinical features

Men are more vulnerable than women and a male preponderance as great as 4:1 has been reported.

The presenting symptom is invariably sore throat leading to dysphagia of such severity in the worst cases that saliva drools from the open mouth. In contrast with the condition in children, dyspnoea is not always severe in adults and stridor, coming on 8–48 hours after the onset of the illness, occurs in no more than 60 per cent. In some 25 per cent, however, respiratory difficulty increases rapidly, needing tracheostomy for its relief. When breathing becomes very difficult, the patient chooses to sit propped up on his extended arms, his mouth open, chin thrust forward looking pale, slightly cyanosed and anxious. Because the vocal cords are not affected, hoarseness is not a feature although the voice may sound muffled. The temperature varies from normal to 39 °C.

Diagnosis

The mode of onset is characteristic but the diagnosis is confirmed by the physical findings. In children, indirect laryngoscopy, even depressing the tongue is likely to provoke an asphyxial attack or even cardiac arrest and so must be undertaken with the greatest caution, but mirror examination is usually possible in the older patient and safe enough unless it threatens to provoke violent coughing and retching in the presence of grave dyspnoea. Very often nothing more can be seen than the enormously swollen, red epiglottis although sometimes the swelling and hyperaemia are more marked in the aryepiglottic and arytenoid regions. Very rarely may the vocal cords be visualized. The neck is often stiff and tender and there may be moderate tender enlargement of the regional lymph nodes. A lateral soft tissue x-ray will confirm the supraglottic swelling when examination fails to reveal it.

Throat swabs must be taken and antibiotic therapy started without waiting for the result. Blood culture may confirm *H. influenzae* bacteraemia even when this organism is not identified from the throat swab.

The differential diagnosis is often difficult and includes a greater range of problems in young patients in whom laryngotracheobronchitis is likely to be suspected initially.

Treatment

Because of the agonizing sore throat, most adult patients will find their way into hospital well before severe respiratory distress calls for urgent tracheostomy. There will be time to institute conservative measures, order confirmatory investigations and observe progress.

Antibiotic treatment must be commenced immediately without waiting for the bacteriological report. Ampicillin intramuscularly is probably still the correct choice although the recent emergence of ampicillin resistance in *H. influenzae* may alter this. If the patient is ill enough to require intravenous fluids, the ampicillin also may be given intravenously.

The place of the corticosteroids in the management of these cases is equivocal. The use of intramuscular or intravenous hydrocortisone may reduce oedema and could be of critical value where tracheostomy is debated. In the presence of progressive respiratory obstruction, its use is recommended. The breathing of cool, humidified oxygen-enriched air is helpful in respiratory distress but the expected advantages must be weighed against the problems arising from nursing the patient in a tent. Sedation is important to allay anxiety but narcotics and atropine are to be avoided.

About half of the cases will experience dyspnoea and of these a proportion will improve rapidly on the regimen outlined. The remainder are candidates for surgical relief. The arguments for nasotracheal intubation as an alternative to tracheostomy are given on p. 367. They apply to the problem as it presents in children and when intervention is judged necessary in the adult, tracheostomy is the recommended method. If an experienced anaesthetist is prepared to give a general anaesthetic the patient will be spared a further ordeal but a bronchoscope may be less difficult to pass through the swollen supraglottic structures than the usual endotracheal tube. The technical considerations are fully set out in Chapter 19.

In conclusion, it is necessary to repeat that a proportion of these cases – in one series (Hawkins *et al.*, 1973) the figure was more than 20 per cent – develop an epiglottic abscess. If the epiglottis remains red and swollen in spite of adequate treatment and general improvement, this possibility has to be considered. The treatment is surgical drainage using a Boyle–Davis gag or a large-lumen suspension laryngoscope of the Kleinsasser sort. If tracheostomy has not proved necessary previously, the need for it as an elective procedure prior to surgery must be given careful consideration.

Prognosis

One in three of the 62 adult cases reported in the literature between 1958 and 1973 died but the 26 cases, reported in two papers since, survived (Hawkins *et al.*, 1973; Richards and Kander, 1977).

With adequate treatment the outlook is good and the duration of the illness, even if tracheostomy has to be resorted to, no longer than two weeks.

Acute infective laryngitis in infancy and childhood

Simple laryngitis

Aetiology and pathology

Three factors are generally considered responsible for the special features of laryngitis in young individuals. The first is that immunity against the common infections is still in process of being acquired and there is no better example of this in the present context than the age incidence of epiglottitis due to *H. influenzae*. The second is anatomical, the areolar tissue of the submucosa being plentiful and delicate, binding the mucous membrane to the underlying cartilage and fibrous membranes far more loosely than in the adult. This feature is especially conspicuous in the structures which bound the laryngeal inlet and in the subglottic region. It is this abundance of loose connective tissue which facilitates swelling due to oedema and inflammatory infiltration. The third is physiological and concerns the brisk reflexes of the very young which permit laryngeal spasm to occur more easily.

The importance of regarding the respiratory system as a whole has already been emphasized (Cawthorne and Edwards, 1966) but this is of even greater consequence in the child. Simple laryngitis may occur in children with colds as it does in adults but at this age is equally likely to complicate the infectious fevers and measles in particular. Measles is no longer as serious an illness in the western world as in many developing countries where the mortality remains high. Measles laryngitis is common in these lands though often as part only of a more extensive respiratory infection, namely laryngotracheobronchitis (p. 355). The high mortality is not only due to such serious pulmonary complications as viral pneumonitis, giant-cell pneumonia or secondary bronchopneumonia but also to grave upper respiratory obstruction with the risk of respiratory and cardiac arrest. Serious malnutrition frequently contributes to lowered resistance and adds to the gravity of the complications.

Histologically the inflammatory changes correspond to those found in the adult (p. 346) but are characteristically most marked in the subglottic region which is the site of the obstruction to breathing when this occurs.

Symptoms and signs

The clinical picture of acute laryngitis in children is significantly different from that in the older age groups, being dominated by the croupy cough. The old name 'croup' lingers on in popular parlance to describe not only this but particularly laryngotracheobronchitis. A degree of huskiness is usually present but persistent stridor is suggestive of tracheobronchial involvement.

An alarming feature occasionally is the sudden suffocating nocturnal stridor which may waken the patient and terrify not only the victim but the parents. It seems to have been commoner in the past when it was described as *laryngitis stridulosa* and more recently *spasmodic laryngitis*. It is probably different from the attacks of laryngeal spasm occurring in the absence of infection and called *laryngismus stridulus* (Volume 3). The attack is usually of short duration but may be repeated a few hours later, probably as the result of laryngeal spasm triggered off by tenacious secretions temporarily obstructing the glottis. However, the symptoms vary widely in degree largely in accordance with the extent to which infection spreads to the lower air passages and, to obtain an overall view, this section should be read in conjunction with the next.

Diagnosis

The practitioner confronted with a previously healthy child who has developed a husky voice and croupy cough in the course of a cold is likely to institute treatment without attempting laryngeal examination and the subsequent uneventful course to recovery will support his diagnosis of 'croup', meaning simple laryngitis. Such cases are unlikely to be referred to the specialist or find their way into hospital. When dyspnoea is a feature or stridor is present or supervenes, the differential diagnosis is immediately widened and includes laryngotracheobronchitis high on the list. Examination and investigation and the exclusion of other causes of stridor then become mandatory and often urgent and is fully considered in the next section. Never forget the possibility of an inhaled foreign body.

Treatment

This too will be found later but management of the sudden paroxysms that characterize so-called laryngitis stridulosa needs mentioning here. They are more likely to occur towards evening or during sleep as in laryngismus stridulus and rarely last more than a few minutes.

More often than not medical aid will arrive when the worst is over and when nothing more than re-assurance, particularly of the parents, is called for. The patient may be helped to breathe by drawing the tongue forward and encouraging him to cough or clear his throat.

Acute laryngotracheobronchitis

Aetiology and pathology

The great majority of these cases occur in the very young between the ages of six months and three years, with the peak incidence in the second year. Boys are more often affected than girls and the major incidence is during the winter months.

A number of viruses have been found to be causative, especially the para-influenzal virus type 1, respiratory syncytial virus and the virus of measles. The importance of the last-named agent in countries where measles remains a major cause of death in childhood is well-illustrated by Hancock's study from Nairobi (1972). Of 800 children admitted to the main hospital between January and June 1970, 74 developed laryngotracheobronchitis and 29 died. Among 72 cases of non-measles laryngotracheobronchitis admitted over the same period there were six deaths.

However, it has to be emphasized that overall the aetiological agent goes unidentified in all but a small proportion, although secondary bacterial invaders are frequently cultured from swabs or sputum.

The slowly progressive respiratory obstruction characteristic of this dangerous disease is caused by two pathological phenomena. The first is the swelling of the mucosa lining the conus elasticus, i.e. the subglottic larynx; and the second, the character of the exudate poured out into the lumen of the trachea and major bronchi. Consisting of mucus, leucocytes, epithelial debris and fibrin, it is curiously tough and tenacious so that the relatively feeble cough of the very young is inadequate to move it. Unless the humidity is high, it tends to become inspissated and to assume a semi-solid consistency. This is particularly liable to occur after tracheostomy. Such secretions tend to block the bronchi and produce areas of pulmonary atelectasis.

Clinical features

At first the course of events suggests nothing more serious than a febrile upper respiratory infection with laryngitis and a croupy cough. There may be little anxiety because the child does not seem ill and not uncommonly there will have been a similar attack before, which has resolved without complications. However, during the ensuing 24–48 hours difficulty in breathing is noticed and stridor sets in and persists. At first inspiratory, it may later occur with expiration also. Increasingly the signs of laryngeal obstruction become evident with the tell-tale movements of the alae nasi and suprasternal and intercostal recession. Cough is rarely troublesome and may be absent but when it occurs the harsh, metallic croupy quality is unmistakable evidence of subglottic swelling. The temperature may be as high as 39–40 °C, feeding is difficult and the fluid balance must be carefully watched if dehydration is to be avoided.

A fulminating variety of the illness has been described with the rapid development of obstructed respiration, hypoxia, acidosis, circulatory failure and death but many of the cases are more likely to have been examples of the supraglottic obstruction due to *H. influenzae* considered on p. 350. Nevertheless, if treatment is not instituted before the signs of severe obstruction with tracheal plunging, rapid pulse and cyanosis occur, a fatal outcome is certainly likely. This is seen frequently in the developing countries where measles and malnutrition are concerned and where tracheostomy attempted too late is, in the words of Arthur Durham, little better than 'the coup-de-grâce.'

Diagnosis

A reliable account of the onset and course of the illness will suggest the correct diagnosis. Respiratory obstruction following rapidly on severe sore throat is characteristic of supraglottic laryngitis (epiglottitis). The abrupt onset of urgent dyspnoea in a child, until then quite well, suggests a laryngeal foreign body. Angioneurotic oedema and other varieties of allergic laryngeal oedema have to be borne in mind but the absence of infection and the history, for example of an insect bite, will be helpful. At one time it would have been of paramount importance to exclude laryngeal diphtheria and even today, it would not do to forget it. An account is given later in this chapter. Further consideration of the differential diagnosis will be found on p. 360.

Finally, however, the diagnosis will rest on the examination and investigations and here something must be said about the examination of the child with stridor. Cases are on record of asphyxiation and cardiac arrest consequent on a struggle to examine the larynx of the child with obstructed breathing where the diagnosis has proved to be epiglottitis. The struggle has resulted in a desperate inspiratory effort either with the impaction of oedematous tissue in the glottis or, more likely, the inhalation of the pharyngeal secretions (Morus Jones, 1970). For this reason paediatricians urge caution when attempting to examine the throat of a child with acute stridor. At the same time, however, there is an argument which has been taken to be in the opposite sense. Laryngologists with paediatric experience since Chevalier Jackson have emphasized that the cause of laryngitis in the young patient must not be a matter of inference but based on the sound foundation of observed signs. Jackson practised direct laryngoscopy and bronchoscopy on the very young without anaesthesia and greatly advanced our knowledge and management of stridor in infancy and childhood. Much more recently Pracy (1965), working with skilled paediatric anaesthetists, has demonstrated that even more can be learned and treatment rendered even more effective by the judicious use of general anaesthesia for these purposes (*see also* Chapter 19). No doubt, if the child has the good fortune to be admitted to a hospital able to call on an anaesthetist skilled and experienced in this highly specialized field, he may be examined and treated as necessary under a general anaesthetic with less risk than if the same procedures are attempted without anaesthesia.

At laryngoscopy the inflamed and swollen subglottic tissues appear as semi-elliptical mounds, usually intensely red, one below each vocal cord. At bronchoscopy the tracheal mucosa is seen to be hyperaemic and velvety and more or less obscured by the tenacious, glue-like exudate.

X-ray examination of the chest will often confirm the presence of scattered areas of pulmonary collapse.

Treatment

The object of treatment is the maintenance or, if necessary, the restoration of adequate respiratory exchange over the several days taken for recovery to occur. If dyspnoea is not severe and not increasing nothing more may be necessary than the nursing of the patient in a cool, moist environment. The type of tent known as a 'croupette' with an ultra-sonic atomizer is ideal and for the more severe case the percentage of oxygen can be increased without difficulty. Restlessness and anxiety must be allayed but the narcotics avoided since they depress the respiratory centre. Chloral hydrate is useful, 5–10 mg/kg. Adequate fluid intake must be ensured and intravenous fluids may be necessary for a day or two.

It is generally held that the other mainstays of conservative treatment are antibiotics and corticosteroids. However, the position is not clear.

We are dealing with an infection caused by a virus and available antibiotics are not effective against viruses. At least one study (Tercero-Talavera and Ropkin, 1974) demonstrated no difference in the course of the illness whether antibiotics were used or not. Moreover, there is evidence to suggest that bacterial superinfection is not prevented by the use of antibiotics either. The matter has been well summarized by Singer and Wilson (1976) who observe that antibiotics though rarely indicated are commonly used.

The place of corticosteroids is even more difficult to evaluate and is by no means settled. Different trials have led to opposite conclusions. However, this form of therapy is not often contra-indicated in the young child and when deterioration has not been arrested by the treatment already outlined, hydrocortisone i.v., 100–200 mg should be given as a therapeutic trial and repeated if improvement appears to result. Massicotte and Tétreault (1973) have found methyl-prednisolone valuable.

The use of adrenaline as a topical vasoconstrictor and bronchodilator is well established but over the past ten years this sympathomimetic has been used in conjunction with intermittent positive pressure breathing (IPPB) to improve the respiratory exchange in patients with laryngotracheobronchitis (Jordan, 1970). Nebulized racemic epinephrine is administered by a suitable respirator and a tight-fitting face-mask for 15 minutes and repeated if necessary. Very often one treatment only is needed to produce marked improvement in the dyspnoea and avert tracheostomy. Singer and Wilson (1976) compared 509 patients treated on the usual conservative lines with 359 patients treated with racemic epinephrine in this way and describe the technique. In the first group 13 patients (2.55 per cent) came to tracheostomy as compared with one case in the second group.

Failure of conservative treatment

In the face of increasing upper airway obstruction, the patient will maintain adequate alveolar ventilation and blood gas tensions only by increased respiratory effort and a rising respiratory rate. However, these compensatory mechanisms may fail suddenly and reliance cannot be placed on blood gas estimations as a means of judging that the time has come to abandon conservative methods in favour of more radical steps to relieve the obstruction (Jones and Owen-Thomas, 1971).

The signs of pending respiratory failure comprise an increase in respiratory rate above 100 per minute in the infant and above 60 per minute in the older child, a marked increase in respiratory effort, growing restlessness and central cyanosis of the lips even in the croupette with 30–45 per cent O_2.

The means of relieving the obstruction must depend on the facilities available and the experience of the medical and nursing staff. In the major paediatric hospitals and departments with Paediatric Intensive Care Units, and particularly anaesthetists familiar with the management of the young patient with croup, tracheostomy will not be the treatment of choice. Instead, an oral endotracheal tube will be passed under general anaesthesia and the tracheobronchial tree thoroughly sucked clear of the obstructing gummy secretions. This will not relieve the subglottic oedema but it may produce sufficient improvement to justify a further period of observation and if necessary it may be repeated.

If suction alone fails, the next step has to be the passage of a nasotracheal tube which will remain for hours or if necessary days depending on the rate of general improvement. If the condition deteriorates after the tube is removed it may be re-introduced. Adherence to certain technical details is critical if damage to the larynx with the risk of stenosis, particularly subglottic stenosis, is to be avoided. The most important relate to the design, size and length of the tube, observance of scrupulous suction discipline and the duration of intubation. For a detailed description of these matters the reader is referred to the appropriate chapters in the *Care of the Critically Ill Child* (Jones and Owen-Thomas, 1971) but it must be emphasized that in the unlikely event of the need for intubation persisting beyond seven days, tracheostomy should be performed and the nasotracheal tube removed.

There will be many localities where the management described in the preceding paragraphs is inappropriate in which case tracheostomy must be undertaken without delay. However, the special hazards of tracheostomy in the very young must not be overlooked (Salmon, 1975) nor must it be forgotten that the problems of management are not at an end once the operation has been performed. The displaced or blocked tracheostomy tube is an ever-present danger of which all grades of staff must be aware and able to attend to. It is as much the surgeon's responsibility to ensure this as it is to take the decision to proceed with the intervention.

After intubation or tracheostomy the young patient must be returned immediately to the cool moist environment of the croupette. Adequate humidification is, if possible, more important after these steps are taken than before. Finally, let it be repeated that the obstruction to the airway is as much a matter of the characteristic tenacious exudate in the tracheobronchial tree as it is of the subglottic swelling and careful regular aspiration of these secretions employing a carefully rehearsed aseptic routine is essential.

Prognosis – complications

As soon as the child can ventilate his lungs adequately and keep his air passages free of secretions without aid, recovery will usually continue uneventfully, to be complete within a few days. There is, however, a small number of young children liable to recurrences of laryngotracheobronchitis who may need admission to hospital on two or three occasions before reaching the age of four or thereabouts when susceptibility usually ceases.

The significant complications are iatrogenic, being those of the intubation e.g. subglottic stenosis, or of the tracheostomy. Tracheostomy continues to be a dangerous operation in the very young in spite of modern methods. Mediastinal emphysema and pneumothorax still occur and are still mis-diagnosed as bronchopneumonia and the mortality from all causes is as high as three per cent even in the well-provided western world.

Acute supraglottic laryngitis (epiglottitis)

Compared with laryngotracheobronchitis this is a rare disease. Figures vary, but on average not more than 1 child in 50 admitted to hospital with acute infective croup proves to be suffering from acute epiglottitis. However, although rare it is highly dangerous with a fatal outcome in 3–4 per cent of cases treated by experienced personnel in ideal conditions (Fearon, 1975). Mortality rates of up to 50 per cent have been reported. Its exceptional occurrence in adults has been described already on pp.350–353 where the aetiology and pathology are included.

Aetiology and pathology

The details given above apply equally to the young patient except that, for reasons already mentioned, the inflammatory changes are more severe in childhood and the prognosis worse. In summary the disease is to be regarded as a local manifestation of a bacteriaemia due to *Haemophilus influenzae* type B. The supraglottic larynx only is attacked, intense swelling of the epiglottis being the principal feature. Blood culture is more likely to reveal the organism than a throat swab.

Clinical features

Acute supraglottic laryngitis occurs in a somewhat older age group than acute laryngotracheobronchitis, with a peak age incidence between the third and sixth years. Its relative rarity means that even a large paediatric hospital is unlikely to admit more than a few cases per annum.

The onset is usually sudden, starting with a mild sore throat that quickly progresses to severe dysphagia with a high fever. Because the inflammatory changes are confined above the glottis the voice though muffled is not hoarse, and the croupy cough typical of subglottic laryngitis usually absent. Dyspnoea is noticed within an hour or two and worsens rapidly. The patient assumes a characteristic posture, leaning forward propped up on the extended arms, the chin thrust out and the mouth open drooling saliva. Stridor is not a marked feature. However, evidence of increasing respiratory effort is more and more apparent, with the alae nasi working, the chest wall particularly at the costal margins being drawn in while the abdomen protrudes and the supraclavicular structures including the trachea being tugged downwards and backwards with each inspiratory effort. The respiratory rate increases, the child's face often expressing the fear of the impending respiratory failure. Pallor, cyanosis and sweating are among the first warnings of circulatory failure. Tachycardia gives way to a slow pulse and cardiac arrest is imminent. Blood gas estimations will reveal severe hypoxia, hypercapnia and acidosis, the high pCO_2 resulting at first in headache and later deepening narcosis. Successful resuscitation at this stage may succeed in saving life but not in avoiding brain damage.

If nothing is done to halt this train of events, the illness may proceed from beginning to end in as little as 6–24 hours. Provided adequate respiratory exchange is ensured, however, spontaneous resolution can be expected to commence within some 72 hours and proceed uneventfully.

Examination; investigations

Whenever possible a specimen for blood culture should be taken as soon as the provisional diagnosis is made as well as throat swabs for bacteriological examination.

The characteristic finding is a red, intensely swollen epiglottis which, on skilful depression of the tongue, can be seen rising out of the hypopharynx like the rising sun. However, as already explained in the sick, stridorous and frightened child, depressing the tongue may lead to struggling, coughing and crying and the deep inspiration associated with such activity may in turn cause laryngeal spasm and, rarely, a fatal outcome from cardiac arrest.

Whether or not to attempt this examination will be a matter of nice judgment, therefore, for an experienced laryngologist who will proceed only if he estimates that the general condition of the patient allows him a margin of safety. Soft tissue, lateral x-rays of the neck to show the swollen epiglottis have been advocated as a less hazardous alternative but in an advanced case the delay may be unacceptable.

Direct examination under an anaesthetic is unquestionably the better method but only where first-class facilities and anaesthetic staff skilled in this type of procedure are available.

Very often the patient will arrive at the hospital already threatened by respiratory and circulatory failure when the measures outlined below for their relief must proceed without delay.

Differential diagnosis

A sudden feverish illness with progressive laryngeal obstruction in a patient of the appropriate age is characteristic of infective croup and many of the other causes of stridor in the infant and young child, such as the congenital diseases described in Chapter 11, will not come in for serious consideration here. Laryngeal foreign body and angioneurotic oedema already mentioned, although of sudden onset, are unlikely to be mistaken for acute infection, nor are the laryngeal neoplasms of the child, multiple papillomas and haemangioma of the larynx. Mediastinal tumours, thymoma, teratoma and so on will run a non-febrile course with an insidious onset. An acute paroxysm of asthma may start abruptly and may occur in the course of an upper respiratory infection but the typical expiratory wheezing, absence of upper respiratory obstruction, characteristic signs and previous history make up a picture quite unlike that of infective croup. An account of the acute and dramatic events of swallowed caustics and inhaled fumes is given below. The circumstances can be expected to make the diagnosis abundantly clear.

The child with a retropharyngeal or parapharyngeal abscess (peritonsillar abscess is not likely to occur in this age group) will have an acute febrile illness with sore throat, complicated sometimes by dyspnoea and may very well be suspected of having acute supraglottic laryngitis. However, careful examination will reveal the obstructing swelling to be elsewhere than in the supraglottic larynx.

Finally, of course, the differential diagnosis must be a matter of deciding whether the child is suffering from acute laryngotracheobronchitis, acute epiglottitis or, in those parts of the world where it is at present occurring, laryngeal diphtheria. *Table 13.1* sets out the principal differential features.

Treatment

This is a bacterial infection, due to an organism still sensitive to a number of antibiotics, so that treatment with the appropriate antibiotic may be regarded as specific therapy. The problem, however, is that the supraglottic swelling develops so rapidly in the child, that grave obstruction to breathing must be anticipated before the effect of the antibiotic is manifest. In the paragraph concerned with the treatment of supraglottic laryngitis in the adult (p. 352) it is stated that there will usually be time to observe the effects of conservative treatment before resorting to surgical measures to by-pass the obstruction. This is almost never so in the young patient and although reports justifying a trial of conservative treatment have appeared (e.g. Strome and Jaffe, 1974), Strong's advice (Strong and Paparella, 1975, p. 264) that 'if the decision to "observe" the patient with epiglottitis is made, it means you will stay by the bedside with a laryngoscope in one hand and an intratracheal tube in the other', (*sic*) while not to be taken literally perhaps, should be borne constantly in mind.

The conservative treatment of acute laryngotracheobronchitis including nursing the patient in a properly humidified croupette is in the main the treatment to be adopted in these cases also, except that the reservations about the value of anti-biotics and corticosteroids do not apply. For acute epiglottitis, ampicillin by the intramuscular route (while the intravenous drip is being set up) is mandatory. Ampicillin-resistant strains of haemophilus have been reported recently and on receipt of the sensitivity report from the bacteriologist, an alternative antibiotic may be indicated.

For these critically ill children, corticosteroid treatment should not be withheld. The intravenous route should again be employed with an initial dose of 100–200 mg of hydrocortisone hemisuccinate, repeated four hours later, half this dose to be given six-hourly over the following 48 hours. Dexamethasone or methyl-prednisolone in the correspondingly smaller dosage may be preferred.

Several reports mention the use of nebulized racemic epinephrine (adrenaline) given by intermittent positive-pressure breathing and claim successes. The technique was referred to in the section dealing with the treatment of acute laryngotracheo-bronchitis (p. 357).

Table 13.1   Differential diagnosis

	Acute laryngotracheo-bronchitis	*Acute supraglottic laryngitis (epiglottitis)*	*Laryngeal diphtheria*
Incidence	Not uncommon	Rare	Generally very rare
Maximum age incidence	6 months to 3 years	2–6 years	6 months to 10 years
Aetiology	Viruses, particularly para-influenza virus type 1	*H. influenzae* type B	*Corynebacterium diphtheria*
Pathology	Subglottic swelling Tenacious exudate obstructing tracheo-bronchial tree	Severe supraglottic swelling Bacteriaemia	Characteristic pseudomembrane in larynx usually spreading from pharynx Severe toxaemia
Chief clinical features	Moderate fever Coryzal onset Slowly progressive upper airway obstruction and stridor Croupy cough	High fever Severe sore throat and dysphagia Voice muffled Rapidly progressive laryngeal obstruction	Fever not conspicuous Slow onset with malaise, headache and sore throat Hoarseness Croupy cough Paroxysmal dyspnoea Stridor Marked cervical adenitis Profound constitutional effects
Prognosis	Spontaneous resolution in days if respiratory exchange maintained	Grave danger from respiratory and circulatory failure Prompt intervention to restore respiratory exchange ensures early recovery	Severe risk of asphyxia, tonic myocarditis with circulatory failure, widespread paralysis etc. in the absence of prompt diagnosis and treatment

Relief of obstruction

In fact many children with supraglottic laryngitis will reach hospital struggling desperately to breathe with a respiratory rate over 60 per minute, anxious, pallid and cyanosed, i.e. poised on the brink of respiratory failure. In such cases immediate steps must be taken to restore the airway either by means of intubation or tracheostomy.

Many such desperate problems present in Casualty or Emergency Departments of hospitals where relatively unskilled doctors may attempt to pass soft endotracheal tubes. The glottis cannot easily be seen beyond the grossly swollen supraglottic structures and extension of the head increases the obstruction. The struggle to pass the tube in vain may precipitate respiratory and circulatory failure. It must again be emphasized that intubation should be attempted only by specialists practised in its use and where facilities are instantly available to proceed with tracheostomy if there should be a problem. Even the most skilled may find intubation with a soft endotracheal tube impossible in severe cases of supraglottic laryngitis but will quickly recognize this and go on to pass a bronchoscope. Sharp pressure on the sternum by an assistant will produce air bubbles from the glottis and indicate the line of approach. Once the bronchoscope is in place, tracheostomy may be undertaken without haste and in such an event is the recommended procedure.

This must not be taken to mean that in the well-equipped and expertly staffed departments of paediatric hospitals and special departments with Paediatric Intensive Care Units, pernasal endotracheal intubation for epiglottitis is not an entirely feasible and safe procedure. This is well illustrated in a paper by Schuller and Birck (1975) dealing with intubation in 86 cases with infective upper airway obstruction including 55 cases of supraglottic laryngitis; 33 of these 55 were successfully intubated without mortality.

From time to time a child with gross laryngeal obstruction will present to a practitioner unskilled in either intubation or tracheostomy and perhaps far away from hospital facilities of any kind. Is there a safe procedure he can undertake to save life and tide the patient over until the more sophisticated treatment described above may be attempted? Such a measure is the introduction of one or more large needles into the trachea. Various needle-mounted plastic cannulae designed for intravascular use are suitable for this purpose and are now widely available. Clarke and Cochrane (1975) have measured the inflow through a No. 12 Medicut cannula and have shown it to be suitable for trans-tracheal cannulation in an emergency.

Laryngotracheal diphtheria

The *Corynebacterium diphtheriae* may infect a variety of sites including uncommonly the nose, conjunctiva, vagina and wounds (surgical diphtheria). The usual locality, however, is the fauces but in one case in four the infection spreads from the pharynx to involve the larynx and trachea. Primary laryngeal diphtheria is known to occur but must be very rare indeed even at the height of epidemics.

The nasal disease is described in Volume 3.

A full and detailed account of diphtheria would be out of place here but the salient features are included for the reader's convenience.

Aetiology

In many parts of the world diphtheria has almost completely disappeared. The great pandemic that swept through Western Europe between the 16th and 19th centuries was beginning to decline before the discovery of the antitoxin and the widespread use of preventive immunization but these advances accelerated the process. Nevertheless, the disease remains endemic and epidemic throughout the world and no one can be sure that serious outbreaks may not occur again.

Three types of the organism are recognized: gravis, intermedius and mitis. The major epidemics have been associated with the gravis strain and the high mortality with the characteristic profound toxaemia. When deaths have occurred in infections due to the mitis strain, they have usually been due to respiratory obstruction consequent on laryngotracheal involvement.

The main incidence is in children between the ages of two and five years and although adults may be affected, it becomes increasingly rare after age ten. It is highly contagious, the first signs appearing after an incubation period of 2–7 days. Convalescents may carry virulent organisms in their noses and throats and spread the disease.

Pathology

The gravity of diphtheria is not due simply to the local lesion with the possibility of upper airway obstruction when the larynx is involved, but particularly to the production of an exotoxin which diffuses widely exposing the patient to the risk of myocarditis and peripheral neuritis. Thus, between them, asphyxia, acute circulatory failure and respiratory paralysis have been responsible for the majority of the deaths.

The local lesion is characteristic. The exotoxin inhibits the inflammatory response and quickly produces epithelial necrosis. An exudate rich in fibrin is poured out and forms together with the necrotic tissues and a great number of bacteria a dense false membrane, pearl grey in colour, with a well-defined edge elevated above the general surface. At first it is glistening and firmly adherent so that attempts to remove it may produce bleeding. At a later stage, its appearance has been likened to wash leather and it separates more easily from the ulcerated surface beneath. When it occurs on the tonsil, patches of exudate as in follicular tonsillitis, coalesce and extend. The membrane may be limited to one side. Bleeding may occur spontaneously into the membrane turning it brown or even black in places. Adherence is less marked when it forms on or spreads onto the respiratory epithelium from which, even at first, it may be easily separated.

The regional lymph nodes are early and often strikingly involved and the surrounding oedema and cellulitis give the bull-neck appearance of the classical descriptions.

Symptoms

Because laryngotracheal diphtheria occurs as part of an infection with local and general manifestations and usually spreads to the larynx and trachea from the pharynx, the symptoms of the laryngotracheal lesion will constitute only part of a wider clinical picture which must be briefly described.

The illness is ushered in by malaise, headache, anorexia, moderate pyrexia and, as a rule, sore throat although the onset may be insidious, pyrexia absent and the discovery of the membrane over the fauces the first intimation of the disease. Usually the evidence of toxaemia is soon apparent and prostration, pallor and a falling blood pressure occur. The regional lymph nodes become swollen with oedema of the skin sometimes spreading to the face. Dysphagia increases in proportion to the pharyngeal involvement, a blood count reveals polymorphonuclear leucocytosis and the urine usually contains albumen. The presence of the membrane in the throat imparts to the breath a distinctive sickly odour which, when the disease was common, experienced clinicians found almost diagnostic.

Spread to the larynx and trachea may take place at an early stage of the disease with symptoms closely resembling those of acute viral laryngotracheobronchitis. These include a hoarse voice, a loud croupy cough and increasing dyspnoea. As the membrane increases in amount and extent all the evidence of increasing upper respiratory obstruction presents. Stridor, chiefly inspiratory and recession of the chest wall and the root of the neck tend to occur in paroxysms often precipitated by bouts of violent croupy coughing. These paroxysms become increasingly frequent and more and more exhausting until, if nothing is done to relieve the obstruction, death from asphyxia and cardiac failure supervenes. However, respiratory failure is not the principal threat to the circulation. More common than this is acute toxic myocarditis, occurring typically during the second week of the illness and leading in most cases to cardiac failure and death.

Paralytic symptoms complicate up to 20 per cent of cases with palatal paralysis the most frequent and the first to appear. It produces a nasal voice and regurgitation of fluids through the nose on swallowing. The nerves of the ocular muscles, the diaphragm and the pharynx and larynx may all become affected while after the fourth week of the disease progressive general paralysis involving the face, neck, trunk and extremities may set in. The paralysed parts may take many weeks to recover.

The mitis strain of *C. diphtheriae*, while causing the typical lesion at the site of infection is not liable to produce severe toxaemia. The stages of cardiac failure and paralysis are often inconspicuous or absent in infections with the mitis strain and when such infections assume a serious form, it is usually because of laryngotracheal involvement. The corollary of this is that many cases of laryngotracheal diphtheria run their course without developing either toxic myocarditis or peripheral neuritis.

Diagnosis

Diphtheria will be suspected when the typical pseudomembrane as described above is observed on one or both tonsils, the faucial pillars, soft palate, posterior pharyngeal wall, post-nasal space, in the nose, mouth or elsewhere or in several of these localities at once but the differentiation from other varieties of ulcero-membranous disease will depend on laboratory tests, chiefly identification of the organism and examination of the blood. If such a case develops laryngeal symptoms the diagnosis is hardly in doubt even before the results of the tests are available. However, laryngotracheal diphtheria may occur before a typical lesion has been found elsewhere or as a primary manifestation and in this event the disease may be confused with other kinds of infective croup, the differential diagnosis of which is considered earlier in this section.

Of course, consideration of such matters as the occurrence of other confirmed cases of diphtheria, the individual's history as to previous active immunization and the result of the Schick test if available must not be overlooked. Finally, as in the case of acute laryngotracheobronchitis and where facilities and experience are available, examination of the larynx under an anaesthetic may be necessary before the nature of the laryngitis is ascertained.

Treatment

It must not be forgotten that diphtheria is now almost unknown over large areas of the world and the practitioner is unlikely to have the diagnosis in mind. All kinds of sore throat and most cases of croup are treated nowadays with antibiotics, probably with one of the newer penicillins. The *C. diphtheriae* is penicillin-sensitive and the organism easily eliminated by this therapy allowing the local lesion to heal and the symptoms caused by it to abate. However, this may be disastrous, particularly in the severe case. The powerful toxin of diphtheria is produced from the outset of the disease, circulates everywhere and is quickly taken up by the vulnerable tissues. Penicillin does not neutralize the toxin so that patients apparently cured by it are still liable to the late complications such as myocarditis and neuritis.

There must therefore be a twofold attack: on the bacteria with penicillin and on the toxin with antitoxin. Both must be given as soon as the disease is diagnosed clinically and a swab of the infected site taken for smear examination and culture but without waiting for the result. The dose of antitoxin should be related not only to the clinical severity of the case but also to the length of time since the onset of symptoms. In the early mild case 10 000 units by the intramuscular route are given but in the delayed severely ill patient as much as 100 000 units may be injected, one half intramuscularly and one half intravenously 30 minutes later. The risk of serum sickness has been largely eliminated since the introduction of enzyme-digested serum. If improvement is not marked within 24 hours, a further injection of antitoxin should be administered.

Benzylpenicillin (penicillin G) is probably the antibiotic of choice given intramuscularly 500 000 units six-hourly for six days, although there is some evidence to suggest that erythromycin may be preferable.

The general management of the obstructed airway will be along the lines already described for a case of non-diphtheritic croup. The child will be nursed in a croupette and the air moistened with an ultra-sonic nebulizer if this is available. Up to 30–45 per cent oxygen may be added if necessary. If respiratory failure appears imminent, adequate respiratory exchange must be ensured by the best means at hand. In a fully equipped paediatric hospital the first step should be laryngoscopy under general anaesthesia at which membrane may be removed by suction or with forceps and a nasotracheal tube passed. Where the facilities and personnel for this kind of management are not available, tracheostomy will be necessary. Neither the nasotracheal tube nor the tracheostomy are likely to be needed for more than a day or two since recovery of the local disease can be expected to proceed rapidly once administration of the appropriate antibiotic has been commenced.

It must not be forgotten, however, that the danger of diphtheritic croup is not over once the threat to the airway is passed. In this respect diphtheritic laryngitis differs significantly from laryngotracheobronchitis. The late complications of the toxaemia, particularly myocarditis, are still liable to occur especially if antitoxin has been given late and this risk demands complete bed rest for from two to four weeks.

Prognosis

Provided the disease is promptly diagnosed and treated the outlook nowadays is excellent. The risk of cardiac failure from myocarditis remains when the true diagnosis is overlooked and the disease treated with antibiotics without antitoxin.

Non-diphtheritic membranous laryngitis

Aetiology

Membranous laryngitis may be due to infection, to the damage caused by the inhalation of certain fumes and gases or to thermal injury from hot steam or the hot gases generated in fires. (The latter causes are considered on p. 376).

Infective membranous laryngitis will prove to be diphtheritic in all but the very occasional case where certain other organisms have been incriminated, particularly haemolytic streptococci and *Pseudomonas aeruginosa*. They are likely to colonize the mucosa already damaged by viruses and the latter organism is known to occur in debilitated infants and children with cystic fibrosis. This rare type of laryngitis, like laryngeal diphtheria, is chiefly a disease of childhood, with its main incidence between the second and eighth years.

Clinical features

The local lesion will resemble that of laryngeal diphtheria and produce a croup-like picture with stridor and obstruction to the laryngeal airway, but the severe constitutional symptoms will be absent as will the faucial involvement characteristic of diphtheria. Even more important, the patient is not at risk from the grave consequences of diptheritic toxaemia, myocarditis and peripheral neuritis.

Treatment

The immediate treatment must be as for other infections threatening the airway, the maintenance or restoration of adequate respiratory exchange and, as explained above, the means of doing so will depend on the facilities. Where these permit, direct examination under an anaesthetic with removal of the membrane if possible should be followed by nasotracheal intubation.

The treatment of the infection will depend on the organism identified and its sensitivities. There will be no problem in the case of streptococcal infection which can be expected to respond to one of the penicillins but where *Ps. aeruginosa* is concerned the antibacterial therapy is likely to present difficulties. This organism will almost certainly prove insensitive to the commoner antibiotics such as may be given orally so that carbenicillin intravenously or one of the aminoglycosides, gentamicin or tobramycin, will be necessary. It is, however, indicative of the rarity of this type of infection that the present writer has been unable to find an account of such a case occurring since these antibiotics have been available.

Acute perichondritis, chondral necrosis and abscess of the larynx

These conditions, now very rarely encountered, are described together because they are usually associated, one leading to the other. When intact the tough fibrous laryngeal perichondrium is not readily infected and in the majority of cases perichondritis and its sequelae occur when the perichondrium has been damaged by trauma, exposed by ulceration or devitalized by interference with its blood supply.

Aetiology

Primary perichondritis of the larynx has probably been rare at all times and even when the larynx is involved in a bacteriaemia such as typhoid fever, perichondritis is likely to be due to secondary infection with pyogenic organisms of the perichondrium exposed by the ulceration.

Whatever disease process exposes or damages the perichondrium, therefore, may give access to pyogenic bacteria and set in train these pathological events. Acute laryngeal perichondritis, cartilage necrosis and abscess formation arose often in the past, and may occur still in ulcerative diseases of the larynx, as the result of spread of a septic process from the pharynx, or when the laryngeal cartilages have been injured (either by accidental or surgical trauma) or their blood supply is impaired by trauma or an excess of ionizing radiation. Anything that impairs the process of inflammation and the control of infection such as, for example, agranulocytosis or nowadays immuno-suppression, may sometimes facilitate the spread of suppuration to the skeletal structures of the larynx. The list of laryngeal diseases in the course of which perichondritis etc. has been recorded is a long one therefore. It includes laryngeal tuberculosis, syphilis, enteric fever, diphtheria, smallpox, measles, advanced laryngeal cancer, all forms of serious injury to the laryngeal cartilages, particularly road traffic accidents and suicidal attempts, surgical encroachment on the laryngeal framework, particularly the cricoid cartilage as in inexpert tracheostomy, injury caused by foreign bodies impacted in the larynx or hypopharynx, ill-planned radiotherapy to the larynx and even such diseases, little feared in this antibiotic era, as Vincents' and Ludwig's angina and peritonsillar abscess.

Accordingly the list of factors responsible for the striking decrease in the incidence of these conditions makes an interesting commentary on the epidemiological, social and therapeutic changes in the current century. It includes the control of tuberculosis, the prevention of the late stages of syphilis, preventive immunization against smallpox, diphtheria and measles, the public health and hygienic measures which have in many places almost eradicated enteric fever, the discovery of chemotherapy and an ever-increasing number of antibiotics and the progress in their use, the advances in the surgery of the larynx and trachea particularly with regard to tracheostomy and accidental trauma, the improvements that have resulted in earlier diagnosis of laryngeal neoplasms and, finally, the advances in the techniques of radiotherapy.

Pathology

Cartilage derives its nutrition from the overlying perichondrium and, although its demands are small, stripping the perichondrium off the underlying cartilage carries the risk of necrosis. If the perichondrium is elevated from both surfaces of the cartilage necrosis is inevitable. While the intact perichondrium constitutes an effective barrier against the occurrence of an inflammatory exudate between it and the cartilage, once infection has broken through it, because it is injured or damaged by adjacent ulceration or by impairment of its blood supply, the common pyogenic organisms may invade this vulnerable plane. Abscess formation may elevate the perichondrium more and more extensively and chondral necrosis will occur with sequestration of the dead tissue as in osteomyelitis. In the larynx of the elderly patient where a great deal of the cartilage has been ossified, the process is truly osteomyelitis rather than chondritis. The abscess may eventually rupture spontaneously and discharge, usually through a mucosal surface though rarely through the skin of the neck.

All the laryngeal cartilages may be involved except the epiglottis, which, partly because of its different structure, is not liable to such pathological changes. Acute epiglottitis may go on to abscess formation however, and this may be regarded as a specific variety of perichondritis. The cricoid cartilage is the most often attacked. Arytenoid necrosis occurred not infrequently in tuberculous laryngitis and sometimes in diphtheria and there are accounts of the exfoliated cartilage being coughed up. In the most severe cases the cricoid, thyroid and arytenoid cartilages have all been involved with disastrous long-term consequences for the laryngeal airway.

The processes of repair familiar in osteomyelitis, with new bone formation a prominent feature, are quite different where cartilage is concerned and in these conditions healing takes place without cartilage regeneration but with extensive fibrosis. The characteristic form of the larynx may then be lost, sometimes completely, and a greater or lesser degree of laryngeal stenosis is inevitable. Sometimes complete atresia results. In conclusion it must be said that the progress of perichondritis to abscess formation and chondritis are not inevitable and the process may stop short of suppuration. This has been noticed in the younger patient and particularly in perichondritis following radiotherapy. Oedema and fibrosis are marked with much thickening of the laryngeal structures and, here too, consequent stenosis.

Clinical features

Perichondritis is likely to occur only when the causative disease is advanced or its treatment neglected so that the clinical features will be obscured by those of the primary disease and may be regarded as due to it alone. In such circumstances, the emergence of the perichondritis and its consequences may then be overlooked until it too is well established.

The leading symptoms are progressive dysphagia, hoarseness and dyspnoea with pain and fever and in general resemble those of supraglottic laryngitis. The signs will depend on which cartilage or cartilages are attacked. External swelling and tenderness occur when the thyroid and cricoid cartilages are involved, but not in arytenoid perichondritis. Abscesses may point into the larynx, trachea, pharynx, upper oesophagus or, rarely, externally.

On laryngoscopy gross swelling, sometimes pallid sometimes red, of parts or all of the larynx will be seen, with pus in the hypopharynx or the larynx if an abscess has discharged. The swelling may be so great as to obscure the underlying disease, e.g. a neoplasm, tuberculous ulceration or even a foreign body (*see Plate 3, facing page 384*).

The value of radiographs not only to exclude a radio-opaque foreign body but also to help assess the extent of the disease should not be forgotten.

Treatment

It must be assumed that perichondritis, chondral necrosis and laryngeal abscess will occur in modern conditions principally when, for whatever reason, the primary disease has been incorrectly diagnosed and treated, signs of pyogenic infection overlooked and the appropriate antibiotic therapy therefore not initiated or delayed. As in the case of the other asphyxiating conditions described in this chapter, for example, supraglottic laryngitis, the first step when necessary must be to restore or maintain an adequate airway. This may mean tracheostomy or, where the cause of the perichondritis is injury of the larynx (usually the cricoid cartilage from a tracheostomy performed too high) the establishment of a lower opening and the abandoning of the faulty one. Intubation will rarely be a safe alternative to tracheostomy in such cases. The swelling and distortion of the larynx will create serious difficulty and if an abscess is present, the attempt may rupture it before the airway is safeguarded.

Vigorous antibiotic treatment must be started at once; flucloxacillin intravenously and benzyl penicillin intramuscularly can be expected to control infection including that due to penicillin-resistant staphylococci pending the result of culture and sensitivity tests. Abscesses that have not already ruptured must be incised and drained under general anaesthesia maintained by way of the tracheostome. If the abscess presents at direct laryngoscopy it may be incised and the pus aspirated. If an abscess points externally it should be opened by external incision and necrotic cartilage removed. The external approach is likely to be the better technique whenever extensive chondral necrosis is suspected. Cases with multiple abscesses and widespread cartilage necrosis – the result of injudicious irradiation – are unlikely to be seen now but have been described in the past. Maxwell Ellis refers to it in the third edition of this book. Laryngectomy proved to be the only solution with sacrifice of the devitalized pre-laryngeal soft tissues and the creation of a pharyngostome. Finally, there remains the management of the primary disorder of which the perichondritis has been a complication. Including such different conditions as carcinoma and tuberculosis, the treatment will be correspondingly disparate and will be found described under the appropriate heading elsewhere.

Prognosis

The outlook will depend not only on that of the perichondritis and its consequences but also on that of the initial disease or injury. However, on the rare occasion when an established case is encountered today, the measures described above can be expected to ensure recovery but not to prevent cicatricial stenosis of the larynx. As mentioned already, the scarring may even result in atresia with, of course, loss of normal voice. Voice may be affected too as the result of crico-arytenoid ankylosis following septic arthritis of the crico-arytenoid joint in perichondritis. It will mimic vocal-cord paralysis.

The treatment of laryngeal stenosis is difficult and not always successful so that a proportion of these patients are never relieved of their tracheostomy cannulae and a few remain to remind us of the gravity of a problem now largely overcome.

Herpes laryngis

Among the many viruses responsible for laryngitis, that of Herpes simplex is usually included. This infection produces the characteristic vesicular eruption on the lips or elsewhere on the face but may involve the mouth or pharynx and, unusually, the larynx and lower airway. The vesicles are very rarely observed in these latter localities because they rupture quickly and give way to shallow ulcers with a whitish base and little surrounding reaction. They are usually small, multiple and rather painful, resembling the ubiquitous aphthous ulcer, the virus origin of which has not been proved. Sometimes they coalesce to form a large ulcer.

When they appear in the larynx they are usually on the epiglottis but have been seen on the arytenoids and ventricular bands. Nash and Foley (1970) found herpes of the larynx in 8 of their 25 patients with herpetic tracheitis and bronchopneumonia.

The disease runs a short self-limiting course and no treatment has been found to accelerate this. The ulceration is always superficial and healing leaves no scar.

Oedema of the larynx

The classification of laryngitis worked out when the aetiological factors were even less well understood than they are today, included categories based on the predominant gross pathological change observed, for instance haemorrhagic laryngitis and oedematous laryngitis. Oedematous laryngitis is not a disease *per se* but oedema of the larynx may be the most conspicuous feature of the inflammatory reaction in a wide range of infective and non-infective diseases of the larynx. These include acute and chronic disorders so that oedema may on the one hand erupt with dramatic rapidity as in angioneurotic oedema or, on the other, occur as an insidious process as in myxoedema. As the last example illustrates, what is often called 'oedema' is better named 'pseudo-oedema' since the swelling may be caused by an inflammatory infiltration with an accumulation of cells as well as fluid in the tissues, or by myxomatous changes.

True oedema of the larynx may occur following major surgery of the tongue and floor of the mouth and the risk of it is the reason why tracheostomy is advocated as an elective procedure in such operations. Before fluid retention was managed by modern means, it was not rare in such conditions as heart failure and nephritis. It is described in this chapter rather than the next since the acute variety is the more important clinically.

Aetiology

Laryngeal oedema occurring as the result of allergy is considered elsewhere, as is angioneurotic oedema. Here it is appropriate to mention the infective causes. They are very many but are nowadays far less common than in the past. The manner in which progress in various fields of medicine has largely eliminated certain complications of laryngitis has been outlined already in connection with perichondritis and laryngeal abscess and the same applies to laryngeal oedema. The time when it was an ever-present threat in such septic conditions as peritonsillar abscess, retropharyngeal abscess and Ludwig's angina is largely past. As a complication of acute fevers such as typhoid, smallpox, scarlet fever and even mumps it is now very rarely encountered although subglottic oedema in measles laryngotracheitis and, indeed, in laryngotracheobronchitis due to other viruses, is still prevalent and important. Oedema and pseudo-oedema of parts of the larynx were common findings in tuberculous laryngitis, e.g. the 'turban' epiglottis, but even when tuberculous laryngitis occurs in parts of the world where tuberculosis is still not controlled, oedematous forms are not often encountered, perhaps because of early treatment. Wherever there is deep ulceration of the larynx or hypopharynx, oedema of the adjacent parts may be observed, for instance of the aryepiglottic fold in pyriform fossa carcinoma, and this is often more severe where secondary infection is present to a marked extent. The severe localized oedema often described in the past in tuberculous and gummatous ulceration was similarly most likely to assume conspicuous proportions where pyogenic infection complicated the primary disease, and particularly where perichondritis and its sequelae had occurred.

Pathology

Oedema occurring in the course of infective laryngitis is seldom simply a matter of fluid distension of the tissue spaces as it is in many examples of non-infective oedema. The intense swelling of the epiglottis in supraglottic laryngitis, for instance, is more a matter of cellulitis than simple oedema with not only lymph and fibrin present in the supraglottic tissues but large numbers of leucocytes and eventually suppuration.

'Oedema glottidis' was once the term used to describe laryngeal airway obstruction caused by laryngeal oedema. In fact the glottis is not involved in these cases, the oedema occurring in the submucosa of the supra- or subglottic tissues.

Symptoms and signs

The extent to which the symptoms can be related to the oedema rather than to the laryngitis of which the oedema is a feature can be determined only by examining the larynx, but in general, because of its location above or below the cords, it will tend to interfere with breathing rather than voice.

In the adult indirect laryngoscopy will usually be possible, but in the child general anaesthesia and direct laryngoscopy not only for examination but also, if necessary, for treatment e.g. intubation, may be judged necessary. Oedema, in the absence of infection will produce a pale shiny swelling but in these cases, secondary to infection, the swelling is likely to be red due to hyperaemia. The arytenoid region, aryepiglottic folds, false cords, epiglottis or all of these structures may be seen to be involved, the distribution being symmetrical or asymmetrical according to the nature of the underlying disease. Sometimes, as in laryngotracheitis, the oedema will be confined to the subglottic larynx.

Treatment

It follows from what has been said that the treatment has to be that of the causative laryngitis along the lines already detailed but, of course, the first consideration as in all cases of a threat to breathing must be attention to the airway. The reader should refer to the treatment section under the heading concerned.

Acute non-infective laryngitis

Aetiology

The causes of acute laryngitis other than infection are misuse of the voice, trauma either accidental or surgical, irritating chemicals generally in the form of gases, thermal damage usually from inhaling hot steam or gases, ionizing radiation and allergic reaction.

Misuse of the voice

Prolonged use of the voice, even prolonged and strenuous use, does no damage to the larynx if the voice is produced correctly. The chief aim of the singing and drama teacher is to enable the professional voice-user to produce voice correctly in this sense. The speech therapist is often asked to do the same with less keenly motivated individuals and in a therapeutic rather than a prophylactic role.

For most of us, however, the need to use the voice for an unaccustomed length of time or with excessive effort carries the risk of a brief bout of huskiness. Many supporters of football teams know what it is to shout – or sing – themselves hoarse, but even short bouts of vocal misuse may have the same effect, particularly if voice is forced out through vocal cords under unnecessary tension. Violent or staccato phonation as in screaming, sobbing, retching or coughing may be considered examples of this and whooping cough is particularly culpable. The small amount of damage to the vocal cords produced by a single incident of this kind can be expected to resolve spontaneously in a matter of hours but if it is often repeated, then chronic changes will occur. It is not always remembered that school children are liable to develop chronic laryngitis from often repeated minor incidents of this kind.

If the larynx should be the site of some other disease, simple infective laryngitis for example, then an amount of voice use that would be insignificant in health, may prove the last straw for the already inflamed cords.

Trauma

Accidental trauma

Injury to the larynx is considered in the previous chapter. Open wounds, even if not complicated by serious infection, are bound to be attended by a greater or lesser degree of inflammation in the damaged laryngeal lining. Incised wounds opening into the larynx are among the causes of laryngeal oedema, sometimes severe. Closed injuries produce oedema or haematoma or both. Not only may the mucosa, e.g. of the vocal cords, be involved but also the laryngeal muscles and even the crico-arytenoid joints.

Foreign bodies lodged in the larynx will produce an inflammatory reaction, the severity of which will depend on the nature of the foreign body and the length of time it is allowed to remain.

Surgical trauma

Endotracheal intubation. This important example of iatrogenic disease has been occurring since the early days of endotracheal anaesthesia. The specialist anaesthetist of today will not be guilty of clumsy technique or the choice of too large a tube but such faults were not unknown when responsibility for the anaesthetic was entrusted to the house surgeon or, in some places, to the nurse. The damage caused with resultant oedema or haematoma required tracheostomy from time to time. Even more recently, however, traumatic laryngitis with a hoarse voice persisting for days after the operation has been a known complication of endotracheal anaesthesia (Blackburn and Salmon, 1961). Granulomas have been found springing up at the site of injury.

Intubation as an alternative to tracheostomy became widely practised after the introduction of the O'Dwyer tube at the end of the last century but was rarely performed except in cases of laryngeal diphtheria. During the past 35 years tracheostomy has been widely used as a means of providing respiratory support and access to the tracheobronchial tree, and often when the larynx is normal. Once again tracheal intubation, usually nasotracheal intubation, has been advocated and employed as an alternative to tracheostomy for this purpose. It has led to laryngeal injury with traumatic laryngitis as the least manifestation and laryngeal, usually subglottic stenosis as the gravest (Abbott, 1968; McGovern, Fitz-Hugh and Edgemon, 1971; Fearon *et al.*, 1966).

Bronchoscopy. Any operation on the larynx will result in inflammatory changes although generally these are not within the scope of this chapter. However, just as prolonged intubation is likely to result in laryngitis, so may bronchoscopy. Here, too, it is the child who is most at risk and particularly from a prolonged attempt to remove an inhaled foreign body – or foreign bodies, e.g. a number of fragments of peanut.

The use of too large an instrument is again important and no one should regard himself as equipped to carry out this type of surgery without the full range of bronchoscopes (four sizes) any more than without the full range of forceps. As usual, in the infant or young child, it is the subglottic larynx that bears the brunt of the injury and subglottic oedema may be severe enough to necessitate nasotracheal intubation or even tracheostomy.

Chemical irritation

Irritant chemicals may reach the larynx by being inhaled or, rarely, via the blood stream, having been swallowed or injected. Swallowed caustics may reach the larynx directly in sufficient quantity to produce laryngitis.

The accidental inhalation of irritant gases such as ammonia, sulphur dioxide or the fumes from concentrated nitric or sulphuric acid may produce laryngotracheo-bronchitis with many of the features of the disease due to infection. The classical examples are chlorine and phosgene used as war gases in 1915. Although the chief effect was on the lungs, many 'gassed' servicemen went on to develop intractable chronic laryngitis. Various irritant smokes have been used as weapons in peacetime too, chiefly however for their action on the eyes and nose. Industry today produces an increasing number of toxic chemicals and accidental exposure to these has happened and is bound to occur. The possibility of injury to the respiratory lining is often present.

By far the most commonly inhaled irritant is tobacco smoke. The tars from the burning tobacco acting over a long period of time have been considered a factor in the aetiology of chronic laryngitis but their importance in relation to acute laryngitis is, to say the least, equivocal.

Of the ingested substances three deserve mention and it is interesting that the mode of action may be different in each case. Various corrosive substances are swallowed accidentally, chiefly by children or rarely in suicidal attempts by older patients. The frequency of this injury varies from one part of the world to another as does the nature of the chemical substance swallowed but acute laryngitis is a not uncommon complication. As a rule it will be the epiglottis and arytenoid eminences that suffer when, as the caustic bolus is propelled through the hypopharynx, these structures come together to keep the fluid out of the air passages, but sometimes coughing and spluttering followed by a deep inspiration will permit the entrance of the corrosive into the larynx and the lower air passages.

Potassium iodide has long been known to produce coryzal symptoms in susceptible individuals. It is rarely prescribed in considerable dosage today so that the modern practitioner is unlikely to be familiar with this complication, but an oedematous laryngitis was often attributed to it when its use in the treatment of syphilis was traditional. The drug reached the vulnerable laryngeal tissues by way of the blood stream.

Thirdly, alcohol must be mentioned although, because like tobacco smoke its effects are insidious, it has to be considered also in connection with chronic laryngitis (Chapter 14). The inflammatory changes observed in the larynx are the result of peripheral vasodilatation while the increase in secretions is probably a reflex phenomenon.

Thermal injuries

These may occur from hot steam, for example when a young child puts the spout of a boiling kettle to its mouth or from hot gases in conflagration injuries. A bad fire will generate toxic fumes so that chemical and thermal damage to the respiratory tract may coexist. Children are often the victims, 15 per cent of the total annual deaths from thermal trauma in London occurring under the age of 15 (Clarkson, 1965). The larynx is affected in a high percentage of cases, these being in general where the face and neck are involved. Moylan *et al.* (1972) found tracheostomy necessary in 18.2 per cent of 1564 burns cases admitted to hospital over a five-year period.

When scorching or scalding of the buccal, palatal and pharyngeal mucosae are observed, it is more than likely that thermal damage to the larynx will have taken place also. In the worst cases the trachea and lungs will share in the injury.

Ionizing radiation

The modern treatment of malignant disease with rays emanating from high-energy sources such as radioactive isotopes (^{60}Co and ^{137}Cs), and particle accelerators (the linear accelerator and betatron) has made it possible to treat malignant disease, in this context malignant disease of the head and neck, with reduced risk of damage to normal tissues. Nevertheless, treatment of this kind – particularly when used in cases of cancer of the larynx and pharynx – still produces a degree of inflammation in the normal tissues, including those of the larynx. This inflammation is the result not only of the destructive capacity of the radiation, but arises in the surrounding tissues in response to the death of the cancer cells.

Oedema is the chief feature of this reaction, which can be expected to subside over the weeks following the termination of treatment. Persistence or increase in the amount of swelling must always suggest the possibility of persistence of tumour. When extra-laryngeal lesions are treated the previously normal larynx may share in this radiation reaction, the patient developing the symptoms and signs of a degree of oedematous laryngitis.

Allergic laryngitis

The antigen–antibody reaction results in the release into the tissues of chemical substances (mediators) which, among other effects, produce contraction of smooth muscle and an increase in vascular permeability with oedema formation. The most familiar of these mediators is histamine. The inflammatory reaction produced by histamine and the other mediators may be widespread but among the organs affected is the larynx. The most severe response of this type due to a specific reaction between the antigen and antibody, in man almost always IgE, is called 'anaphylaxis'. It is usually so acute and severe that immediate emergency measures are called for.

The list of allergens incriminated is long and includes various foodstuffs, penicillin, horse serum, the venoms of insects and snakes, injected gamma-globulins and preparations of pollens, dust and all sorts of protein used in allergy hyposensitization. There is reason to think that exposure to cold may produce substances that lead to acute allergic reactions.

A special paragraph must be devoted to angioneurotic oedema. The true form of this, Quincke's disease, is a genetic disease with autosomal dominant inheritance. Sixty affected families are known and the absence of an alpha-2-globulin in the serum is considered the cause. Recurrent episodes of giant urticaria and circumscribed oedema of the genito-urinary and respiratory tracts occur, beginning in childhood. Trauma seems to be a precipitating factor. Almost 20 per cent of the known cases have died of asphyxia from acute supraglottic oedema (Patterson, 1972).

Pathology of non-infective laryngitis

Because the causes range widely so do the pathological changes. Certain points have emerged already in the general descriptions above but a number of details remain to be mentioned.

Secondary bacterial infection is not a feature of the lesion in acute vocal abuse nor in the allergic reactions but may complicate the other diseases and is almost inevitable in the burns cases.

Acute misuse or over-use of the voice may result not only in swelling and hyperaemia of the vocal cords, often most apparent in the middle parts, but sometimes in haemorrhages. These may be diffuse or localized. Violent coughing, e.g. whooping cough, is especially blameworthy in this respect. Such haematomas will usually absorb without trace but may organize as small or larger areas of submucous fibrosis, once again diffuse or localized. Some vocal nodules may be organized haematomas.

As stated on p. 374 traumatic instrumentation of the larynx may result in granulomas (*Plate 5, facing page 432*).

Blistering of the larynx particularly the supraglottis, an early feature in severe burns, will quickly give way to ulceration, sloughs and membrane formation. A similar chain of events may occur in some chemical injuries.

The risk of perichondritis and its consequences in certain kinds of accidental trauma has been described on p. 368.

The laryngeal oedema in anaphylaxis and angioneurotic oedema is commonly called 'oedema of the glottis'. This is a misnomer. The oedema affects the supraglottic structures and occasionally the subglottic tissues.

Treatment

The varieties of laryngitis listed above include on the one hand the minor consequences of shouting and on the other the potentially lethal attack of angioneurotic oedema. The treatment will vary widely too. The husky supporter the day after the football match is unlikely to seek medical advice but will recover within a short time, particularly if he has the sense to rest his voice.

The more severe examples of thermal and chemical injury are, however, quite another matter. Infection is common and in burns cases antibiotics will almost always be indicated and not only for the larynx. Conflagration burns involving the face and the front of the neck will lead to severe upper respiratory obstruction in such a high proportion that prophylactic tracheostomy has been urged for all these (Clarkson, 1965). The obstruction is by no means always due to the swollen laryngeal tissues only or even chiefly, since the burns of the mouth and nose may close-off the airway proximal to the larynx. The serious mortality in these cases is not usually the result of airway obstruction but due to the effects of the extensive burns elsewhere with such grave complications as renal failure and septicaemia high on the list. Intubation as an alternative to tracheostomy has not been advocated for burns and may present difficulties where severe swelling and blistering of the lips and mouth are present.

Severe upper airway obstruction following endotracheal anaesthesia is most uncommon nowadays although the writer recalls children intubated inexpertly and with too large a tube who subsequently needed tracheostomy. Cases of severe subglottic oedema after prolonged bronchoscopy in the child still occur, however, and may cause anxiety. The treatment will be as for a case of infective croup including nursing in a croupette with careful attention to humidification. Corticosteroids are almost certainly useful and should be administered as described on p. 362. Tracheostomy or nasotracheal intubation should not be necessary but must be undertaken at once if signs of pending respiratory failure are observed.

The treatment of allergic laryngitis calls for special mention. In anaphylaxis and angioneurotic oedema with laryngeal involvement the onset of asphyxia may be so sudden that urgent surgical measures cannot be put off while conservative treatment is tried. As has been explained, the choice between tracheostomy, intubation and trans-tracheal cannulation will depend on the facilities available, but one of these steps must be taken as soon as there is evidence of increasing laryngeal obstruction. Because the oedema can be expected to subside quickly with prompt medical treatment, nasotracheal intubation is considered the method of choice.

Conservative treatment relies upon three drugs. First and most urgent is adrenaline, 0.3–0.5 ml adrenaline injection (1:1000) to be given intramuscularly and repeated every 15 minutes if necessary. Secondly, hydrocortisone which acts more slowly and should be injected intravenously as the hemisuccinate, 100–250 mg at once and repeated four hours later if necessary. A smaller dose may be given six-hourly for a day or two if the oedema persists. The antihistamines are more suitable for long-term rather than emergency treatment but may be given by slow intravenous injection, for example promethazine hydrochloride (Phenergan), 25–50 mg. Unfortunately in hereditary angioneurotic oedema conservative treatment is unlikely to have a considerable effect on the oedematous larynx and intubation or tracheostomy should be resorted to as soon as the cause of the obstructed breathing has been diagnosed.

A patient with a known history of anaphylaxis is well advised to have available at all times certain First Aid supplies. These are ampoules of adrenaline injection and the syringe to inject it, oral antihistamines – and a tourniquet to localize the antigen in the event of a sting from the insect concerned.

References

Abbott, T. R. (1968). *British Journal of Anaesthesia*, **40,** 347

Blackburn, G. and Salmon, L. F. W. (1961). *British Journal of Surgery*, **48,** 371

Cawthorne, T. and Edwards, W. (1966). *Proceedings of the Royal Society of Medicine*, **80,** 359

Clarke, S. W. and Cochrane, G. M. (1975). *Practitioner*, **215,** 340

Clarkson, P. W. (1965). *Annals of the Royal College of Surgeons of England*, **37,** 207

Eggston, A. A. and Wolff, D. (1947). *Histopathology of the Ear, Nose and Throat*; The Williams and Wilkins Co., Baltimore

Fearon, B. W. (1975). *Canadian Medical Association Journal*, **112,** 760

Fearon, B. W., MacDonald, R. E., Smith, C. and Mitchell, D. (1966). *Annals of Otolaryngology, Rhinology and Laryngology*, **75,** 975

Hancock, B. D. (1972). *Journal of Laryngology and Otology*, **86,** 23

Hawkins, D. B., Miller, A. H., Sachs, G. B. and Benj, R. T. (1973). *Laryngoscope*, **83,** 1211

Jones, H. Morus (1970). *Proceedings of the Royal Society of Medicine*, **63,** 706

Jones, R. S. and Owen-Thomas, J. B. (1971). *Care of the Critically Ill Child*; Edward Arnold, London

Jordan, W. S. (1970). *Journal of the American Medical Association*, **212,** 585

Mackenzie, Morell (1880). *A Manual of Diseases of the Throat and Nose*, Churchill-Livingstone, Edinburgh

Massicotte, P. and Tétreault, L. (1973). *Union of Medicine, Canada*, **102,** 2064

McGovern, F. H., Fitz-Hugh, G. S. and Edgemon, L. J. (1971). *Annals of Otolaryngology*, **80,** 556

Moylan, J. A., West, J. T., Nash, G., Bowen, J. A. and Pruitt, B. A. (1972). *American Surgery*, **38,** 119

Patterson, R. (Ed.) (1972). *Allergic Diseases: Diagnosis and Management*; Lippincott, Philadelphia and Toronto

Pracy, R. (1965). *Proceedings of the Royal Society of Medicine*, **58,** 19

Richards, S. H. and Kander, P. L. (1977). *Journal of Laryngology*, **91,** 295

Salmon, L. F. W. (1975). *Proceedings of the Royal Society of Medicine*, **68,** 347

Schuller, D. E. and Birck, H. G. (1975). *Laryngoscope*, **85,** 33

Sinclair, S. E. (1941). *Journal of the American Medical Association*, **117,** 170

Singer, O. P. and Wilson, W. J. (1976). *Canadian Medical Association Journal*, **115,** 132

Strome, M. and Jaffe, B. (1974). *Laryngoscope*, **84,** 921

Strong, M. S. and Paparella, M. M. (1975). *The Year Book of the Ear, Nose and Throat*; Year Book Medical Publishers, Inc., Chicago

Tercero-Talavera, F. I. and Ropkin, R. H. (1974). *Clinical Pediatrics, Philadelphia*, **13,** 1074

Thiesen, D. F. (1900). *Albany Medical Annals*, **21,** 395

14 **Chronic laryngitis**
L F W Salmon

Introduction

Except for the infective granulomata, the aetiological factors at work in the production of chronic inflammatory changes in the larynx are more difficult to identify precisely than they are in acute laryngitis. There, although more than one factor is often seen to be concerned, the relative importance of infection, vocal misuse, environmental irritants and so on, is usually apparent. Here, at any rate in the case of the diseases described as non-specific chronic laryngitis, the position is far from clear.

The problem is greatest with regard to the conditions characterized by keratin formation. A considerable proportion of such cases proceed through stages to the development of invasive carcinoma, although many of them, included here as chronic hyperplastic laryngitis, are certainly inflammatory in origin. At the other end of the scale, however, are certain circumscribed keratin-producing lesions about which the evidence is insufficient for us to class them certainly either as examples of inflammatory hyperplasia or as benign neoplasms.

Another group is that which includes the polyps and polypoid degeneration. No one regards these as neoplasms and yet the basis for listing them as examples of chronic laryngitis is, to say the least, unsure.

Friedmann and Osborn (1976), pathologists with special experience in this field, are worried by what they consider to be the misuse of the term 'laryngitis' to include both keratosis and the polyps. The present writer shares this concern and includes these conditions in this chapter only with this acknowledgment.

The next difficulty to be faced is the question of terminology and again this arises chiefly in connection with hyperplasia and keratosis. Laryngologists writing on these matters always feel obliged to define their terms and deplore the ambiguous use of words like hyperplasia, hypertrophy, keratosis, leucoplakia, pachydermia and so on. The classification of these conditions employed in this chapter cannot avoid being to some extent controversial therefore, and this too is acknowledged.

In the previous chapter a large section was devoted to the special problems of acute infection of the upper – and lower – air passages in infants and young children. Chronic laryngitis affects the adult chiefly, although something has to be said about the chronic changes in the young larynx as the result of misuse of the voice. It is necessary also to mention the question of multiple papillomata of the larynx in children. Although it has now been shown that these are due to a virus as in the case of ordinary cutaneous warts and so might earn a place here, they are in fact described in Chapter 15 (p. 426).

Chronic non-specific laryngitis

Chronic laryngitis without hyperplasia

Aetiology

Like chronic hyperplastic laryngitis and pachydermia laryngis this is a disease of adult life with the main incidence in the fifth decade. Nowadays there is probably little difference in the incidence between the sexes.

Usually by the time the patient with chronic laryngitis is seen by the laryngologist, metaplastic and hyperplastic changes in the laryngeal epithelium of greater or lesser extent are already established. Indeed, on the basis of many micro-laryngoscopic examinations Kleinsasser considers that most cases of chronic laryngitis assume a chronic course from the outset. Nevertheless, from time to time cases will occur where chronic diffuse inflammation is observed in the absence of such hyperplastic change and where the history suggests preceding acute infective laryngitis.

Most cases of simple acute laryngitis recover spontaneously within a week or two but in some the disease tends to persist, even throughout the winter months. The existence of a group of patients with an unexplained liability to recurrent simple laryngitis has been mentioned in Chapter 13; a proportion of these will go on to develop chronic laryngitis.

A number of causes for the emergence of these chronic changes have been suspected and most of the textbook descriptions in the past have listed them as a matter of fact. They include over-use and misuse of the voice, chronic or repeated infection elsewhere in the upper or lower respiratory tract, occupational factors such as exposure to dust and fumes, the abuse of alcohol and tobacco, and the coexistence of other diseases regarded as in different ways predisposing, such as diabetes, renal disease, anaemia and many others.

In a controlled study of chronic diffuse laryngitis, Stell and McLaughlin (1976) attempted to assess the respective importance of these factors. Only infection of the upper and lower respiratory tracts proved to be statistically significant, inasmuch as it was found to be present in more than half the 58 patients investigated.

No doubt the long list of supposed aetiological agents cited in the past has come about as the result of including in this limited and less important category, cases of polyposis and keratosis of the larynx where almost certainly other irritants than infection are concerned and these are considered in the corresponding sections below.

The sort of changes found in the larynx in nephritis, cardiac failure and myxoedema have been mentioned already and are irrelevant here. Non-specific reaction in the tissues surrounding neoplasms and the granulomata are surely to be regarded as an essential part of the disease concerned. The special pathological processes at work in the larynx in rheumatoid arthritis, gout and other systemic illnesses are considered on p. 415 *et seq.*

Pathology

In general the inflammation is diffuse and symmetrical, being most marked in the true cords, ventricular bands, interarytenoid region and root of the epiglottis. The free part of the epiglottis is relatively spared.

Histological preparations show chronic non-specific inflammatory changes with vasodilatation and infiltration with leucocytes, chiefly round cells. In more severe cases the submucosa and even the intrinsic muscles are seen to be involved. Where there is respiratory epithelium, the mucous glands may undergo hypertrophy, giving rise to a granular appearance.

Clinical features

Hoarseness persisting for weeks or months is the characteristic complaint. Usually it is worse on waking but the voice tires easily, becomes weak and, rarely, aphonic towards the end of the day. Dryness and intermittent tickling are often troublesome. The patient feels compelled to clear his throat frequently. The onomatopoeic term 'ahem' is descriptive of this. However, cough is not a feature unless the lower air passages are involved. Expectoration is not marked although a little grey gelatinous mucus may be produced when the throat is cleared, particularly in the morning. Sore throat is not complained of although the effort to produce voice may lead to an ache in the throat towards evening. The sensation of a lump in the throat is sometimes mentioned.

Very much has been written comparing and contrasting the appearance of the larynx in acute simple laryngitis and chronic non-specific laryngitis. In fact, according to the duration and severity of the condition, the appearance will resemble that of acute laryngitis at one end of the scale and early chronic hyperplastic laryngitis at the other. It is at the latter end of the scale that the differential diagnosis needs most consideration.

Diagnosis

In a high proportion of cases, infection in the para-nasal sinuses, mouth, pharynx or lower air passages will be found to coexist, so that the physical signs will not often be confined to the larynx only. The finding of pus in the nose or post-nasal space, or clinging to or dried on the posterior pharyngeal wall may lead to the diagnosis of chronic sinusitis and will require x-ray confirmation. The mouth may be unhealthy with neglected carious teeth, gingival infection and a dry and coated tongue. Examination and radiography of the chest may reveal evidence of lower respiratory infection. Sputum culture and blood examination should be ordered. The chance discovery of pulmonary tuberculosis, at one time by no means uncommon, is a rare event today, except perhaps in the developing world.

Direct laryngoscopy, of major importance in hyperplastic laryngitis, will be required only occasionally, chiefly when mirror examination proves difficult and unsatisfactory. If hyperplastic changes are found, biopsy must be considered to exclude early carcinoma.

Diffuse inflammatory changes may occur in secondary or in the early stage of tertiary syphilis but these late manifestations nowadays seldom come the way of the laryngologist. However, serological tests should be included among the investigations.

Treatment

It must be repeated that hyperplastic changes, with squamous metaplasia and keratosis are frequently present when the case is first seen and that their presence almost certainly precludes recovery unless surgical treatment is undertaken. However, in the absence of hyperplasia chronic non-specific laryngitis may be expected to recover if the following measures are strenuously pursued.

First, attention must be paid to infection elsewhere in the respiratory tract. Chronic sinusitis is the condition most often calling for active steps and these may include surgery, for example the Caldwell–Luc operation, in obstinate cases. Badly carious teeth or recurrently infected tonsils may require operative treatment also. Reference to a general physician for help with infection of the lower air passages and for advice about the general health will be necessary from time to time. Indeed, not infrequently the case will have been referred from the physician who is already investigating or treating the patient's chest.

Secondly, and while these matters are in train, voice rest must be imposed. Although in contrast with certain of the other kinds of chronic laryngitis considered in the following sections, over-use or misuse of the voice may not play a major aetiological role here, nevertheless its avoidance once the disease is established is of paramount importance. The difficulties met with in practice are however considerable. It will usually prove impossible to keep the patient at work while resting his voice sufficiently and whereas a few days at home may suffice in acute infective laryngitis, a few days only are quite useless in this case. Sometimes the investigation and management of respiratory infection may require admission to hospital which will then provide the opportunity for the strict enforcement of silence at least for a time, although this too will prove in vain unless it is followed up by effective voice rest perhaps for weeks. During these the help of the speech therapist may be invaluable, not only in encouraging the patient to persevere with voice rest but also in training him to produce voice with less wear and tear on the vocal cords.

It has to be admitted, however, that many patients will find such measures unacceptable for what they regard as no more than a nuisance and, even when this is not so, are unwilling to face the economic and other consequences or risk the loss of a job.

What has been said about the aetiological importance of vocal abuse probably applies as much to the abuse of tobacco and alcohol but equally the avoidance of these irritants as a measure of treatment has to be urged. The difficulties of persuading the patient to adopt this degree of self-control and self-denial are of course no less than the difficulties of ensuring voice rest, and failure to obtain the admittedly considerable

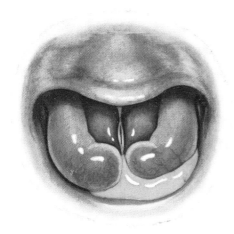

Plate 3 Radionecrosis and perichon-dritis with abscess formation. The in-flammatory infiltration and oedema almost occluded the airway and a tracheotomy was necessary

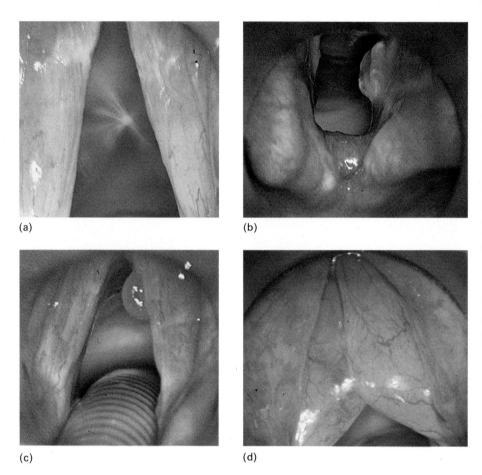

(a)

(b)

(c)

(d)

Plate 4   (a) Early hyperplastic laryngitis with keratinization appearing towards the front of the left vocal cord; (b) early contact pachydermia; (c) a typical vocal cord polyp; (d) polypoid degeneration of the vocal cords (Reinke oedema). (Intra-operative photographs taken by direct laryngoscopy.) Photographs made by Professor O. Kleinsasser, University of Marburg, West Germany, reproduced with his kind permission

measure of cooperation demanded of the patient is a main reason for the poor results obtained.

Of rather less therapeutic significance, if contrarily more acceptable to the patient, are a number of medicaments. Antibiotics need considering inasmuch as they relate to coexisting infection in the respiratory tract apart from the larynx. Sputum culture may give help in identifying the antibiotic to employ. Nasal swabs almost never do. Various sprays have been advocated although their value is, to say the least, equivocal; some, like the once popular silver nitrate, must have been harmful as were the various oily sprays. The latter when persisted with over a long period were sometimes responsible for lipoid pneumonia. Expectorants, for instance mixtures containing ammonium carbonate and ipecacuanha, loosen clinging secretions but in a chronic illness are to be employed only intermittently. The various proprietary preparations have no greater potency.

Finally, something must be said about inhalations. The supportive value of medicated steam inhalations was mentioned in the last chapter in connection with acute infective laryngitis. The occasional use of this treatment over the few days sufficient for recovery of that disease, cannot be expected to influence the course of chronic laryngitis. However, in many European countries patients seek treatment of this kind, sometimes over an extended period, in various spas and watering places catering specially for chronic respiratory illnesses, for example Sirmione on Lake Garda. Many successes are claimed but these are probably related more to the fresh air and the change to a disciplined way of life than to the sulphuretted steam.

Chronic hyperplastic laryngitis

Pathology

The problems of terminology involved in the description of chronic non-specific laryngitis have been referred to already. The words keratosis, hyperkeratosis, leucoplakia and pachydermia have been used in different contexts by different authors and have given rise to considerable confusion. The use of the operating microscope to examine the chronically inflamed larynx and the correlation of the appearances observed with the histological changes in tissue removed have helped towards a more rational terminology. The work of Kleinsasser (1968) in this connection has been particularly important.

The section on pathology is put first here not only to define at once what is meant by chronic hyperplastic laryngitis but equally to make clear what is *not* comprised under this heading.

The healthy larynx, although part of the respiratory tract, is not lined everywhere with respiratory (i.e. ciliated columnar) epithelium. The free part of the epiglottis, the aryepiglottic folds and the vocal cords are covered with non-keratinized squamous epithelium. So far as the vocal cords are concerned the junction of the respiratory with the squamous epithelium is clear-cut where the upper surfaces join the floor of the ventricles as the superior arcuate lines but beneath the glottis, the border on either side, the inferior arcuate line, is not so clear. The extent to which the squamous covering of the upper part of the epiglottis and the aryepiglottic folds encroaches on the lower part of the laryngeal surface of the epiglottis and the false cords is variable but in general, as the individual grows older, the squamous epithelium creeps further into the interior of the larynx. However, in health, squamous epithelium will not be found over the false cords, the petiolus of the epiglottis or in the laryngeal ventricles, nor is keratinization of the squamous epithelium ever observed.

It is typical of chronic hyperplastic laryngitis that both these distinctive features may be lost. The ciliated epithelium on the false cords and on the lower part of the epiglottis becomes liable to metaplasia into squamous epithelium, and the squamous epithelium of the cords and, less commonly the metaplastic epithelium, may become keratinized to a greater or lesser extent. This assumption by the laryngeal epithelium of a skin-like character has been called *epidermization*.

The process is essentially a diffuse and symmetrical one and can be discerned sometimes as proceeding from chronic laryngitis without hyperplasia of the sort described in the preceding section. More often, however, the hyperplastic character of the disease seems to be present from the outset. The changes are first seen in the vocal cords which become hyperaemic and swollen. The swelling is smooth initially but soon becomes irregular, granular or nodular. The earliest appearance of keratinization, usually seen again in the true cords, has been likened to frosted glass. It tends to be patchy and obscures the underlying capillaries which previously could be seen with the operating microscope through the still translucent epithelium. It is often bilateral and confined at first to the part of the cord in front of the vocal process. So-called collateral oedema of the ventricular lining may appear, also often bilaterally, producing the appearance that has, in the past, been mistakenly regarded as prolapse or eversion of the ventricle. As the degree of hyperplasia increases the cords may become increasingly bulky, irregular and pale and the worse affected side may be moulded by the more normal one to produce what Kleinsasser has described as duplication of the cord.

a simple inflammatory kind, but when metaplasia commences a more complicated pathological process is set in train. The metaplasia of ciliated into squamous epithelium in this region involves the ducts of the mucous glands, so that the mucus blanket typical of respiratory epithelium is lost in places. This produces further destruction of ciliated epithelium and the metaplastic process extends further over the ventricular bands, onto the epiglottis and downwards into the subglottic larynx. The few remaining mucous glands are inadequate to moisten the laryngeal lining adequately and it becomes dry, what viscid mucus there is clinging to the inflamed tissues. The obstruction of the ducts may lead to the formation of small retention cysts.

Histologically, changes are first apparent in the glottic region with capillary dilatation, oedema and cellular infiltration of the submucosa. This is followed by hyperplasia of the prickle-cell layer of the epithelium and, in many cases, keratinization. The basal-cell layer sends down-growths into the stroma but the basement membrane remains intact and the cell arrangement orderly.

In later cases the respiratory epithelium is seen to be replaced more or less extensively by squamous epithelium which may in turn show hyperplasia and keratinization. The lamina propria becomes increasingly hyperaemic and heavily infiltrated with lymphocytes, plasma cells and macrophages. A degree of fibrosis is often observed but the amount is variable.

Although it is now widely accepted that the macroscopic appearance or even the micro-laryngoscopic appearance of the lesion gives no certain evidence of the presence or absence of malignant potential or early malignant change, the histological evidence with regard to this is clearer, if still, on occasion equivocal. Several attempts have been made to classify it and to link the histological features to clinically descriptive terms. Thus, in the USA the histological section is scrutinized for signs of 'atypia'. These signs include, among others, crowding and disorderly arrangement of the cells in the prickle-cell layer, nuclear swelling and irregularity, an increase in mitotic figures and dyskeratosis. When atypia is present in a case showing keratinization it is called *leucoplakia* (Norris and Peale, 1963). Kleinsasser (1968) classifies the histological characteristics of epithelial hyperplasia into three grades, the first showing no evidence of atypia, the second corresponding to what Norris calls leucoplakia, and the third to what most pathologists would class as carcinoma *in situ*.

It will be seen that this account of the pathology of chronic hyperplastic laryngitis does not encompass certain localized forms of hyperplasia. They seem to be distinct entities and are described separately below. They are:

(1) Contact pachydermia (often misleadingly called 'contact ulcers').
(2) Interarytenoid pachydermia.
(3) Circumscribed epithelial hyperplasia.

No excuse is made for the use of the term 'pachydermia', introduced by Virchow in 1860 and well understood. The terms 'leucoplakia' and 'hyperkeratosis' will not be used. Clinically speaking leucoplakia is not distinguishable from keratinization in general and hyperkeratosis is meaningful only when applied to normally keratinized epithelia.

Aetiology

The matters considered on p. 382 with regard to chronic laryngitis without hyperplasia are also relevant here and the reader may wish to refer back to that section.

There is general agreement that the changes in the epithelia in hyperplastic laryngitis are brought about by irritation acting over a considerable period of time. Chronic infection elsewhere in the respiratory tract cannot be identified in many of these cases and other factors are certainly concerned. Abuse of tobacco, if not this alone, is certainly one of them. Ryan, McDonald and Devine (1955) demonstrated that the changes found in the larynx after prolonged smoking were precisely those of this disease. They included epithelial hyperplasia, metaplasia and keratinization as well as oedema and round-cell infiltration of the submucosa.

Since hyperplastic laryngitis is a pre-cancerous state, it is probable that the same irritants are concerned in both diseases. Auerbach, Hammond and Garfinkel (1970) have shown that there is a relationship between the amount smoked and the incidence of metaplasia and malignant disease of the larynx. Considering this question in Chapter 15 (p. 440), Shaw draws attention to the particular liability to laryngeal cancer of Asians, especially Indians, and to the possibility that chewing tobacco and betel-nut could be involved.

However, proof of the identity of the irritant or irritants responsible for chronic hyperplastic laryngitis is still lacking.

Clinical features

There is no special symptom which distinguishes this type of laryngitis from the other sorts of non-specific inflammation of the larynx nor indeed, and most significantly, from carcinoma of the larynx. The account given on p. 383, therefore, of the symptoms of chronic laryngitis without hyperplasia, serves equally as an account of the symptoms of this disease.

The age incidence is similar but most references to the hyperplastic cases show a male preponderance sometimes as great as 8:1.

The need for careful general examination but with special emphasis on the upper and lower air passages applies very much here and evidence of infection of the paranasal sinuses, pharynx and lower respiratory tract will often come to light. Palpable neck nodes are not a feature and their presence must seriously raise the question of malignant change.

Careful inspection of the larynx is crucial, of course, but these patients often find indirect laryngoscopy almost intolerable and may need to be examined under general anaesthesia if the necessary thorough assessment of the extent and nature of the disease process is to be made. This direct examination should be made under the operating microscope as described in Chapter 10.

The appearance with regard both to the extent and nature of the condition will vary considerably as the description of the pathology indicates. In the early case the inflammation may be confined to the vocal cords but in what may be described as hyperplastic panlaryngitis, the whole larynx from the subglottis to the false cords and root of the epiglottis may be involved. At first there is no more than a somewhat irregular swelling of the cords with evident capillary injection, as in the left cord in *Plate 4a (facing page 384)* but later keratinization will appear as on the right cord in the plate. Even before keratinization is seen, the cords may appear red, boggy and nodular. The collateral oedema and infiltration of the mucosa in the ventricle may be so marked as to produce a florid inflammatory mass hiding the cord altogether. Epidermization of the false cord will be seen as pallid, nodular patches on the swollen and inflamed mucosa. Viscid mucus and fibrinous exudate may be in evidence, clinging to the surface. At this stage, or even earlier, the vocal cords may appear severely altered, bulky and grey, the normal smooth, straight profile replaced by an irregular or nodular outline. Patchy keratinization may extend backward over the vocal processes towards the interarytenoid commissure. A longitudinal groove on one side may produce the appearance of duplication mentioned above. Rarely small cysts may be observed, particularly in the subglottic region.

Diagnosis

The points made when the diagnosis of chronic laryngitis was considered (p. 383) apply just as much here, but central to the question in cases with hyperplasia is the need to identify early malignancy. The facilities should be available for every case to be submitted to micro-laryngoscopy. Nodularity, induration and ulceration are suggestive features and Kleinsasser has drawn attention to the significance of atypical capillaries. These are most likely to be observed where the malignant and simple hyperplastic tissues adjoin. The straight uniform capillaries seen in inflammatory states give way to tortuous, cork-screw like vessels, liable to abrupt changes in calibre. It must be emphasized, however, that histological evidence only is to be considered conclusive and must always be sought.

The possibility of mistaking tuberculous laryngitis for non-specific chronic hyperplasia has been well known for more than 50 years but nowadays when tuberculosis rarely involves the larynx, it is more likely to be overlooked (*see also* p. 402). The same is true of syphilis although in this case the lesion is even more unlikely to mimic the symmetrical non-ulcerated appearance of chronic hyperplastic laryngitis.

Treatment

Conventional treatment
The various therapeutic measures recommended above for chronic non-hyperplastic laryngitis must be considered and where appropriate applied to these cases also. They include:

(1) Attempts to eliminate infection elsewhere in the respiratory tract.
(2) Voice rest and speech therapy.
(3) Attempts to protect the patient from noxious environmental factors.
(4) Advice to avoid smoking, alcohol and any other ingested or inhaled irritant.
(5) The prescription of antibiotics when indicated, expectorants and inhalations.

On p. 384, the difficulties to be expected in implementing such a programme were discussed and the frequency of failure mentioned. Where hyperplastic changes are present and particularly where there is squamous metaplasia and keratinization, the chance of success from such treatment, even when the patient is willing and able to follow it through, is very small indeed. Fortunately, however, the outlook has been improved since the introduction of micro-laryngoscopy and laryngeal micro-surgery and increased experience in the use of these new tools. Advances are still being made in this direction and more are likely (Dedo, 1976).

Surgical treatment
This should be considered as soon as it is evident that conventional means are not succeeding. The object is the removal of all or most of the diseased *epithelium* in anticipation of healing with healthy tissue. Its importance is not only that it offers a prospect of cure but also that it removes a pre-cancerous lesion. A secondary but still important indication is that by removing all of the worst affected parts of the laryngeal lining, the chance of finding any locality in which malignant transformation has already occurred is altogether greater than if a small area only is selected for biopsy.

Needless to say, if the irritation that caused the original laryngitis continues after recovery, it is probable that in course of time the condition will recur and may become as bad as or worse than ever. Accordingly, what has been called the conventional management must not be abandoned because it failed to reverse the established laryngitis; instead, whatever parts of it are relevant must be persisted with after the operation to prevent a relapse. This may mean helping the patient to find different employment, persisting with speech therapy to prevent a return to a hyperkinetic manner of vocalization and discouraging a return to dependence on tobacco and alcohol. These are all very difficult matters and will not always prove possible or succeed with every case.

The operation
This consists of decortication usually of the vocal cords but sometimes of the false cords as well. It is performed under a general anaesthetic using a laryngoscope of the Jako or Kleinsasser pattern. General experience of these instruments has been that they are ideal when the patient is easy to examine, for example if he is edentulous with a mobile head and neck, but that in some five per cent or more, the anterior part of the larynx cannot be satisfactorily exposed. Dedo (1976) reports that his modification of the Holinger anterior commissure laryngoscope overcomes this problem in all but the exceptional case.

Another difficulty relates to the anaesthetic. This has been maintained until recently using a specially designed, armoured endotracheal tube which obscures a large part of the field. The Venturi method of insufflation has been successfully used in many centres for long enough to establish its value. Adequate oxygenation in the apnoeic patient is achieved by using a so-called 'jet needle' through which oxygen may be forced at a pressure of between 30–60 lb/in^2. This small cannula in no way obscures the view or access to any part of the larynx (Norton *et al.*, 1976; Urban, 1976).

The stripping of the diseased epithelium is carried out under the operating microscope with a set of special instruments – scissors, forceps, suction-cautery and knives – all with long (27 cm) rigid shafts which can be used, one in each hand when necessary, through the specially widened laryngoscope. The decortication of the vocal cords makes use of the well-defined subepithelial plane described in 1895 by the German anatomist Reinke (*see also* p. 397). An incision is made along the superior arcuate line curving medially just short of the anterior commissure in front and just short of the vocal process behind to reach the edge of the vocal cord. The D-shaped flap so-defined is then carefully raised from the subjacent vocal ligament and turned medially over the edge of the cord until its attachment along the inferior arcuate line is reached. The diseased epithelium is then trimmed off using scissors along the inferior arcuate line from behind forward. If both cords are involved as is usual, the more hyperplastic one is dealt with first, the less affected one being operated on after an interval of 3–4 weeks, i.e. when the first side has healed completely.

Great care must be exercised close to the anterior commissure since the removal of too much tissue here will result in blunting of the glottis with permanent dysphonia. For this reason the operation must never be attempted unless full exposure of the anterior commissure can be achieved and it is in this respect that advantages are claimed for the new fibre-optic anterior commissure laryngoscope designed by Dedo. Equally, great care must be taken to remain strictly in the subepithelial plane and avoid damage to the fibrous edge of the vocal ligament. A mistake here may result in a weak, so-called 'breathy' voice. The definition of the subepithelial plane is aided by the subepithelial injection before decortication is commenced of a 1:200 000 solution of adrenaline in Normal saline.

For a day or two after the operation while the patient remains in hospital he should not attempt to speak and, even more not to whisper. On discharge and for one month when healing is complete, he should use his voice sparingly and never raise it above a quiet conversational tone. The importance of avoiding thereafter whatever irritants may have been judged responsible for the laryngitis in the first place, has been emphasized already but cannot be repeated too often.

Contact pachydermia *(see also* p. 393)

In 1860 Rudolf Virchow, the great German pathologist, conferred the descriptive title 'pachydermia verrucosa laryngis' on a sort of laryngitis characterized by annular epithelial over-growth centred on the vocal processes of the arytenoid cartilages. He considered the cause to be gross vocal abuse. Morrell Mackenzie (1880) and, nearly 50 years later, Chevalier Jackson (1928) and others regarded the lesion as an ulcer. Chevalier Jackson identified exposed cartilage in the base of the ulcer in some cases and gave the weight of his authority to the name 'contact ulcer'. Examination of many of these lesions under the microscope has not confirmed the presence of ulceration or perichondritis and 'contact pachydermia' would seem the proper description for the condition as seen nowadays (Kleinsasser, 1963). In the UK it is now a rare disease.

Aetiology

Virchow's opinion that this disease occurs as the result of serious misuse of the voice has been endorsed by most writers on the subject since his time. It is not the amount of voice use that is significant but the quality of the voice produced. These patients usually exemplify what is called 'hyperkinetic dysphonia', vocalizing in a loud, harsh and staccato manner, the voice forced out between cords held adducted with unnecessary tension. Virchow's patient was a Prussian lieutenant barking orders at the troops he commanded. Jackson's patients included a foreman, a salesman and a huckster *(sic)*. Almost all the recorded cases have been in adult males and it has been suggested that the use of a deep, 'manly' voice of a pitch lower than is natural may be relevant. The writer has encountered the reverse of this, a tall strong man whose voice had never 'broken' at puberty and who later developed typical contact pachydermia. A speech therapist taught him how to produce a bass voice and the pachydermia quickly resolved. Other factors are frequently mentioned, particularly smoking and occupational hazards of different kinds. Jackson regarded abuse of alcohol as an important source of the disease. The typical patient described in the older texts is the bawling drunkard.

However, the one constant factor is vocal abuse. The foundry worker exposed to heat and fumes has to raise his voice above the noise. The barman, drinking short-ones in the smoky atmosphere of the pub must do the same. Very likely it was the bawling not the drink that was to blame in the typical case.

Pathology

The gross appearance of the developed condition is entirely characteristic. The principal changes are confined to the vicinity of the vocal processes. At first circumscribed injected oedematous swellings appear but as a rule by the time the patient reaches the laryngologist the typical lesions are found. They lie opposite each other, the hyperplastic epithelium being heaped up round a crater, beneath the floor of which lies the vocal process. Frequently some degree of keratinization is present and may be marked (*Plate 4b, facing page 384*). Very often when the cords are adducted, an elevated part of the edge of one lesion fits into the depression on the other so that, seen in the laryngeal mirror, the appearance is of a prominence on one side corresponding to a pit on the other. Usually some degree of inflammation is apparent in the membranous part of the cords, which look a little swollen and hyperaemic.

The presence of these bulky lesions over the vocal processes introduces something like a vicious circle into the pathogenesis of the disease. Early in its course they will prevent proper apposition of the cords thereby provoking a greater effort to phonate clearly. This further misuse of the voice added to the other harmful vocal activities will aggravate the situation, lead to further hyperplasia and so on.

As already mentioned, descriptions of this condition written three or four decades ago, refer to ulceration in the floor of the crater with the necrotic tip of the vocal process of the arytenoid exposed at the centre. This must have been due to localized perichondritis but observers in recent times have not found this complication to be present.

Histologically, the thickened tissues are seen to be the site of localized hyperplasia demonstrating at different stages the changes found in chronic hyperplastic laryngitis but stopping short of the disorderly cellular arrangement and other atypical features of the pre-cancerous state. This is entirely in accord with the clinical course of contact pachydermia since carcinoma almost never develops in this part of the larynx.

Symptoms

The complaint is of a rough hoarse voice with a frequent desire to clear the throat, in vain. However, in the sort of patient likely to develop the disease, these symptoms may be accepted without complaint. Pain is uncommon but may occur after prolonged use of the damaged cords. It has been known to be referred to the ear, a worrying symptom since this is a feature also of carcinoma of the larynx. More often, after prolonged vocalization, an ache may develop in the throat as with other kinds of laryngitis.

Diagnosis

There is therefore nothing in the symptomatology that will in the least indicate the nature of the diagnosis but this will be made with reasonable certainty on examination. Indirect laryngoscopy will serve in the majority of cases since even in the difficult patient the posterior part of the larynx with its entirely pathognomonic appearance is likely to be seen, but where there is any doubt, direct examination under anaesthesia must be made, preferably using the microscope. This is important not only for a thorough inspection but also to exclude coexistent disease elsewhere in the larynx. Jackson and Jackson (1937) refer to typical contact ulcers (*sic*) occurring in patients with tuberculous laryngitis, a coincidence admittedly most unlikely nowadays.

Treatment

An early case in a well-motivated patient may do well on conservative treatment. A period, as long as possible, of absolute voice rest should be followed by regular treatment from a speech therapist. If the patient understands the need to lose his hyperkinetic voice production and can be taught to produce voice of the correct pitch and amplitude with relaxation, he may be cured of his pachydermia in a surprisingly short time. This happy outcome is not usual, however, and where it fails only surgery will offer a reasonable prospect of cure.

The operation is micro-surgical excision carried out in the same manner as the operation described previously for diffuse hyperplastic laryngitis but in this case the exposure will be easier and the larger laryngoscopes suitable. If an endotracheal tube is used it must be positioned to lie at the anterior commissure but the Venturi technique overcomes this difficulty. The aim is to excise the heaped-up hyperplastic epithelium forming the rim of the crater. The base need not be touched.

As in the case of surgery for hyperplastic laryngitis, success will depend as much on the post-operative measures as on the operation itself. A period of silence followed by voice rest is imperative and the speech therapist must not relax in efforts to maintain a high standard of voice production.

Interarytenoid pachydermia

This is a very rare disease accounting for perhaps one per cent of all cases of chronic laryngitis as described in this chapter. A brief account will suffice therefore.

When tuberculosis of the larynx was common, interarytenoid mammilation, indicative of tuberculous ulceration at the posterior commissure was often seen. Now, to find laryngeal inflammation in this area is altogether unusual.

The cause of non-specific interarytenoid hyperplasia is unknown.

The symptoms are significantly different from those of contact pachydermia. In that condition, because of the location of the epithelial thickening over the vocal processes, hoarseness is the leading complaint. In this case the cords are at first normal and voice is little affected, but metaplasia of the respiratory epithelium on the posterior laryngeal wall with loss of cilia will hinder the passage of mucus and produce the need frequently to clear the throat. Mucus clinging to the altered tissues may cause intermittent huskiness. It is only when the lesion reaches a certain size and severity that it will hinder full adduction of the arytenoid cartilages and so cause a persistent hoarseness which becomes worse as the day wears on.

The appearance is curious and unlikely to be mistaken for anything else except perhaps laryngeal tuberculosis. During quiet respiration the lesion appears as a heaping-up of the epithelium between the posterior ends of the aryepiglottic folds at the laryngeal inlet. In the laryngeal mirror, it seems indeed to lie between the arytenoids although in fact it is proximal to this region. On phonation, the thickened tissues are compressed into a number of corrugations as the arytenoids come together and present as a sort of cock's comb, preventing full approximation of the cords posteriorly. Deep fissures (Stoerk's fissures) separate the elevations so formed.

Treatment has proved ineffective in this condition since surgical removal of the hyperplastic epithelium is not easy and is likely to result in scarring and failure to improve the voice.

Circumscribed epithelial hyperplasia

It has been emphasized already that the changes of chronic hyperplastic laryngitis are essentially diffuse and that where a patch of keratinization occurs, it shades off into the adjacent inflamed and hyperplastic epithelium. From time to time, however, a circumscribed keratinized lesion will be observed, sharply demarcated from the relatively normal lining elsewhere in the larynx. It is precisely such examples of keratosis that pathologists have wished to see excluded from the laryngitis category. Because doubt about its true identity is conceded, it will be described briefly here, rather than with 'Tumours of the larynx' (Chapter 15).

Pathology

Localized white patches appearing on normally non-keratinized squamous epithelium occur in a number of localities including the vulva, tongue, palate and inner aspect of the cheek. The disease is variously spoken of as leucoplakia, keratosis and hyperkeratosis. Atypical keratin formation is stimulated at these sites by different sorts of chronic irritation not always easy to define.

It is such patches as these that may occur in the larynx, usually on the membranous vocal cords. They vary in size and gross appearance from a small prominent white wart to an extensive nodular plaque involving the entire free edge of the cord and with the general texture and colour of cauliflower. They may be papilliferous, the keratin presenting as a sort of shaggy beard.

On histological examination the same variations may be found. The lesion may be described as a keratinized squamous papilloma or as inflamed hyperplastic epithelium showing keratinization. Not infrequently the pathologist will report difficulty in excluding early malignant change since cellular and nuclear atypia suggestive of carcinoma-*in-situ* is not uncommonly observed.

Moreover, apart from this, cases diagnosed on sound histological grounds have been found to undergo malignant transformation in course of time (McGavran, Bauer and Ogura, 1960).

Diagnosis

Here it must be said again, as elsewhere in this chapter, that there is nothing in the symptoms to differentiate this condition from the different sorts of laryngitis on the one hand and laryngeal carcinoma on the other. Similarly, the appearance on mirror examination may reasonably be taken for papilloma or carcinoma, the only characteristic being the striking degree and extent of the keratin formation. Even when the larynx is examined under the microscope the same is true and the eventual decision will depend on the histologist's opinion.

Treatment

Conservative treatment has no place in the management, the only course being careful excision of the whole lesion under the operating microscope. The complete specimen, so removed, will be submitted for histological examination and it is only on the basis of this report rather than the report on a small forceps' biopsy, that a confident diagnosis may be made.

Atrophic laryngitis

The older textbooks contain accounts of laryngitis sicca and ozaenatous laryngitis, conditions of the larynx characterized by atrophy of the laryngeal mucous membrane and crust formation. The Jacksons in their classical account of the diseases of the larynx, published in 1937, describe these diseases as different entities, the latter being regarded as a complication of ozaena of the nose. Nasal ozaena has become increasingly rare in most parts of the western world in the past three or four decades and it is generally supposed that this is the reason for the lack of descriptions of atrophic laryngitis in the laryngeal literature in recent times. On the occasions when nasal ozaena is encountered nowadays, crusting of the pharynx is often found to coexist but laryngeal involvement is uncommon. Crusting of the larynx is extremely rare and laryngeal ozaena in the literal sense of evil-smelling crusts occurring in the larynx is outside the experience of most contemporary laryngologists.

   Chronic laryngitis typified by lack of lubrication of the inflamed cords which appear dry and glazed is noted often enough but it is doubtful if it calls for a separate description or if atrophy of the laryngeal mucosa is the basic pathology. When drying of this kind is conspicuous, traces of dried blood may be noticed on the surface of the cords.

   Treatment will be along the lines advocated above for chronic diffuse laryngitis but where atrophic rhinitis is present with or without sinusitis, an attempt must first be made to cure these conditions.

Vocal cord polyps

These, together with the cases of so-called polypoid degeneration of the cords constitute the commonest cause of chronic hoarseness. They are rare in the young and the very old, commonest in the fifth decade, and affect men twice as frequently as women.

Aetiology

The cause has not been certainly identified although in the majority of cases misuse of the voice is apparent. It is not only the amount of voice use that is concerned but the manner of voice production. Polyps are particularly likely to occur in patients with hyperkinetic dysphonia i.e. who phonate in a shrill or strident way with unnecessary tension. This kind of vocalization when persistent injures the connective tissue of the vocal cords probably by severely distorting it. Vascular engorgement and micro-haemorrhages occur followed by oedema and the other changes described in the next section. Once such a process starts, even normal phonation will aggravate it.

Pathology

The condition under consideration here is clinically different from the diffuse polypoid degeneration involving the whole length of both cords and also from the symmetrical vocal nodules known often as singer's nodes, preacher's nodes and so on according to the occupation of the patient. Accounts of these two clinical entities will be found in the following sections.

The vocal polyp is usually a translucent, sessile lesion arising close to the anterior commissure from the subglottic aspect of one vocal cord (*Plate 4c, facing page 384*). In about 20 per cent of cases the condition is bilateral. The size varies from a few millimetres across the base to as much as a centimetre in which case the polyp extends from the anterior commissure almost to the vocal process and resembles the polypoid degeneration described below. The surrounding epithelium and the fragile epithelial envelope of the polyp show no sign of inflammatory change although on micro-laryngoscopy fine capillary marking is seen. The stroma is as a rule scanty, relatively acellular and distended with glairy yellow-grey exudate. Sometimes, however, it is more vascular when small haemorrhages may occur or more fibrous when hyalinization may be a conspicuous feature. In such cases the polyp may lose its usual translucency and appear opaque and hyperaemic or opaque and white. The epithelium investing a polyp which has been present for a long time may show a degree of hyperplasia or even some keratinization. Because of this range of histological features, polyps have often been mistakenly regarded as fibromas, angiomas or myxomas.

It is not unknown for a polyp to assume an uncharacteristic multilobed form or to produce a degree of contact hyperplasia on the opposite vocal cord.

Clinical features

A constantly hoarse voice is almost always the only complaint although a large mobile polyp may be responsible for choking attacks and diplophonia.

On indirect or direct laryngoscopy a lesion corresponding to one or other of the conditions described above will be found. A pendulous polyp may be difficult to see with a mirror during inspiration but will be propelled between the cords to lie on top of them during phonation.

Diagnosis

The appearance of the typical gelatinous polyp is diagnostic, particularly when well observed under the operating microscope, but in all cases the excised specimen must be sent for histological examination to confirm its true pathological status. Friedmann and Osborn (1976) have found amyloid foci, squamous papillomas, keratotic nodules or even early squamous carcinomas masquerading clinically as simple polypi.

Treatment

When polyps were removed by tugging them off the cord with large cup forceps, the result was not uncommonly disappointing because of scarring from injury to the vocal ligament, adhesions blunting the anterior commissure or incomplete removal. Where facilities do not exist for laryngeal micro-surgery, these cases should be referred to a larger centre where this technique is available. The polyp should be grasped by suitable small forceps, pulled medially and carefully trimmed off using the scissors designed for the purpose.

A week or ten days' voice rest should be followed by a course of speech therapy with the object of correcting faulty voice production.

Polypoid degeneration of the vocal cords (Reinke oedema)

Bilateral symmetrical polypoid swelling of the whole length of the membranous part of the vocal cords, although seen less often than vocal cord polyps, is still one of the commoner laryngeal lesions. It occurs most often in the middle-aged and affects both sexes.

Aetiology

Here again the cause is uncertain but as with the polyps there is reason to suspect misuse of the voice in the majority of cases. Kleinsasser (1968) states that these patients are usually heavy cigarette smokers and cites Hünermann (1958) in support of the frequent coexistence of sinusitis.

Pathology

Professor Hajek of Vienna proposed that this disease should be named after the German anatomist Reinke (Hajek, 1925/6). In 1895 Reinke described for the first time the existence of the loose subepithelial connective tissue of the vocal cords, the presence of which permits the ripple-like motion of the mucosa during phonation. This subepithelial plane is limited by the superior and inferior arcuate lines on the upper and subglottic surfaces of the cords, by the anterior commissure in front and the vocal processes posteriorly. It is this connective tissue that is the site of the swelling and the anatomical limits of Reinke's space that determine the characteristic appearance of the cords in this condition. It is not often that tissue finds its way to the pathologist in significant amount. The strips of epithelium that are removed (*see below*) are likely to show no pathological change and the fluid exudate leaks away from the featureless submucosa. In the long-standing case the oedematous cords may become a little shrunken, lax and hyperaemic and the epithelium somewhat, but never considerably, hyperplastic.

Clinical features

At first the patient has a weak and slightly husky voice but if nothing is done, and in course of time, a rather coarser quality is noticed. Often this is an intermittent change and may be due to what is called *dysphonia plicae ventricularis* (*see* p. 523). In an effort to produce a greater volume of sound, the patient will discover how to phonate using the false cords. This produces a low-pitched, rough but often quite loud voice and if this is resorted to frequently or becomes habitual, the ventricular bands will undergo marked hyperplasia and hyperaemia and may become so bulky that they hide the polypoid true cords almost completely.

Examination early in the course of the disease will show the entirely typical pale translucent fusiform swelling of the cords. These loose swellings will meet in a straight line in front separating towards the vocal processes so that the diamond-shaped opening of the glottis is reduced to a greater or lesser extent in the antero-posterior dimension (*Plate 4d, facing page 384*). Phonation will produce a limp, fluttering movement in the oedematous rolls of tissue. Later, the changes in the false cords may be observed and in time the cords themselves will be largely hidden from view. However, where specialist advice is readily available most cases are seen before these late changes have commenced.

Treatment

Conservative treatment is almost always ineffective and the condition is best treated by micro-surgery. It is important that a view is obtained of the whole length of the cords and when this cannot be achieved with the large Kleinsasser laryngoscope the use of the recently introduced Dedo–Pilling micro-laryngoscope may make a significant difference. The operation consists in the excision of an oval strip of epithelium extending from front to back of the swollen cord. On one side the strip should be removed from the upper surface of the oedematous roll, on the other from the caudal aspect, thereby avoiding the risk of an adhesion forming at the anterior commissure. If for technical reasons, this degree of precision is not possible, the second cord should be operated on three or four weeks after the first when healing is complete. The operation must never be attempted unless the full range of specially designed instruments is available.

Voice rest is important while healing is proceeding and as with vocal nodules and polyps, the help of a speech therapist should be enlisted in the hope of teaching the patient to produce voice with greater relaxation.

Vocal nodules

Symmetrical vocal cord nodules are common occurrences but among certain sections of the population only. They are popularly known by a variety of names indicating not only the sort of people liable to develop them but also the current view of their aetiology. The synonyms include among others, singer's, ranter's, preacher's, heckler's, teacher's, hawker's and screamer's nodes.

Aetiology

However, these synonyms are not all well chosen since the hecklers, hawkers and ranters are more likely to develop contact pachydermia and polyps than nodules. Nodules occur more frequently in females than males and more often in children than in adult males. The writer's experience leads him to favour singers, teachers and screamers rather than the others as candidates for the development of these lesions. Khambata (Chapter 16) gives an account of the aetiology of nodes in professional voice-users based on close observation of their problems and the reader should turn to those pages. It is generally agreed that misuse of the voice is the invariable cause and while it may be readily understood why the pop singer is liable to develop this disease, it may seem surprising that the well-trained product of the great musical academies and conservatoires should do so. Of course, even these use their voices for purposes other than singing and it is likely that patterns of vocalization acquired long before a career as a singer was first dreamt of may be relevant. Professional singers are often extrovert and gregarious and perhaps more damage to the vocal cords occurs off the stage or concert platform than on it.

With regard to the personality and psychological make-up of these patients certain characteristics emerge and adults liable to form nodes have been classed as hyperkinetic, vociferous and aggressive.

Pathology and pathogenesis

The nodules are almost always symmetrical, occurring on both cords at the junction of the anterior with the middle one-third. They rarely exceed a millimetre or two in size. It is the anterior part of the cord which is active in the production of high-pitched sound and the dynamics of phonation appear to expose this point on the cords to traumatizing pressures during the loud sounding of high notes. It seems that this point of the cords is even more liable to trauma when loud vocalization is attempted at the end of expiration. The cords must then be held more firmly in adduction if a loud high note is to be produced with falling subglottic air pressure. The trained singer learns correct breathing and is accordingly better equipped to avoid this injurious circumstance than the untrained performer.

At first the nodules are strictly localized and limited areas of oedema, vascular engorgement and, sometimes, focal haemorrhage occur in the connective tissue immediately beneath the epithelium of the free edge of the cord. In established cases, the overlying epithelium is seen to have undergone a degree of hyperplastic thickening. In time a variable amount of subepithelial fibrosis may appear, the collagen undergoing in turn a greater or lesser degree of hyalinization. However, the nodule remains entirely superficial and does not hinder the rhythmical flowing movement of the epithelium during phonation.

Symptoms and signs

To begin with the speaking voice is scarcely affected though in time it may come to have a slight 'throaty' quality made universally familiar by one or two famous film stars. It is the soprano singer who is most likely to complain in the early stages, however; she finds that when she sings up the scale she reaches a point where it requires an extra amount of pressure from the pulmonary bellows to produce the note. At this point therefore her voice may fail, only to break through again but with greater volume. An inability to sing high notes softly is almost diagnostic. The voice tires easily and after prolonged use an ache develops in the throat. In long-standing cases hoarseness becomes a constant feature during speech and singing becomes impossible.

The diagnosis is confirmed as a rule at indirect laryngoscopy when the typical white sessile nodules are observed at the typical site (p. 426). If an adequate inspection of the front part of the glottis with the laryngeal mirror or fibrescope is not possible direct examination under general anaesthetic is necessary.

Treatment

In many cases of chronic non-specific laryngitis, conservative treatment fails because the cause cannot be certainly identified or easily eliminated, or because the patient cannot or will not comply with the advice offered. In this condition the main, often the sole aetiological agent is misuse of the voice. Moreover, the determination of the patient, at least the adult patient, to undergo whatever rigours are demanded to regain the normal use of what is often her source of livelihood is great. There is a good chance therefore that conservative measures will succeed, at any rate where professional voice-users are concerned and these should be given every chance to benefit from such treatment before surgery is contemplated. In the first place voice rest may be necessary for anything from weeks to months and the patient may have to cancel engagements and even radically re-organize her way of life for some time ahead. During this period the health of the nose, para-nasal sinuses, mouth or pharynx may need attention and smoking is forbidden.

As often as not the patient will have been trained to use her voice by a teacher held in high regard or maybe consider herself as being in some measure *in statu pupillari*. Where this is so, to introduce a speech therapist into the scheme of management will be quite impossible and the laryngologist may find it necessary or prudent to discuss the way ahead with the teacher in whom the patient has confidence. In other cases, the help of the speech therapist will be welcomed and in this event speech therapy has an important part to play in what amounts to the rehabilitation of the case. The special problems of the child with this sort of laryngeal disorder are considered in the next section.

When these measures fail or seem likely to fail, micro-surgical removal of the nodes must be considered. It should not be undertaken unless post-operative voice rest can be assured and then only if there is a reasonable prospect that the condition will not relapse because faulty voice production continues uncorrected.

The operation is not easy particularly when, as usual, the nodes are small and hard to grasp. A small incision is made close to the base of the nodule. The medial lip of the incision may then be seized without too much difficulty, the nodule pulled medially and trimmed off with the curved scissors. Both sides may be dealt with at the same time but silence must be insisted on while the patient remains in hospital, and voice rest for a few days more. The speech therapist or singing teacher then resumes the care of the patient for as long as the laryngologist judges necessary.

Regrettably and despite every care recurrence is not uncommon.

Chronic laryngitis in childhood

Considering the particular vulnerability of the child's larynx to acute laryngitis it is perhaps surprising that chronic laryngitis is not more common in children. In fact, most chronically hoarse children will be found to be suffering from multiple laryngeal papillomata, a disease usually classified as neoplastic, although now known to be due to a virus. An account appears on p. 426.

Chronic infective laryngitis in this age group was not rare in the early decades of this century chiefly because of tuberculous laryngitis in the young and congenital syphilis, but these occurrences have now become unknown at least in the developed parts of the world. Non-specific infective laryngitis is not liable to become chronic at this age because the irritants responsible for the disease in the adult are not at work. However, misuse of the voice certainly is and a surprisingly large number of schoolchildren suffer from its effects. Senturia and Wilson (1969) found six per cent of 32 500 St Louis schoolchildren to be suffering from laryngitis so caused, and Fitz-Hugh, Smith and Chiang (1958) reported four per cent of 300 benign vocal cord lesions in children under ten years of age.

Nearly all chronic cases are cases of vocal nodules and Toohill (1975) has studied 77 of these. The peak incidence was between five and ten years of age, and boys were affected three times as often as girls. Sixty-two were described as screamers or as incessant or loud talkers and the same psychological traits as those already mentioned in adult cases were noted among these children. However, as well as aggression and hyperactivity, tension, frustration and emotional disturbance are listed.

Conservative treatment as outlined above for the adult cannot be expected to succeed in the child since prolonged voice rest is clearly not practicable and the patient's cooperation in meaningful speech therapy hard to maintain. The involvement of the parents must be sought and counselling by an experienced therapist or psychologist arranged if possible. However, such measures will frequently fail.

Surgical removal is disappointing also and is likely to be followed by early recurrence because the cause persists. However, it should be recommended if the nodes are large, of long standing and the voice badly affected. Fortunately, spontaneous improvement takes place in most cases with the arrival of puberty and the maturing of the voice and the parents will be re-assured to be told this.

Chronic specific infective laryngitis

Micro-organisms like the *Mycobacterium tuberculosis* and the *Treponema pallidum* which once were able to persist unchecked by the defences of the body over long periods, are now almost always controlled by antibiotics and rarely produce the classical protracted disseminated disease patterns of the past. Moreover, particularly in the case of tuberculosis, changes in social conditions, public health measures and other factors have dramatically reduced the incidence. Now over large areas of the world, many of the complications, such as laryngeal involvement for instance, have become clinical rarities. The pride of place once accorded to these great epidemic diseases, the infective granulomata, must be yielded now to the pathologically less exciting but far commoner conditions described above.

Tuberculosis of the larynx

Incidence

Tuberculous laryngitis is a consequence of tuberculosis of the lungs and its incidence is related to that of the pulmonary infection. The spectacular decrease in the number of cases of the latter and the improvement in the prognosis is one of the great success stories of modern medicine. In 1923, 59 172 cases of tuberculosis of the lungs were notified for England and Wales compared with 11 180 in 1973. Even more remarkably, the 50 000 deaths attributed to this disease in 1860 had been reduced by 1973 to only 801, although over these years the population had increased two-and-a-half times. Clearly, this astonishing decline in the mortality is not to be explained simply by the diminished incidence but by the fact that from 1945 onwards there was available for the first time effective specific treatment.

Thomson (1924) estimated that at the end of the second decade of this century one in three patients with active phthisis suffered from laryngeal tuberculosis and, on this basis, Scott Stevenson (1935) concluded that there were 75 925 such cases in England and Wales. By 1950, according to Ormerod the percentage had fallen to 2.5. Figures are no longer available but a case seen recently by the present writer, the first for many years, was regarded as a remarkable curiosity.

However, it would not do to forget that pulmonary tuberculosis is, throughout the world, still one of the most prevalent communicable diseases, accounting still for many deaths (35.4 per 100 000 in Hong Kong in 1968), and that laryngeal infection must be looked for and will be encountered in many of its less fortunate or overcrowded corners.

Aetiology

Almost all cases of respiratory tuberculosis nowadays are due to *Mycobacterium tuberculosis* (i.e. the human type) and in only a small proportion have *Mycobacterium avis*, *Mycobacterium kansasii* and *Mycobacterium bovis* been identified.

The larynx is infected by the bacilli in the sputum coughed up from the diseased lungs and the more there are, the greater the risk of the disease taking hold. From time to time reports of cases thought to be examples of primary laryngeal tuberculosis have appeared but have been received with scepticism.

Caseating tuberculous foci including hilar lymph nodes may ulcerate into blood vessels and cause a tuberculous bacillaemia or the blood stream may be invaded by way of the lymphatics. In these events miliary tuberculosis will usually occur but it is rare for the larynx to be involved.

The factors predisposing to respiratory tuberculosis such as inadequate housing and diet, particularly a shortage of first-class protein, have been thoroughly studied but will not be considered here. Why some patients with advanced open phthisis escaped laryngeal infection, while others succumbed was a matter of frequent speculation at one time (*see* the discussion in Blegvad, 1937) but there has been no general agreement on the answer.

Nowadays, the sexes are equally vulnerable, the disease being most common between the ages of 20 and 40 years.

Pathology

The *tubercles* characteristic of the disease form in the subepithelial tissue. The invading organisms are first engulfed but not destroyed by polymorphonuclear leucocytes and this transient stage is critical inasmuch as it localizes the infection. Within 24 hours mononuclear cells and macrophages of the reticulo-endothelial system appear in large numbers. The subsequent destruction of the engulfed bacilli by the macrophages results in the formation of the typical epithelioid cells. Soon the cells at the centre of the tubercle undergo necrosis and the surrounding epithelioid cells coalesce to form giant cells. Lymphocytes and fibroblasts accumulate round the tubercle as if to wall it off from the surrounding connective tissue. The presence of tubercles sets up low-grade inflammation with the formation of tuberculous granulation tissue. Coagulation necrosis occurs in the larger tubercles, a process known as *caseation*. However, this is not a constant feature and is often absent when the host resistance is high. As the disease advances, there is a tendency for the parts affected earlier to heal by fibrosis, the processes of destruction and repair often proceeding at one and the same time. The submucosa of the epiglottis and aryepiglottic folds is particularly likely to undergo fibrous infiltration producing the pallid swelling called 'pseudo-oedema'. Finally, the epithelium overlying areas of active inflammation becomes involved. Small shallow ulcers may occur or considerable hyperplasia, even keratinization.

In the past great attention was paid to the mode of onset and the nature of the early lesions of laryngeal tuberculosis. The isolated redness of one vocal cord, swelling and redness of the epithelium over the vocal processes, interarytenoid thickening, the 'prolapse' of hyperaemic swollen mucosa from one or both laryngeal ventricles and subglottic swelling have all been cited among the early signs. In the established case, there is a tendency for the different pathological features described above to become manifest in characteristic localities. Thus, ulceration is most often seen where the epithelium is more closely applied to the underlying membrane or cartilage as over the vocal cords or arytenoid cartilages. Infiltration with tuberculous granulation tissue is most apparent on the posterior laryngeal wall and in the laryngeal ventricles, whereas the pallid pseudo-oedema is seen typically in the free part of the epiglottis and the posterior ends of the aryepiglottic folds.

Clinical features

In the third and fourth decades of this century, a number of extensive and authoritative accounts of laryngeal tuberculosis were written by laryngologists who had accumulated a large experience of this disease in the major sanatoria and chest hospitals (e.g. Ormerod, 1939). All cases admitted with pulmonary tuberculosis would be subjected to laryngoscopy and were often found to exhibit signs of laryngitis before laryngeal symptoms were manifest (Thomson and Negus, 1948). These special circumstances apart, however, patients with tuberculosis of the lungs would not infrequently attend hospital with a hoarse or weak voice unaware of any chest infection and with laryngeal changes revealed by indirect laryngoscopy. These changes might or might not be considered diagnostic of tuberculosis but x-ray of the chest was a routine matter and would reveal the causative pulmonary disease. The identification of tuberculous laryngitis in this way is quite exceptional now in the western world but by no means rare elsewhere.

The earliest *symptoms* are those of laryngitis from whatever cause but the classical descriptions all emphasize weakness of the voice as a typical feature. A rough whisper was considered characteristic.

As soon as the supraglottic larynx becomes heavily attacked, pain becomes a feature. At first it amounts to no more than discomfort on swallowing but as the lesions progress, pain in the larynx and pharynx may become very severe with radiation to the ear. In the worst cases, dysphagia may become almost intolerable.

At laryngoscopy, the observer must expect to find a great variety of abnormalities as already indicated above. Among the most suggestive are the single red vocal cord, what has been called interarytenoid mammillation, asymmetrical distribution of redness and induration, the so-called pyriform arytenoids – pale often symmetrical swellings of the posterior ends of the aryepiglottic folds – the turban epiglottis and shallow ragged ulceration of the vocal cord or over the infiltrated interarytenoid tissues. Pallor of the surrounding mucosa is often a striking finding, even extending to the fauces and soft palate.

In the advanced case where the ventricular bands are heavily infiltrated, *dysphonia plicae ventricularis* may be present with the corresponding very rough, low-pitched vocalization. Sometimes in long-standing cases, impaired mobility of the cords may be seen. Various causes for this have been suggested including involvement of the crico-arytenoid joints, infiltration of the laryngeal muscles, the presence of the interarytenoid swelling and even pressure on or other involvement of the laryngeal nerve supply.

Diagnosis

Because of the protean aspect of the larynx in this condition, the need to consider the other major causes of gross laryngeal pathology in this connection has always been emphasized. Thus chronic hyperplastic laryngitis, the pachydermias, carcinoma of the larynx and syphilitic laryngitis have always to be borne in mind and the necessary investigations arranged. A particular hazard of differential diagnosis presents rarely in patients with pulmonary tuberculosis who happen to develop carcinoma of the larynx. The presence of a suggestive chest x-ray and positive sputum make the diagnosis of tuberculosis of the larynx entirely probable but prudent biopsy confirms the double diagnosis.

The differential diagnosis from lupus laryngis is considered in the following section (p. 406).

Treatment

Writing in the last edition of this book Maxwell Ellis states, 'The management of cases of tuberculous laryngitis has in the past called for considerable experience and judgment in the use of the various forms of treatment available.... However, the greatly lessened incidence of the disease and its earlier diagnosis, together with the administration of modern antibiotics has, within the last few years, completely altered the clinical picture and considerably reduced the active role of the laryngologist.'

The various forms of treatment referred to included such widely different measures as the application of chaulmoogra oil and formaldehyde, galvanocautery, helio-therapy, gastrostomy, tracheostomy, alcohol injection of the superior laryngeal nerve and even unilateral section of the recurrent laryngeal nerve. The laryngologist today is indeed fortunate to be spared the need to select and subject his patient to such radical therapy.

Streptomycin was introduced in 1945 but did not become widely available until two or three years later. The many reports of its use in tuberculous laryngitis over the following ten years or more gave unequivocal evidence of its specific action and its superiority over all the forms of treatment previously employed. Not unexpectedly it was found to be most effective in early, acute and spreading lesions and even when it failed to control the pulmonary disease it often cured the laryngeal complication. The emergence of streptomycin-resistant strains of the bacillus was quickly followed by the introduction of sodium aminosalicylate (PAS) and isoniazid, and the realization that drug-resistance could be avoided by the use of more than one drug at a time. Besides these three drugs there are now available ethambutol and rifampicin.

The treatment of laryngeal tuberculosis is now the treatment of the pulmonary infection with appropriate combinations of anti-tuberculous drugs and will be in the hands of the chest physician. In general terms an initial phase of treatment lasting two or three months with three drugs, e.g. rifampicin, ethambutol and isoniazid, is followed by a continuation phase using two drugs, perhaps for a year or more.

Complications and prognosis

In the pre-streptomycin years, perichondritis usually due to secondary infection with pyogenic organisms was not uncommon, the arytenoids being more often affected than the other laryngeal cartilages.

Before the advent of artificial pneumothorax, the prognosis of patients with severe laryngeal tuberculosis was extremely grave but this operation and the other surgical means of collapsing the lung which followed, greatly improved the outlook not only for the pulmonary disease but of the laryngeal infection. The laryngeal lesions were often found to recover even when the pulmonary ones did not, so that artificial pneumothorax came to be advocated as treatment for tuberculosis of the larynx as well as for tuberculosis of the lung (Scott Stevenson, 1933). An increasing number of cases were known, therefore, where recovery even from the severer forms of tuberculous laryngitis had occurred. These cases revealed the extent to which tuberculosis in this site heals by fibrosis, contracting scar tissue resulting often in severe deformity and stenosis.

On the occasions nowadays when tuberculosis of the larynx is diagnosed, full recovery on drug therapy, usually without significant scarring, can be expected. However, late cases still occur, usually in the remoter parts of the world, but sometimes elsewhere because the rarity of the disease causes it to be overlooked. These too are likely to be cured of the tuberculous infection but may not avoid the scars.

Laryngeal lupus

Lupus vulgaris of the face and nose has been known to spread back into the nasopharynx, sometimes involving the palate and, exceptionally, the larynx. The main features of the condition as it affects the nose are given in Volume 3.

Briefly, lupus vulgaris is an indolent tuberculous infection of the skin and mucosae, histologically identical with the usual form of tuberculosis. It is now a rare disease. Affecting females twice as often as males, it is confined in the majority of cases to the skin of the nares and the mucous membrane at the front of the nose. The diagnostic feature is the presence of apple-jelly nodules, pin-head sized red spots which do not blanch when compressed, for instance with a glass slide. It is slowly destructive, producing characteristically loss of the edges of the alae nasi and perforation of the cartilaginous part of the nasal septum.

It never occurs in the larynx except as the result of spread from the nose but it may be active in the larynx after the nasal lesion has healed. The free part of the epiglottis is the initial site of the laryngeal disease but from here it may spread along the aryepiglottic folds as far back as the arytenoids. It has been known to encroach onto the false cords. Ulceration results in more or less destruction, chiefly of the epiglottis.

It is painless, indeed often entirely symptomless, but examination of the larynx may be prompted by the nasal condition. Routine examination of the larynx has sometimes revealed the scarred evidence of the past disease.

Lupus is not likely to be confused with laryngeal tuberculosis principally because of its characteristic distribution, the absence of pulmonary disease and the presence of active or burnt-out lupus of the nose.

Spontaneous healing, but only after years, is the rule. If it is encountered in the active, treatment with anti-tuberculous drugs is indicated and can be expected to result in sound healing.

Laryngeal syphilis

Despite the fact that effective treatment for syphilis has been available for more than 30 years, the worldwide incidence of the disease has risen steadily since the late 1950s. However, year by year, the late manifestations have become increasingly less common and, thanks to the almost universal availability of ante-natal care, congenital syphilis is disappearing. In these days the majority of cases will be seen in the early, highly infectious secondary stage and it is at this stage that hoarseness and sore throat, evidence of laryngeal and pharyngeal involvement, may occur. However, it is entirely unusual for such cases to come the way of the laryngologist.

Aetiology and pathology

An account of the aetiology and pathology of syphilis in general is not called for here but certain points need to be made. The infecting organism, *Treponema pallidum*, becomes dispersed throughout the body within hours of the initial infection and therefore long before the appearance of the primary sore. The subsequent occurrence of lesions in the various systems is due to hypersensitivity which develops in different areas after varying intervals. The skin rash and mucosal ulceration of the secondary stage appear within 2–3 months, clearing up in the untreated case after a few weeks. However, mucocutaneous relapses are likely to occur, sometimes over years (Grimble, 1975). The late (tertiary) lesions emerge from the secondary stage from three to thirty or more years after infection and no system in the body is spared. A syphilitic infant born alive may show signs of early disease at birth but the mucosal manifestations including laryngitis do not appear before three weeks. In the congenital cases, tertiary lesions may occur early or not until as late as the seventh to twentieth year.

The treponemes gain access to the blood stream by way of the perivascular lymphatics where they excite a characteristic granulomatous reaction. Lymphocytes and plasma cells accumulate like a cuff around the vessel and excite swelling of the endothelium, sufficient to narrow or obstruct the lumen (obliterative endarteritis).

In late lesions necrosis occurs and giant cells appear though less plentifully than in tuberculosis. Fibroblasts proliferate, encapsulating the lesion which, when large, constitutes the gumma typical of the tertiary stage. Healing leads to the formation of dense scar tissue with distortion of the affected part.

Clinical features

The secondary stage of the acquired disease is usually a mild illness today. The appearance of the rash is often accompanied by sore throat but hoarseness is no longer common. When it occurs and the opportunity for examination is offered, the first sign is seen to be hyperaemia. This may be generalized as in simple laryngitis or patchy and uneven; for instance one cord may be affected only, as in tuberculous laryngitis. The 'mucous patches', typical of this stage and pathognomonic when seen in the mouth and pharynx, may be observed also in the larynx. The Jacksons writing in 1937 claim to have seen them often in this locality, usually on the vocal cords, sometimes on the anterior surface of the epiglottis and, in a few instances, on the ventricular bands. They appear as superficial smooth, pearl grey, oval areas with fine red margins and heal without scarring. Secondary lymphadenitis, often persisting for months, is an invariable finding. The same authors claim also to have found laryngitis present in every congenital case examined with 'snuffles' but the changes observed were limited to hyperaemia. Very few laryngologists in practice nowadays will have heard or be likely to hear the 'hoarse raucous cry' of the syphilitic infant once considered characteristic.

Late syphilis is becoming increasingly rare and in recent years isolated cases of gummatous laryngitis have been reported occasionally as curiosities (e.g. Ismail, 1966). Two sorts have been described; the once-familiar localized gumma, breaking down to form a painless, deep, punched-out ulcer with a gummy base resembling wash-leather in appearance; and gummatous infiltration producing a nodular appearance, either diffuse or localized, with a rather bluish colouration. The epiglottis is the favoured site but the disease may spread throughout the larynx though usually remaining asymmetrical.

The extent and quality of the voice change produced will depend on the site and extent of the lesion.

Diagnosis

In early syphilis the appearance of the rash and the mucosal ulcers together with the regional lymphadenitis will be diagnostic. In confirmation the organism may be identified in swabs taken from the mucous patches.

The late manifestations must be differentiated from tuberculosis and carcinoma. The Wasserman and Kahn tests have now given way to specific antibody tests, such as the TPI test (Treponema Immobilization) or serological investigation, the VDRL test (VD Reference Laboratory).

Treatment

Benzylpenicillin is the antibiotic of choice. It is given as a daily intramuscular injection, 900 000 units of procaine penicillin, for 10 days in the early case but for 14 days in the late case. If treatment is started in the sero-negative phase, that is within two weeks of infection, the outlook is uniformly good. However, cases of laryngeal syphilis will be diagnosed later, perhaps much later and the course may have to be repeated. Patients known to be allergic to penicillin may be treated with tetracycline or erythromycin.

Complications and prognosis

When gummata of the larynx occurred more frequently and before the introduction of antimicrobial treatment, secondary infection would from time to time lead to perichondritis and chondral necrosis. If and when healing finally took place, deformity of the larynx with a greater or lesser degree of laryngeal stenosis was the rule and such patients were sometimes doomed to wear a tracheostomy tube for the rest of their lives. With late syphilis of the larynx now rare and perichondritis even rarer, such cases are no longer met with. Nevertheless, marked cicatricial distortion of the laryngeal structures with some degree of upper airway obstruction may follow laryngeal gumma without the supervention of perichondritis, and cases with these features may still be found, particularly in the developing countries.

Leprosy of the larynx

Like tuberculosis and syphilis, leprosy is a chronic granulomatous infection which may on occasions spread to the larynx. To the European reader it is an exotic disease although at the end of the last century it was widespread in Europe particularly in Norway and Portugal. It remains a disease of first importance in many parts of the East, over large areas of Africa and in Central America. As with the other infective granulomata, the organism, in this case *Mycobacterium leprae*, becomes widely distributed throughout the body although in leprosy the systems chiefly affected are the skin and the peripheral nerves.

The cellular granulation tissue formed is mainly composed of large mononuclear cells having a pale, foamy appearance. They are often crowded with organisms and are known as lepra cells. There is no evidence of caseation or necrosis.

When mucosal involvement occurs it is the nose which is at first and often exclusively affected (*see* Volume 3) but in a proportion of these cases there is spread to the larynx, probably by way of the lymphatics. The only part to be at all commonly implicated is the epiglottis and sometimes the aryepiglottic folds. However, in advanced cases of the lepromatous form of the disease, the larynx may become more extensively infiltrated resulting in a degree of laryngeal obstruction.

The early laryngeal changes produce little in the way of symptoms and probably go undiagnosed. Voice changes indicate spread to the glottis and so must be looked upon as a feature of the well-established case. Dyspnoea and stridor are exceptional complications not only of the active lepromatous condition but also of the healed lesion. Healing as in the other granulomatous infections is accompanied by marked fibrosis and, in these cases, laryngeal stenosis.

The appearance of the larynx varies according to the extent and stage of the disease. Usually the epiglottis will be seen to be nodular and deformed. The early nodules look inflamed but later become pallid and may ulcerate. Healing occurs in one area while activity is present in another, rather as in laryngeal lupus. The scarred areas look conspicuously white. Not uncommonly, the epiglottis will have been altogether destroyed. Nodules and scarring elsewhere in the larynx are less often observed but will be a prominent feature of cases which have advanced to the stage of dyspnoea. The Jacksons (1937) point out the ease with which direct laryngoscopy may be undertaken since, they observed, the larynx and pharynx are typically anaesthetic.

D-amino-diphenysulphone (dapsone) given in increasing doses up to 300 mg weekly for as long as four years is the standard treatment but the management must be the responsibility of an expert and other drugs may be indicated. Rifampicin, used now for the treatment of tuberculosis, has been shown recently to be bactericidal against *M. leprae* and may have an important role in the future.

From time to time tracheostomy has to be undertaken for the relief of laryngeal obstruction.

Laryngeal scleroma

Scleroma is an unusual disease affecting chiefly the nose and indeed named rhinoscleroma by Hebra (1870) in his original description. It is endemic in Eastern Europe particularly but also in some countries bordering the Mediterranean, in parts of Asia and Africa and in Central America. Sporadic cases occur elsewhere but very rarely.

Aetiology and pathology

A more detailed account of these aspects will be found in the article in Volume 3, but, in summary, it occurs where there is a low standard of domestic hygiene and is considered to be due to infection with *Klebsiella rhinoscleromatis*. The characteristic lesion is a nodular granuloma found at the front of the nose but liable to spread slowly backwards to involve the sinuses and pharynx and sometimes the larynx and tracheobronchial tree.

Nothing has been published on the laryngeal disease in recent times but the older texts agree that although lesions may occur in any part of the larynx, the usual site is the subglottic region.

The tissues are at first indurated and considerable obstruction to the airway is mentioned. Crusts may form on the affected parts. Ulceration and offensive discharge, common in the nasal disease, seem not to occur in the larynx. As in the other infective granulomas, healing tends to occur with marked scarring and distortion.

Clinical features

The dominant symptoms and signs will be those of the nasal disease (*see* Volume 3), spread to the larynx being indicated by the onset of cough and hoarseness. Stridor and increasing dyspnoea, if they occur, are likely to be late manifestations. The expectoration of crusts has been mentioned.

Treatment

Treatment should not be commenced until the diagnosis has been confirmed by nasal biopsy. Successes have been claimed for prolonged courses of either streptomycin or tetracycline. Corticosteroids have been advocated as a means of lessening the risk of scarring. In the unlikely event of progressive dyspnoea, tracheostomy will have to be considered.

Maxwell Ellis, writing in the last edition of this book, described the submucosal resection of indurated tissue by the laryngofissure route as a means of improving the laryngeal airway in obstructed cases. An elective tracheostomy is necessary and a course of streptomycin and cortisone is advocated lasting a month or more. By this time, the disease being controlled and the laryngeal airway restored, the tracheostome may be allowed to close.

If indeed scleroma is a specific bacterial infection, it is most unlikely that it will continue to be a problem once the appropriate antibiotic has been identified.

The laryngeal mycoses

Of all the tens of thousands of fungi known to biologists, only a very few are parasitic in man and no more than ten are certainly responsible for disease of the larynx. Laryngeal mycosis is extremely rare even when all the varieties mentioned below are taken together. Certain of them, like coccidioidomycosis, will occur only in regions where the environment will support the saprophytic stage of the organism but travellers to such parts may contract the disease and present with it in non-endemic areas. Others, like candidosis (moniliasis) appear as opportunistic infections, breaking out when local or general resistance is lowered by some other illness or circumstance. Mycosis laryngis assumes particular importance when the organism invades the tissues deeply to produce a granuloma and mycotic granulomatous laryngitis, when it is exceptionally encountered, is likely to be mistaken at first for one or other of the infective granulomas described above. Often the larynx is involved as part of a disseminated infection which may add to the confusion.

The different kinds of laryngeal mycosis are mentioned below in alphabetical order to avoid the need to judge their relative significance.

Actinomycosis

It is a matter of debate whether the diseases caused by *Actinomyces bovis* and *Actinomyces israelii* should be considered as fungal or bacterial infections. These organisms belong to a species related to the mycobacteria (e.g. *M. tuberculosis* and *M. leprae*) invariably classified as bacteria. However, it is a time-honoured convention to speak of actinomycosis as a fungal disease and of the organism as the ray fungus.

It is difficult to ascertain how many cases of actinomycosis of the larynx have been confirmed but certainly the Jacksons described one in their treatise (1937), and a case of A. J. Wright is quoted by Thomson and Negus (1948). It has been stated that the disease is not a primary laryngeal infection but whether it is secondary to the rare cervico-facial variety due to *Actinomyces bovis* or the rather less rare respiratory variety due to *Actinomyces israelii*, the writer is not prepared to judge.

The Jacksons' case developed a granuloma on the left ventricular band and adjacent part of the epiglottis on which yellow spots ('sulphur granules') appeared. These proved to be clumps of the fungus.

Actinomycosis usually responds to penicillin but the treatment should be continued for several weeks.

Blastomycosis

This is another rare manifestation of a rare disease. Most of the cases have occurred in America and are presumably due to infection with *Blastomyces dermatitidis* (North American blastomycosis – although the organism is now known to be common throughout Africa also). The related disease due to *Cryptococcus neoformans*, a fungus distributed throughout the world, and *Paracoccidiodes brasiliensis* found in South America, may also be concerned.

These are true yeast-like fungi with a saprophytic phase in the soil. Infection of the lungs is by inhalation but the disease may become disseminated by the blood stream, foci appearing in any part of the body. The skin is regularly involved in infection with *Blastomyces dermatitidis* and the central nervous system in cryptococcosis.

Laryngeal blastomycosis is usually secondary to the pulmonary disease but has been thought sometimes to be primary (Jackson and Jackson, 1937). The lesion is granulomatous and likely to be confused either with tuberculosis of the larynx, particularly in view of the pulmonary involvement, or even with carcinoma.

The diagnosis is confirmed by biopsy, the histological preparation revealing tuberculoid granulomas within which the typical round, thick-walled fungal cells may be seen. Single buds protruding from parent cells are characteristic.

Treatment consists of amphotericin B given daily by intravenous infusion in increasing doses and in accordance with a strict protocol (*see* manufacturer's literature). The concomitant administration of 25–50 mg of hydrocortisone may be expected to control side-effects. Flucytosine has been used along with amphotericin B for its supposed synergistic effect.

Candidosis (moniliasis)

Infection of the mouth with the yeast-like fungus, *Candida albicans*, is a common condition in sick children and debilitated adults, particularly the elderly. It is popularly known as thrush, producing milky-white patches on the mucous membrane of the cheeks, tongue and palate. It often complicates the later stages of radiotherapy directed at neoplasms in these areas.

Rarely it may spread to the respiratory tract, infecting the lungs and, exceptionally the larynx. Perrone (1970) has described laryngeal obstruction in a neonate due to candida. It is unlikely to occur in the larynx except as the result of direct spread from extensive involvement of the mouth and pharynx and the present writer has treated such a case.

The diagnosis is suspected from the typical appearance and confirmed by the bacteriologist who is usually able to detect the organism in scrapings or swabs from the patches.

The anti-fungal agents, nystatin, amphotericin B and clotrimazole are all likely to be effective treatment, although resistance sometimes occurs. The first two of these are effective only locally and cannot be given systemically. In laryngeal candidosis, Nystatin Mixture BPC or Amphotericin Mixture should be sprayed into the larynx four times a day. A preparation of clotrimazole (Canesten) for oral administration and capable of producing therapeutic blood levels is on clinical trial.

Coccidioidomycosis

This uncommon condition due to a dimorphic fungus, *Coccidioides immittis*, is endemic in the seaboard region of the south-western United States where the critical environmental conditions for the survival of the saprophytic form of the organism obtain. It is called San Joaquin Valley fever after the valley in Southern California where it is particularly prevalent. It is an important disease because of its high infectivity and because the desert areas where it occurs are popular holiday locations. Thus visitors become infected and return with the condition to their homes as far away as Western Europe. Recently, four cases have been reported where the disease presented in the larynx, and the possibility that laryngeal involvement is more common than previously supposed suggests itself (Ward *et al.*, 1977).

The spores of the fungus are inhaled in dust and set up a primary pulmonary focus in susceptible individuals. The primary infection may be symptomless or it may cause a fever, typically accompanied by erythema nodosum.

The secondary disseminated form of the disease is uncommon and may present as a single lesion or as multiple lesions in almost any part of the body. In the larynx the extent and distribution of the granulomatous changes are variable. The appearance in the more florid case has been reported to resemble carcinoma; that in the less extensive examples, tuberculosis of the larynx. Even where the infection is endemic and the cause suspected, the diagnosis will be made only as the result of laboratory investigations, including skin sensitivity tests and serological tests. Where the true diagnosis is not suspected, biopsy is likely to be resorted to and will reveal a granulomatous type of inflammation which may or may not be diagnostic. If the sporangium of the fungus – a spherical structure packed with spores – is observed, however, the diagnosis is likely to be apparent.

The treatment of the disseminated case is with amphotericin B, bearing in mind the need to observe the strict precautions mentioned in the section on blastomycosis. Amphotericin B is a very toxic antibiotic and in children must be used only when the extent of systemic dissemination justifies it.

Histoplasmosis

The common variety of histoplasmosis due to infection with the yeast-like diphasic *Histoplasma capsulatum* is another fungal disease endemic in areas which favour the existence of the saprophytic form of the organism. This proliferates in dust enriched by bird and bat droppings. The disease is endemic in many parts of North America, particularly in the valleys of the Ohio and Mississippi rivers but also in parts of Central and South America, Africa and Asia.

Like coccidioidomycosis (q.v.), the disease is caused by inhaling dust containing the spores and the majority of those infected develop a subclinical infection. A primary focus occurs in the lungs from which the infection is disseminated by the blood stream widely throughout the body. Generally these foci heal uneventfully but in about one per cent of cases symptomatic manifestations appear (Schwarz, 1971). Some of these patients become gravely, even fatally ill. Among the lesions of the serious, disseminated form of the disease are granulomatous ulcers in the larynx. Biopsy specimens are likely to show histiocytes containing the typical fungal cells, often in large numbers.

The difficulty of differential diagnosis from other granulomatous lesions, particularly tuberculosis, or even from carcinoma, arises from the fact that when patients infected abroad develop clinical histoplasmosis in countries where the disease is not endemic (e.g. in Europe) it is unlikely to be suspected.

Treatment is with amphotericin B as for blastomycosis and coccidioidomycosis. The dangers of this toxic antibiotic are mentioned earlier (p. 413).

Leptothricosis

Among the common commensals found frequently in the mouth is a fungus named *Leptothrix buccalis*. It was sometimes regarded in the past as responsible for the disease called keratosis pharyngis although when present in the lesions of this disease it is almost certainly saprophytic and non-pathogenic. The same is probably true when the organism is occasionally found in the larynx in association with a similar kind of keratosis.

Rhinosporidiosis

As the name implies, this is typically a nasal mycosis and an account of it will be found in Volume 3. Briefly, it is an exophytic infective granuloma caused by *Rhinosporidium seeberi*. It is a common disease in Sri Lanka and in Kerala, in Southern India, but occurs also in Central and South America. Neither its source nor the route of infection is known with certainty, although the inhalation of contaminated dust is suspected. Involvement of the larynx is secondary to the disease in the nose and post-nasal space and must be exceptionally rare.

Two cases, claimed to be the first on record, were described by Radhakrishna Pillai in 1974. Both gave a history of nasal obstruction going back many years and a more recent history of voice change and slight dyspnoea. Both sides of the nose were totally obstructed by the characteristic polypoid masses and the mass in the post-nasal space could be seen hanging down into the oropharynx. A similar lesion was found in the larynx in each case. It arose from the neighbourhood of the ventricular band on one side and hung down below the vocal cords. The 'polyps' measured some 1.5 × 1.5 cm and were pedunculated with a lobular and rather papilliferous structure.

The lesions in the larynx as well as those in the nose and nasopharynx were successfully avulsed with symptomatic relief.

Histologically, the granulomatous tissue consists mainly of lymphocytes and plasma cells with, here and there, fungus cells (rhinosporidial spherules) and occasionally the unmistakable, very large spherical sporangium. A remarkable micro-photograph may be seen in the chapter by Friedmann and Osborn on the nose and nasal sinuses in Symmer's *Systemic Pathology* (1976).

Sporotrichosis

This is an occupational disease of professional nurserymen, florists and gardeners, usually confined to the skin but rarely disseminating to other regions. Baum *et al.* (1969) have described pulmonary sporotrichosis and Eggston and Wolff (1947) state that its occurrence in the larynx may be mistaken for tuberculosis.

It is caused by *Sporotrichium schenckii*, a biphasic fungus with a yeast-like form in the tissues of the body. The saprophytic form, a mould, grows on a variety of plants, especially thorny bushes. The spores are present in the soil. The skin may be infected when pricked or scratched by infected thorns producing sores, often widespread and obstinately chronic. It may occur as a primary pulmonary disease with apical cavitation, presumably from inhaling infected dust.

The typical lesion is a granuloma, liable to undergo caseation and rarely revealing the causative organism. However, this may be cultured from biopsy specimens and sometimes from the sputum or gastric aspirate. Its pathogenicity may be demonstrated by animal inoculation.

Amphotericin B is specific treatment but it must be employed with care as mentioned earlier.

The larynx in some chronic diseases of uncertain aetiology

The larynx is found to be affected more or less infrequently in a number of chronic diseases, usually systemic in distribution, where the aetiology is obscure. It is not possible to assert that they are inflammatory diseases and that the laryngeal involvement is strictly laryngitis, and yet it may be argued that these important conditions are better considered here than elsewhere. A measure of justification of this is the fact that the basic pathological process in at least two or three of the diseases to be considered is a granulomatous reaction strikingly similar to that found in the infective granulomas considered previously.

Sarcoidosis of the larynx

Sarcoidosis typifies the problem of classification referred to above. It resembles tuberculosis in so many ways that it has been called 'non-caseating tuberculosis'. However, tubercle bacilli are never found, the Mantoux test is frequently negative and the disease does not respond to anti-tuberculous drugs. Many explanations of its true nature have been advanced but they are only theories.

It is a chronic granulomatous disease, the typical lesion being a tubercle like that of tuberculosis. Epithelioid cells and multinucleate giant cells containing refractive bodies are constant features but even when large the tubercles rarely show caseation. The active process tends to heal by fibrosis and hyalinization.

Sometimes one organ only may be affected but as a rule the disease is widely disseminated. Every system in the body has been known to become involved but the lungs, skin, eyes and bones, particularly the bones of the extremities, are the common sites.

Often there is little or no constitutional upset although a fairly frequent mode of onset comprises fever, bilateral hilar lymphadenopathy, erythema nodosum and arthropathy of the wrists, knees and ankles. The illness is characterized by its chronicity and the occurrence of relapses, first in one system, then another. In the majority of cases it resolves spontaneously over many years and leaves little if any disability.

The question of laryngeal involvement has been studied very thoroughly by Devine (1965). The incidence has been differently assessed in different reported series but seems likely to be in the region of 3–5 cases per 100.

The true cords are infrequently affected, the supraglottic structures and occasionally the subglottis being the usual sites invaded. Consequently, changes need to be considerably advanced before the voice is much affected and the earliest symptom is likely to be a degree of dyspnoea. When there is considerable huskiness, nocturnal stridor or dyspnoea on exertion, paralysis of one or both recurrent laryngeal nerves may be discovered.

The reports of the appearance of the larynx on laryngoscopy are consistent and describe pale, diffuse oedema-like thickening of the affected parts, chiefly the epiglottis, aryepiglottic folds and arytenoid eminences. Rarely the same sort of change has been observed in the subglottis. Nodular and polypoid changes have also been noted.

The diagnosis will rest on the demonstration of non-caseating granulomatous infiltration of biopsy material but confirmation may be had from the history of suggestive incidents from the past, such as erythema nodosum, migratory polyarthritis or some other spontaneously remitting occurrence. The typical changes of present or past disease may be found on chest x-ray or on x-ray of the hands or feet. Some laboratories may be able to undertake the skin test described by Kveim *et al.* (1957). Not uncommonly, however, the diagnosis is reached or considered only after the exclusion of other less rare chronic granulomatous diseases, such as tuberculosis, syphilis, histoplasmosis and so on. Amyloidosis, myxoedema and lipoid proteinosis may produce changes resembling laryngeal sarcoidosis.

There is no known specific treatment for sarcoidosis although the use of corticosteroids produces marked regression of symptoms and signs. However, these may return if the treatment is suspended so that most clinicians reserve this therapy for the more serious cases.

Tracheostomy has been necessary for the relief of increasing obstruction of the laryngeal airway (five out of Devine's eight cases). Surgical removal of polypoid or nodular masses may be indicated and Devine reports the use of steroids injected directly into the swollen laryngeal tissues.

Wegener's granulomatosis

This disease is considered at length in Volume 3 under the heading 'Non-healing granuloma'. It is the Wegener type of this destructive granulomatous disorder that may occasionally involve the larynx (Friedmann, 1964). Its aetiology is controversial but Friedmann makes out a case for regarding it as an auto-immune disease analogous to systemic lupus erythematosus.

Although the lesion is usually present in the nose and cases commonly present with nasal bleeding and crusting, a form of periarteritis (polyarteritis nodosa) affects the vasculature of the lungs, kidneys and other organs and is responsible for the systemic nature of the disease.

The principal histopathological features include multinucleate giant cells and fibrinoid necrosis of the small arteries and arterioles.

It occurs in young or middle-aged men and women and is likely to run a fatal course terminating in respiratory or renal failure.

The onset of hoarseness in such a case will suggest laryngeal involvement and direct examination will confirm the extent and usually the nature of the granulomatous changes.

The treatment is considered in Volume 3. It is now generally agreed that the essence of effective therapy is immuno-suppression, whether by the corticosteroids or by such drugs as azathioprine (Imuran) and cyclophosphamide. Frequently the steroids will be administered together with the cytotoxic agent chosen. Successes have been claimed where the treatment has been persisted with for long periods. In large centres with a specialist in immunology on the staff, his help should be sought before treatment is planned.

Rheumatoid arthritis

The estimate of the incidence of laryngeal involvement in this crippling disease varies but it may be as high as 25–30 per cent (Grossman, Martin and Root, 1961; Lofgren and Montgomery, 1962). When it is considered that between one and three per cent of the population suffer from rheumatoid arthritis, it will be seen that 'laryngitis' from this cause is not an uncommon condition.

Rheumatoid arthritis (rheumatoid disease) is a systemic disease of unknown cause in which the predominance and magnitude of the articular manifestations make it easy to overlook its frequently widespread nature. There is usually found diffuse necrotizing arteritis indistinguishable from polyarteritis nodosa, and the lungs, heart, skin, muscles and nerves are all involved from time to time.

Wolman, Darke and Young (1965) studied the larynx *post-mortem* in eight cases of advanced rheumatoid arthritis; all but one had complained of dyspnoea and stridor; dysphagia was present in two. Changes were found not only in the crico-arytenoid joints but, significantly, also in the laryngeal muscles. The joint changes consisted of marked thickening of the synovial membrane, as the result of infiltration by chronic inflammatory cells, and erosion of the adjoining articular surfaces of both cricoid and arytenoid cartilages. However, there was no ankylosis and, although movement was restricted, the arytenoids remained mobile in all cases. The myopathy was particularly interesting and was considered to be the result of rheumatoid neuropathy and secondary muscular atrophy. The essential lesion was thought to be arteritis of the vasa nervorum. Indirect laryngoscopy in these cases will reveal more or less redness and swelling adjacent to the arytenoid cartilages together with a degree of impaired mobility.

The classical basis for differentiation from recurrent laryngeal nerve paralysis, that is the demonstration of crico-arytenoid ankylosis at direct laryngoscopy, would not seem to be valid therefore, but rheumatoid disease of the larynx will be seen only when the other evidence of rheumatoid arthritis is advanced and the patient long under treatment for it. Crico-arytenoid ankylosis occurs as the result of previous severe infections such as syphilis or tuberculosis often with consequent perichondritis or chondral necrosis or may follow various kinds of trauma. The history should be diagnostic. Gout is sometimes cited as a cause of crico-arytenoid swelling and even ankylosis, but such cases must be very rare today.

The treatment is that of the generalized disease and should be undertaken by a rheumatologist. No attempt will be made to summarize it here. If, rarely, dyspnoea is progressive and adequate respiratory exchange threatened, tracheostomy may have to be considered.

The larynx in certain severe skin diseases

The justification for referring in a chapter on chronic laryngitis to the following rare conditions is that the lesions are of an inflammatory kind and that it may be considered that they fit better here than elsewhere.

Scleroderma

Like rheumatoid arthritis this is a connective tissue (collagen) disease of uncertain aetiology, often systemic and progressive and in which arterial lesions, like those of Wegener's granulomatosis and rheumatoid arthritis, also occur. The skin is chiefly involved but the mucous membranes, for instance of the mouth and oesophagus, may also be affected. Laryngeal lesions have been described presenting as firm white plaques somewhat depressed beneath the general level, for instance on the ventricular bands or aryepiglottic folds. The aim of treatment is the preservation of function since nothing has been found to alter the course of the disease significantly.

Pemphigus vulgaris

This is now regarded as an auto-immune disease characterized by a bullous eruption of the skin and mucous membranes with a relatively high incidence in people of Jewish and Mediterranean ancestry. The oropharynx and larynx are involved at some stage in 50 per cent of cases. The lesions in the larynx are not always seen in the bullous stage, the rupture of the blister leaving a shallow ulcer – an erosion – covered with yellow fibrinous exudate. Bullae and erosion may coexist, eventually healing but only to recur at irregular intervals. The almost uniform mortality that once attended such cases has been remarkably changed since the use of corticosteroids. Large doses are necessary and often for a long time.

Epidermolysis bullosa

Epidermolysis bullosa is a rare hereditary disorder with either autosomal dominant or recessive inheritance. The former variety tends to produce only slight mucosal lesions whereas in the latter the mucous membranes are extensively involved. The disease appears soon after birth and the severe dystrophic cases do not survive. It is characterized by extensive blistering of the skin and sometimes of the mucosae which may leave the affected surfaces denuded of epithelium.

Golding-Wood (1963) has described granulomatous lesions resembling plasmacytomas arising in the mouths and larynxes of two affected children.

Once again, the use of corticosteroids has dramatically improved the prognosis.

References

Auerbach, O., Hammond, E. C. and Garfinkel, L. (1970). *Cancer*, **25**, 92

Baum, G. L., Donnerberg, R. L., Stewart, D., Mulligan, W. J. and Putnam, L. R. (1969) *New England Journal of Medicine*, **280**, 410

Blegvad, N. Rh. (1937). *Proceedings of the Royal Society of Medicine*, **30**, 221

Dedo, H. H. (1976). *Transactions of the American Academy of Ophthalmology and Otolaryngology*, **82**, 91

Devine, K. D. (1965). *Laryngoscope*, **75**, 533

Eggston, A. A. and Wolff, D. (1947). *Histopathology of the Ear, Nose and Throat*, The Williams and Wilkins Co., Baltimore

Fitz-Hugh, G. S., Smith, D. E. and Chiang, A. T. (1958). *Laryngoscope*, **68**, 855

Friedmann, I. (1964). *Proceedings of the Royal Society of Medicine*, **57**, 289

Friedmann, I. and Osborn, D. A. (1976). In: *Systemic Pathology*, (Ed. W. St. C. Symmers) 2nd edn; Churchill-Livingstone, Edinburgh

Golding-Wood, P. H. (1963). *Proceedings of the Royal Society of Medicine*, **56**, 890

Grimble, A. S. (1975). In: *Conybeare's Textbook of Medicine* (Ed. W. N. Mann); Churchill-Livingstone, Edinburgh

Grossman, A., Martin, J. R. and Root, H. S. (1961). *Laryngoscope*, **71**, 530

Hajek, M. (1925/6). *Zeitschrift der Halsen Nasen-Ohrenheilkliniken*, **13**, 161

Hebra, F. (1870). *Wiener medizinische Wochenschrift*, **20**, 1

Hünermann, Th. (1958). *Zeitschrift der Laryngologie und Rhinologie*, **37**, 182

Ismail, H. K. (1966). *Proceedings of the Royal Society of Medicine*, **80**, 638

Jackson, Chevalier (1928). *Annals of Otology, Rhinology and Laryngology*, **37**, 227

Jackson, Chevalier and Jackson, Chevalier L. (1937). *The Larynx and its Diseases*; Saunders, Philadelphia and London

Kleinsasser, O. (1963) *Zeitschrift der Laryngologie und Rhinologie*, **42**, 339

Kleinsasser, O. (1968). *Microlaryngoscopy and Endolaryngeal Microsurgery*; Saunders, Philadelphia and London

Kveim, A. (1957). Cited by Nelson, C. Y. and Schwimmer, B., *Journal of Investigative Dermatology*, **28**, 55

Lofgren, R. H. and Montgomery, W. W. (1962). *New England Journal of Medicine*, **267**, 193

Mackenzie, Morrell (1880). *A Manual of Diseases of the Throat and Nose*; Churchill-Livingstone, Edinburgh

McGavran, M. H., Bauer, W. C. and Ogura, J. H. (1960). *Laryngoscope*, **70**, 932

Norris, C. M. and Peale, A. R. (1963). *Journal of Laryngology*, **77**, 635

Norton, M. L., Strong, M. S., Vaughan, C. W., Snow, J. C. and Kripke, B. J. (1976). *Annals of Otology, Rhinology and Laryngology*, **85**, 650

Ormerod, F. C. (1939). *Tuberculosis of the Upper Respiratory Tracts*; John Bale Co., London

Ormerod, F. C. (1950). *Proceedings of the Royal Society of Medicine*, **43**, 1099

Perrone, J. A. (1970). *Laryngoscope*, **80**, 288

Radhakrishna Pillai, O. S. (1974). *Journal of Laryngology*, **88**, 277

Reinke, F. (1895) *Fortschritte der Medizin*, **13**, 469

Ryan, R. F., McDonald, J. R. and Devine, K. D. (1955). *Archives of Pathology, Chicago*, **60**, 472

Schwarz, J. (1971). In: *Human Infection with Fungi, Actinomyces and Algae* (Ed. R. D. Baker); Springer, New York, Heidelberg, Berlin

Scott Stevenson, R. (1933). *British Medical Journal*, 2, 960

Scott Stevenson, R. (1935). *Recent Advances in Otolaryngology*; J. & A. Churchill Ltd., London

Senturia, B. H. and Wilson, F. B. (1969). Cited by McWilliams, B. J., Bluestone, C. D. and Musgrave, R. H., *Laryngoscope*, **79,** 2072

Stell, P. M. and McLaughlin, M. P. (1976). *Clinical Otolaryngology*, **1,** 265

Thomson, Sir St. Clair (1924). 'Tuberculosis of the larynx; etc.', *Medical Research Council Special Report Series*, No. 83

Thomson, Sir St. Clair and Negus, V. E. (1948).

Diseases of the Nose and Throat, 5th edn; Cassell, London

Toohill, R. J. (1975). *Archives of Otolaryngology*, **101,** 591

Urban, G. E. Jr. (1976). *Southern Medical Journal*, **69,** 828

Virchow, R. (1860). *Allgemeine medizinische Centralzeitung*, **29,** 760

Ward, P. H., Berci, G. Morledge, D. and Schwartz, H. (1977). *Annals of Otology, Rhinology and Laryngology*, **86,** 655

Wolman, L., Darke, C. S. and Young, A. (1965). *Journal of Laryngology*, **79,** 403

15 Tumours of the larynx
Henry Shaw

Benign tumours

Simple laryngeal tumours are not uncommon, occurring in an approximate ratio of 2:3 with malignant lesions in adult males, while in women the ratio is reversed. It is, however, important to note that the great majority of cordal benign 'tumours' are non-neoplastic, usually in a ratio of about 6:1, thus emphasizing the comparative rarity of true benign neoplasms at this site. Statistics given by Friedmann (1974) are illustrated in *Table 15.1*.

Table 15.1 **Benign tumours of the larynx seen at the Institute of Laryngology and Otology, London 1948–69**

Non-neoplastic		*Neoplastic*	
Vocal cord polyps	1122	Papilloma*	170*
Retention cysts	72	Adenoma	16
Tuberculous granuloma	44	Chondroma	3
Intubation granuloma	18	Miscellaneous (includes	16
Contact ulcer granuloma	14	fibroma, haemangioma, lipoma,	
Amyloid deposit	13	and neuro-fibroma)	
Wegeners' granuloma	8		
Granular cell myoblastoma	6		
Miscellaneous	3		
Total	1300 (86%)	Total	205 (14%)

* Approximately 25 per cent were multiple juvenile papillomas.

In the larynx simple tumours exhibit certain anomalous features which must be carefully noted. There is often difficulty in deciding clinically whether a swelling is neoplastic, inflammatory, degenerate or traumatic in nature, and even histological appearances may be confusing.

A swelling which appears clinically to be a simple fibroma, may on histology, prove to be a tuberculoma; while a cordal haematoma due to vocal abuse may organize and develop into a fibro-angioma on histological examination.

Following the use of endotracheal anaesthetic tubes, especially after a prolonged operation, small granulomas may sometimes arise on the vocal processes of the arytenoids. If they are not removed at an early stage they may later closely resemble a typical fibroma on section.

Again, the common bilateral condition of 'singer's nodules' is certainly due to misuse of the voice and may disappear with complete rest of the voice, but histological appearances may range from simple polypoid degeneration of the cordal margin through vascular fibrous tissue to what is impossible to differentiate from a true fibroma.

Symptoms

The location and size of the tumour will mainly determine the presence and type of symptoms. Small swellings or even those of some size in areas such as the outer side of the aryepiglottic folds or around the epiglottis, may produce no symptoms and may only be discovered accidentally on routine inspection of the larynx.

Tumours large enough to displace muscle fibres may cause a feeling of discomfort in the throat, especially on speaking or swallowing, and also variable alterations in the timbre of the voice.

Since the majority of simple tumours are found on the vocal cords, hoarseness will be an early symptom in many cases. Quite a small tumour in the anterior commissure or a small sessile swelling on the cordal margin may cause marked dysphonia, whereas a larger but pedunculated tumour on the upper or lower cord surfaces can be displaced upward or downward on phonation and may produce only slight weakness of the voice or intermittent hoarseness.

Pain as opposed to discomfort is a rare symptom, as also is dysphagia. An irritating or paroxysmal cough sometimes occurs with pedunculated tumours. Dyspnoea and stridor are predominant symptoms in the more bulky benign tumours, especially in multiple papillomas of childhood and, more rarely, with large chondromas or adenomas in the adult.

Diagnosis

After consideration of the history this can usually be made by simple inspection with a laryngeal mirror or fibre-optic laryngoscope. However, confirmation of the diagnosis by histological examination must be sought whenever possible.

Direct laryngoscopy

This technique remains the essential means of performing any intralaryngeal operation, especially where tissue must be removed for biopsy. In young children where mirror examination of the larynx is usually impossible, there should be no hesitation in proceeding to direct laryngoscopy under general anaesthesia, both for establishing a diagnosis and very often for regular treatment of multiple papillomas.

Micro-laryngoscopy

During the past ten years the technique of direct inspection under general anaesthesia has been taken a stage further in the interests of greater accuracy of observation and surgical precision. Kleinsasser (1965) adapted the Zeiss operating microscope, fitted with a 400 mm objective lens to work with wide calibre tapered laryngoscopes of his own design and held in place by a suspension system supported on the patient's anterior chest wall. General anaesthesia with relaxants and a small calibre endotracheal tube are employed.

The method has proved extremely successful, being also particularly useful for endoscopic photography and accurate surgical manipulations within the larynx. Both hands of the surgeon are free to work with a special set of small instruments designed for use under magnification.

Earlier investigators have also given thought to developments of this kind and it was Broyles of Baltimore (1941) who first linked a fibre-optic lighting system with built-in (× 6) magnification to an anterior commissure pattern laryngoscope.

Both of these refinements in the basic technique of direct laryngoscopy have a valuable application and also some limitations. In certain aspects they are complementary, the Kleinsasser method being invaluable for photography and operative intervention but having problems in application to the 'anatomically difficult' throat, whereas the Broyles' instrument is ideal for inspection of the 'difficult' throat, but less suitable for surgical intervention other than simple biopsy. Other instruments of this type are also available.

Papillomas

These are the most common true benign neoplasms in the larynx; even so they are relatively infrequent. In the large Mayo Clinic series of benign laryngeal tumours (New and Erich, 1938) they formed approximately 25 per cent of the total; whereas Winston and Epstein (1958) give their incidence as roughly 10 per cent (*Table 15.1*). They may be single or multiple. The solitary types are more common in adults and the multiple more frequent in children. Of 39 cases reported by the latter authors 31 were single and in adults (*Plate 5a, e* and *f, facing page 432*), and 8 were multiple and in children (*Plate 6a, facing page 432*).

Solitary papillomas

These usually grow from the edge of the vocal cord in its anterior two-thirds, but they may also arise from the ventricular band or subglottic region. They are twice as common in males and are most frequent in the 30–50 age group.

Sites of occurrence
When pedunculated and growing from the edge of the vocal cord, papillomas may be difficult to see on quiet respiration because they hang down into the subglottic region.

However, on phonation they are immediately displaced upward and may then appear to lie on the upper surface of the cord (*Plate 5e* and *f, facing page 432*).

They occasionally arise in the anterior commissure but are very rarely found growing from the posterior part of the larynx. They range from pink to deep red in colour with a warty or papillary surface and vary in size from a millet seed to a walnut (*Figure 15.1*). In the condition called 'pachydermia of the larynx' there may be multiple areas of hypertrophy of the posterior part of the cord and the interarytenoid region. These areas of papillary keratosis are very similar in appearance to papillomas and often most difficult to distinguish histologically.

Treatment

If small, removal is easily accomplished by using sharp cup forceps with direct laryngoscopy. The use of micro-laryngoscopy can be most helpful in treating many of these small tumours. The occasional large papilloma may require careful excision via the laryngofissure approach.

Danger of recurrence

If removal is incomplete, a small proportion of solitary papillomas will recur. A further and more serious feature is a definite tendency for a small number, probably not more than three or four per cent of these tumours, to undergo eventual malignant change. Winston and Epstein (1958) found definite carcinoma in only one of the 31

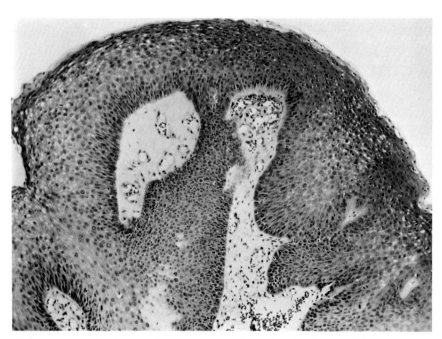

Figure 15.1   Massive but regular squamous cell proliferation in a papilloma with intact basement membrane. (× 160, reduced to three-quarters on reproduction)

adult papillomas they described, but gradations of cell atypia in several others may well be significant. All tissue removed from the cords must therefore be subjected to microscopic scrutiny.

Multiple juvenile papillomas

These interesting tumours, by reason of their multiplicity, tendency to spontaneous regression and alleged response to the tetracyclines have, by analogy with the common infective wart, a suspected viral aetiology (Holinger, Johnson and Anison, 1950).

In 1956, Bjork and Weber claimed to have produced clinical evidence of this and also of a possibly significant amino-acid dietary deficiency in their patients. Inclusion bodies have also been demonstrated. Further support for a viral aetiology comes from a number of more recent authors, notably Szpunar (1977).

The tumours appear in childhood chiefly between the ages of 5 and 15 but may commence in infancy. Their incidence is about equal in the sexes and there is generally a tendency to regression at puberty or before (*Plate 6a, facing page 432* and *Figure 15.2*). Although uncommon, they make a regular appearance in ENT Clinics

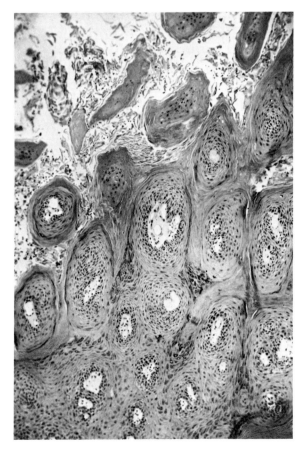

Figure 15.2 Papilloma of childhood showing papillary processes surrounded by whorls of desquamating keratin. (× 125, reduced to three-quarters on reproduction)

and in the recent decade 1968–78, 30 cases were seen and treated at the Royal National Throat, Nose and Ear Hospital in London.

Danger of recurrence

Unfortunately these tumours show a tendency to recur with spread to almost any site in the larynx, pharynx or trachea. Sometimes they may also reach an external tracheostomy orifice. Histologically, unlike adult papillomas they normally show no tendency to become malignant however frequently removed. Even so, Capps (1957) quoted three cases of a laryngeal cancer in adults who had suffered recurrent papillomas in childhood. All had had irradiation to their larynges in childhood with subsequent malignant change 18–20 years later.

Further resemblance to skin warts is shown by their sudden spontaneous disappearance after years of recurrence. Since this may occur about puberty and because of the natural limitation of the disease it is very desirable to damage the mucosa as little as possible by surgical intervention.

Treatment

The principal method of treatment remains that of micro-surgical excision by 'scalping' with sharp cup forceps (Szpunar, 1977) or by a diathermy/suction technique, also under microscopy (Pracy, 1970). Such intervention should always be conservative, requiring repeated sessions at appropriate intervals.

Medical treatment using tetracyclines (Holinger, Johnson and Anison, 1950), systemic hormones, bovine wart vaccine (Moffitt, 1959) and especially autogenous papilloma vaccine (Gross and Hubbard, 1974), have been useful in a number of cases. In attempts to stimulate cellular immunity the use of transfer factor has lately been advocated (Quick et al., 1975).

Local applications

Caustics such as silver nitrate or podophyllin are traditional and have been at times helpful (Holinger, Johnson and Anison, 1950). Painting with oestrogens after removal is also historical (Broyles, 1941) and still advocated (Szpunar, 1977). Recently the application of the anti-viral agent idoxuridine after micro-surgical removal has been reported (Bone et al., 1976; Cook et al., 1973).

Ultra-sound. This method of treatment has been claimed to have some success with repeated applications (Birck and Manhart, 1962; Fairman, 1972).

Cryosurgery. Destruction of the papillomas by this technique is also under trial (Miller, 1973).

Irradiation. This is mentioned only to be condemned as being completely unjustified (Capps, 1957). The tumours are seldom radio-sensitive and the risks of later malignant change are very great.

Tracheostomy must be carried out without hesitation if indicated. It should always be placed low, about the 4th tracheal ring, being sited as far as possible from the papillomas. It may be required for some months or even years and a decision to decannulate should not be made until months have elapsed after the last recurrence has been successfully removed. A speaking valve will generally be fitted to the inner tube.

Fibromas

The true neoplasm, as distinct from a fibrous polyp or node, is rare. Stewart (1957) found only nine cases over a 12-year period at the Royal Infirmary, Edinburgh. In a nine-year survey at the Royal National Throat, Nose and Ear Hospital, London (*Table 15.1*) only eight were reported. It may occur in any age group, but mainly in adults between the ages of 30 and 50, and most commonly on the edge of the vocal cord at the junction of the middle and anterior thirds (*Plate 5b, facing page 432*). However, they may also occur at any other laryngeal site. Off the cords they may well go undetected owing to their small size and the absence of symptoms.

Treatment

They are usually round, firm, smooth and sessile. Their treatment is by complete endoscopic removal with suitable forceps under general anaesthesia.

Cysts

Those cysts that have origin within the larynx may be usefully divided into:

(1) True cysts, having a secretory lining epithelium of columnar or cubical cells interspersed with goblet cells, as in congenital cysts and the retention cysts of seromucinous glands.
(2) Pseudocysts, due to degeneration of simple tumours such as polypi or fibromas, and those due to trauma such as lymph or blood cysts.

Congenital cysts

Congenital cysts are very rare. New and Erich (1938) reported only one out of 35 laryngeal cysts of all types. They conclude that these cysts originate from a sequestration of embryonic cells in the saccule or appendix of the laryngeal ventricle. It is also possible that some of them are of branchiogenic origin from the third branchial pouch (Wilson, 1955). Among laryngeal tumours they are relatively rare, and most likely to be encountered in early infancy. Asherson (1957) refers to the congenital cyst as 'a benign lesion which belies its deadly nature'. They are most commonly diagnosed *post-mortem* and their sinister repute gives emphasis to the importance of early endoscopic examination in all cases of infantile stridor. These cysts are found even less frequently in adults, and by this time they tend to be larger, sometimes extending through the thyrohyoid membrane into the anterior triangle of the neck.

Retention cysts

Retention cysts of seromucinous glands are easily the most common. They form the great majority of all adult cysts and at least 50 per cent are located on or adjacent to the epiglottis, although they are sometimes found in the ventricles and on the ventricular bands or aryepiglottic folds (*Plates 5c, and 6f, facing page 432*). They are typically lined by columnar epithelium, and are thin-walled, smooth, submucous, translucent grey swellings compared with congenital cysts which are deeper, have thicker walls and are therefore less easy to identify (*Figure 15.3*). In young children they can also be extremely dangerous, although perhaps less so than the congenital variety.

Pseudocysts

Pseudocysts, whether due to simple tumour degeneration or traumatic implantation, and blood or lymph cysts are also rare. They may occur in any part of the larynx, although the vocal cords and immediately adjacent areas are the more frequent sites. They are usually small and their differential diagnosis presents little difficulty if there is an accurate history.

Symptoms and signs usually point to airway obstruction of variable degree in childhood, often with added huskiness or stridorous 'cry'. In adults interference with the airway may well be apparent but hoarseness and a fluctuant swelling in the anterior triangle of the neck may also be found.

Diagnosis and treatment should always be prompt owing to their great potential danger. Endoscopic inspection and diagnosis followed by marsupialization, using diathermy, or removal by snare excision, may be effective in children. External removal via pharyngotomy or thyrotomy is sometimes required in adults.

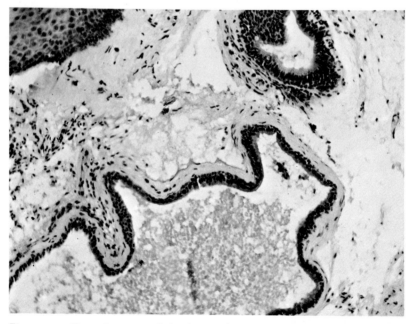

Figure 15.3 Retention cyst of the larynx lined by columnar epithelium with occasional goblet cells. (× 160, reduced to three-quarters on reproduction)

Laryngocoele

Essentially a laryngocoele is an air-filled sac – neither a cyst nor a tumour. It may, however, become a 'pseudo-cyst' after its neck is obliterated by inflammatory changes, and it may mimic neoplasm by causing voice changes together with visible swelling in the supraglottic larynx, vallecula, or anterior triangle of the neck.

This rare dilatation of the ventricular saccule of the larynx is usually found in adult males, particularly in glass blowers and players of wind instruments. Although the laryngeal saccule is vestigial in man, it is dilated to form an air sac in many of the higher apes and other mammals; these air sacs are expansile and it is believed that they are used for re-breathing of air at times of physical stress (Negus, 1949).

Laryngocoeles may project internally into the larynx as a swelling beneath the ventricular band and aryepiglottic fold resembling a cyst; or alternatively, they present as external subcutaneous swellings in the subhyoid region, having expanded through the thyrohyoid membrane (*Figure 15.4*). They are often bilateral and can be seen and felt to bulge on coughing or performing the Valsalva manoeuvre (*Figure 15.5*), but completely disappear on pressure. They can be demonstrated radiologically by taking an x-ray during forcible Valsalva expiration. Differential diagnosis of the internal variety from ventricular cysts must be considered.

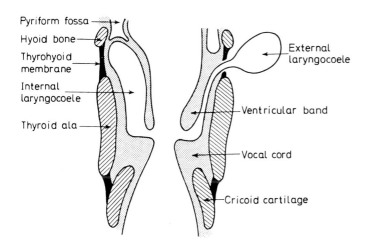

Figure 15.4 Laryngocoeles. (From Simpson *et al.* (1960), reproduced by courtesy of John Wright)

Symptoms
Internal laryngocoele if large may cause voice changes or attacks of dyspnoea. The external type may present as a large acutely inflamed cyst in the neck, if its narrow communication through the thyrohyoid membrane becomes obliterated by infection. Perhaps the majority of both types are asymptomatic and are only discovered accidentally in the course of routine laryngological or x-ray examination.

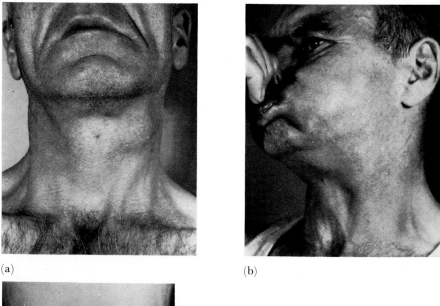

(a)   (b)

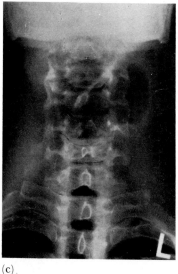

(c).

Figure 15.5 (a) and (b) Patient demonstrating large external laryngocoele; (c) postero-anterior x-ray of
the same case

Treatment

Treatment is only indicated if symptoms are troublesome, and consists of excision by
an external approach to the thyrohyoid membrane. It may be necessary to divide the
thyroid cartilage vertically to obtain access to the intralaryngeal portion of the sac.
The laryngocoele is dissected free, excised, and its stump closed and invaginated. The
thyrohyoid membrane is meticulously repaired with sutures.

Angiomas

Three different conditions are described under this name and must be carefully
distinguished.

Pseudo-angiomas or vascular polyps

Such lesions are produced by trauma to the vocal cords causing subepithelial rupture of a small blood vessel. The resulting haematoma soon becomes converted into vascular reparative tissue with distended blood spaces, and then takes on an angiomatous appearance both clinically and histologically. As previously mentioned these tumours are simply a variety of cordal polyp. Any collection of blood occurring as a result of vocal stress should be evacuated rather than allowed to form a submucous haematoma.

Congenital telangiectasia (Osler-Rendu disease)

These small swellings are usually multiple, occurring diffusely in the skin and in mucous membranes. They are familial in nature. The face, neck and fingers are common sites on the skin; while the mucosa of the lips, nose, tongue, cheeks, palate, epiglottis and interior of the larynx may be variously involved (*Plate 6c, facing page 432*). Hoarseness is not a usual symptom, but bleeding may occur on very slight trauma and this is one of the causes of haemoptysis for which the help of the laryngologist may be sought. If bleeding is persistent it may be necessary to cauterize the bleeding point electrically.

True angiomas

These are rare tumours compared with the pseudo-angiomas. In the well-known series of 722 benign laryngeal tumours reported by New and Erich in 1938, there were only 25 true angiomas and one lymphangioma. The capillary cavernous variant may be represented separately or combined in any haemangioma. Two definite types are recognized: the infantile and the adult. The former usually presents in the first three months of life and both sexes seem equally affected. It tends to grow rapidly after birth, is usually subglottic, may be associated with dermal angiomas and causes a febrile episodic laryngeal obstruction. Diagnosis may be difficult owing to the depth of the tumour beneath normal mucosa, and biopsy confirmation is certainly dangerous. Despite possible risk of later carcinoma, the only effective treatment is by small doses (200–500 rad of irradiation. This is only justified by the high mortality of the untreated condition. Holborow (1958) and Mawson (1961) give good descriptions of the hazards involved.

Adult haemangiomas appear as rather large sessile purplish tumours usually in the supraglottic region and often extending submucosally into the laryngopharynx (*Plate 6d, facing page 432*). They do not project into the lumen, do not grow and as a rule there are no symptoms. If possible they should be left untreated.

Chondromas

These are also rare. Little more than 100 have so far been reported in the literature. They chiefly affect men in the 40–60 age group. They are slow-growing, smooth, hard, sessile and generally subglottic, often growing from the posterior plate of the cricoid cartilage. They may also arise from other laryngeal cartilages, for example the arytenoid, as described by Salmon (1957) (*Plate 6e, facing page 432*). They vary from the size of a cherry to that of an orange. The smaller variety are the most numerous and consist equally of enchondromas and ecchondromas; the larger are usually mixed (Capps, 1957). They can grow to a large size and, by causing dyspnoea, may necessitate tracheostomy (*Figure 15.6*). Bronchopneumonia and asphyxia are the less common complications which may endanger life. In some cases calcification and myxomatous degeneration may occur. Sarcomatous degeneration has also been described but this appears extremely rare.

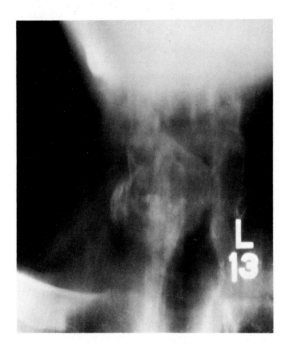

Figure 15.6 Tomogram to show position of a massive chondroma of the cricoid cartilage causing gross obstruction of the airway and distortion of the whole larynx

Treatment
Treatment is by laryngofissure and local removal of the tumour if not too large. At times the whole larynx may become so involved that total laryngectomy will be required but surgery should be as conservative as possible.

Amyloidosis

The classical description of homogeneous intercellular amyloid material states it to be a well-known secondary manifestation in generalized chronic toxaemia. In the primary disease without any apparent precipitating condition, there is maximal diffuse involvement of the heart and striated muscles with less striking abdominal involvement. Many cases of a third type in which local 'amyloid tumours' occur typically in the upper air passages or bladder may sometimes be found at *post-mortem* to have more widespread primary disease. Nevertheless, in such cases the local deposit is often solitary.

These local amyloid tumours are usually found in the larynx and trachea, but may

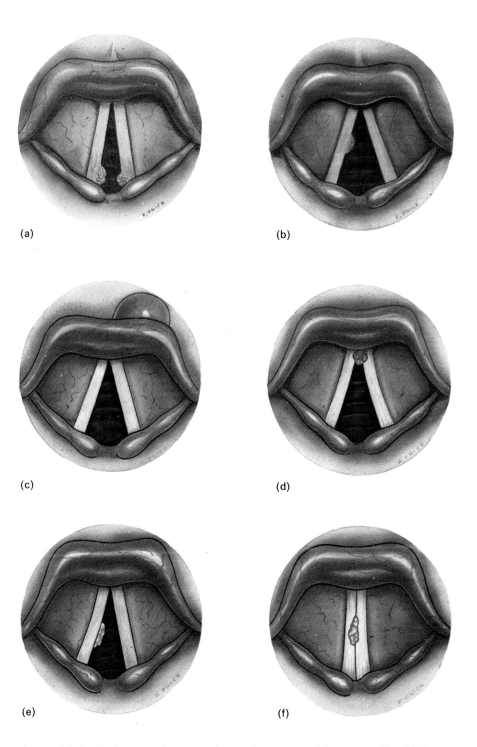

Plate 5   (a) Intubation granulomas on the vocal processes of the arytenoids; (b) fibroma growing from the edge of the right vocal cord; (c) retention cyst of the left vallecula; (d) pedunculated papilloma growing from the anterior commissure; (e) single papilloma of the right vocal cord in quiet respiration; (f) effect of phonation on the papilloma shown in (e)

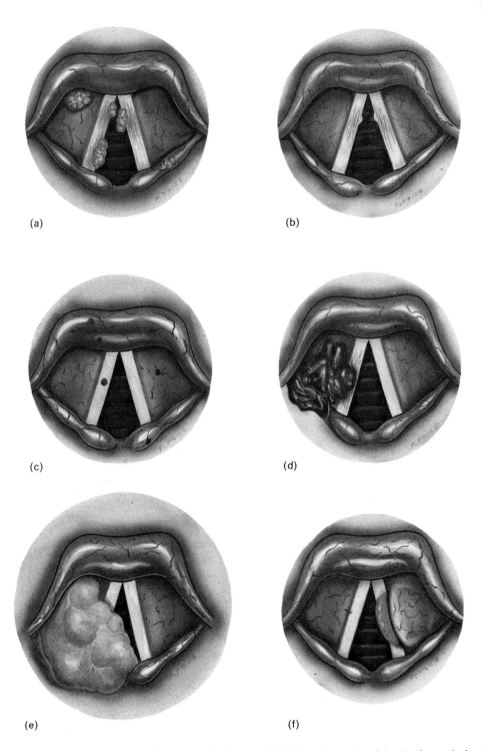

Plate 6 (a) Multiple papillomas in the larynx; (b) bilateral vocal nodules in the typical position; (c) multiple congenital telangiectases in the larynx (Osler-Rendu disease); (d) large angioma of the right ventricular band and the aryepiglottic fold; (e) chondroma growing from the right arytenoid; (f) retention cyst of left laryngeal ventricle projecting into the larynx between the left vocal cord and ventricular band

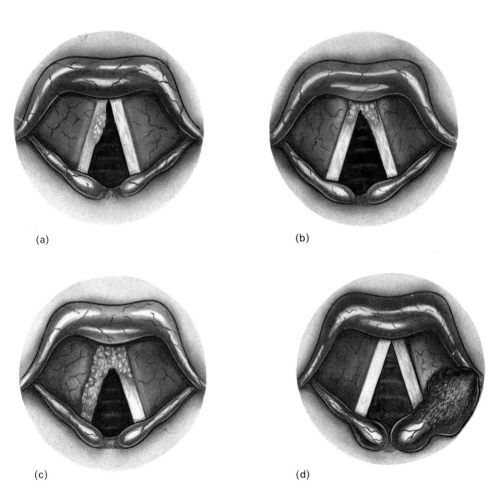

(a)　　　　　　　　　　　　　　(b)

(c)　　　　　　　　　　　　　　(d)

Plate 7　(a) Stage 1 carcinoma limited to the membranous right vocal cord. (Irradiation is the treatment of choice.) (b) Carcinoma involving the anterior commissure and anterior thirds of both vocal cords (stage 2). (Irradiation preferable to partial laryngectomy.) (c) Stage 3 carcinoma involving the anterior third of the left cord, the anterior commissure, the base of the epiglottis and the whole length of the right vocal cord to include the arytenoid. Some reduced mobility of the right cord. Total laryngectomy would be the treatment of choice. (d) Early stage 1 carcinoma of left aryepiglottic fold. (Treatment by irradiation or partial laryngectomy.) (*continued*)

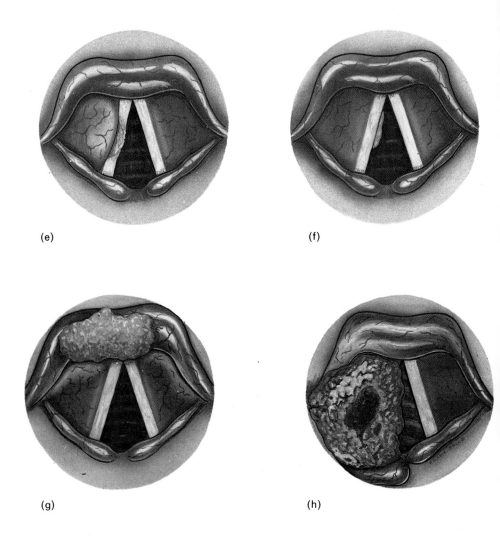

(e)

(f)

(g)

(h)

Plate 7 (*continued*)   (e) Stage 2 carcinoma of right ventricle involving the middle third of the right vocal cord. (Treatment by irradiation or total laryngectomy.) (f) Subglottic (stage 1) carcinoma beneath mobile right vocal cord. No posterior extension. (Irradiation is the treatment of choice.) (g) Extensive epiglottic carcinoma (stage 2). (Treatment by total laryngectomy.) (h) Massive carcinoma involving whole fixed right hemilarynx with subglottic extension and two mobile palpable homolateral neck nodes (stage 3). (Treatment by total laryngectomy with right radical block dissection in continuity.)

also occur in the tongue, nose, pharynx and elsewhere in the respiratory tract (McAlpine, Radcliffe and Friedmann, 1963; Payling Wright, 1958). The sex incidence is about equal, although with a slight male preponderance, and they are generally found in adults in the 40–70 age range. The vocal cords are the most common site, although any intralaryngeal structure may be involved. Appearances are variable, but two types are recognized: the localized swelling or subepithelial deposit seen as a slightly raised smooth pink nodule or plaque, and the diffuse infiltrative variety (*Figure 15.7*).

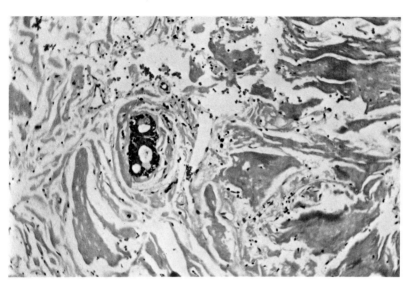

Figure 15.7 Hyaline intercellular amyloid material surrounding mucous gland ducts. (× 160, reduced to three-quarters on reproduction)

The aetiology of primary localized amyloidosis is obscure. Experimental studies have suggested that the formation of amyloid is a perverted phase of protein synthesis, the initiation of which is still hypothetical. Chronic local infection or irritation is a suspected but unproven cause (Holinger and Delgado, 1959).

Symptoms
Symptoms arise entirely from the mechanical effects of the lesions depending upon their precise situation in the larynx. Hoarseness, irritation and dry cough are therefore usual.

Treatment
Treatment of the localized variety is by simple endoscopic removal; if complete, recurrence is rare. The diffuse type requires more consideration since medical measures and irradiation are ineffective, despite some claims for corticosteroid therapy (Creston, 1961). It would seem that simple excision of as much affected tissue as possible via a laryngofissure approach probably with free skin grafts to the raw surface is the most effective. However, such treatment should be reserved only for those cases in which the airway is significantly reduced. No case of malignant change has yet been reported.

Adenomas

These tumours are very rare, few having been described since Moore's description of 13 cases in 1920. Stewart (1960) stated that only about 20 cases had been reported in the English literature in the past 30 years, and the recent large series referred to in *Table 15.1* (page 421) lists only 16.

They are found occasionally throughout the mucosa of the respiratory tract, more commonly below the larynx, Willis (1953) stating that they account for about five per cent of bronchial tumours. In the larynx they usually arise in the supraglottic region, frequently in the ventricles where mucous gland aggregates are most numerous. Growth is slow and symptoms are those of mechanical interference. They are mostly sessile, with well-defined margins, covered with an intact epithelium, and having a congested, smooth or mammillary appearance. They have a slight preponderance in men and vary greatly in size from a millet seed to a hen's egg.

Pathology
Histologically, they are a distinct entity arising from the mucus-secreting glands of the air passages. There is thus no need to invoke the presence of ectopic salivary tissue. They range from the typically solid variety resembling a benign 'mixed salivary'

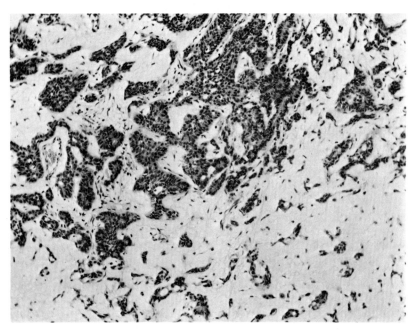

Figure 15.8   Laryngeal adenoma showing epithelial cells and tubule formation lying in a soft fibrous stroma

tumour to an extremely cystic tumour akin to the adenolymphoma of Warthin, the main distinction being the usual absence of lymphoid tissue in the laryngeal tumour (*Figure 15.8*). A further variant is an eosinophilic glandular cell cystadenoma.

Treatment

Treatment is by surgical removal via an external approach where the tumour is of any size, since excision must be complete if recurrence is to be avoided. Prognosis remains excellent if removal has been adequate.

Myoblastoma

This unique and rare tumour was first described on the vocal cord by Abrikossoff in 1931, although it had been described quite frequently in the tongue, also in skeletal muscle and a few subcutaneous sites, some years before. At least 59 cases have been recorded up to 1970 (Booth and Osborn, 1970), with a peak age incidence in the fourth decade and a male:female ratio of 2:1; occasional appearance in childhood is also noted. The fourth decade has furnished the highest frequency. They appear as small flat or nodular submucous plaques, pink or yellow in colour, with a poorly defined margin. They tend to arise in the posterior half of the larynx and are of slow growth. Symptoms again result entirely from their size and situation.

Pathology

The aetiology of these tumours is not known with certainty. Willis (1953) regarded lingual myoblastomas as degenerative lesions of muscle fibres and not true neoplasms. Others have considered them to be a type of neurofibroma, since there is alleged evidence of a possible neural origin (Fust and Custer, 1949).

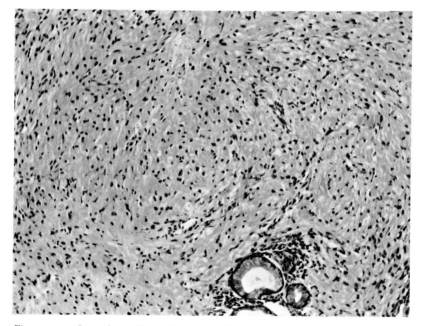

Figure 15.9 Granular cell myoblastoma of the larynx, showing typical fibrillar streaming pattern and incorporating mucous glands. (× 160, reduced to three-quarters on reproduction)

Histologically, the most important feature is the marked pseudo-epitheliomatous hyperplasia of the overlying squamous epithelium. Not infrequently this results in a mistaken diagnosis of squamous carcinoma. However, no true case of malignant change has yet been reported (*Figure 15.9*).

Treatment
Treatment is by endoscopic removal for the majority of small tumours. Larger lesions or recurrences may require excision via laryngofissure. Prognosis is excellent although the tendency to recurrence through poor clearance of margins imposes a necessity for prolonged follow-up.

Neurofibromas, lipomas, rhabdomyomas, plasmacytomas, xanthomas and thyroid gland rests occur so rarely in the larynx as to need no detailed discussion here, except to state the possibility of their appearance. Cummings, Montgomery and Balogh (1969) give a good account of neurofibroma, noting that 15 per cent of cases reported were associated with Von Recklinghausen's disease. Batsakis and Fox (1970) note the reporting of 86 cases of neurogenous tumours in the larynx, none of which were malignant.

Malignant tumours

Classification

Cancer of the larynx accounts for about two per cent of all reported cases of malignant disease, but there is still some difficulty in assessing its relative frequency because full accord has not yet been reached on terminology and classification. Nevertheless, in recent years a greater appreciation of the natural history and surgical pathology of laryngeal cancer has resulted in growing agreement. This has been much helped since 1954 by the International Union Against Cancer, which then accepted the task of drafting a precise classification for cancer of the breast, cervix uteri and larynx. A further scheme was later added to include the oral cavity, pharynx and bladder (UICC report, 1962). Since then the latest UICC report and *Livre de poche* third edition (1978) offers full classification for 27 main anatomical sites which, in the head and neck include the oral cavity, oropharynx, lips, nasopharynx, hypopharynx, larynx and thyroid gland. Complete agreement has now been reached with the American Joint Committee and other national bodies for these proposals which are now intended to remain unchanged for at least ten years.

The earliest and most important attempts at classification were made by Isambert (1876) and Krishaber (1879) who separated tumours into two main groups – intrinsic and extrinsic – although Isambert also suggested that subglottic growths should constitute a distinct subdivision. Many years later, Thomson suggested four main subdivisions: (a) intrinsic; (b) subglottic; (c) extrinsic; and (d) mixed (Thomson and Colledge, 1930).

From pathological and therapeutic viewpoints there is basic soundness in Krishaber's original division into intrinsic and extrinsic lesions, in view of the very different behaviour of growths arising within the larynx, especially on the vocal cords, and those arising outside. However, there was much dispute as to the precise topographical limits of these areas, intrinsic often being held to include the true cord, ventricle and ventricular band, and extrinsic to include those growths arising in the laryngopharynx. Consequently these terms are now in decline and today the distinction survives in some measure as cordal and non-cordal laryngeal cancer.

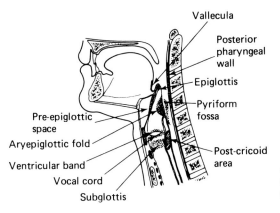

Figure 15.10 Sagittal section to show common sites of origin of laryngeal and laryngopharyngeal carcinoma

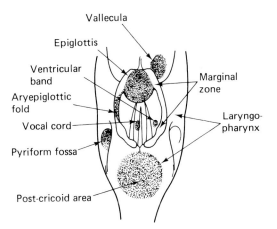

Figure 15.11 Posterior view to show common sites of tumour origin; also the marginal zone between the larynx and laryngopharynx

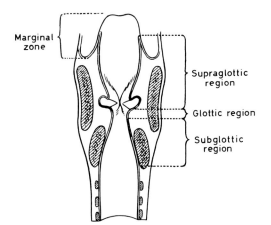

Figure 15.12 Coronal section to show the division into laryngeal regions and marginal zone

The scheme of classification of the larynx and laryngopharynx shown in *Table 15.2* was first proposed in 1972. It has now been fully discussed and finally confirmed by the UICC, AJC and other bodies in 1978. It would seem to meet all reasonable requirements by dividing the larynx into precise anatomical regions and sites (*Figures 15.10, 15.11* and *15.12*).

Table 15.2

Regions	Sites
Larynx	
Supraglottis	
(a) Epilarynx (including marginal zone)	Posterior surface of the suprahyoid epiglottis (including the tip)
	Aryepiglottic folds
	Arytenoids
(b) Supraglottis (excluding epilarynx)	Infrahyoid epiglottis
	Ventricular bands
	Ventricular cavities
Glottis	Vocal cords
	Anterior commissure
	Posterior commissure
Subglottis	Walls of the subglottis
Laryngopharynx	Pyriform fossae
	Post-cricoid area
	Posterior pharyngeal wall

In 1954 the Committee on Clinical Classification and Applied Statistics of the International Union Against Cancer also proposed the 'TNM' system as a universal method of classification for each anatomical site. This defines the extent of the disease in terms of its three main components: T = extent of primary tumour; N = condition of regional lymph nodes; M = distant metastases.

Variation or degrees of local extension are designated by numbers (for example, T1, T2 as below). The same procedure may then be used for the clinical condition of the regional lymph nodes (N) and distant metastases (M).

After trial over the years, a wide measure of international agreement has now been reached for the latest UICC and AJC proposals confirmed in 1978 and set out in *Table 15.3* as a pre-treatment clinical classification for laryngeal tumours.

In agreement with the AJC a system of Staging has also been adopted as set out in *Table 15.4*, although the UICC generally regards the use of TNM as more desirable in the interests of precision.

Table 15.3

	Supraglottis	Glottis	Subglottis
T =	*Primary tumour*		
TiS	Pre-invasive carcinomas (carcinoma *in situ*)	Pre-invasive carcinomas (carcinoma *in situ*)	Pre-invasive carcinomas (carcinoma *in situ*)
To	No evidence of primary tumour	No evidence of primary tumour	No evidence of primary tumour
Ti	Tumour confined to the region with normal mobility	Tumour confined to the region with normal mobility	Tumour confined to the region
Tia	Tumour confined to the laryngeal surface of the epiglottis *or* to an aryepiglottic fold *or* to a ventricular cavity *or* to a ventricular band	Tumour confined to one vocal cord	Tumour confined to one side of the region
Tib	Tumour involving the epiglottis and extending to the ventricular cavities or bands	Tumour involving both vocal cords	Tumour with extension to both sides of the region
T2	Tumour with extension to adjacent sites or to the glottis without fixation	Tumour extending to either the supraglottis or the subglottis with normal or impaired mobility	Tumour confined to the larynx with extension to one or both cords with normal or impaired mobility
T3	Tumour confined to the larynx with fixation and/or other evidence of deep invasion	Tumour confined to the larynx with fixation of one *or* both cords	Tumour confined to the larynx with fixation of one *or* both cords
T4	Tumour with direct extension beyond the larynx	Tumour with direct extension beyond the larynx	Tumour with destruction of cartilage *and/or* with direct extension beyond the larynx
TX	The minimum requirements to assess the primary tumour cannot be met	The minimum requirements to assess the primary tumour cannot be met	The minimum requirements to assess the primary tumour cannot be met

N = *Regional lymph nodes*
No No evidence of regional lymph node involvement
N1 Evidence of involvement of movable homolateral regional lymph nodes
N2 Evidence of involvement of movable contralateral or bilateral regional lymph nodes
N3 Evidence of involvement of fixed regional lymph nodes
NX The minimum requirements to assess the regional lymph nodes cannot be met

M = *Distant metastases*
Mo No evidence of distant metastases
M1 Evidence of distant metastases
MX The minimum requirements to assess the presence of distant metastases cannot be met

Table 15.4

Stage I	TI	No	Mo
Stage II	T2	No	Mo
Stage III	T3	No	Mo
	TI, T2, T3	NI	Mo
Stage IV	T4	No, NI	Mo
	Any T	N2, N3	Mo
	Any T	Any N	MI

General features

There is evidence of a very slow increase in the incidence of this disease in males throughout the world, the highest incidence and rate of increase in Europe being in Scandinavia (Barclay and Rao, 1974). Recent Annual Reports of the South Thames Cancer Registry (1960–76) would also confirm a very slightly rising incidence both in males and females, more significantly in the latter which may correspond to a recent rise in bronchial cancer in females.

Shumrick (1969, 1971) gives some evidence that the frequency of laryngeal cancer may be increasing by as much as four per cent per annum and with a proportionately greater increase among females. By far the highest rates are among Asian races, particularly Indians, in whom the incidence is more than double that of Western races.

No definite causes are yet known although it is likely that chronic mucosal irritation by heavy smoking, excessive intake of alcohol (especially spirits) and the

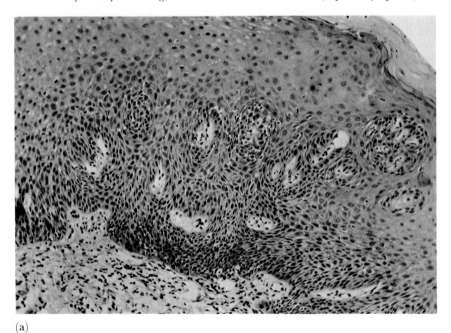

(a)

Figure 15.13   (a) Hyperkeratosis of a vocal cord showing acanthosis in deeper layers but intact basement membrane

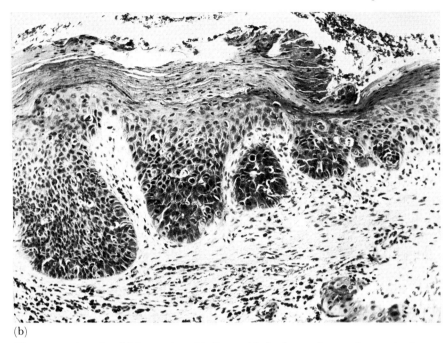

(b)

Figure 15.13 (contd)   (b) keratotic epithelium with *in situ* carcinoma changes in deeper layers but no penetration of basement membrane

chewing of tobacco or aromatic nuts in Asian countries play significant roles in its aetiology. The US Surgeon–General's report on Smoking and Health (1964) specifically finds a definite correlation between heavy smoking and laryngeal cancer. Auerbach, Hammond and Garfinkel (1970) have now shown that metaplasia and malignant change in human laryngeal epithelium develop in proportion to tobacco smoke exposure, especially cigarettes, and that the changes may be reversed by abstention. Very prolonged vocal strain with severe chronic laryngitis and also previous irradiation of the neck may be additional contributory causes, although it must be doubted whether chronic respiratory infection alone plays any real part. More recently, Stell and McGill (1973) have noted a highly significant association between laryngeal cancer and asbestos dust exposure.

   Throughout the larynx and pharynx the disease predominantly affects men in the approximate ratio of 8:1, with the sole exception of the post-cricoid type of tumour where the sex incidence is reversed and is often associated with the pre-cancerous mucosal changes of the Paterson–Kelly syndrome. Laryngeal cancer may occur at any age, although it is rare in young people under 30. One of the youngest cases reported was a boy of ten (Crookes, 1953). In males the sixth and seventh decades are most affected; in females usually one decade younger.

Histopathology

By far the most common type of tumour is the squamous cell carcinoma. It is generally well differentiated but there is often a difference according to the region

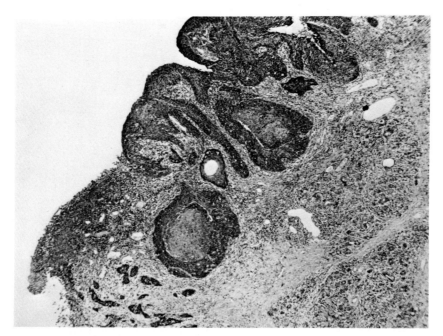

Figure 15.14 Low-power view of well-differentiated squamous carcinoma of the vocal cord, showing general features, cell nest formation and invasion of the stroma. (× 50, reduced to three-quarters on reproduction)

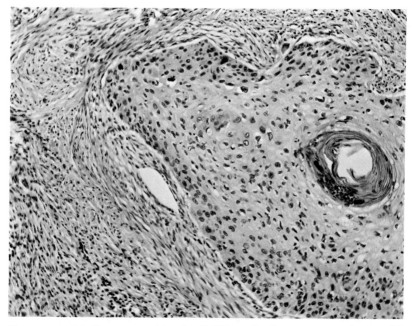

Figure 15.15 Medium-power view of well-differentiated squamous carcinoma of the supraglottic region, showing nuclear irregularity, cell mitosis and pearl formation. (× 160, reduced to three-quarters on reproduction)

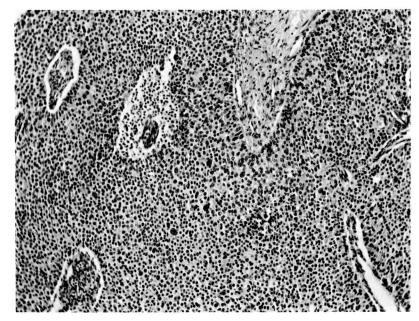

Figure 15.16 Undifferentiated laryngeal carcinoma, showing nuclear pleomorphism and hyperchromasia. (× 160, reduced to three-quarters on reproduction)

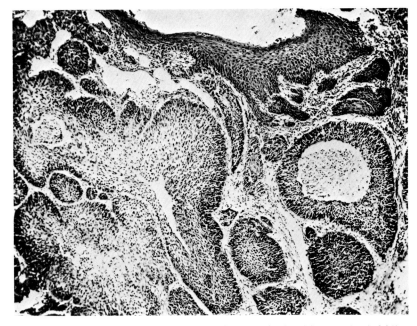

Figure 15.17 Transitional cell carcinoma of the epiglottis with extensive infolding and cystic pseudonecrosis

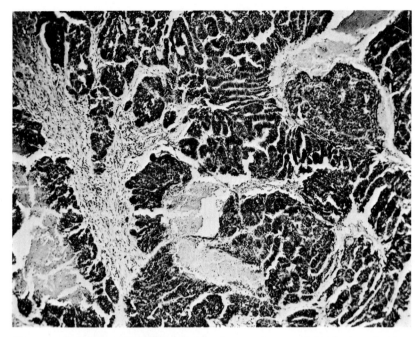

Figure 15.18 Moderately differentiated adenocarcinoma of the larynx showing invasion of stroma by hyperchromatic masses of columnar epithelium. (× 85, reduced to three-quarters on reproduction)

affected. Cordal tumours show a high degree of differentiation, 80 per cent in one series, whereas in a parallel extra-cordal and laryngopharyngeal series there was only a 55 per cent proportion of well-differentiated tumours (Shaw, 1965) (*Figures 15.14, 15.15* and *15.16*).

In any large series it is usually found that 96–98 per cent are squamous cell carcinomas with the occasional transitional cell carcinoma of the epiglottis (*Figure 15.17*). Adenocarcinoma of mucous glands (*Figure 15.18*) and basal cell carcinoma also occur. A good review of the former by Whicker *et al.* (1974) reports poor response to treatment and a serious prognosis in the majority. Cady, Rippey and Frazell (1968) reported a series of 31 cases of non-epidermoid cancer of the larynx out of a total 2500 cases of laryngeal cancer seen at Memorial Center, New York. Of these, 17 were adenocarcinomas.

At the Royal Marsden Hospital, London, during the period 1948–77, out of a total of 2784 new patients with laryngeal cancer, 19 cases of non-epidermoid cancer were seen and are listed as follows:

Adenocarcinoma	6
Malignant lymphoma	4
Chondrosarcoma	2
Plasmacytoma	2
Fibrosarcoma (*Figure 15.19*)	2
Spindle cell sarcoma	1
Muco-epidermoid carcinoma	1
Malignant melanoma	1

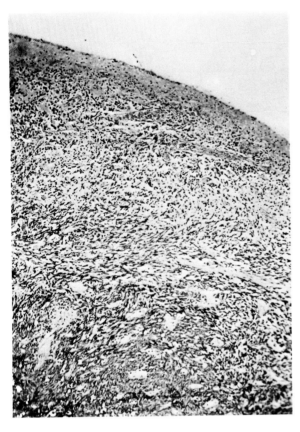

Figure 15.19 Fibrosarcoma of larynx, showing spindle cell patterns. Post-radiation changes are present

Fourteen cases of pseudosarcoma were seen in the same period (*Figure 15.20*). Although the stromal cells of this lesion have a sarcomatous appearance, the tumour is epithelial in origin and contains inconspicuous and often intramucosal elements of squamous carcinoma. It must be treated as such.

Another rare variant is verrucous carcinoma, now being reported more frequently (*Figure 15.21*). Burns, van Nostrand and Bryce (1976) state that it may account for 1–2 per cent of primary laryngeal cancers. There is still some controversy regarding its propensity to anaplastic change with radiotherapy. However, these authors regard the risk as small.

True sarcomas are very rare (Batsakis and Fox, 1970) and apart from those listed above, rhabdosarcoma and reticulosarcoma may occasionally be found. Malignant melanoma also occurs very rarely in the larynx (Conley and Pack, 1974).

Since Broders proposed his scheme for histological grading of squamous carcinoma of the lip in 1920, it has been customary to use the system of four grades applied to the larynx as indicated in *Table 15.5*.

However, in the UK Broders' grading is generally used in the modified form of three categories: 'well', 'moderately', and 'poorly' differentiated – expressions that are descriptively adequate providing precise statements are included regarding *in situ* or *invasive* (*Figures 15.13* and *15.20*). The description *in situ* carcinoma is now generally accepted to indicate intra-epithelial malignant change without penetration of the basement membrane. Added significance also lies in the fact that its natural history is

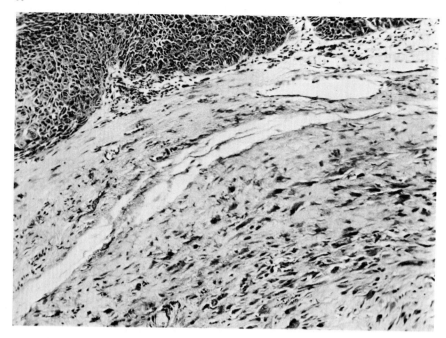

Figure 15.20 Pseudosarcoma of larynx. Lying beneath the surface layer of *in situ* carcinoma is the so-called pseudosarcomatous stroma. (× 160, reduced to three-quarters on reproduction)

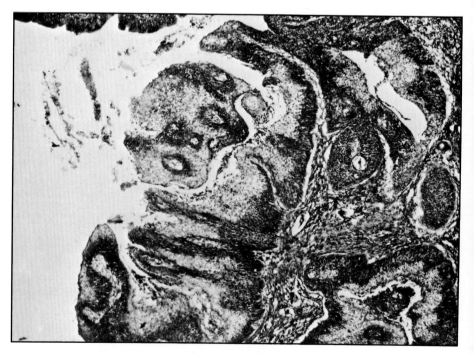

Figure 15.21 Verrucous carcinoma of the larynx to show gross keratin formation with reduced stroma and surface shedding. (× 50, reduced to three-quarters on reproduction)

not rapidly or necessarily progressive. However, Kleinsasser (1963) reports that if untreated, 90 per cent of cases will sooner or later develop invasive tendencies. Its existence adjacent to an area of invasive carcinoma must also be considered. Most cases of *in situ* carcinoma develop as a progressive change from keratosis with atypia.

Table 15.5

Grades	% of cells undifferentiated
1	0–25
2	25–50
3	50–75
4	75–100

Glottic region

Glottic cancer is generally the most common type of laryngeal neoplasm in the adult. It is also the most frequent variety of laryngeal cancer, estimates varying from 50 to 85 per cent being quoted by Negus and Thomson (1955). This is fortunate since its diagnosis is quicker, its treatment usually simpler and prognosis, when limited to the vocal cord, infinitely better than that of cancer in other regions of the larynx or of most other sites in the head and neck.

It usually arises on the free margin or upper surface of the true vocal cord in its middle or anterior third – the area of maximal work-load (*Plate 7a, facing page 432*). Local spread along the cord in both directions is slow, owing to the dense layers of elastic and fibrous tissue present, and metastasis to cervical lymph nodes is uncommon owing to the absence of any lymphatics in Reinke's subepithelial connective tissue layer. Ten cases only out of a total of 306 consecutive cases of glottic cancer seen at the Royal National Throat, Nose and Ear Hospital during the years 1947–56, were found to have clinically positive neck nodes on first attendance (Shaw, 1965).

Tumours arising in the anterior commissure are uncommon and also treacherous in behaviour (*Plate 7b, facing page 432*). Only five were encountered in the above series. Growths in the posterior commissure are almost unknown.

Subglottic region

Although this area is frequently involved to some degree by tumours spreading downwards from the true cords – at least one-fifth of the above series having had some evidence of this type of spread – it is uncommon for cancer to arise *de novo* in the subglottic region (eight per cent: Lederman, 1970; less than one per cent: Bryce, 1972). When it does, it is usually in the anterior half of the subglottis, often spreading anteriorly across the midline, and may be difficult to detect clinically (*Plate 7b, facing page 432*). It differs significantly from cordal lesions in that it gains early access to lymphatics draining directly into the pre-laryngeal, para-tracheal and lower deep cervical chains of nodes. A further danger is of direct spread through the cricothyroid membrane into the thyroid gland or deep fascia and strap muscles. Diagnosis and treatment are always correspondingly more difficult and prognosis must be serious.

Supraglottic region

Ventricles and ventricular bands

These are uncommon sites of origin for laryngeal cancer. They are most often involved by tumours spreading upward from the true cords. Disease is generally extensive by the time the diagnosis is made owing to lack of early symptoms. The laryngeal ventricle has a bad reputation as it may conceal early lesions and often leads to delayed diagnosis and an underestimate of the situation (*Plate 7e, facing page 432*).

Infrahyoid epiglottis

This is the most frequently involved area of the epiglottis and amounted to 12 per cent of a large series of laryngeal tumours at all sites (Shaw and Epstein, 1959). Even so, this is a low incidence compared with reports from Continental and US authorities. Early diagnosis is again difficult owing to the 'silent' nature of small lesions, which may be hypertrophic and proliferative in type, or more often may form a slow but deeply penetrating ulcer just above the petiolus. On a backward curling epiglottis they are easily missed at mirror examination.

   These tumours have a particularly sinister repute owing to their midline position, easy access to bilateral deep cervical lymphatics and tendency to early invasion of the pre-epiglottic space (*Plate 7g, facing page 432* and *Figure 15.10*).

   In Lederman's large series reported in 1970 the total incidence of supraglottic lesions was given as 18 per cent.

Epilarynx (Marginal zone)

Suprahyoid epiglottis

The projecting or free part of the epiglottis is a much less common site for the origin of laryngeal cancer, although it is often involved by spread from neighbouring areas. It generally appears as a slowly growing superficial ulcer associated with gradual erosion of the tip and with minimal symptoms. Alternatively a proliferative granular lesion is sometimes found. Owing to the presence of fewer lymphatics in the area and its comparative isolation, a tumour confined to this site is more amenable to treatment and has a better prognosis than on the infrahyoid epiglottis.

Aryepiglottic folds

These tumours are usually large when diagnosed because there are few early symptoms. In the relative frequency of primary tumours of this region, they occupy a position midway between the ventricular bands and epiglottis. However, the area is commonly involved by tumours that have spread from the vallecula or epiglottis and from the lateral pharyngeal wall or pyriform fossa, or even from the upward extension of an advanced cordal tumour (*Plate 7d* and *h, facing page 432*). In appearance they are usually nodular and proliferative, and although accessible to treatment they generally carry a poor prognosis due to their extent and the frequent invasion of the rich lymphatic field.

Again, Lederman (1970) reports a total incidence of 14 per cent epilaryngeal tumours.

Spread of malignant disease

The spread of malignant disease in this area is exactly the same as in other parts of the body by: (a) direct extension; (b) lymphatic spread; and (c) blood stream metastases.

Direct extension

Inside the larynx extension occurs for the most part along the mucosal surface or by submucous infiltration. The presence of the surrounding cartilage seems to limit its spread beyond these borders in many cases.

On the vocal cord the general direction of spread is antero-posteriorly; there is some tendency to invade the false cord but spread readily occurs backwards to the tip of the arytenoid and forwards to the commissure, and from there along the opposite cord (Kirchner, 1974). In the case of subglottic tumours, the spread may be downwards into the trachea or horizontally around the anterior wall, affecting the subglottic region of the opposite side before there is any invasion of the edge of the cord. This is a bad point in the prognosis of such tumours, which frequently prove to be extensive before any symptoms are apparent.

Significantly a subglottic tumour will spread through the cricothyroid membrane and a glottic lesion may penetrate the thyroid cartilage, but this is unusual unless it is extensive or arises in the anterior commissure. Similarly, a tumour commencing on one surface of the epiglottis may spread around the tip and invade the other surface before it invades the epiglottic cartilage. Reference has already been made to the tendency for epiglottic cancer to invade the pre-epiglottic space.

Tumours in the region of the anterior commissure, especially on the epiglottis in the neighbourhood of the petiolus, frequently invade the thyroid cartilage and there may be deep burrowing ulceration in this area at an unexpectedly early stage with extra-laryngeal extension into the deep neck tissues and thyroid gland. Tumours of the aryepiglottic fold and edge of the epiglottis often spread along the fold very rapidly and also spread along the pharyngo-epiglottic fold to the lateral wall of the pharynx.

It is uncommon for supraglottic tumours to spread downwards across the vocal cord so that most trans-glottic lesions are likely to be of cordal origin.

Direct invasion of small veins or nerve sheaths passing through the thyrohyoid or cricothyroid membranes may sometimes take place; this causes rapid permeation of these minute channels leading to separate involvement of structures well outside the larynx.

The work of Kirchner and his associates in serial sectioning of laryngeal specimens has done much to emphasize the routes of spread from different points of origin. In his paper of 1974 he demonstrated the high incidence of involvement of the laryngeal framework in cancer crossing the ventricle or in the anterior commissure.

Lymphatic spread

This is of great importance from the point of view of treatment and prognosis. There are practically no lymph vessels in the true vocal cord and, while a tumour is limited to the cord, there is very little tendency for involvement of neck nodes. It is because of this feature that it is possible to remove an early neoplasm of the vocal cord by a limited local excision, with a very good prospect of cure. This fact, combined with the early onset of symptoms of hoarseness in carcinoma of the vocal cord, makes the prognosis of such lesions more favourable than anywhere else in the body cavities. Below the vocal cord, in the anterior subglottic region, the lymphatic supply is again not very rich. The lymph vessels drain into the cricothyroid, pre-tracheal and para-tracheal nodes. Unfortunately the prognosis is generally poor because symptoms occur later and therefore cases may not come under observation until the tumour has already become extensive. In addition, involvement of the para-tracheal lymphatics may be bilateral and may pass undetected until the disease has reached adjacent structures in the mediastinum.

The lymphatics of the ventricle drain upwards through the thyrohyoid membrane with those of the supraglottic region to the lymph nodes of the upper and middle deep cervical groups. Neoplasms of the epiglottis metastasize into the same group of nodes but may occasionally affect the submaxillary and submental nodes. Always of importance in a midline area such as the epiglottis is the likelihood of bilateral lymphatic involvement.

The work of Pressman and Simon (1961) has indicated that the vocal cords may be considered almost a 'lymphatic divide', there being virtually no trans-glottic lymph channels. This is of great importance when considering the theoretical basis of supraglottic partial laryngectomy. Nevertheless, trans-glottic tumours are not infrequent, and it would therefore seem likely that direct growth in two directions from the vocal cord is responsible.

Metastatic spread

Metastatic spread by the blood stream is not common, and cases have been reported with deposits in the lungs, liver, bones and occasional other sites, sometimes three or four years after operations on the larynx and when there has been no evidence of local recurrence. The disease as a rule remains localized to the head and neck throughout its course, and upon this are based the concepts of effective radical treatment.

Symptoms

Hoarseness is the main early symptom of malignant disease of the larynx. This will occur with very early lesions of the vocal cord but usually at a late stage with supraglottic tumours, and will probably be absent or slight in those of the epilarynx.

There are no early symptoms of any constancy in tumours in these last two situations.

Other symptoms of laryngeal cancer are sensations of discomfort in the throat, some increased expectoration, a thickness rather than huskiness of the voice and occasionally an irritable cough, but the disease is usually already well established before these symptoms appear.

It might be expected that cough would be an early symptom of glottic carcinoma of the larynx, but this is not the case. It is, in fact, more common as a symptom of marginal zone tumours.

Alteration of the voice and possibly some dyspnoea on exertion may be two of the early symptoms to become evident in subglottic disease. This is due to infiltration of the vocal cord from below and limitation of its movement before the tumour can be seen by mirror examination.

Discussion of late symptoms is of no great value; they generally include earache, dyspnoea, dysphagia, loss of appetite, cachexia, foetor of the breath and bleeding. They will depend on the situation of the tumour, its direction of spread and its extent.

Diagnosis

A diagnosis of cancer will be made after consideration of:

(1) The history.
(2) Examination of the larynx and pharynx by both indirect and direct methods.
(3) Examination of the neck.
(4) General examination of the patient, which may include examination of blood and sputum for bacteriology and cytology.
(5) Radiological examination of the chest, neck and larynx.
(6) Histological examination of a biopsy specimen.

History

The symptoms have already been considered and nothing more need be said than that practically any other disease affecting the larynx may exhibit symptoms compatible with malignant disease; the converse is also true. Again, cancer may co-exist with other diseases such as tuberculosis or syphilis, and a condition such as leucoplakia of the larynx may undergo malignant change without any apparent change in the symptoms.

Examination of the larynx and pharynx

The appearance of the lesion will, of course, vary with the site but may also vary in any one situation on the vocal cord. A typical raised nodule may be seen with a flat rather rough surface, or a hypertrophic papillary growth; in other cases there may be a local thickening of one vocal cord or sometimes a typical neoplastic ulcer (*Figure 15.22*). If there is much keratinization of the surface the appearance will be pale or

white; in other cases it may be pink or red, particularly if there is associated
inflammation.

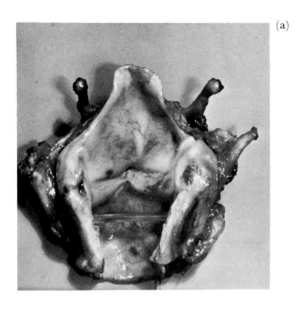

(a)

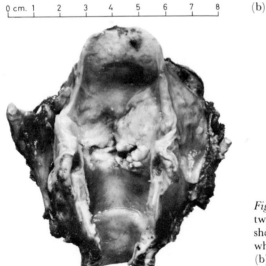

(b)

Figure 15.22 Surgical specimens of
two larynges split open posteriorly to
show: (a) carcinoma involving the
whole right vocal cord with fixation;
(b) extensive trans-glottic carcinoma
of the right side of the larynx

A tumour originating at the anterior commissure may appear as a small bud of
granulation tissue, whereas in the subglottic region a lesion may be quite extensive
and yet not be seen on indirect laryngoscopy because it is hidden by the overlying
edge of the vocal cord (*Figure 15.24*). A tumour in the commissure, or one arising just
above the commissure on the epiglottis, may fail to be seen by mirror examination
because it is hidden by the backward curve of its tip.

Impaired mobility of the vocal cord is not an early sign of malignant disease since it

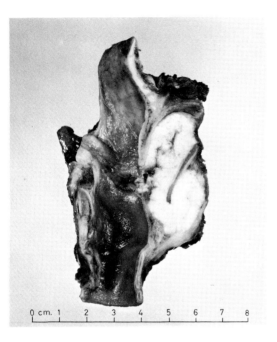

Figure 15.23 Specimen of larynx split sagittally to show gross penetration by tumour through thyroid cartilage into the pre-epiglottic space and soft tissues of the neck

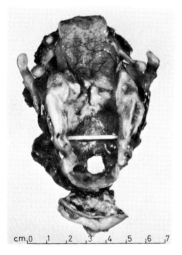

Figure 15.24 Extensive subglottic infiltration by carcinoma of both vocal cords, especially left, with bilateral midline fixation, in female aged 72 years. Tumour found microscopically in strap muscles. Tracheostomy fistula completely excised

is usually due to invasion of the thyro-arytenoid muscle and often the adjacent cartilages; nevertheless, it is present in many patients when first attending and is therefore an important sign in the clinical staging of lesions and prognosis. It is particularly important in the case of a subglottic lesion as this may not produce any symptoms in the early stages and will only cause some alteration in the voice when it begins to infiltrate the submucous tissues and produces limitation of cord movement. This impaired mobility is mostly a limitation of full abduction together with some sluggishness in adduction. It is a sign of deeper extension of disease.

When a tumour commences in the ventricle the only indication of its presence in the early stage may be a slight fullness of the ventricular band on that side, and later, an appearance suggesting some oedema or prolapse of the mucosa of the ventricle. If the ventricular band is then pushed outwards it may be seen to be hiding a comparatively large tumour. In all cases of doubt it is wise to pass a direct laryngoscope and the subglottic region must also be inspected. In such cases micro-laryngoscopy and the use of a right-angled endoscope are often valuable.

In the aryepiglottic region the appearance is usually that of a localized swelling of the fold with ulceration – generally of the outer or upper surface (*Plate 7d, facing page 432*). Occasionally a small indurated ulcer, without much swelling is seen most commonly on the postero-lateral aspect of the arytenoid. Less commonly a pedunculated tumour is found which may obscure the whole field of view and cause doubt as to the true site of origin.

Similar variations occur on the epiglottis; the most common type is a nodular ulcerating tumour arising more frequently from one edge than from the tip, or as a secondary extension from a carcinoma of the vallecula. Less commonly a cauliflower type of tumour is seen completely hiding the glottis and yet surprisingly causing very little dyspnoea. Rarely a deeply infiltrating tumour of the petiolus may be found; this does not cause symptoms early and may be missed on examination for reasons already given.

Examination of the neck

As already mentioned, involvement of the internal jugular chain of lymph nodes occurs rarely with carcinoma of the vocal cords and seldom occurs early with subglottic tumours. If nodes are affected in cordal tumours, it is frequently the small

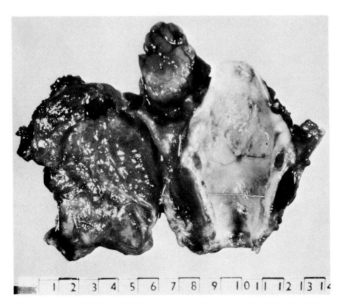

Figure 15.25 Advanced Stage 3 carcinoma of epiglottis, left ventricular band and aryepiglottic fold. Specimen showing combined total laryngectomy and left radical neck dissection

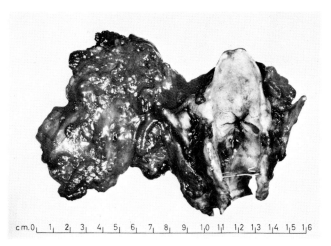

cm.0 1 2 3 4 5 6 7 8 9 10 11 12 13 14 15 16

Figure 15.26   Massive Stage 3 carcinoma involving left subglottic region with fixation of left vocal cord. Specimen to show combined total laryngectomy and elective left radical neck dissection

pre-laryngeal node on the cricothyroid membrane and in subglottic growths the pre-tracheal and para-tracheal nodes that are first involved.

There may be some swelling of the larynx which can be felt on palpation. This is due either to associated perichondritis, when the cartilage will be tender on pressure, or to a mass of tumour infiltrating directly through the cricothyroid membrane. This occurs only at a late stage and with extensive lesions.

Occasionally an aggressive tumour of the anterior commissure invading thyroid cartilage or with some subglottic spread will produce a midline indurated swelling beneath the skin over the lower border of the thyroid cartilage at the junction with the cricothyroid membrane.

With supraglottic and epilaryngeal tumours the nodes most frequently affected are the homolateral upper and middle deep cervical groups. In tumours of the epiglottis similar deep cervical node groups may be affected, often bilaterally, and spread may occasionally take place to the submaxillary or submental nodes of either side.

General examination

General physical examination of any patient suspected of malignant disease of the larynx or laryngopharynx should always be carried out as a routine measure. It is essential to perform serological tests for syphilis and, if in doubt, the sputum should be examined for tubercle bacilli. Also, a haemoglobin estimation and white-cell count with routine biochemistry and electrocardiogram are minimal requirements. The coexistence of diabetes mellitus, renal, hepatic, chronic pulmonary or cardiovascular disease may well modify the line of treatment to be advised.

456

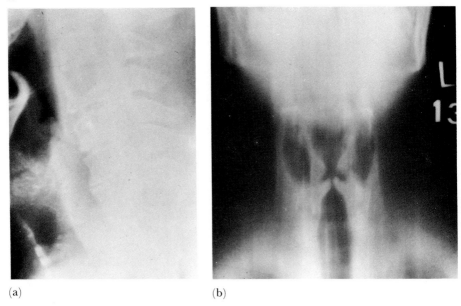

(a)   (b)

Figure 15.27 (a) Normal soft-tissue lateral radiograph of larynx showing calcification in laryngeal cartilages and tracheal rings; (b) normal tomograph of larynx showing vocal cords, ventricular bands, ventricles and pyriform fossae

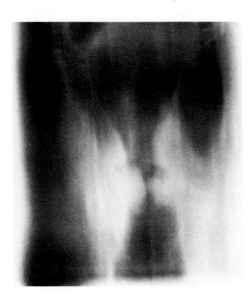

Figure 15.28 Tomograph to show tumour of right vocal cord with partial obliteration of the right ventricle

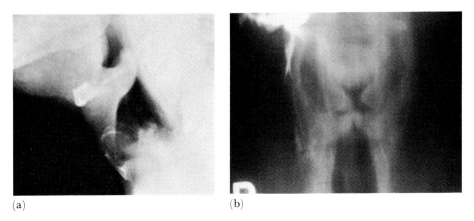

(a) (b)

Figure 15.29 (a) Lateral radiograph to show tumour of epiglottis and vallecula with invasion of the pre-epiglottic space; (b) tomograph of similar epiglottic tumour

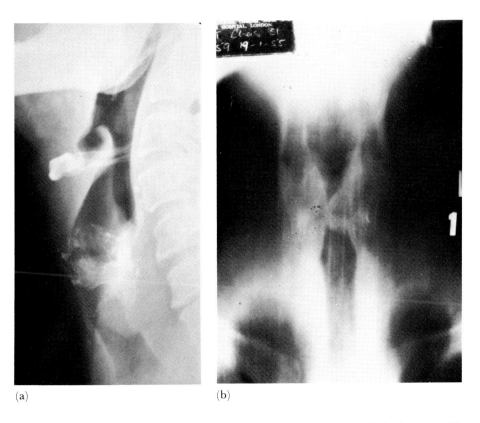

(a) (b)

Figure 15.30 (a) Lateral radiograph to show growth on posterior wall of subglottic region; (b) tomograph of fibrosarcoma of left hemilarynx

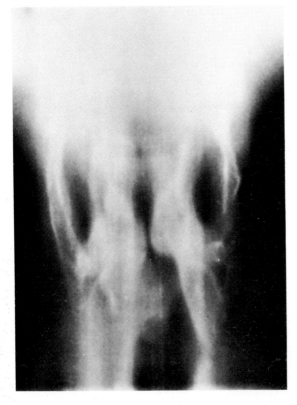

Figure 15.31 Tomograph to show extensive right subglottic tumour

Radiological examination

The chest should be examined radiologically before treatment is undertaken in order to:

(1) Eliminate or verify the coexistence of a tuberculous infection or other lesion.
(2) Note the presence of any retro-sternal mass of nodes in the mediastinum or pulmonary hilum.
(3) Detect any metastatic disease in the lung fields themselves.

Radiological examination of the neck is also of considerable value, partly as an aid to diagnosis but more especially in assessing the extent of a tumour which can only be seen from above, before planning treatment. Lateral and postero-anterior plain films of the larynx will often demonstrate the presence of a tumour of the epiglottis with possible invasion of the pre-epiglottic space, the approximate extent of the tumour mass within the larynx or the presence of a subglottic neoplasm growing in the anterior or lateral part of that region.

Tomographic techniques are of additional value in certain situations, particularly for suspected tumours in the ventricular and subglottic regions. Positive contrast laryngography and pharyngography using Dionosil and local anaesthesia can also be of the greatest value, especially in determining the lower extent of supraglottic tumours and the integrity of the ventricles, subglottic region and pyriform fossae

(Brindle and Stell, 1968; Samuel, 1974). However, it must be remembered that the use of these techniques should be selective and that none of them is reliable in evaluating the post-irradiation larynx (*Figures 15.32, 15.33* and *15.34*).

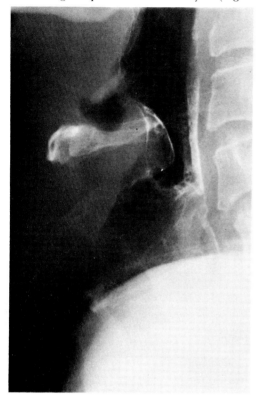

Figure 15.32 Laryngogram to outline large tumour of laryngeal surface of the epiglottis. Probable involvement of pre-epiglottic space but not reaching anterior commissure

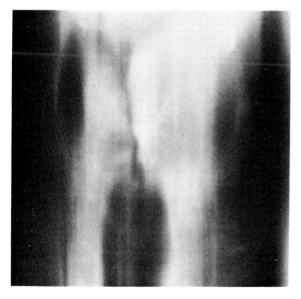

Figure 15.33 Tomograph showing massive trans-glottic tumour of left hemilarynx

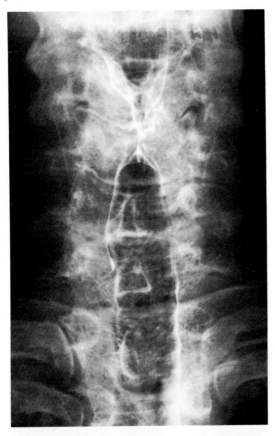

Figure 15.34 Laryngogram during phonation to reveal crater of small recurrent tumour on left ventricular band

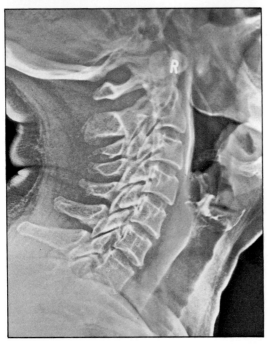

Figure 15.35 Lateral xerogram to show gross involvement of epiglottis by tumour and probable invasion of pre-epiglottic space

More recently the value of xero-radiographic techniques in producing positive prints of the larynx (*Figure 15.35*) with very clear definition has been reported especially in the lateral projection (Samuel, 1974; Woesner, Braun and Sanders, 1974). The use of computerized tomography is also being investigated relative to the larynx and other structures in the head and neck.

Histological examination

Histological examination of any tumour or ulcer is essential before treatment can be considered. Nowadays the removal of a sample of tissue for microscopical examination will almost invariably be done by direct laryngoscopy, using the pattern of laryngoscope that seems most suitable for the particular case. It has been suggested that the removal of a specimen for histological examination was undesirable (a) because it made metastatic dissemination of the growth more probable, although this is not borne out by practical experience, and (b) because a diagnosis could rarely be made from the material removed. This objection may sometimes have applied in the days of removal of tissue by indirect laryngoscopy, but has ceased to be true if adequate portions of tissue are removed by direct laryngoscopy. It is generally agreed by now that histological examination is essential for the following reasons.

For definitive diagnosis
Even the most experienced of laryngologists has been guilty of diagnosing a tuberculous laryngitis as cancer, and a carcinoma of the vocal cord may occur in a patient with obvious signs of pulmonary tuberculosis. Again, it may be impossible to know whether keratosis has not undergone malignant change without microscopic examination, and to what extent such change may show invasive disease or be confined to carcinoma *in situ*.

For the selection of treatment
In well-differentiated tumours it may be reasonable to advise conservative surgery for a borderline case, whereas in cases with poor differentiation and active mitosis conservative surgery should not be attempted in other than very favourable circumstances and an alternative line of treatment by radical surgery or radiotherapy or both would be advised.

Multiple primary tumours

The incidence of multiple primary carcinoma in the air and upper food passages is slowly increasing with the rising cure rates of cancer and the rising age of the population. At present it is about ten per cent of all patients who have been successfully treated for any one lesion in this area. Especially significant is the high incidence of bronchial carcinoma associated with preceding primary cancer in the upper air and food passages (Epstein and Shaw, 1958). This reflects a tendency to widespread mucosal degenerative changes throughout the air passages in general. The occurrence of mucosal field changes and multiple tumours within the larynx itself has also been noted (Auerbach, 1956).

It is interesting to find that there is now evidence for an increased frequency of carcinoma of the larynx in patients successfully treated for bronchial carcinoma (Lavelle, 1969). If such treatment were more successful it seems likely that there would be a corresponding increase in laryngeal cancer.

These facts emphasize the necessity for prolonged follow-up of all surviving patients, if possible throughout their natural life.

Differential diagnosis

Confusion with malignant tumours can arise mainly from four conditions affecting the larynx. These are: chronic laryngitis, benign tumours, tuberculosis and syphilis.

Less frequently the chronic benign lesions of pachydermia and leucoplakia may give rise to doubt, and more rarely still such conditions as scleroma, inflammation of the crico-arytenoid joint, or prolapse of a ventricle may cause difficulty. When a well-established lesion is present on first examination a tentative diagnosis will be made by consideration of the history, by routine examination, by examination of the neck, by examination of the nose and pharynx and by indirect laryngoscopy.

Final diagnosis will be by histological examination of a sample of tissue removed at direct laryngoscopy.

Other investigations may exclude or confirm associated conditions and will be undertaken at the discretion of the physician. In cases of doubt it may be wise to keep a patient under observation for a few weeks. It is necessary to forbid tobacco and alcohol during such a period and to avoid vocal stress. A course of wide-spectrum systemic antibiotics may also be desirable.

A more difficult question is to decide if and when a previously benign lesion has become malignant. The question arises most commonly in cases of cordal carcinoma supervening on keratosis. The keratotic condition may have been present for some years and the patient probably kept under quarterly observation (*Figure 15.13*). The change to malignancy is insidious and may occur in only one part of the keratotic area. A single biopsy may well be misleading in these circumstances.

It is therefore necessary to examine the patient at more frequent intervals, remove specimens whenever it might be thought necessary and, if doubt persists, resort to stripping of the vocal cord.

Persistent and asymmetric oedema in the larynx or localized perichondritis may also give rise to doubt as to whether residual disease is present or not in cases following treatment by irradiation. However, where the larynx has returned to normal as a result of this treatment, and some months later persistent hoarseness recurs with further oedematous swelling of the arytenoid region or of the false cord, there are much greater grounds for suspicion of recurrent cancer. Prompt imposition of absolute voice rest and the use of antibiotics and oral steroids may alter the picture favourably, but if it does not respond within two or three weeks resort must be made to careful biopsy under antibiotic cover. In these difficult cases one negative biopsy alone is insufficient evidence since residual tumour is often deeply buried as isolated cell nests in oedematous and fibrotic tissue beneath a healed mucosal surface (Olofsson and van Nostrand, 1973).

Nevertheless, it is also well recognized that such oedema may persist for six months or more following irradiation, the larynx eventually returning to normal without recurrent disease.

Curative treatment

There are still only two principal methods of curative treatment in use today: surgery and irradiation. They have complementary roles in the treatment of laryngeal cancer. In the last 30 years considerable changes have occurred involving both indications for, and the application of, these methods.

From 1920 to 1935, following the introduction of Coutard's technique of fractionated external irradiation, the larger tumours were treated by this method and the smaller Stage 1 and 2 lesions by surgery. A phase of disillusionment then set in, and shortly after the Second World War, with its rapid development of newer surgical aids, it was realized that irradiation with preservation of function was more effective in the smaller tumours, whereas the safer use of radical surgery could give greatly improved results in the more extensive tumours. This trend continues and the more recent developments are towards greater safety with preservation of function in the application of both methods.

During the past five years the value of cytotoxic chemotherapy has begun to be intensively investigated in an adjunctive role to conventional treatment. Early results are promising and sometimes remarkable but its future awaits continued trial.

Immunotherapy as yet has no specific place in treatment, but the study of immune competence may prove helpful in identifying individuals especially at risk and for planning treatment and follow-up (Chretien, 1974).

Surgery

Resection of primary tumour

The operation of vocal-cord excision by partial lateral laryngectomy via the 'laryngofissure' approach has had much popularity over the years and gives excellent results, although at the price of permanent voice impairment (Jackson, 1940; Thomson and Colledge, 1930). For this reason and because radiotherapy gives similar results in such cases, it is seldom performed today except for irradiation failures. The main indications are that the tumour shall be superficial and limited to one vocal cord without involvement of the mucosa of the arytenoid or anterior commissure and without impaired movement of the cord. However, various modifications or extensions of this procedure, for example, fronto-lateral resection, may be used when the tumour extends to the anterior commissure or on to the opposite cord. Involvement of the arytenoid vocal process by tumour with or without some impaired cordal movement may also be dealt with by a conservation procedure of somewhat greater extent – with good results. These operations are all based upon the concept of Hautant's original hemilaryngectomy and are well described by Leroux-Robert (1956) and others (Alonso, 1957; Leonard and Litton, 1971; Norris, 1958; Norris, 1974; Ogura *et al.*, 1969; Ogura, 1974; Shumrick, 1971).

Where the tumour is confined to the epiglottis and laryngeal vestibule above the vocal cords, supraglottic partial laryngectomy may be carried out today via a pharyngotomy with good results and preservation of the voice (Bocca, Pignatoro and Mosciaro, 1968; Cachin, 1974; Leroux-Robert, 1956 and 1974; Ogura *et al.*, 1969; Som, 1970). Probably the simplest example of this technique is amputation of the epiglottis via a transverse pharyngotomy for a tumour confined to its tip (Martin, 1957).

These conservation operations are often difficult; suitable cases are few and must be selected with care. Restoration of the normal swallow may give much anxiety after some supraglottic procedures. There is also the danger that preservation of vocal function may obscure the main objective – to give a patient the best initial chance of a cure by complete resection of the tumour. All these hazards are increased after irradiation; nevertheless, partial resections are still possible (Radcliffe and Shaw, 1978). For tumours causing complete fixation of one vocal cord, marked subglottic or trans-glottic spread, wide extension to the opposite cord or involvement of the anterior or posterior commissure, total laryngectomy is the only safe operation.

The disadvantages of total laryngectomy are that it involves the loss of the natural voice, interruption of the normal airways with substitution of a permanent tracheal stoma in the neck, and definite limitations on some forms of physical activity such as swimming and heavy manual work. Nevertheless, a reasonable oesophageal voice can be developed after operation in about two-thirds of patients, while the remainder today can be fitted with effective speech aids. The operation itself is not technically difficult. It now has a low mortality rate of 1–3 per cent, equivalent to other major head and neck operations, and healing is usually rapid, unless previous irradiation has been given.

Neck dissection

The place of radical block dissection of the neck in laryngeal cancer has been much debated in recent years. Where palpable evidence of metastatic disease to one or both sides of the neck exists in the absence of distant metastases, there is no doubt that dissection of one or both sides in continuity with excision of the primary disease is mandatory if a cure is to be attempted. There is also conflicting evidence that courses of pre- or post-operative irradiation for palpable and resectable cervical metastases will give some improvement in cure rates (Fletcher, Jesse and Koons, 1970; Lindberg and Jesse, 1968; Strong *et al.*, 1969).

In the past this was the only indication for neck dissection, but the detailed work of Kuhn, Devine and McDonald (1957), McGavran, Bauer and Ogura (1961) Ogura (1951), Pietrantoni and Fior (1958) and others in the past 25 years have demonstrated the existence of a high percentage of impalpable metastatic deposits in the cervical lymphatics of patients with extensive supraglottic, epilaryngeal and laryngopharyngeal cancer. As a result, the concept of elective block dissection of the neck has evolved. Accordingly, it is felt by some that elective in-continuity neck dissection should today be carried out for most extensive well-lateralized primary carcinomas at these sites (*Figures 15.47* and *15.49*) (Ogura, Sessions and Spector, 1974).

A modification of the original Crile radical neck dissection may also be made by preservation of the spinal accessory nerve in many elective dissections. This imposes little extra risk of failure and functionally gives a much better result.

Where bilateral neck dissection is required it is better carried out with an interval of three to four weeks between operations. Nevertheless, if necessary, bilateral simultaneous dissection with sacrifice of both internal jugular veins involves no increased operative risk to life, although morbidity may be severe and prolonged in some patients (Ewing and Martin, 1952). In selected cases one vein may be spared.

If neck dissection is required on one or both sides without surgery to the larynx, but where the larynx or neck has been previously irradiated, a temporary elective tracheostomy must always be performed.

Irradiation

The greatest single benefit of recent developments in radiotherapy is the increasing ability to direct high cancer-lethal dosage into the tumour while causing minimal damage to the surrounding normal tissues. In the last few years the achievement of even greater accuracy by the introduction of the linear accelerator, giving energy output up to 35 MV or more, does not yet appear to have produced much better results than by using the more modest supervoltage techniques (Lederman, 1970).

Because modern irradiation can achieve a high percentage of cures in limited glottic cancer there is a tendency to justify its initial application to all cases in the cause of preserving function, the subsequent argument being that all failures have a 'second chance' of cure by surgery. Although beguiling, this is an over-simplification for the following reasons:

(1) The true extent of the tumour cannot always be established.
(2) It may progress locally and remain undetected during treatment.
(3) It may metastasize during treatment.
(4) Deceptive appearance at follow-up or inability of the patient to attend for follow-up leads to:
(5) Delay in surgery.
(6) Increased chance of local and general post-operative complications.

For example, in supraglottic cancer where it has now been shown that adequate surgery can give better survival rates with functional conservation than irradiation, continued preference for the latter as initial therapy may result in greater loss of function owing to the probable necessity of radical surgery for the failures (De Santo, Willie and Devine, 1976). It is a long-established principle that the most effective initial treatment gives the best chance of a permanent cure.

For more extensive laryngeal and pharyngeal tumours (T3 and T4) there is evidence in recent years that pre-operative irradiation to the primary lesion and appropriate neck fields up to 3000–4000 rad can give a slightly increased survival rate and better control of neck recurrences (Biller *et al.*, 1969; Lederman, 1970). Radical resection should follow in 3–4 weeks, although there may occasionally be the chance of cure, especially in women, by completion of the course to 6000 or 7000 rad with careful follow-up.

More recent experience has apparently shown good results in extensive disease using a programme of rigid adherence to high-dosage irradiation (up to 7000 rad) followed invariably by radical surgery (Goldman *et al.*, 1972; Goldman, 1974).

Careful assessment of surgical specimens, however, revealed 34 per cent free of tumour.

Other experienced opinion has given recent evidence of improved results using post-operative full-dosage irradiation to neck fields (Fletcher, Jesse and Koons, 1970; Schneider, Lindberg and Jesse, 1975). It is clear that agreement has yet to be reached.

Chemotherapy

Single drug cytotoxic chemotherapy has been used biochemically via the intravenous and intra-arterial routes for head and neck cancer during the past 20 years or more. This method involved small doses of the drugs over periods of weeks and gave equivocal results with often serious local and general complications. However, following the successful use of multi-drug protocols based biologically on cell kinetics in the treatment of leukaemias and lymphoma, protocols have been devised using high doses of four or five drugs pulsed in short intravenous courses over about 20 hours for head and neck squamous carcinoma. These have now been in use for five or six years in this country (O'Connor *et al.*, 1977; Price and Hill, 1977) and are at present under intensive study here and elsewhere. It has been found that reduction in tumour bulk by at least 50 per cent can be achieved in 75 per cent of untreated patients with minimal complications, roughly twice the response rate of the single-drug protocols.

The drugs now used at the Royal Marsden Hospital include Vincristine, Methotrexate, Bleomycin, Cyclophosphamide, 5-Fluorouracil and Hydroxyurea. Three independent trials are in progress to establish the value of chemotherapy as an adjuvant to conventional cancer therapy at all head and neck sites. The Price–Hill 'A' protocol is used in two or three courses prior to irradiation or surgery or both in T3 or T4 laryngeal tumours. The Clifford VBM protocol is integrated by alternate weeks with a full course of irradiation. In addition, a modified Price–Hill protocol is also on trial as a follow-up adjuvant for 5–6 months in patients who have had successful treatment for T3 and T4 tumours, but remain at high risk.

Preliminary initial results for both types of protocol are encouraging for most sites including the larynx, but more time is required for a full evaluation.

Choice of treatment

The initial method of treatment will depend on the facilities available, the site and size of the tumour and upon its histology. In addition the physiological age, general health, psychology and personal factors pertaining to each patient must be weighed. Calendar age itself is no bar to surgery and physicians or anaesthetists should not be asked whether a patient is fit for operation. They should be requested to help in achieving optimum fitness. Where there is doubt as to the most suitable method, a report of poor histological differentiation should weigh in favour of irradiation or combined treatment.

Carcinoma *in situ* (T1S) has been much discussed in recent years. There would now seem to be a consensus that stripping of the affected vocal cord under microscopy with careful follow-up is the wisest initial treatment for small single lesions (Miller, 1974;

Miller and Fisher, 1971). Where the changes are multiple or recurrent irradiation will be the choice, bearing in mind the consequences of failure (Lederman, 1963).

External teleradiation is at present the choice for small T1 tumours of the vocal cord and anterior commissure. For similar limited lesions of the supraglottis and epilarynx (T1 and early T2) it is felt that the best initial treatment is by partial laryngectomy, as already described, possibly also giving post-operative irradiation to the neck. In the former case recurrent disease can still be treated by conservation surgery (Radcliffe and Shaw, 1978; Shaw, 1966). In the latter local recurrence will probably require total laryngectomy.

For late T2 tumours of all sites with or without palpable mobile neck nodes or cord fixation, and the majority of T3 tumours, radical surgery is the best choice of treatment combined with a preliminary modified course of 4000 rad teleradiation. This may also be preceded by or integrated with cytotoxic chemotherapy. A wide-field total laryngectomy will be required, often with radical neck dissection as a monobloc operation.

The majority of T4 tumours are suitable only for palliation although it is occasionally possible to salvage a few by using the combination of chemotherapy, irradiation and radical surgery.

Effective support for the above clinical indications for partial or total laryngectomy is given as already stated, in the serial sectioning of surgical specimens. This especially relates to the significance of cord fixation, cartilage involvement, and anterior commissure and subglottic lesions (Kirchner, 1969, 1974; Olofsson and van Nostrand, 1973).

If for any reason surgery is used as initial treatment of any T3 or T4 lesion without preliminary irradiation, especially in subglottic or trans-glottic tumours, it is felt that a full course of irradiation to the neck fields and stomal area must be given as soon as healing is complete (Bryce, 1972; Harrison, 1971). An adjuvant follow-up course of chemotherapy should also be considered.

In summary, small T1 tumours confined to one vocal cord are today best treated by irradiation alone and regular follow-up. Similar small T1 or early T2 tumours confined to the epilarynx or supraglottis, with or without palpable nodes, are probably best treated by primary conservation surgery. With few exceptions all more extensive tumours of the larynx are best treated by wide-field resection with neck dissection in a high proportion and usually preceded by chemotherapy and irradiation. It is clear that treatment must be highly selective to obtain the best results.

Palliative treatment

Surgery

If there is any reasonable possibility of removing surgically an ulcerated tumour in the throat with immediate healing and re-establishment of the natural swallow in an otherwise fit individual this should be done, providing any untreatable metastases are small and symptomless. In this way the worst features of terminal disease may be avoided. Otherwise surgery is generally limited to essential tracheostomy or gastrostomy, and then only with good palliative prospects.

Chemotherapy

The use of cytotoxic drugs has greatly increased since Bierman (1951) and Klopp (1950) independently noted in 1950 that the intra-arterial administration of nitrogen mustard produced profound local effects on a variety of tumours.

Although there have been only a few useful additions to the number of drugs effective against squamous carcinoma in the last 20 years, we do know more about the uses and limitations of those which are of value. The main indications for their palliative use are pain and interference with function. For this they can be effective for limited periods and preferably given on an out-patient basis by oral or intravenous routes. The most reliable and least generally toxic single drugs are considered to be cyclophosphamide and methotrexate. The use of these agents is described in more detail in Volume 1.

Irradiation

Short, well-spaced courses of 250 kV grid x-ray therapy or occasionally even supervoltage irradiation, and the carefully planned insertion of radioactive implants can often produce marked regression of inoperable growths, even in a previously irradiated field. Probably the most useful effect of irradiation in these cases lies in the reduction of pain and prevention of fungation. Cytotoxic therapy can also be used effectively when integrated with short courses of external irradiation.

Symptomatic relief

Dyspnoea
This can be very distressing, and if a tracheostomy must be performed it is better that it should be done before the stage of urgency is reached. It is usually carried out under local anaesthesia and should be as low as is convenient, especially when there is any likelihood of subglottic spread.

Dysphagia
All efforts must be directed to preserving the natural swallow by treatment and by judicious variation in the pattern of diet. But in terminal cases where tube feeding becomes inevitable, an effective early gastrostomy avoids the unpleasant features of the continuous use of a naso-oesophageal feeding tube.

Infection
This will tend to aggravate both of the preceding conditions and will also cause increased pain. Careful attention to local hygiene, especially in the mouth, is essential. The use of oral antiseptic sprays and mouth-washes with short courses of systemic wide-spectrum antibiotics can do much to improve the situation.

Salivation
Increased salivation is not uncommon in uncontrolled cancer of the larynx or pharynx, and if the patient has had irradiation the secretions are more likely to be highly viscid and distressing. Mouth-washes of one per cent bicarbonate of soda or

potassium chlorate and phenol, with plenty of watery or milky drinks and simple-flavoured glycerin lozenges can be helpful. In excessive secretion small doses of belladonna or Probanthine may be useful.

Pain

Most commonly this is a referred otalgia or pain in the side of the neck. It can be extremely severe, especially in growths with involvement of the internal laryngeal or glossopharyngeal nerves. It is seldom possible to divide the internal laryngeal nerve surgically as it is often involved in the growth, but a well-placed nerve block infiltration can sometimes be most helpful. Occasionally it may be justifiable to perform a pre-frontal leucotomy for really severe and prolonged pain. In general, however, reliance must be placed first on the aspirin group of drugs often combined with a tranquillizer, such as diazepam (Valium), before proceeding to pethidine and eventually to chlorpromazine (Largactil) and the morphine group, of which heroin is by far the most effective drug in terminal cases. A standard mixture of aspirin and nepenthe can also be most effective. Other useful substitutes are methadone (Physeptone), levorphanol (Dromoran), dextromoramide (Palfium) and pentazocine (Fortral).

The use of anaesthetic powders and local anaesthetic lozenges, emulsions or sprays may help especially if used before meals, but generally they tend to be disappointing owing to the involvement of nerve trunks. A patient should be allowed to decide for himself whether he takes alcohol or tobacco in reasonable quantity. For ensuring sleep, alcohol is the best choice at night for many elderly people once pain has been controlled. Glutethimide (Doriden) or chloral compounds are to be preferred to the barbiturates. Combinations of nepenthe and cocaine with additives such as gin and honey often give the best results. Severe secondary haemorrhage in these patients is better dealt with by sedation than by active interference. When simple drug relief of pain seems ineffective consideration should be given to cytotoxic chemotherapy.

Treatment by irradiation

Those who treat laryngeal cancer by this method should also have facility in clinical examination of the larynx. Only in this way can a radiotherapist achieve the best results and, in view of the comparative infrequency of the disease, there is much to be gained by treating these patients in large centres. Close cooperation with a laryngologist and if possible with a chemotherapist is essential in regular joint clinics.

As soon as the diagnosis has been confirmed histologically, further investigations may be required to ascertain as accurately as possible the site of origin within the larynx and the extent of the growth. A clear idea of the latter is important in planning irradiation not only to include the whole tumour within the treated area but also to minimize the amount of normal tissue irradiated.

Selection of cases

This is discussed in Volume 1. Apart from the indications discussed therein, irradiation may also be used in the presence of coexisting disease which makes surgery too hazardous; when operation is refused; or when surgical resection of the primary tumour is technically impossible, or non-resectable nodes are present. In a few cases a good response to irradiation may make a successful resection possible.

Irradiation, possibly with cytotoxic therapy, should also be considered: (a) whenever biopsy shows the tumour to be poorly differentiated; (b) after surgical resection if there is good reason to suspect that removal of disease has been incomplete; or (c) in overt and inoperable recurrence following radical surgery. In the latter case it is unlikely to be curative.

Irradiation is generally contra-indicated: (a) where there is fixation of a vocal cord by tumour; (b) where there is cartilage invasion; and (c) when established perichondritis is present.

Methods of treatment

Irradiation to the larynx may be given as follows.

External irradiation

The many varieties of apparatus which are now available to the radiotherapist, together with the more important advantages and disadvantages of each, are described in Volume 1.

In cancer of the larynx, there is much to be said for using a convenient means of gamma-radiation in the medium supervoltage range, such as the small telecurie

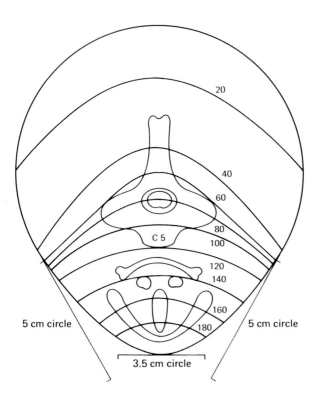

Figure 15.36 Cross-section through the neck at the level of the vocal cords with a radiation distribution superimposed. The 150 curie cobalt-60 unit is applied through three portals at a source-to-skin distance of 8 cm

therapy unit especially designed for treatment of head and neck tumours. Radioactive cobalt-60 and caesium-137 are highly satisfactory and relatively cheap sources of energy for these units. Two or three fields are planned to give a homogeneous dose to the whole volume of tissue involved. A fractional dose of 200–300 rad/day is usually given for 5–6 days per week, the total tumour dose varying from 5500 rad to 8000 rad in 6–8 weeks (*Figure 15.36*). It must be emphasized that the patient's best chance of cure is proportional to the skill and practical experience of the radiotherapist in day-to-day observation of the clinical response to treatment. Adjustments to the fields and decisions regarding fractionation and total dosage can thus be made according to local and general progress (Lederman, 1970).

In recent years much research effort has gone into conventional supervoltage irradiation under hyperbaric oxygen in the hope of increasing tumour sensitivity. So far the small improvement in results is outweighed by the complexity of treatment (Hurley, Richter and Torrens, 1972).

Interstitial irradiation
The Finzi–Harmer operation. This is mentioned mainly because of its historical importance, since it is now little used. By exposing the thyroid cartilage, partially resecting the ala adjacent to the tumour, and inserting a palisade of radium needles for a period of 6–8 days, it is possible to deliver a high dose of about 10 000 rad to the tumour without damaging the skin. It was suitable only for limited Stage 1 cordal growths before the advent of efficient external telecurie therapy, and was an excellent substitute for 250 kV x-radiation. In skilled hands it gave equal results to partial laryngectomy without impairment of the voice. A possible application today is in the treatment of poor-risk elderly patients in situations where skilled supervoltage therapy is not available or might prove too arduous for them.

Radio-active gold grain implants. Using a special type of 'gun' these tiny pellets can be inserted in any suitable pattern into a metastatic tumour mass in the neck. If planned and inserted with surgical exposure under direct vision they can deliver a depth dose of up to 10 000 rad at 1 cm distance without excessive skin damage, despite a previous full course of external irradiation. For this reason they are particularly valuable in the palliation of small tumour masses considered to be unresectable. Occasionally they can even be curative. Another valuable implant technique is by using radioactive iridium wire (Pierquin, Chassaque and Perez, 1964).

Reactions and complications

The degree of morbidity after external irradiation is very variable. It depends upon the relative biological sensitivity of the tumour and host tissues, the total dosage and the total area of tissue irradiated; for example, whether large neck fields are included and upon the individual tolerance of the patient. Very few patients require hospitalization during, or as a result of, their treatment, and those in poor general health or whose daily attendance involves much travel are usually boarded as hostel patients from the start.

In the third or fourth week of treatment some erythema of the skin and oedema of the laryngeal tissues will appear which may cause enough pain, dysphagia and dysphonia to require full hospitalization for the last one or two weeks of treatment and for about a similar period after its termination.

True perichondritis during or following irradiation today is rare and generally occurs in advanced disease with cartilage invasion or is due to an error in dosage. It may well indicate the need for a change to surgical treatment but, if slight, it is often feasible to continue irradiation under an antibiotic cover and with modified dosage. A mild subacute perichondritis is occasionally encountered as evidenced by localized tenderness, earache and laryngeal oedema. It occurs towards the end of treatment or shortly afterwards and usually responds well to voice rest and antibiotics which may be required for several weeks. This type of perichondritis may also occur some years after irradiation and may be provoked by respiratory infections.

Persistent localized laryngeal oedema, often with some degree of cervical subcutaneous oedema, is occasionally seen when high dosage has been given. The presence of residual disease is especially difficult to rule out in these cases as already discussed (p. 462).

Tracheostomy for radiation-induced oedema is now a rare event and, if it occurs, may be due to faulty radiotherapy technique. With large and infected tumours, nevertheless, laryngeal oedema is often difficult to avoid, however much care is taken. Post-radiation tracheostomy is usually a result of failure to control the disease.

Moist skin desquamation is now most uncommon but may occur in patients with especially sensitive skins. Other forms of tissue necrosis are rare and would again indicate errors or failure in treatment.

Among minor sequelae, dryness of the mouth and throat with bizarre aberrations of taste may cause discomfort for some months, but they partially resolve in time. By the fourth week dry desquamation of the skin with some atrophy and tanning are usually present. Telangiectasia and subcutaneous fibrosis will appear later.

General symptoms such as malaise, insomnia, anorexia and some loss of weight by dehydration and dysphagia are much less frequent today, but may occur if large cervical fields are used. Dietary measures to increase the fluid intake to six pints daily and to adjust the semi-solid nature of food intake may be required towards the end of treatment. The use of an aspirin or benzocaine emulsion before swallowing is often very useful. Breathing exercises, mouth hygiene and the maximum possible movement are important, especially in older patients in whom bronchopneumonia is always a risk.

A patient undergoing modern irradiation for laryngeal cancer may therefore expect a mild local and general reaction to therapy which is transient and which usually allows a return to work about four weeks after completing treatment. He must, however, take great care of the voice, no shouting or excessive strains – and no smoking – are permitted for at least three months after the end of treatment. Ideally this abstinence should continue.

Surgical techniques

Many different techniques for surgical treatment of laryngeal cancer have been devised since Gordon Buck in 1851 first performed a successful partial laryngectomy by laryngofissure for this disease in the United States; and Billroth of Vienna carried out the first total laryngectomy for cancer in 1873. All the subsequent techniques, however, have derived from the work of these early pioneers, and later modifications have concerned mainly such details as anaesthesia, skin incisions, succession of stages and methods of closure.

In the early years of the present century although these operations were increasingly used, serious complications were the rule and operative mortality due to haemorrhage, wound infection and bronchopneumonia was at times as high as 25 per cent for the smaller procedures and 50 per cent or more after complete removal of the larynx.

From about 1910 onward this toll was gradually reduced through the work of pioneers such as Gluck (1914), MacKenty (1925), Thomson and Colledge (1930). Their achievements were obtained not merely by technical skill, but by a realization of the importance of adequate preparation of the patient before surgery and careful post-operative nursing to combat the dangers of infection.

After 1940, with the advent of surgical aids such as antibiotics, safer anaesthetics and blood transfusion, the whole scene changed. There are now few definite contra-indications to laryngeal surgery and serious complications are rare. Operative mortality for major laryngeal operations is no more than 2–3 per cent.

The following types of procedure are now used:

(1) *Vertical partial resection.*
　(a) Cordectomy.
　(b) Frontal partial laryngectomy.
　(c) Lateral partial laryngectomy.
　(d) Fronto-lateral partial laryngectomy.　}　'Hemilaryngectomy'
　(e) Extended fronto-lateral partial laryngectomy.
(2) *Horizontal partial resection.*
　(a) Epiglottectomy.
　(b) Supraglottic partial laryngectomy.
　(c) Extended supraglottic partial laryngectomy.
(3) *Total resection.*
　(a) Total laryngectomy alone.
　(b) Total laryngectomy with partial pharyngectomy or partial glossectomy.
　(c) Total laryngo-pharyngo-oesophagectomy.

The operation of radical block dissection of cervical lymphatics on one or both sides may need to be combined with any of these procedures (*Figure 15.47* and *15.49*). It is seldom required in the first two owing to the absence of lymphatics in the true cords and therefore the improbability of metastatic spread. In addition, partial or total thyroidectomy may be obligatory in the major resections.

Lateral partial laryngectomy (*Figure 15.37a, b*), often termed 'laryngofissure', is today performed less frequently, owing to the equally effective results achieved by teleradiation in suitable cases. However, it still has a very definite place in situations where good radiation is not available, in some cases of irradiation failure and possibly for limited cordal tumours in young adults, where irradiation may be liable to provoke future neoplastic changes; perhaps also in a few older patients unsuitable for prolonged irradiation. Primarily it is indicated for T1a lesions of one vocal cord which should not extend into the anterior commissure or onto the arytenoid cartilage. It is also a suitable operation for the removal of many large benign laryngeal tumours.

Fronto-lateral partial laryngectomy may be useful where a glottic tumour crosses

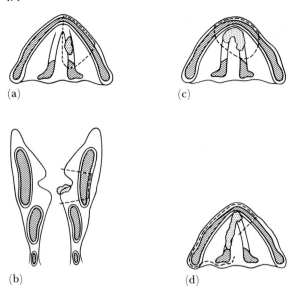

(a)

(c)

(b)

(d)

Figure 15.37 Diagram in transverse section (a) and coronal section (b) through the larynx to show the extent of tissue removed by lateral partial laryngectomy (laryngofissure) for Stage 1 growth of the vocal cord. (c) In transverse section to show extent of tissue removed by fronto-lateral partial laryngectomy for growth involving the anterior commissure; also (d) to show extended fronto-lateral resection

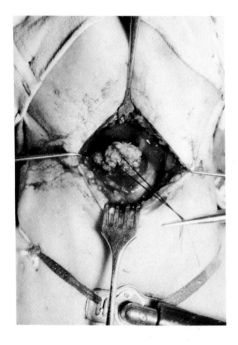

Figure 15.38 Tumour of suprahyoid epiglottis being removed through anterior pharyngotomy

the anterior commissure to involve the anterior third of the opposite cord and without any reduction of mobility ('horseshoe tumour', *Figure 15.37c*) (Som and Silver, 1968).

The older more anatomical hemilaryngectomy of Hautant (1937) is no longer employed, but providing there is no evidence of deep infiltration, an extension of the lateral partial laryngectomy technique to include the whole ventricular band and arytenoid cartilage may on occasion be used in highly selected cases (Ogura and Mallen, 1965), and is often termed 'hemilaryngectomy'. This term is also rather loosely applied to other types of partial resection (*see above*).

Pharyngotomy, either by the anterior transverse approach or by the lateral route (Trotter, 1926), provides a satisfactory access to limited Stage 1 or 2 supraglottic tumours. The anterior pharyngotomy approach is also useful in excising small tumours of the tip of the epiglottis and marginal aryepiglottic folds (Martin, 1957) (*Figure 15.38*). The larger operation of supraglottic partial laryngectomy for T1 and T2 lesions of the epiglottis and laryngeal vestibule is more modern in concept. Although growing in popularity in Continental and US Centres (Alonso, 1957; Bocca, Pignatoro and Mosciaro, 1968; Cachin, 1974; Leroux-Robert, 1974; Ogura *et al.*, 1969; Som, 1970), it is still not widely practised in Britain partly due to the relative rarity of suitable cases. However, it deserves greater acceptance in view of the consistently good results published in contrast to those of irradiation. Primarily it is indicated for T1a or T1b lesions confined to the supraglottis. Trans-glottic extension or involvement of the tongue base usually contra-indicates the procedure. It is also · inadvisable in poorly-differentiated lesions, in patients over 65 years and those with reduced pulmonary function (Som, 1970).

Consent for total laryngectomy must always be obtained before attempting any type of partial resection and the operation prudently should start with a direct endoscopy. Previous full-dosage irradiation is certainly no bar to lateral partial laryngectomy but greatly increases the hazards of the horizontal supraglottic operations. Also it should not be performed without a precise knowledge of the extent of the lesion before irradiation (Radcliffe and Shaw, 1978; Stell and Ranger, 1974).

Lateral partial laryngectomy (Laryngofissure)

Using this technique it is possible to remove completely many tumours confined to the vocal cord, with an adequate margin of healthy tissue and without removal of the arytenoid cartilage. The principles involved in operative surgery for malignant disease elsewhere will apply, with the exception that it is unnecessary to remove the associated cervical lymph nodes for reasons already given.

The tumour must be removed in one piece with as wide a margin of apparently healthy tissue as is practicable. It has been suggested that this margin should be at least 0.5 cm and although this suggestion is of some practical value the tissue removed must be as much as is possible and prudent. Even in the earliest case it should consist of the whole of the side of the larynx anterior to the arytenoid cartilage, including its tip; and from the upper border of the cricoid cartilage below to the upper border of the thyroid ala above. It may be more than 1 cm above, but may be less anteriorly if the tumour approaches the commissure, or less posteriorly if it approaches the tip of the arytenoid cartilage.

Naturally, the smaller the margin of healthy tissue removed, the less satisfactory are the results likely to be, and it is only by the judgment of the individual surgeon that a decision can be taken as to whether this method is satisfactory in any particular case.

If, on histological examination of the specimen removed at operation, any doubt exists as to the complete removal of the lesion with an adequate margin of healthy tissue, a full course of irradiation should at once be given if the larynx has not previously been irradiated. However, in the latter event, vigilant follow-up alone is permissible with recourse to total laryngectomy at the first sign of recurrent disease.

Preparation for surgery

The most important pre-operative measure in this type of surgery is to ensure as far as possible the cleanliness of the mouth. All carious teeth should be filled or removed and, in particular, attention must be paid to the gums. Gingivitis or pyorrhoea are more important even than caries of the teeth. Operation should not be undertaken until the mouth has completely healed. Nasal sepsis should be eliminated as far as is practicable and it is wise to forbid alcohol and smoking for at least two weeks before operation. Attention to general health, a normal haemoglobin level, chest film and cell count with control of other medical conditions is advisable.

From a psychological point of view the surgeon will naturally assess each case individually and will tell the patient as much or as little about the operative procedure as he thinks wise. His attitude will be encouraging, sympathetic and optimistic; and rightly so, for if optimism is not justified it is doubtful if partial laryngectomy is the correct line of treatment. The surgeon should always obtain the patient's permission for total laryngectomy in case it should prove necessary.

Anaesthesia

The operation can be performed under local anaesthesia or a combination of local with general anaesthesia. The choice will depend upon the surgeon's own particular preference, upon the availability of an experienced anaesthetist and upon the suitability of the patient for either a local or a general anaesthetic.

Whichever form of anaesthetic is used it is important that the cough reflex shall return immediately after the operation. Pre-operative medication other than atropine or scopolamine may be disadvantageous and morphine should not be used before or after surgery.

For local anaesthesia, xylocaine two per cent with adrenalin 1:200 000 is used for infiltration of the skin and tissues superficial to the larynx, while five per cent cocaine is used for intralaryngeal surface application.

For general anaesthesia after induction with thiopentone and relaxant, halothane with nitrous oxide and oxygen via a small calibre cuffed peroral endotracheal tube is satisfactory.

Where the resting airway is seriously reduced by the tumour, there should be no hesitation in carrying out a preliminary tracheostomy under local anaesthesia with insertion of a right-angled cuffed anaesthetic tube. As soon as the trachea is exposed, a few drops of five per cent cocaine solution are injected into the lumen before insertion of the cuffed tube and induction of general anaesthesia.

Position of the patient

This should be similar to that used for tracheostomy; the head is extended by placing a sandbag or a flat firm pillow beneath the shoulders. The degree of extension will vary with the individual patient and must not be so great as to cause dyspnoea. It is important that the pillow or sandbag be evenly placed under the two shoulders; if it is not, one shoulder may be higher than the other and the neck will tend to be rotated so that the trachea and larynx may not be exactly in the midline.

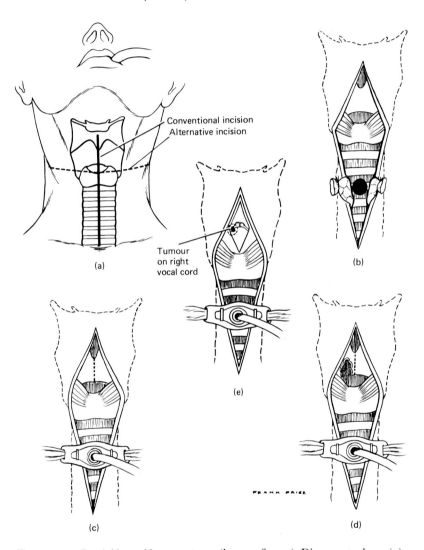

Figure 15.39 Partial lateral laryngectomy (laryngofissure). Diagram to show: (a) the incisions; (b) infrahyoid muscles retracted, larynx exposed, thyroid isthmus divided and trachea opened; (c) tracheostomy tube inserted. Dotted line shows saw cut groove in thyroid cartilage; (d) ala of thyroid cartilage being removed on the side of the tumour, up to the midline groove and back to the area of muscle attachments, prior to incision of cricothyroid membrane and internal perichondrium; (e) larynx opened to expose tumour for excision

Operative technique (*Figures 15.37* and *15.39*)

Exposure of the larynx
The classical incision is vertical in the midline and extends from the hyoid bone to a finger's breadth above the sternum. However, adequate exposure can also be obtained through a transverse curved incision centred on the border of the cricoid cartilage. A separate lower stab incision will then be required for tracheostomy. The upper flaps are developed, strap muscles exposed and skin separated mainly by blunt dissection, and at some point below the cricoid cartilage the isthmus of the thyroid gland is identified. Up to this stage the only difficulties encountered will be the division of one or two transverse connecting veins, and occasionally some difficulty in deciding the line of separation between the muscles; hence the importance of the head and neck being in the correct position.

The strap muscles should be separated in the midline to just below the lower border of the thyroid isthmus. The thyroid isthmus is now elevated from the anterior surface of the trachea. It may be necessary to incise the pre-tracheal fascia immediately above the isthmus for this purpose, but there is usually no difficulty in separating it from the trachea.

The isthmus of the gland is now clamped and divided between haemostats. Although bleeding is not usually marked, there may be large veins which will cause trouble later and for this reason it is wise to ligate the divided ends of the isthmus by trans-fixion. The front of the larynx and upper part of the trachea should now be well exposed.

Injection of the larynx and trachea
The next step will be to inject 0.5 ml of a five per cent solution of cocaine into the trachea between the second and third rings and then a similar amount through the cricothyroid membrane. The object of this is to anaesthetize the mucosa and so avoid coughing spasms on exposure of the lumen. As soon as the injections have been made, all remaining ligatures are tied and the trachea is then opened.

Tracheostomy
The tracheostomy opening is made by excising a small circular disc of the anterior tracheal wall at the second or third ring and then laterally splitting the wall with a small scalpel. This will allow the insertion of a large-sized cuffed and right-angled plastic tracheostomy tube, which is inserted as the peroral tube is withdrawn, and then connected to the anaesthetic circuit after inflation of its cuff. Ordinarily the tube is retained for 12–24 hours after operation but may then be safely removed in the absence of complications and after adequate corking for five or six hours. When the operation is performed after full-dosage irradiation, retention of the tube for about one week may be required.

Excision of the thyroid ala
It was formerly the practice to leave the thyroid ala on the affected side intact, the perichondrium on the outer surface not being touched. This method leaves the bare inner surface of the cartilage to line the larynx on the side from which the growth has

been removed. Healing over such an exposed surface is necessarily slow and some sequestration or necrosis of cartilage is possible, with formation of granulomas and prolonged subsequent healing. The present accepted practice is to excise almost the whole ala on the affected side, leaving the larynx to be lined by the external perichondrium. This removal of the thyroid ala is not followed by falling in of the soft parts but healing occurs more rapidly than if bare cartilage is left exposed. Additional advantages are that the removal of the growth is made easier and haemorrhage in the deeper part of the larynx after removal of the growth is more easily dealt with.

The external perichondrium should therefore be separated laterally on the affected side using a blunt elevator as far as possible. The most adherent part, where a sharp dissector may be needed, is at the oblique line where the inferior constrictor, sternothyroid and thyrohyoid muscles are attached, and is the usual limit of this dissection. A sharp elevator is next used to separate the perichondrium of the deeper surface at the upper and lower edges of the ala, care being taken not to separate more than about 0.6 cm. The middle line of the cartilage is next outlined by a small saw. No attempt should be made to divide the whole thickness of the cartilage but merely to make a vertical groove in the midline. The cartilage is now removed piecemeal on the involved side using a small pair of bone nibbling forceps.

After each bite the internal perichondrium is separated for another 0.6 cm, until a column of cartilage has been removed to one side of the saw-cut groove. The internal perichondrium can now be separated quite easily from the cartilage which is then removed as far back as necessary, usually back to the region of the muscular attachments.

The soft tissues of the larynx are now exposed and if the growth, as previously examined by direct laryngoscopy, approaches the anterior commissure then some of the cartilage on the unaffected side must be similarly removed.

Opening of the larynx
A vertical incision is now made in the cricothyroid membrane in the midline extending from the upper edge of the cricoid cartilage to the lower border of the thyroid cartilage.

This incision is now carried upward in the midline through the internal perichondrium of the thyroid cartilage using a pair of angled blunt-pointed scissors, and carried upwards for a distance of about 2.5 cm, the upper end probably reaching the petiolus of the epiglottis.

When the larynx has been opened in this manner the interior can easily be inspected by distracting the edges of the incision. A flat type of self-retaining mastoid retractor is most useful at this stage for exposing the lumen, leaving the assistant with two hands free.

Excision of the growth
If the tumour proves to be more extensive than was first thought, it may be necessary to carry out a total laryngectomy, the patient's consent having previously been obtained.

Careful preliminary examination, especially by tomography or laryngography, should enable such a possibility to be avoided, but it sometimes happens that the growth extends further downwards into the subglottic region than had been suspected. In such a case very fine judgment is required to decide the correct surgical

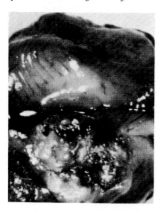

Figure 15.40   Specimen following lateral partial laryngectomy for limited cordal cancer

procedure. Hemilaryngectomy is contra-indicated if the tumour extends more than
5 mm below the vocal cord.

After packing normal-saline-moistened 2.5 cm ribbon gauze down onto the
tracheostomy tube the excision of the growth is carried out with sharp scissors.
Horizontal cuts are first made well above and well below the growth for a sufficient
distance posteriorly. The upper cut will always be through the ventricular band and
the lower one will be about 1 cm below the apparent lower border of the growth.
These incisions are best made with short straight-pointed scissors.

A troublesome vessel is usually opened at the back of the lower incision and it is wise
to secure this before removing the growth. Well-placed suction is essential at this stage
of the operation. The specimen posteriorly is best excised with a pair of scissors curved
on the flat. It should be pulled well forwards with forceps and the tip of the vocal
process of the arytenoid cartilage must always be included. Troublesome haemorrhage may be encountered in the bed of the resection close to the arytenoid. This will
need prompt diathermy coagulation.

Haemostasis and closure

All packing should now be removed and bleeding points carefully controlled. A
further proof of haemostasis is to allow the cough reflex to return at this time.

After spraying the raw surface in the larynx with a suitable antibiotic the external
perichondrium is sutured vertically with a few stitches of 1/o chromic catgut and the
wound then carefully closed in layers and again sprayed with antibiotic. A drain is
not usually required. Simple gauze dressings with a crêpe bandage are applied and
the tracheostomy tube checked and secured with tapes.

Post-operative care

The main complications to be feared after operation are haemorrhage from the
larynx, and chest infections due to aspiration of blood or inability to expectorate
blood or mucus. Both these conditions are preventable. If care is taken in ligation of
bleeding vessels, particularly subcutaneous veins, and the patient is allowed to cough
before the incision is sutured, then there is little likelihood of severe post-operative
haemorrhage. If this should occur the wound is re-opened, blood clots are removed
by suction and the bleeding points cauterized or ligated. If the bleeding cannot be

fully controlled, it may be necessary to pack the larynx, and the tracheostomy must be retained as required.

Freedom from chest complications depends upon avoiding aspiration of blood and the preservation of an active cough reflex. This, again, is one of the advantages of tracheostomy as part of the operation, since the trachea can then be packed off from the larynx during surgery. The effect of cocaine in the trachea and larynx will have worn off by the end of the operation and the patient should not be allowed to leave the operating table until his cough reflex has returned. Morphine should be avoided both before and after the operation and no analgesic other than aspirin compounds or pethidine should be necessary. The patient must be sat up as soon as possible after return to bed as it is easier for him to cough in this position. A further essential is the administration of a systemic antibiotic in full doses, starting if possible the day before surgery. Tetracycline or ampicillin and cloxacillin are usually appropriate.

The patient should not be left alone during the first five or six hours and should be in an Intensive Care Unit for the first 24 hours after operation. A nurse must be in constant attendance to make sure the tracheostomy tube is in position, and to wipe away or aspirate any mucus or blood that is coughed out. If necessary, the tracheostomy tube can be occluded by the finger to allow the patient to cough occasionally through the larynx and so clear away any blood-stained mucus which may have collected. He should be allowed to have frequent mouth-washes of iced water to keep the mouth moist, but should not at this stage swallow.

The surgeon should visit the patient some five or six hours after operation and the patient may then be given a few sips of water to swallow. Swallowing is usually a little painful and occasionally a drop or two may trickle into the larynx and cause a spasm of coughing, or be coughed out through the tracheostomy. This is only temporary and swallowing should be fairly satisfactory after 24 hours, although slightly painful for the first day or two.

If the swallow is satisfactory, two or three tablets of codeine compound in solution may be given and may be repeated later during the night if necessary. The patient may now have sips of water throughout the night as needed.

If there is no evidence of glottic oedema, the tracheostomy tube can be removed next morning, but if any doubt exists it should be left in for 24–48 hours and for about one week if the larynx has been irradiated. The throat may be examined with a mirror, but the best test is to put a finger over the tracheostomy tube and see if the patient can breathe comfortably with the tube occluded.

A dry gauze dressing is all that is required for the wound, which will usually heal without any trouble. If the tracheal fistula is moist it should be dusted with antibiotic powder at each change of dressing.

If he wishes, the patient may be allowed to get up to pass water and should be encouraged to sit out of bed the day after operation. Infection is not a likely complication if the operative and post-operative technique has been sound, but if local sepsis does occur it should be treated on conventional lines. Semi-solid food may be given the day after operation and normal diet on the third or fourth day.

Attempted use of the voice must be banned for the first 14 days. Thereafter gradual resumption of speech will be supervised by the speech therapist.

It may be two months before the interior of the larynx is completely healed. When the operation is performed after irradiation the importance of continuing antibiotic cover up to three weeks after operation should be stressed. In such circumstances healing inside and outside the larynx is delayed. Occasionally, a granuloma appears in the region of the commissure or at the site of resection a few weeks after operation. It may grow to a size sufficient to cause some dyspnoea but usually is quite small. If left alone it tends to disappear after two or three months, but it is better to remove it trans-orally and it must then be examined microscopically after removal. It is probably due to a small area of necrosis of the cut edge of the thyroid cartilage.

The patient can usually leave hospital at the end of 7–14 days but must be examined at monthly intervals for the first year after operation and at three-monthly intervals during the second year, with continued regular review.

Late results of operation

That part of the larynx from which tissue has been removed heals by slow fibrosis and epithelialization. This does not result in stenosis of the larynx, especially if the thyroid ala has been removed. It is usually found, however, that at the level of the glottis the scarring is more pronounced and that a fibrous replica of the cord is produced which, after a year, may become a very passable substitute for the true cord. Conley (1961) claims better healing and an improved voice by fashioning a new cord from an inturned flap of cervical skin used to line the raw side of the larynx. Other reconstructive techniques have been tried.

There is no satisfactory movement of this band of scar tissue and, although the voice will be useful, it is husky, variable in strength and usually cannot be said to approach the normal. Singing is impossible. There is often some stenosis if the anterior part of the opposite cord has been removed as in the fronto-lateral operation. In such cases the voice is seldom as good as in those in which the operation has been limited to one cord.

Local recurrence of growth is uncommon but may take place in the scar, or in any tissue adjacent to the area of resection. If a growth later occurs on the opposite cord it is difficult to decide whether it is a recurrence or a second primary growth.

Metastasis is rare but may become evident in the cervical or mediastinal lymph nodes months or years after operation and with no evidence of local recurrence in the larynx.

Supraglottic partial laryngectomy

Most of the general aspects of this type of surgery have already been covered in the previous pages relating to lateral partial laryngectomy. It is therefore intended to limit the description to relevant differences of detail and technique.

As regards preparation, anaesthesia and position for surgery, there is nothing to add except that general anaesthesia with relaxation is essential for this delicate and precise operation.

Slight variations in the incisions favoured in the past for anterior or lateral pharyngotomy are usually employed, an essential being that they can be rapidly extended for purposes of total laryngectomy or neck dissection. It is also preferable that the tracheostomy should be made through a separate transverse incision. The T-shaped incision illustrated in *Figure 15.44a* and described by Som (1970) is recommended.

Approach to the supraglottis

After elevation of the flaps the strap muscles are exposed and divided close to the hyoid bone. The thyrohyoid membrane should then be exposed and the upper border of the thyroid cartilage identified. The larynx should be gently rotated and the superior laryngeal vascular bundle identified and ligated. The superior cornu and posterior border of the thyroid cartilage can now be defined, displacing the superior thyroid pedicle as necessary. An opportunity is now taken to palpate the jugular chain of lymph nodes and if necessary specimens are sent for cryostat section. If neck dissection is indicated it should be done at this stage.

The external perichondrium on the upper border of the thyroid cartilage must now be incised and stripped downward to the oblique line muscle insertions until the

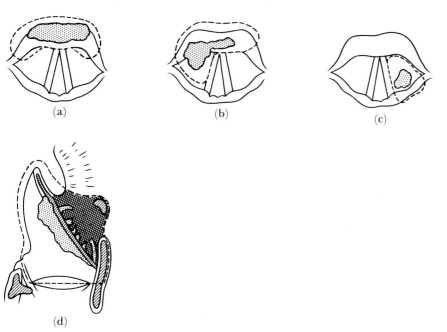

Figure 15.41   (a), (b), (c), The larynx from above to show approximate lines of resection for supraglottic tumours with sparing of the vocal cords; (d) sagittal section showing resection to include the pre-epiglottic space

upper half of the cartilage can be divided horizontally by saw cut as shown (*Figure 15.44b, c*), with the anterior end of the incision crossing the midline on a slightly upward bevel to facilitate closure. The upper half of the cartilage is now dissected away from the internal perichondrium which remains intact. At this point it is convenient to carry out a tracheostomy and to continue anaesthesia through a cuffed right-angled plastic tube, the peroral tube being withdrawn.

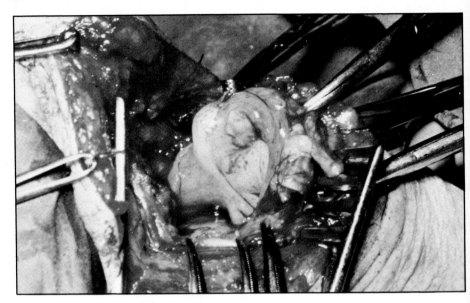

Figure 15.42   Pharyngotomy with exposure of tumour on epiglottis just before resection

Exposure of the tumour

The pharynx is now entered through a horizontal incision about 2 cm above the cut margin of the thyroid cartilage. This will pass through the lateral pharyngeal wall just above the pyriform fossa and should be continued forwards towards the epiglottis until a good view of the tumour is obtained. The tip of a laryngoscope placed by an assistant is helpful in determining the precise point of entry.

Excision of the tumour

Assuming that a resection of the whole supraglottis including the ventricular bands is required, incisions are now carried posteriorly along the summit of the aryepiglottic folds of both sides, then across the front of the arytenoid cartilages and forwards along the lateral walls of the ventricles to meet just above the anterior commissure of the vocal cords. The anterior end of the original incision opening into the pharynx is then continued slightly upwards dividing the mucosa of the pharyngo-epiglottic fold, across the floor of the vallecula and then joining the incision on the aryepiglottic fold of the opposite side. The supraglottis is now surgically encompassed but it must be removed *en bloc* with the pre-epiglottic space and body of the hyoid bone. In this region a surgical margin of 3–5 mm is considered adequate (Som, 1970).

The next and final stage of the resection is therefore division of the hyoid body from its cornua and superior muscle attachments. It is then grasped with a vulsellum and the whole specimen of hyoid body, thyrohyoid membrane, pre-epiglottic tissues and supraglottis bearing the tumour, together with the related area of the thyroid internal perichondrium, is removed.

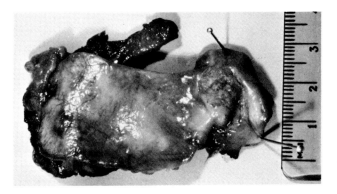

Figure 15.43 Specimen following supraglottic partial laryngectomy to include epiglottis, hyoid bone, left ventricular band, left ventricle and part of left vocal cord

Cricopharyngeal myotomy

At this stage it is convenient to displace the upper pole of the thyroid gland and expose the lower pharyngeal constrictor muscle. This is facilitated by the vertical limb of the T incision. With one finger in the hypopharynx as a guide, the fibres of the cricopharyngeus are vertically and completely divided down to the submucosa posteriorly. Following this a No 12 or 14 FG plastic naso-oesophageal feeding tube should be passed.

Closure

After haemostasis is secured, with tracheostomy and feeding tube in place, the site of resection is sprayed with antibiotic and the sandbag removed from beneath the patient's shoulders. The first step in closure is to eliminate raw surfaces within the larynx. In most cases this is achieved by approximating the cut edge of mucosa at the top of the medial wall of the pyriform fossae and valleculae to the divided laryngeal mucosa in the walls of the ventricles. Occasionally it may be possible to 'borrow' mucosa from the pyriform fossae by simple undermining and advancement or by local rotation flaps using interrupted atraumatic sutures of 2/0 chromic catgut. If raw surfaces cannot easily be covered, undue tension or distortion should be avoided and they must be left to epithelialize.

When this is completed attention is directed to closure of the pharynx. Three or four strong sutures of 1/0 chromic catgut on each side are used to approximate without excess tension the tongue base muscle, pharyngeal mucosa and cut edge of thyroid cartilage as composite stitches. Precise drill holes may be required in the cartilage if this is ossified. The head and neck are gently flexed by the assistant as these sutures are tied securely. The flap of thyroid external perichondrium is then brought up as a second layer and tacked down to the cut lower ends of the suprahyoid muscles with interrupted 2/0 chromic catgut sutures. A third layer of the divided infrahyoid strap muscles is now similarly secured to the suprahyoid muscles and hyoid cornua.

The wound is again sprayed with antibiotic, the skin flaps are approximated and a drain of Paul's tubing inserted to lie across the field in preference to suction drainage. A large gauze, wool and crêpe bandage is applied separate from the tracheostomy dressings and tapes. The nasal feeding catheter is secured and the patient moved to the Intensive Care Unit.

Post-operative care

A similar routine to that following lateral partial laryngectomy is followed at first. The drain is removed in 24 hours and the wound redressed. After 2–3 days the cuffed plastic tracheostomy tube is changed and it is emphasized that during this time the cuff must be deflated for five minutes every 1–2 hours at least.

Aspiration of tracheal secretions must be regular and thorough as some laryngeal spillover of saliva is bound to occur during the first week despite the use of a cuffed tube. All being well small naso-oesophageal tube feeds may be gradually started 24 hours after surgery. However, if regurgitation or coughing occurs it is better to continue intravenous feeding alone for the first few days.

The patient should remain in the Intensive Care Unit for about 48 hours or longer if there is any great problem with spillover or managing the tracheostomy. After the first week, skin sutures can be gradually removed and dressings reduced. The tracheostomy tube is changed every 3–4 days. At the second change a metal tube may be inserted if spillover is not great and the patient encouraged to clear his larynx and trachea by coughing.

Rehabilitation

After about ten days, gradual use of the voice is allowed under the care of a speech therapist, and if spillover is well controlled first attempts at normal swallowing are begun. Ice-cream, jellies, soft-boiled eggs and puréed foods are usually easiest and will be better swallowed if the tracheostomy tube can be plugged during eating. The biggest problem lies in the taking of fluids by mouth. In the early stages drinking with a straw or feeding cup may be helpful, and weeks or months may sometimes be necessary before complete control in this respect is achieved. As soon as there is an adequate fluid intake by mouth the nasal feeding tube can be removed.

Usually the patient will be able to return home in 3–4 weeks although full control of normal swallowing may take longer especially in older patients.

Contra-indications

This technique is precluded by any established trans-glottic disease or gross extension of tumour into the anterior commissure; any major involvement of arytenoid or posterior commissure mucosa; any marked involvement of the pyriform fossa. In general, the tumour must be confined to the supraglottis and/or vallecula, although extended operations are being developed (Ogura, Sesson and Spector, 1974).

In addition to the usual general medical and surgical contra-indications, it is felt with experience that this type of operation should not be carried out on patients who have reduced pulmonary function or who are over the age of 65. Previous full-dosage

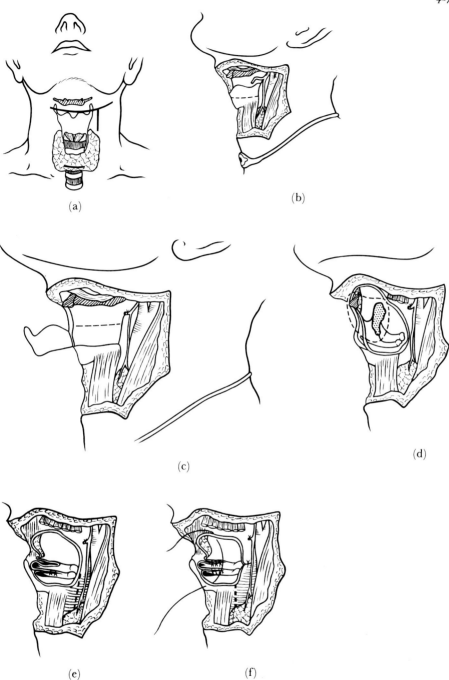

Figure 15.44 Serial diagrams to show steps in supraglottic partial laryngectomy. (a) Incisions, easily adaptable to include radical neck dissection; (b) and (c) exposure of larynx and excision of the upper part of thyroid cartilage; (d) opening pharynx, exposure of tumour with extent of excision; (e) covering of raw surfaces by suturing of laryngeal mucosa; (f) first-stage closure, laryngeal sutures completed and first pharyngeal stitch placed. The dotted line indicates the site of cricopharyngeal myotomy

irradiation to the larynx is also a relative contra-indication (Radcliffe and Shaw, 1978).

Total laryngectomy

History

It is to a Scottish surgeon, Patrick Heron Watson, that the honour of first performing total laryngectomy belongs. But on that occasion the operation was performed for syphilis (Foulis, 1866). It was Billroth of Vienna who first removed the larynx for cancer (Billroth, 1874).

At first, the results of operation were bad and not a single patient survived for one year in the first 25 cases recorded. Post-operative complications were frequent and severe, the most common causes of death being general septicaemia, spreading cellulitis or mediastinitis, septic pulmonary complications, haemorrhage and shock.

An attempt to improve on these poor results was made by performing the operation in two stages, the first consisting of the establishment of a tracheostomy, the larynx being removed a few weeks later.

In 1905, le Bec used this technique, dividing the trachea and suturing it to the skin, while the cut lower end of the larynx was drained by a rubber tube brought through the skin above and to one side of the tracheostomy. The larynx was removed two or three weeks later when the tracheal opening had united with the skin. At this second operation the skin incision did not involve the trachea and the larynx was removed from below upwards.

Single-stage laryngectomy was suggested in 1921 by both Moure and Portmann and, since that time, most surgeons have practised a one-stage operation with increasing safety.

Preparation for surgery

This does not differ essentially from that required for partial laryngectomy (p. 476). The patient should have a general medical examination which should include an electrocardiogram, chest x-ray, blood urea, complete blood count, serological tests, haemoglobin estimation, biochemistry and blood grouping.

If any general condition coexists which might adversely affect the result, the operation should be postponed until the patient can be as fit as possible. His post-operative condition must be kindly and optimistically explained to the patient and to his relatives. The speech therapist introduces herself and the physiotherapist starts simple breathing exercises. At this time it often gives a patient further confidence if he can meet another suitable individual who has achieved a good oesophageal voice after laryngectomy.

Anaesthesia

Very few surgeons may still prefer to perform the operation entirely under local anaesthesia and may attribute their low mortality to its use. Nonetheless, the results obtained today by surgeons using modern general anaesthesia are in most respects superior to those obtained by using local anaesthesia alone. Any post-operative complications which can be attributed to the general anaesthetic as such are extremely rare if a skilled anaesthetist is employed. Where the standard of general anaesthesia available is unreliable, it is possible that careful sedation and local anaesthesia may be preferable.

There is no objection to a suitable pre-medication with omnopon and scopolamine or atropine an hour before operation; any depressing effect it may have on respiration will have worn off before the end of the operation.

Local anaesthesia
This will be best obtained by using lignocaine 1–2 per cent with the addition of a small amount of adrenaline – a strength of 1:200 000 is sufficient.

The lines of the proposed skin incisions should first be infiltrated and then the region of the superior laryngeal nerves between the tip of the greater cornu of the hyoid bone and the superior cornu of the thyroid cartilage. During the course of the operation further injections of this anaesthetic can be used around the trachea and in the neighbourhood of the recurrent laryngeal nerves, or in any other situation when anaesthesia seems to be incomplete.

A solution of five per cent cocaine on a pledget of cotton wool may be applied to mucous membranes both before and after opening of the pharynx.

Alternatively, regional anaesthesia of the cervical nerve trunks may be employed, together with the use of cocaine applied locally on a swab for the superior and inferior laryngeal nerves.

General anaesthesia
This will usually be induced by an intravenous barbiturate, such as thiopentone, with a suitable relaxant, followed by whatever inhalation anaesthetic is considered best for the particular patient. Today it is frequently halothane with nitrous oxide and oxygen. Hypotensive techniques are also applicable.

If a preliminary tracheostomy has been performed, the anaesthetic will be given by this route, using a short right-angled cuffed plastic tube. If the natural airway is adequate the anaesthetist may use an endotracheal tube (nasal or oral) which will be withdrawn when the larynx is mobilized by dissection and the right-angled plastic tube is then inserted directly into the trachea via a tracheostomy before the operation proceeds further. It should be noted that there are some who hold the view that oral intubation of the cancerous larynx carries the danger of tracheal implantation of malignant cells, and for this reason it may be considered preferable to start all anaesthetic proceedings for laryngectomy with a preliminary tracheostomy using local infiltration. If the laryngeal airway is poor, then a preliminary tracheostomy under local anaesthesia is certainly essential for safety before the induction of general anaesthesia.

Technique of operation

There are many variations in technique which can be employed and it is not possible here to go into all their details. It must suffice to describe the essential steps and to indicate briefly some of the more important alternative methods of procedure.

Position
The neck is extended as for partial laryngectomy, with a sandbag beneath the shoulders.

Incisions
The classic approach of Gluck (1914) may still be used with slight modifications (*Figure 15.45*). It comprises a gently curved horizontal incision, convex downwards, at the level of the hyoid bone, extending laterally as far as the anterior border of the sternomastoid on each side. A vertical incision is now carried downwards about 2.5 cm offset from the midline to the level of the first or second ring of the trachea. This incision should be made on the side where the maximum dissection is likely to take place; for example, if radical neck dissection is to be combined with resection of the larynx, so that both skin flaps retain a good blood supply.

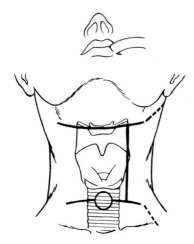

Figure 15.45 Total laryngectomy; Gluck incision modified by offsetting the vertical component. Dotted lines show extensions required if neck dissection becomes necessary; also showing position of tracheostomy

A shorter convex upward horizontal incision is then made across the lower end of the vertical incision, extending across the surface of the sternomastoid muscle for roughly half its width on either side. These incisions mark out two unequal lateral skin flaps which are dissected up to their bases and reflected. The flaps include all the superficial fascia, the platysma muscle and a few subcutaneous veins. These veins should be carefully secured and ligated as they are the most common source of a reactionary haemorrhage. In particular, the anterior jugular veins should be identified and tied. The flaps should then be covered in gauze moistened with normal saline solution.

This approach gives an excellent exposure for removal of the larynx and, with only slight modification, for pharyngolaryngectomy. The blood supply of the flaps is satisfactory, and adequate drainage can be obtained at the extremities of the horizontal incisions as far from the tracheal orifice as possible. The main disadvantage of the incision is that the vertical component is close to the pharyngeal suture line and carotid vessels. If this should break down a serious pharyngeal fistula will generally result.

An alternative incision is illustrated in *Figure 15.46*. This was first advocated by Francesco Durante (1908) and subsequently recommended by Gluck (1914) and by Sorenson (1930). The incision commences on the anterior border of the sternomastoid muscle about the level of the hyoid bone, passes down along the anterior border of the muscle for about 6–7 cm and then curves across the midline at the level of the second or third ring of the trachea.

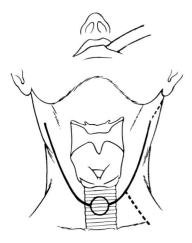

Figure 15.46   Total laryngectomy; Sorensen U flap incision with extensions for neck dissection

The advantages of this approach are that it gives adequate exposure, the suturing of the skin around the trachea is rather simpler than with two lateral flaps and there is no three-point junction. Adequate drainage can be provided on each side, well away from the trachea, the skin incisions are not so close to the pharyngeal suture line, and there is less scarring of neck tissues. This is a very satisfactory incision and preferable after irradiation although occasionally slight necrosis of the tip has been known if the flap is long.

If it should be found necessary to combine a radical neck dissection with either of these incisions, straight extensions can be produced from the nearest points to the mastoid process and to the centre of the clavicle (*Figure 15.46*).

A single vertical incision was at one time advocated (Jackson, 1940) and widely used. In theory ideal, and certainly practicable, it may not give sufficient exposure for the modern wide-field operation and it lies over the pharyngeal suture line.

Other incisions illustrated (*Figure 15.47*) are used especially for combined total laryngectomy and radical neck dissection. The double Y incision of Martin (1957) is very effective and the exposure of neck and larynx good. Its one weakness is after a full course of irradiation to the neck. In such cases there is a tendency for skin breakdown at the upper and sometimes the lower three-point skin junctions. This may result in the carotid arteries being at risk from exposure and delayed healing, the situation being further aggravated by any fistulous breakdown.

The Schobinger flap as modified by Conley has proved useful although the laryngeal exposure may be awkward. The three-point skin junction is placed posterior to the carotid vessels.

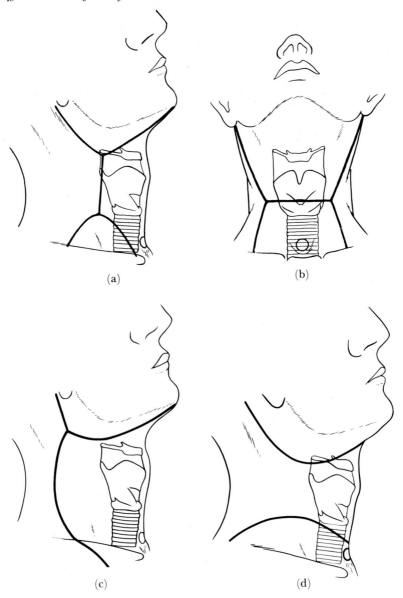

(a)

(b)

(c)

(d)

Figure 15.47 (a) Incision for combined total laryngectomy and unilateral radical neck dissection (Martin); (b) incision for combined total laryngectomy and bilateral simultaneous radical neck dissection (Martin); (c) Schobinger incision modified by Conley; (d) McFee incision modified to include total laryngectomy and neck dissection

More recently the McFee type of incision for neck dissection has been modified for total laryngectomy and laryngopharyngectomy (*Figure 15.47d*). The dissection may also be cramped but there are no weak points with consequent good healing after irradiation. The anterior end of the lower incision may also be brought below the tracheostome as in *Figure 15.47a*.

Exposure of the larynx (Figure 15.48)
After raising skin flaps the first step is to incise the deep fascia at the level of the hyoid bone vertically down the midline and to the level of the upper tracheal rings. A similar incision of the fascia along the anterior border of each sternomastoid muscle is also made. The major strap muscles, sternohyoid and sternothyroid, are now defined and divided low in the neck on each side with exposure of the thyroid gland. The sternomastoid muscles are now retracted laterally, the deep fascia covering the carotid sheath is incised and the inferior belly of the omohyoid muscle is divided. This fascia together with areolar tissue and contained lymph nodes is stripped medially towards the thyroid cartilage. As the fascia is carried medially and forward, the inferior constrictor muscle covering the posterior half of the thyroid ala will be identified. The fibres will be found to be running backwards and upwards and care must be taken not to damage the muscle unduly as it will form an important component of pharyngeal repair.

At this stage it will be convenient to define the upper border of the hyoid bone by dividing the attachments of the suprahyoid muscles close to the bone and then clearing the fascial and ligamentous attachments to the cornua on each side. The larynx can now be rotated using a sharp hook and the neurovascular bundle containing the internal laryngeal nerve and vessels isolated and divided between ligatures as they pass towards the thyrohyoid membrane on either side.

The lateral lobe of the thyroid gland on the side opposite the laryngeal tumour is now peeled away from the larynx and trachea with preservation of its blood supply. The thyroid lobe on the side of the tumour remains attached and will be removed with the larynx and para-tracheal lymphatics in most cases. Identification, ligation and division of the superior, middle and inferior thyroid vessels on this side is then carried out. It will now be necessary to divide the thyroid isthmus and expose the first five or six rings of the trachea. This completes the exposure of the larynx which will need to be freed from its posterior attachments.

Opening of the trachea
At this stage it is convenient to transfer the anaesthetic delivery tube from mouth to trachea, so that it is well free of the field during removal of the larynx.

The anaesthetist must be informed of this intention and should have prepared a sterile cuffed right-angled tracheostomy tube with a suitable connection to the main anaesthetic circuit. In addition, suction apparatus must be switched on and held ready.

Between its third and fourth rings the trachea is now opened through half its diameter, a black silk traction suture placed through the lower anterior cut edge, and the cuffed right-angle tube inserted as soon as the anaesthetist has withdrawn the original oral tube. During this manoeuvre opportunity is taken to remove all excess secretions from the trachea by adequate catheter suction. The cuff on the fresh tube is inflated and the tube itself rapidly connected to the anaesthetic circuit, being anchored in place by one or two skin stitches. Fresh sterile towels are placed in position and a small dry gauze pack inserted above the cuff in the cut end of the trachea.

Freeing the larynx
The initial step is to divide the attachment of the inferior constrictor muscle to the

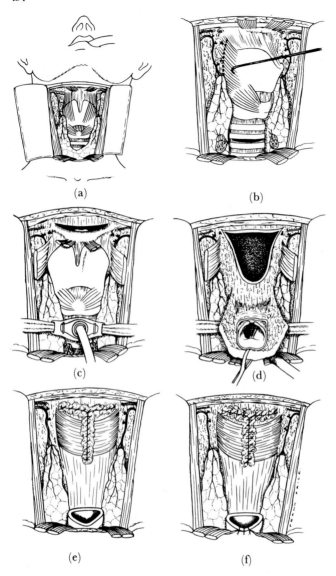

Figure 15.48 Steps in total laryngectomy. (a) Incision, division of strap muscles and exposure of larynx, thyroid gland and upper trachea; (b) rotation of larynx to expose lateral muscular attachments – dotted line showing division of inferior constrictor muscle. Superior laryngeal vessels ligated and thyroid gland isthmus divided. (c) Trachea opened, anaesthetic tube inserted via tracheostomy; (d) pharynx opened through valleculae, above and behind hyoid bone and whole larynx with hyoid bone drawn downward and forwards to expose tumour. Post-cricoid mucosa then divided transversely and pharyngeal mucosa peeled away from cricoid cartilage and out of pyriform fossae; (e) closure of pharynx after removal of larynx from stump of trachea. First layer of continuous chromic catgut to incorporate mucosal and muscle layers; (f) second layer of interrupted chromic catgut stitches binding all available connective tissues to re-inforce first layer. Commencing suture of skin margin to cut edge of trachea

thyroid cartilage while rotating the larynx first to one side and then to the other. This is done with a scalpel, cutting vertically down to the cartilage, and the muscle is then dissected free from the lateral surface of the ala with a sharp dissector. There is some advantage in separating the inferior constrictor muscle together with the perichondrium in one layer, as the stylopharyngeus muscle, which is intimately associated with the inferior constrictor, is attached to the posterior border of the cartilage and should be removed from its attachment to the thyroid cartilage with the

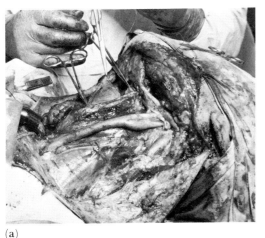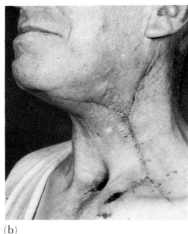

(a)   (b)

Figure 15.49   (a) Left radical neck dissection in continuity with total laryngectomy. The mucosal defect is identified by haemostat tips. The left vagus nerve has been sacrificed, but it and all other structures shown are normally preserved; (b) patient two weeks after the operation. No previous irradiation

inferior constrictor muscle. This can be done more easily if the dissection at this point is subperichondrial. When the posterior border of the cartilage has been freed it is a good plan to divide the superior cornu and remove it, taking care not to perforate the mucosa in so doing. The postero-superior border of the ala then forms a convenient angle for retraction. The deep aspect of the pyriform fossa mucosa is exposed when the posterior border of the cartilage is reached and, by drawing the cartilage well across to the opposite side, the mucous membrane of the outer wall of the fossa can be easily separated from the medial surface of the cartilage.

Removal of the larynx

The larynx can now be removed either from above downwards or from below upwards (method of Perier). There is not much difference between the two methods as regards technical accomplishment, but most surgeons prefer the former method as the growth can be seen more clearly from above and it is therefore easier to decide upon the precise margins required.

It is preferable to remove the hyoid bone with the larynx, since it ensures better clearance of the important pre-epiglottic space and also facilitates the final closure of the pharynx. Accordingly, sharp dissection is carried back through the muscle attachments along the upper surface of the bone until the submucosal layer in the valleculae is reached. This can be stripped upwards off the anterior surface of the epiglottis with a swab. The mucous membrane is then divided transversely with scissors passing across the midline just at the tip of the epiglottis in such a manner that the epiglottis is removed but the mucous membrane of the valleculae is retained for purposes of suture. If the growth is invading the epiglottis the incision in the mucous membrane will need to be modified.

As soon as the pharynx has been widely opened by this transverse incision, the epiglottis is gripped securely with vulsellum forceps and drawn forwards. A careful direct inspection is now made of the larynx to assess the size and extent of the growth and to decide whether any modification is necessary in the plan of resection. The whole larynx is now drawn forward by forceps on the hyoid bone or epiglottis. The mucous membrane on the upper part of the post-cricoid area is undermined by lateral tunnelling and divided transversely. The exact level of the incision will depend upon how much of the mucous membrane it is desired to remove.

This division of the mucous membrane will pass across the top of each pyriform fossa the mucous membrane of which was separated from the deeper surface of the thyroid ala at a previous stage. The mucous membrane from the pyriform fossae together with the mucous membrane from the post-cricoid area is now peeled away by careful gauze and occasional sharp dissection. This mucosal stripping is carried downwards as far as the third or fourth tracheal ring. No more mucous membrane should be separated than is necessary to allow division of the trachea at the desired level.

The larynx with its attached hyoid bone and muscle remnants is now removed by completing the tracheal division, if possible on a slightly forward bevel. The specimen should then be laid open posteriorly for inspection and photography before being immersed in fixative solution.

Closure of the pharynx

The opening into the pharynx is of roughly triangular shape and it is usually convenient to suture it so that the resulting scar takes the approximate shape of the letters I or Y, depending upon the amount of mucosa available. For good healing it is preferable to close the gap in a vertical straight line. There should be at least two layers of sutures; the first should aim at inverting the edge of the mucosa, and the second row of sutures should cover and re-inforce the first row, if possible completely. The best suture material is probably 2/0 chromic catgut on an atraumatic intestinal needle, although individual surgeons will have their own preferences. At this stage the extension of the head and neck should be reduced by removal of the sandbag and a nasogastric feeding tube inserted by the anaesthetist.

If ample mucosa is available, the first or mucosal suture layer should consist of a continuous inverting and locking Connell stitch inserted extramucosally as far as possible. Each bite should also incorporate the divided constrictor muscles, adjacent connective tissue and fascia so that all dead space is eliminated and firm backing is given to the mucous membrane.

Where insufficient mucosa is available for a straight line closure, a Y or T pattern should be the aim. Two similar Connell stitches are again used, the first starting inferiorly and crossing to the patient's right, while the second starts on the patient's left and crosses to the right, joining the ascending line at the middle of the Y.

A second re-inforcing layer of interrupted chromic catgut or nylon stitches is then inserted, binding any remaining remnants of muscle and connective tissue firmly on to the reconstructed pharynx.

This part of the operation may be tedious but it is important that it should not be hurried, since careful suturing of the pharyngeal wall will make all the difference to good healing. When the pharynx has been sutured the surface should be lightly sprayed with a suitable antibiotic solution or powder.

Creation of tracheostome and skin closure
The anaesthetist should now ensure that the blood pressure is brought back to normal limits. When all bleeding points have been controlled, the gauze pack is removed from around the tracheostomy tube and a suction catheter is inserted to remove any inhaled blood or mucus. If any doubt exists a bronchoscope can be passed and direct aspiration carried out.

The wound is again sprayed with antibiotic powder and the skin flaps are approximated. The remainder of the divided tracheal edge is now sutured to the skin, every endeavour being made to leave no raw margin exposed. Careful skin-to-mucosal suture of the tracheal edge will promote rapid healing and prevent subsequent cicatricial contraction of the tracheal orifice.

If the larynx is removed from below upwards, the trachea is divided as already described and is tethered to the skin by two fixation sutures. The larynx is then separated from the anterior wall of the gullet and hypopharynx by blunt dissection from below as far up as the arytenoids, and the pharynx opened at this point. The mucous membrane is then divided with scissors along the same lines as already described and the pharyngeal opening is sutured in the same way.

The suture material for the skin and the tracheal orifice is a matter of personal choice but 2/0 and 1/0 black silk is recommended after the skin flaps are carefully secured with subcutaneous catgut.

Adequate drainage of the wound is extremely important and is best dealt with by using soft latex tubing of the Paul or Penrose type at the lower lateral extremities of the incisions. These should be sutured to the skin and should project about 2.5 cm beyond it in order to conduct any exudate as far away from the tracheal orifice as possible. If continuous suction drainage is to be used, large-calibre perforated plastic aspiration tubes are inserted in place of the drains and should be connected to a pump in preference to vacuum bottles.

Where a previous tracheostomy has been performed, the whole fistula including the surrounding skin must be excised with the laryngeal specimen. The siting of the main skin incisions at the start of the operation should be planned accordingly.

Post-operative care

This must be carried out under the personal supervision of the operating surgeon. For the first two days it is essential that a nurse be in constant attendance and preferably in an Intensive Care Unit.

The immediate post-operative dressing using simple drainage, should include a crêpe bandage with a heavy-pressure dressing of gauze and wool over the area of operation above the tracheal orifice. This will eliminate the dead space, ensure immobilization, tend to prevent exudates from collecting beneath the flaps and encourage their adherence to the pharynx. Alternatively, if continuous suction drainage has been used only a light gauze dressing will be necessary.

A suitable size of laryngectomy cannula such as the Colledge pattern, modified to hold an extra-long inner tube to carry it free of the heavy dressings anteriorly, should be used for the first few days (*Figure 15.50*). After the first three or four days, the inner

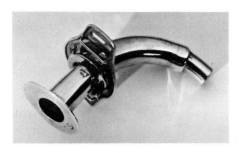

Figure 15.50   Colledge pattern laryngectomy cannula modified to hold temporary long inner tube for use with post-operative dressings

tube can be omitted, although the cannula will need regular changing at least once daily. This has been found to be an improvement on the older Moure–Lombard cannula, which causes pressure damage to the trachea/skin junction.

Care of the tracheostome

The nurse will be provided with a bedside suction apparatus with sterile catheters for keeping the tracheostome free of mucus without disturbing the patient by having to wipe it away. Handling of all suction tubing by the nurses must be as clean as possible. Catheters should be whistle-tipped and of soft rubber or plastic. They are used once only and then discarded into a separate receiver for sterilization or disposal.

The inner tube should be removed every hour or two for cleaning but the nurse must not interfere with the outer cannula; this should be removed by the surgeon himself, for purposes of cleaning or change of dressing. After the first two or three days instructions for changing the tube may be given to the nursing staff. Before operation,

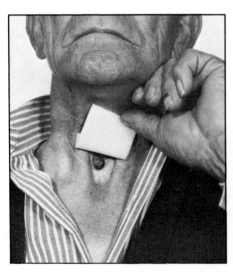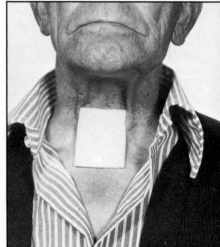

Figure 15.51   Adhesive foam plastic filter/shield for tracheostome

all nurses who are to be in attendance should be fully acquainted with the type of cannula to be used and have a duplicate demonstrated to them. A spare should be available at all times in the ward for changes of dressing.

After the stitches have been removed, in about 6–10 days, a simple metal laryngectomy cannula of the Colledge type, omitting an inner tube, can be used, or a large-size plastic cannula may be worn. The patient must be instructed how to clean and change these for himself. When it is evident that there is no tendency for the tracheal orifice to contract, usually after about 6–8 weeks, the cannula may be discarded completely in most cases and a buckle-shaped shield holding a disposable gauze swab can be worn round the neck to cover and protect the stoma (*Figure 15.52*).

(a)

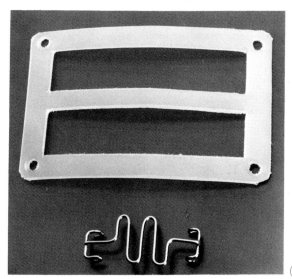

(b)

Figure 15.52 Tracheostome shields. (a) Soft plastic buckle held by tapes around neck and covered with disposable gauze; (b) spring wire baffle clipped to flange of laryngectomy cannula

Another useful device is a foam plastic square with an adhesive upper margin applied just above the stoma and acting as an air filter and moisture absorbent (*Figure 15.51*). Alternatively, a wire mesh shield can be clipped on to the front of a laryngectomy cannula if this must continue to be worn (*Figure 15.51*). A thin gauze veil may then be worn around the neck beneath the shirt.

Care of the wound

If reasonable care has been taken at all stages, and with full antibiotic cover, there is nowadays an excellent chance of healing by first intention. The drainage tubes must be removed after two or three days, if there is no longer any discharge of blood-stained serum. Where there is doubt, as in post-radiotherapy cases, the drainage tubes are best left in position for an extra day or two. If the wound is going to break down, the most critical time is about the tenth day, when the pharyngeal sutures will begin to slough out. The only sign of this may be a small leakage of saliva from one of the drainage areas. Within a day or two the other side may also leak and a large part of the incision quietly open without many signs of inflammation. The leaking saliva would appear in such cases to exert some sort of digestive action on the young fibrous tissue of the wound. Fortunately by this time the tracheal stoma is often firmly healed and does not usually separate.

If leakage occurs, it is important that the nurse changes the dressings frequently, often three or four times daily, and that suction is regularly applied. Although plain dry dressings are most useful together with a suitable antibiotic spray to the wound itself, sloughing and infected wounds will require the additional use of antiseptics and cleansing agents. Freshly-prepared zinc peroxide cream after irrigation with half-strength Eusol solution has been found to be very effective in such cases. The drainage and removal of dead tissue is also essential.

With modern antibiotics, sepsis is no longer the bugbear it was and the large fistulae associated with septic sloughing of the flaps, which were at one time not uncommon, now rarely occur. In the majority of cases and even after irradiation, fistulae will heal within a few weeks. Occasionally, however, a fistula will persist, usually about the midline and requiring secondary closure by a suitable recon-structive procedure. No attempt at direct repair should be made until all infection has resolved and the skin and mucous membrane in the fistula are healed without intervening raw surfaces (Maw and Lavelle, 1974).

Antibiotic cover

Change occurs so rapidly in the use of these agents that it is not easy to lay down any permanent rules. At the present time, however, the safest routine would appear to be a polymyxin-bacitracin spray to the wound at the time of operation and at subsequent dressings, while a routine course of systemic tetracycline or ampicillin with cloxacillin is also given six-hourly, commencing the day before operation and going on for at least two weeks afterwards, even if there is no pyrexia and the wound is healing well.

Naso-oesophageal feeding tube

This should be of soft rubber or plastic. The most practical size is a No 12 or 14 FG whistle-tipped urethral catheter with a washer-type disc mounted at its proximal end to prevent its disappearing into the nose, but very narrow-gauge plastic tubes are now being developed for drip-feed techniques which are more comfortable. They are passed trans-nasally at the time of operation and should be left in until such time as the wound is healed, usually 6–7 days, but often longer in irradiated cases. Saliva can be swallowed quite comfortably and the tube should be fixed to the nose with a strip of adhesive tape or a silk suture. The nurse in attendance must take care to see that the patient does not pull out the tube while he is coming round from the anaesthetic or subsequently.

Chest complications

These depend almost entirely upon the presence of blood or inspissated secretions in the bronchi and are more often in the nature of a partial collapse with mild infection than an established bronchopneumonia. With careful technique they are now uncommon.

Treatment is, in the main, preventive. Omnopon may be given an hour before operation but should not be given after this time because of its depressant effect on the respiratory system.

Cocaine in a five per cent solution may be employed conservatively on the tracheal mucosa but not so liberally that it runs down into the bronchi.

If there is any likelihood of blood in quantity having entered the trachea during operation a bronchoscope should be passed before the patient leaves the table and thorough aspiration carried out. If the operation is being done under general anaesthesia this must always be lightened before the end of the operation so that the cough reflex is present before dressings are applied.

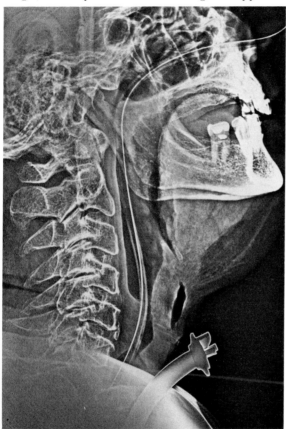

Figure 15.53 Lateral xerogram to show fistula formation from tongue base downward beneath skin flap — after total laryngectomy

The patient should be sat up as soon as possible after operation since coughing is much easier and more effective in this position than if the patient is recumbent. If there are any signs of post-operative pulmonary collapse or obstruction, a bronchoscope should again be passed for direct aspiration, while if bronchopneumonia does develop it should be treated on general medical lines. A portable chest x-ray on the first day after operation is a wise routine measure.

Other complications

Reactionary haemorrhage may occur, particularly from veins in the skin flaps or in the region of the thyroid gland. If necessary the wound must be re-opened at once and the bleeding vessel ligated.

Wound infection is now uncommon and if it arises it must be controlled on a routine bacteriological and suitable antibiotic basis.

Pulmonary and cerebral embolism have been recorded but although serious they are not of especial frequency. Probably the most serious complication which usually occurs without warning is cardiac infarction. A post-operative electrocardiograph the day after operation may well be useful.

Pharyngeal fistula is the most common complication which must be avoided if possible. It occurs in at least 20 per cent of patients. The main factors in its prevention have already been considered.

In the majority of cases the fistula is small and heals within a few weeks without interference. If it persists, it may be closed by a simple plastic operation, in which the skin and mucosal surfaces are separated from each other, the mucosal layer carefully sutured so that the edges are turned into the pharynx and the skin sutured to cover it so that the edges are slightly everted. If possible the two suture lines should not lie over each other. If the opening is of larger size it may be necessary to incise the skin around the fistula and turn the skin inwards so that the anterior wall of the pharynx is now lined by skin. The raw surface remaining may be closed by turning down a rotation flap of skin from beneath the chin or from the side of the neck. If this is not possible or if the tissues are severely devitalized by irradiation the skin cover must be provided from elsewhere, usually by a delto-pectoral skin flap from the anterior chest wall.

Crusting in the trachea is also a common post-operative complication. This is due to the excess drying of the secretions in the trachea from the loss of air-conditioning by the nose and throat. The crusts may be removed by cotton-wool swabs moistened with dilute bicarbonate of soda, and the tracheal surface should be sprayed every two or three hours with a similar one per cent solution, sometimes combined with Alevaire or Varidase if crusting is severe. Some degree of infective tracheitis is also frequently present and may require the further use of systemic and local antibiotics. Care must be taken to see that inspired air is adequately humidified.

The late complication of stomal recurrence is usually associated with subglottic extension of disease either at the primary site or in para-tracheal lymphatics. It is also associated with previous tracheostomy, the site of which must be excised with the specimen. In high-risk cases immediate post-operative irradiation to the stoma and superior mediastinum is advised.

Swallowing after total laryngectomy

As a rule this presents no difficulty. Even while a nasal feeding tube is in position a patient can swallow his saliva and drink fluids quite satisfactorily, although the act of swallowing is painful for the first few days. If healing has proceeded well and a fistula is not anticipated, it is possible to remove the feeding tube after about six days, but if there has been previous irradiation it is much wiser to leave the tube in position for about ten days, since it is often not until the tenth day or later that the pharyngeal wound tends to break down. If the wound does break down, the tube should be left in position until the full extent and size of the fistula are revealed. If the fistula is small, it can probably be controlled during swallowing by pressure from the gauze pack, and if so the tube can be removed. If a large fistula persists, however, it is much wiser to continue using a tube until the fistula is closed, although it may be more convenient to withdraw the tube and insert it for each feed. Occasionally a temporary gastrostomy may be less tiresome for the patient and may facilitate healing in the neck until plastic closure can be completed.

Functional rehabilitation

All operations on the larynx and pharynx imply at least temporary interference with function, depending upon the amount of anatomical and neurological disruption. When the act of swallowing is deranged it is usually due to immediate mechanical factors, such as oedema and distortion of the lumen with neuromuscular in-coordination added to the discomfort of local movement. As healing proceeds these factors resolve and the patient quickly re-educates himself with minimum assistance, although the swallow may remain more of a voluntary effort than formerly.

When the voice is impaired by operations on the larynx, the aid of a speech therapist is essential in restoring its quality and strength. After total laryngectomy a fair though gruff voice can be regained by learning oesophageal speech. This requires using the oesophagus as an air reservoir filled by voluntary effort from the pharynx or even by inflation through a prepared tracheo-oesophageal fistula, as was first suggested by Conley, de Amesti and Pierce (1958). The air is then passed rapidly upward at will, causing the narrower parts of the lower pharynx to vibrate with the production of a low-pitched sound.

Recently several further attempts have been made to aid voice production by means of a tracheo-oesophageal fistula carefully constructed in stages (Asai, 1965; Edwards, 1976; Shedd, 1974). When successful this can certainly produce a stronger voice, but problems of management of the fistula with leakage from the pharynx have been encountered, and there is the necessity to close the tracheostome when speaking, generally by means of a valved tube.

Despite occasional reports there is at present no record of any effective and successful total laryngeal transplant having been carried out in the human. Work continues in animals but so far without lasting success.

Alternatively, a patient may prefer or be obliged to use one of various types of mechanical speech aid now on the market. These include the portable transistorized electrolarynx acting through a vibrating disc placed against the skin of the neck (*Figure 15.54*). Modifications of the original Tapia artificial reed larynx operating from the tracheostome such as the van Hunen nylon membrane vibrator may be used, and also electrically-operated mouth resonators activated by a small wire from pocket batteries, either carried externally, such as the Ticchioni pipe, or built into the upper denture (Edwards, 1976; Tait, 1959).

To a large extent restoration of function depends upon the age, intelligence and determination of the patient, whatever aids may or may not be available. About 60 per cent of all 'laryngectomees' achieve a useful oesophageal voice without artificial aids. However, any good speech rehabilitation programme must give instruction in

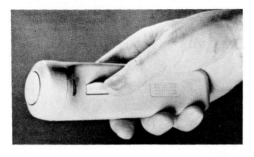

Figure 15.54 The Bell system transistorized electrolarynx to show the vibrating disc operated by thumb switch

artificial aids to those who require them in order to help prevent the lowering of morale and drift into depression that can easily occur in some of these patients (Gilchrist, 1973).

Disability after total laryngectomy

The main disability from which the patient will suffer after operation is naturally the loss of his normal voice. The sense of smell is also impaired only because there is no regular air current through the nose, but taste and the appreciation of flavours remain during eating and there is usually no complaint on this account.

The patient must take care when having a bath or washing that water does not enter the tracheostome, and swimming must be prohibited.

Heavy lifting or strenuous digging is not possible as these actions entail fixation of the chest wall by closure of the larynx, but light physical work is possible and occasionally the patient can partially close the tracheostome by contracting any muscle remnants surrounding it. Some young women who have undergone this operation have subsequently married and borne children without difficulty (Shaw, 1965).

If radical neck dissection has been necessary, some reduction in the usefulness of the arm at the shoulder level may be expected, especially in the later age groups together with a variable amount of persistent discomfort more evident in those whose range of movement is most impaired (Ewing and Martin, 1952).

Apart from these disadvantages, patients generally come to terms with their disabilities, adaptation being usually good in age groups up to 65. Unfortunately many patients are older and less adaptable but with instruction and encouragement from surgeons, speech therapists, laryngectomee clubs and associations, the majority lead happy and useful lives although often socially limited.

Summary and selection of treatment

Assessment of the relative value of differing treatment methods for laryngeal cancer is not easy. Despite the gradual international adoption of the TNM Classification System, now confirmed in 1978 for the larynx, and greater uniformity in end-result reporting, the majority of accounts are still based on retrospective studies. Adequate conclusions by randomized controlled prospective studies are still principally lacking, in part due to their difficult application in cancer therapy. Despite this, much knowledge has been gained in recent years by extensive clinical experience using increasingly refined methods of surgery and irradiation; also by the histological study of serially-sectioned laryngeal specimens (Kirchner, 1969; McDonald, De Santo and Weiland, 1976; Olofsson and van Nostrand, 1973). Important knowledge of lymphatic pathways within the larynx (Pressman and Simon, 1961) and patterns of local spread and cervical lymph node involvement have also been gained (Kirschner, 1974; Olofsson and van Nostrand, 1973).

Forty years ago radiotherapy was condemned even for limited cordal cancer (Colledge, 1940). Today it is established as the treatment of choice in such lesions. In early glottic cancer (T1 and T2) modern irradiation techniques still allow the surgeon to perform partial or total laryngectomy for failures with good salvage rates (Bryce, 1972; Lederman, 1970; Ormerod, 1958). In support of irradiation for early glottic lesions, Lederman (1970) gives five-year survival rates of at least 77 per cent in his large series. Recurrence of glottic cancer after irradiation and still treatable by lateral partial laryngectomy, can give a salvage of about 60 per cent three-year survivals with preservation of voice and natural airway (Radcliffe and Shaw, 1978). In more advanced recurrent glottic or trans-glottic cancer after irradiation a five-year survival rate of 47 per cent by total laryngectomy can still be obtained (Sheehan and Shaw, 1979).

On the other hand, recent five-year survival results for initial treatment by irradiation of early supraglottic and epilaryngeal cancer without nodal spread seldom exceed 50 per cent (Lederman, 1970) and salvage for failures will generally require total laryngectomy. By contrast, such cases treated today by supraglottic partial laryngectomy techniques give five-year survival rates of at least 70 per cent with normal voice preservation and equally good chances of salvage by total laryngectomy for the fewer failures (Leroux-Robert, 1974; Ogura and Mallen, 1965; Shumrick, 1971; Som, 1970). Primary conservation surgery therefore favours vocal cord preservation in such lesions compared with treatment by initial irradiation (De Santo, Willie and Devine, 1976).

In more advanced glottic and trans-glottic lesions (T3 and T4) treatment has come to be based on a planned combination of radical surgery usually preceded by a modified or full dosage of irradiation to the larynx and neck (Constable *et al.*, 1972; Goldman *et al.*, 1972; Lederman, 1970; Sisson, 1974). Most authorities favour pre-operative irradiation in this group of tumours, but Fletcher, Jesse and Koons (1970) and others at MD Anderson Hospital are impressed by the value of post-operative irradiation in their patients.

The rare cases of true subglottic cancer are generally advanced when diagnosed and it is agreed that planned combined treatment by ultra-radical surgery with post-operative irradiation to the lower neck and mediastinum probably gives the best chance of a cure (Bryce, 1972; Harrison, 1971). However, Lederman (1970) has shown that where the disease is limited to the anterior half of the subglottic space with no palpable neck nodes and no vocal cord fixation, a five-year survival rate of 60 per cent can be obtained by irradiation, particularly in women.

A more recently emerging treatment apparently of value when used as an adjuvant method in advanced lesions (T3 and T4) is cytotoxic chemotherapy (*see also* Volume 1). Since 1974, the use of a kinetically based multi-drug protocol has been on trial either before or after conventional therapy (Price and Hill, 1977) or integrated with irradiation (Clifford *et al.*, 1978). Hopeful results are beginning to emerge from both techniques with minimal side-effects. The former authors show a 70 per cent initial response rate in laryngeal cancers so far treated. The latter method of integrated therapy has recently shown a survival rate of 52 per cent up to 24 months, exactly double that of the control series.

These results illustrate certain definite trends in the management of laryngeal cancer. First, that irradiation gives excellent results in the early glottic lesions with absolute preservation of function. Secondly, that the balance of judgment between conservation and radical surgery of the larynx is becoming more refined with the results of the former approximating the latter for supraglottic tumours and surpassing the results of irradiation. Thirdly, that the attack on cancer at the molecular level through cytotoxic drugs is now being applied to the larynx as an aid to conventional methods or combined treatment, again with cure and functional conservation as the objectives.

In conclusion, the ultimate results of treatment still depend on the known clinical and pathological features of the tumour, the biological resistance of the host tissues and upon the patient's sex, age and psychology.

References

Abrikossoff, A. (1931). *Virchows Archiv für pathologische Anatomie und Physiologie und für klinische Medizin*, **280,** 723

Alonso, J. M. (1957). *Annals of Otolaryngology, Paris*, **74,** 75

Annual Reports (1960–76). South Thames Cancer Registry, London

Asai, R. (1965). *Proceedings of the Eighth International Congress of Otolaryngology*, Excerpta Medica ICS No. 113; Tokyo

Asherson, N. (1957). *Journal of Laryngology*, **71,** 730

Auerbach, O. (1956). *New England Journal of Medicine*, **256,** 97

Auerbach, O., Hammond, E. C. and Garfinkel, L. (1970). *Cancer*, **25,** 92

Barclay, T. H. C. and Rao, N. N. (1974). *Laryngoscope*, **85,** 254

Barsocchini, L. M. and McCoy, G. (1968). *Annals of Otology*, **77,** 146

Batsakis, J. G. and Fox, J. E. (1970). *Surgery, Gynaecology and Obstetrics*, **131,** 989

Bierman, H. R. (1951). *Journal of the National Cancer Institute*, **11,** 891

Biller, H. F., Davis, W. H., Powers, W. E. and Ogura, J. H. (1969). *Laryngoscope*, **79,** 1387

Billroth, T. (1874). *Archiv Klinische Chirurgie*, **17,** 343

Birck, H. G. and Manhart, H. E. (1962). *Archives of Otolaryngology*, **77,** 603

Bjork, H. and Weber, C. (1956). *Acta oto-rhino-laryngolica*, **46,** 499

Bocca, E., Pignatoro, O. and Mosciaro, O. (1968). *Annals of Otology*, **77,** 1005

Bone, R. C., Feren, A. P., Nahum, A. M. and Winkelhake, B. G. (1976). *Laryngoscope*, **86,** 341

Booth, J. B. and Osborn, D. A. (1970). *Acta Otolaryngolica*, **70,** 279

Brindle, M. J. and Stell, P. M. (1968). *Clinical Radiology*, **19,** 257

Broders, A. C. (1920). *Journal of the American Medical Association*, **74,** 656

Broyles, E. N. (1941). *Southern Medical Journal*, **3,** 239

Bryce, D. P. (1972). *Journal of Laryngology and Otology*, **86,** 669

Burns, H. P., van Nostrand, A. W. and Bryce, D. P. (1976). *Annals of Otology, Rhinology and Laryngology*, **85,** 538

Cachin, Y. (1974). *Tumori*, **60,** 591

Cady, B., Rippey, J. H. and Frazell, E. L. (1968). *Annals of Surgery*, **167,** 116

Capps, F. C. W. (1957). *Journal of Laryngology*, **71,** 709

Chretien, P. B. (1974). *Centennial Conference on Laryngeal Cancer, Workshop No. 5 Toronto.* (Eds P. W. Alberti and D. P. Bryce, 1976); Appleton Century Crofts, New York

Clifford, P., O'Connor, A. D., Durden-Smith, J., Hollis, B. A. B., Edwards, W. G. and Dalley, V. M. (1978). In: *Antibiotics and Chemotherapy*, Vol. 24, p. 60; Karger, Basle

Colledge, L. (1940). *Journal of Laryngology*, **55,** 443

Conley, J. J. (1961). *Archives of Otolaryngology*, **74,** 21

Conley, J. J., de Amesti, F. and Pierce, M. K. (1958). *Annals of Otology*, **67,** 655

Conley, J. J. and Pack, G. T. (1974). *Archives of Otolaryngology*, **99,** 315

Constable, W. C., Marks, R. D., Robbins, J. P. and Fitz-Hugh, G. S. (1972). *Laryngoscope*, **82,** 1861

Cook, T. A., Brunschwig, J. P., Butel, J. S., Cohn, A. M., Goepfert, H. and Rawls, W. E. (1973). *Annals of Otology, Rhinology and Laryngology*, **82,** 649

Coutard, H. (1939). *Surgery, Gynaecology and Obstetrics*, **68,** 467

Creston, J. E. (1961). *Archives of Otolaryngology*, **74,** 556

Crookes, J. (1953). *Journal of Laryngology*, **67**, 433

Cummings, C. W., Montgomery, W. W. and Balogh, K. (1969). *Annals of Otology*, **78**, 76

Curwen, M. P., Kennaway, E. L. and Kennaway, N. M. (1954). *British Journal of Cancer*, **8**, 181

De Santo, L. W., Willie, J. D. and Devine, K. D. (1976). *Laryngoscope*, **86**, 649

Durante, F. (1908). *International Clinics*, **1**, 122

Edwards, N. (1976). *British Journal of Hospital Medicine*, **17/8**, 145

Epstein, S. S. and Shaw, H. J. (1958). *Cancer, New York*, **11**, 326

Epstein, S. S. and Winston, P. (1957). *Journal of Laryngology*, **72**, 452

Epstein, S. S., Winston, P., Friedmann, I. and Ormerod, F. C. (1957). *Journal of Laryngology*, **71**, 673

Ewing, M. R. and Martin, H. (1952). *Cancer, New York*, **5**, 873

Fairman, H. D. (1972). *Proceedings of the Royal Society of Medicine*, **65**, 619

Finzi, N. S. and Harmer, D. (1928). *British Medical Journal*, **2**, 886

Fletcher, G. H., Jesse, R. H. and Koons, C. R. (1970). *American Journal of Roentgenology*, **108**, 269

Foulis, D. (1866). *Transactions of the International Medical Congress London*, **11**, 25

Friedmann, I. (1974). *Centennial Conference on Laryngeal Cancer, Workshop No. 7 Toronto* (Eds P. W. Alberti and D. P. Bryce, 1976); Appleton Century Crofts, New York

Fust, J. A. and Custer, R. P. (1949). *American Journal of Clinical Pathology*, **19**, 522

Gilchrist, A. G. (1973). *Acta Otolaryngolica*, **75**, 511

Gluck, T. (1914). In: *Handbuch der Speziellen Chirurgie* (Eds Katz, Preysing and Blumefield); Kabitzch, Würzburg

Goldman, J. L. (1974). *Centennial Conference on Laryngeal Cancer, Workshop No. 5 Toronto* (Eds P. W. Alberti and D. P. Bryce, 1976); Appleton Century Crofts, New York

Goldman, J. L., Zak, F. C., Roffman, J. D. and Birken, E. A. (1972). *Annals of Otolaryngology*, **81**, 488

Gross, C. W. and Hubbard, R. (1974). *Laryngoscope*, **84**, 1090

Harrison, D. F. N. (1964). *Quarterly Journal of Medicine*, **33**, 25

Harrison, D. F. N. (1971). *Journal of Laryngology and Otology*, **86**, 669

Hautant, A. (1937). *Journal of Laryngology*, **52**, 65

Holborow, C. A. (1958). *Archives of Diseases of Children*, **53**, 210

Holinger, P. H. (1962). *Archives of Otolaryngology*, **75**, 105

Holinger, P. H. and Delgado, A. (1959). *Archives of Otolaryngology*, **70**, 555

Holinger, P. H., Johnson, K. C. and Anison, C. C. (1950). *Annals of Otology*, **59**, 547

Hollingsworth, J. B., Kohmoos, H. W. and McNaught, R. C. (1956). *Archives of Otolaryngology*, **52**, 82

Hurley, R. A., Richter, W. and Torrens, L.

(1972). *British Journal of Radiology*, **45**, 98

Isambert, A. (1876). *Annales des maladies de l'oreille et du larynx*, **2**, 1

Jackson, C. L. (1940a) *Archives of Otolaryngology*, **31**, 23

Jackson, C. L. (1940b). *Surgery, Gynaecology and Obstetrics*, **70**, 537

Kirchner, J. A. (1969). *Annals of Otology*, **78**, 689

Kirchner, J. A. (1974). *Canadian Journal of Otolaryngology*, **3**, 460

Kirchner, J. A. (1974). *Centennial Conference on Laryngeal Cancer, Workshop No. 10 Toronto* (Eds P. W. Alberti and D. P. Bryce, 1976); Appleton Century Crofts, New York

Kleinsasser, O. (1963). *Zeitschrift für Laryngologie, Rhinologie und Otologie*, **42**, 541

Kleinsasser, O. (1965). *Zeitschrift für Laryngologie und Rhinologie*, **44**, 711

Klopp, C. T. (1950). *Annals of Surgery*, **132**, 811

Krishaber, L. (1879). *Gazette Hebdomadaire de médicine et de chirurgie*, **16**, 518

Kuhn, A. J., Devine, K. D. and McDonald, J. R. (1957). *Laryngoscope*, **67**, 518

Lavelle, R. J. (1969). *British Journal of Cancer*, **23**, 709

Le Bec, E. (1905). *Annales des maladies de l'oreille et du larynx*, **31**, 375

Lederman, M. (1963). *Journal of Laryngology and Otology*, **77**, 651

Lederman, M. (1970). *Journal of Laryngology and Otology*, **84**, 867

Leonard, J. R. and Litton, W. B. (1971). *Laryngoscope*, **81**, 232

Leroux-Robert, J. (1956). *Annals of Otology*, **65**, 137

Leroux-Robert, J. (1974). *Tumori*, **60**, 479

Lindberg, R. and Jesse, R. H. (1968). *American Journal of Roentgenology*, **102**, 132

McAlpine, J. C., Radcliffe, A. and Friedmann, I. (1963). *Journal of Laryngology*, **77**, 1

McDonald, T. J., De Santo, L. W. and Weiland, L. H. (1976). *Laryngoscope*, **86**, 635

McGavran, M. H., Bauer, W. E. and Ogura, J. H. (1961). *Cancer, New York*, **14**, 55

Mackenty, J. E. (1925). *Annals of Otology*, **30**, 599

MacNaughton, I. P. J. and Fraser, M. S. (1954). *Journal of Laryngology*, **68**, 680

Martin, H. (1957). *Surgery of Head and Neck Tumours*; Hoeber-Harper, New York

Maw, A. R. and Lavelle, R. J. (1974). *Minerva Otolaryngologica*, **24**, 75

Mawson, S. (1961). *Journal of Laryngology*, **75**, 1076

Miller, A. H. (1974). *Centennial Conference on Laryngeal Cancer, Workshop No. 2 Toronto* (Eds P. W. Alberti and D. P. Bryce, 1976); Appleton Century Crofts, New York

Miller, A. H. and Fisher, H. R. (1971). *Laryngoscope*, **81**, 1475

Miller, D. (1973). *Annals of Otolaryngology*, **82**, 656

Moffitt, O. P. (1959). *Laryngoscope*, **69**, 1421

Moore, I. (1920). *Journal of Laryngology*, **36**, 49

Moure, E. J. (1921). *Presse Medicale*, **57**, 561

Negus, V. E. (1949). *Comparative Anatomy and Physiology of the Larynx*; Heinemann, London

Negus, V. E. and Thomson, St. C. (1955).

Diseases of the Nose and Throat, 6th edn; Cassell, London

New, G. B. and Erich, J. B. (1938). *Archives of Otolaryngology*, **28,** 841

Norris, C. M. (1958). *Laryngoscope*, **68,** 1240

Norris, C. M. (1974). *Centennial Conference on Laryngeal Cancer, Workshop No. 6 Toronto* (Eds P. W. Alberti and D. P. Bryce, 1976); Appleton Century Crofts, New York

O'Connor, A. D., Clifford, P., Durden-Smith, D. J. and Edwards, W. (1977). *Clinical Otolaryngology*, **2,** 347

Ogura, J. H. (1951). *Transactions of the American Academy of Ophthalmology and Otology*, **55,** 786

Ogura, J. H. (1955). *Laryngoscope*, **65,** 867

Ogura, J. H. (1974). *Centennial Conference on Laryngeal Cancer, Workshop No. 6 Toronto* (Eds P. W. Alberti and D. P. Bryce, 1976); Appleton Century Crofts, New York

Ogura, J. H., Biller, H. F., Calcaterra, T. C. and Davis, W. H. (1969). *International Surgery*, **52,** 29

Ogura, J. H. and Mallen, R. W. (1965). *Transactions of the American Academy of Ophthalmology and Otolaryngology*, **69,** 832

Ogura, J. H., Sessions, D. G. and Spector, G. J. (1974). *Laryngoscope*, **85,** 1808

Olofsson, J. and van Nostrand, A. W. P. (1973). *Acta Otolaryngolica* (Suppl.), **308**

Omerod, F. C. (1958). *Acta Oto-rhino-laryngolica belgique*, **6,** 527

Payling Wright, G. (1958). *Introduction to Pathology*; Longmans, London

Pierquin, B., Chassaque, D. and Perez, R. (1964). *Précis de Curietherapie*; Masson et Cie, Paris

Pietrantoni, L. and Fior, R. (1958). *Acta Otolaryngolica*, **67,** 268

Portmann, G. (1921). *Presse Medicale*, **57,** 561

Portmann, G. (1939). *Treatise on Surgical Technique in Otolaryngology*; Williams and Wilkins, Baltimore

Pracy, R. (1970). *Journal of Laryngology*, **84,** 37

Pressman, J. J. and Simon, M. B. (1961). *Laryngoscope*, **71,** 1019

Price, L. A. and Hill, B. T. (1977). *Clinical Otolaryngology*, **2,** 339

Quick, C. A., Behrens, H. W., Brinton-Damell, M. and Good, R. A. (1975). *Annals of Otolaryngology*, **84,** 607

Radcliffe, G. and Shaw, H. J. (1978). *Clinical Otolaryngology*, **1,** 49

Salmon, L. F. (1957). *Journal of Laryngology*, **71,** 766

Samuel, E. (1974). *Centennial Conference on Laryngeal Cancer, Workshop No. 4 Toronto* (Eds P. W. Alberti and D. P. Bryce, 1976); Appleton Century Crofts, New York

Schneider, J. J., Lindberg, R. D. and Jesse, R. H. (1975). *Journal of Surgical Oncology*, **7,** 187

Shaw, H. J. (1957). *Annals of the Royal College of Surgeons of England*, **21,** 290

Shaw, H. J. (1965). *Journal of Laryngology*, **79,** 1

Shaw, H. J. (1966). *Journal of Laryngology*, **80,** 839

Shaw, H. J. and Epstein, S. S. (1959). *Cancer, New York*, **12,** 246

Shedd, D. P. (1974). *Journal of Surgical Oncology*, **6,** 269

Sheehan, A. J. and Shaw, H. J. (1979). In press

Shumrick, D. A. (1969). *Archives of Otolaryngology*, **89,** 629

Shumrick, D. A. (1971). *American Journal of Surgery*, **122,** 440

Sisson, G. A. (1974). *Centennial Conference on Laryngeal Cancer, Workshop No. 5 Toronto* (Eds P. W. Alberti and D. P. Bryce, 1976); Appleton Century Crofts, New York

Smith, R. R. (1961). *Surgery, Gynaecology and Obstetrics*, **113,** 435

Som, M. L. (1970). *Journal of Laryngology and Otology*, **84,** 655

Som, M. L. and Silver, C. E. (1968). *Archives of Otolaryngology*, **87,** 138

Sorensen, J. (1930). Quoted by Thomson St. C. and Colledge, L. (1930)

Stell, P. M. and McGill, T. (1973). *Lancet*, **2,** 416

Stell, P. and Ranger, D. (1974). *Centennial Conference on Laryngeal Cancer, Workshop No. 6, Discussion, Toronto* (Eds P. W. Alberti and D. P. Bryce, 1976); Appleton Century Crofts, New York

Stewart, E. F. (1960). *Journal of Laryngology*, **74,** 525

Stewart, J. P. (1957). *Journal of Laryngology*, **71,** 718

Strong, E. W., Hensche, U. K., Nickson, J. J., Frazell, E. L., Tollefsen, H. R. and Hilaris, B. S. (1969). *Cancer*, **19,** 1509

Sullivan, R. D. (1960). *Cancer Chemotherapy Reports*, **10,** 39

Szpunar, J. (1977). *Otolaryngology Clinics of North America*, **10,** 67

Tait, R. V. (1959). *Proceedings of the Royal Society of Medicine*, **52,** 747

Thomson, St. C. and Colledge, L. (1930). *Cancer of the Larynx*; Routledge, Kegan Paul, London

Trotter, W. (1926). *British Medical Journal*, **1,** 269

UICC (1962). *Report of Committee on Clinical Stage Classification*, p. 17; Geneva

UICC (1968). *Report of Committee on TNM Classification*; Geneva

UICC (1978). *Report of Committee on TNM Classification*; Geneva

Ungerecht, M. (1951). *Archiv der Ohren-Nasen-Kehlkopf Heilklinik*, **160,** 158

US Department of Health, Education and Welfare (1964). *Smoking and Health*; A report of the Advisory Committee to the Surgeon General of the Public Health Service

Whicker, J. H., Weiland, L. H., Neel, H. B. and Devine, K. D. (1974). *Annals of Otolaryngology*, **83,** 487

Willis, R. A. (1953). *The Pathology of Tumours*, 2nd edn; Butterworths, London and Boston

Wilson, C. P. (1955). *Annals of the Royal College of Surgeons of England*, **17,** 1

Winston, P. and Epstein, S. S. (1958). *Journal of Laryngology*, **72,** 452

Woesner, M. E., Braun, E. J. and Sanders, I. (1974). *Annals of Otology, Rhinology and Laryngology*, **83,** 42

16 Laryngeal disorders in singers and other voice users

A S Khambata

Singers and other professional voice users, by virtue of the very nature of their occupations, are at greater risk of laryngeal misuse, abuse and injury, just as an athlete may be at risk of muscular injury. But whereas the latter is more or less immediately aware of his disability and generally is obliged by his management to rest until fully recovered, a singer often minimizes his disability to avoid cancelling performances, or is obliged to carry on for fear of losing future engagements. The singer, of all such voice users, is more exposed to the possibility of laryngeal injury as he is often called upon and unwisely agrees to undertake roles for which his vocal material or technique is unsuited. The laryngologist is at an advantage, therefore, if he has some knowledge of music and the mechanics of singing. Furthermore, an insight into each particular singer's vocal mechanism is of invaluable help in the assessment and treatment of his disability. For it is the duty of the laryngologist to enable the singer to continue his work when possible, or resume his singing as soon as possible, as long as there is no risk of permanent or serious damage to his vocal organ.

The majority of theatres and concert halls and rehearsal rooms in which singers and actors have to pass the greater part of their waking and working hours tend to be over- or under-heated; the atmosphere is often dry and dusty – conditions which are the very opposite of those conducive to good vocal health. Many successful singers have to move from one city to another between engagements, often singing two vocally disparate roles during the same week in different centres, travelling in over-heated trains or in the air-conditioned dryness of aeroplanes – all factors conducive to physical and mental strain with subsequent effects on the voice; whereas previously, in the so-called 'Golden age of opera', singers were engaged for a season at one particular opera house, and led fairly settled lives over the course of a few months, even when singing a number of demanding roles in the course of a season. There is certainly no dearth of magnificent vocal material available, though standards of vocal training may have deteriorated over the past 50 years; and pressures placed on these singers have increased, as have the size of the orchestras they sing with – all factors exposing the singer to the risk of vocal strain and, frequently, premature vocal decline.

The muscles of the larynx, and the movements produced by them, are described in Volume 1, as also is the mechanism of speech and the physiological mechanism of voice production. But to understand fully the problems encountered by singers, it is necessary to have some understanding of the singing voice.

The singing voice is essentially a wind instrument and arguably the most beautiful of them; it has three essential parts: the bellows, the reeds, and the resonators.

The respiratory bellows

All good singing is based on correct breathing and cannot exist without it. This has been taught and accepted by all teachers of singing and singers. Many a singer's vocal difficulties are due to faulty breathing which has not been recognized and corrected early on during his training; and treatment of the laryngeal disorder must therefore be supplemented by a retraining involving these basic principles if a recurrence of these disorders is to be avoided. The 'bellows' are constituted by the lungs and muscles of the thorax, the diaphragm, and the muscles of the abdominal wall. In order to produce the singing voice, a controlled act of respiration is of prime importance, the lungs being capable of filling rapidly and emptying at a steady controlled rate. The upward expiratory movement of the diaphragm is sustained and re-inforced by the controlled contraction of the muscles of the abdominal wall.

All good teachers of singing agree that, apart from articulation, breathing should be the only active part in singing, hence 'to breathe correctly is to lay the foundation for good singing, technically and artistically. It is not the size, but the flexible strength of the breathing machinery that counts' (E. Herbert Caesari, 1951). 'Correct breathing, strange as it may sound, is even more essential than a beautiful voice ... Phrasing, tone, resonance, expression all depend upon respiration' (Dame Nellie Melba, 1926).

The reeds

The reeds in the human voice are the vocal cords but, unlike those in other wind instruments, these reeds are mobile and alterable in dimension and shape. Consequently, a wide range of notes can be produced with rapid changes in pitch, intensity and quality. The vocal cords, and in particular their free edges, are set in vibration as the air stream supplied by the bellows is forced through the narrow aperture of the glottis. This produces the fundamental pitch of the basic tone. Segmental vibration of the cords adds harmonics to the basic tone.

Husson (1950) postulated a 'neurochronaxie theory', which purported that vibrations of the vocal cords were initiated and maintained entirely by nerve stimuli and not by the physical passage of air through the 'reeds' from the 'bellows', but von Leden (1960), using ultra-slow-motion cinematography by indirect laryngoscopy, demonstrated that the passage of air under pressure was a pre-requisite for normal laryngeal vibrations and voice production. In one patient with a tracheostomy, vibrations of the vocal cords ceased as soon as his breath by-passed the larynx, thus supporting the 'aerodynamic theory' of phonation.

Punt (1968) states that as the vocal cords vibrate, the air stream is converted into a rapid series of puffs which consequently form a tone.

The resonators

The pure laryngeal sound formed by the vibrating cords is in itself thin and weak but, by passing through the natural resonators, this fundamental tone and various overtones are amplified selectively to varying degrees and the primary laryngeal sound is endowed with resonance and 'timbre'. The most important of these resonators are the pharynx, oral cavity, nose and nasopharynx and to some extent the chest cavity. The dimensions of the hard palate particularly affect the quality of the voice. Erbstein (1929) in particular correlates the form and size of the hard palate with the qualities of the sound produced. Perhaps all parts of the thoracic wall and particularly the sternum act as sounding boards. Hence, anatomical defects such as a deviated nasal septum or inflammatory processes can affect the timbre of the voice. The para-nasal sinuses themselves probably do not appreciably alter the resonance of the voice (Negus, 1929; Punt, 1968) though singing teachers and singers for many generations have talked about 'sinus tone' in singers. The latter term probably best describes the sensation felt by the singer in the mask of the face during the production of certain tones.

Pitch

There is nowadays more or less universal agreement that the pitch of the human voice is determined by the frequency of vibration of the vocal cords, but there is still much confusion about the way in which these variations in frequency are brought about. It has already been said that there is little support for the 'neuro-chronaxie theory' of a certain French school which maintains that the vibrations of the vocal cords are initiated entirely by nervous stimuli, and the very great majority of investigators support the 'aerodynamic theory' which postulates that the passage of air through the glottis under pressure is essential for normal vibrations of the cords. What is less certain is the role played by variations in the subglottic air pressure in the control of pitch.

Negus (1962) expressed the view that vocal pitch appears to depend on the relationship between the elasticity of the glottal margins and the pressure of air expelled from the trachea; and he believes that pitch can be increased by an increase in air pressure alone, the elasticity of the cords remaining almost unchanged. He even goes so far as to say that, in the higher notes, a rise in pitch may be produced principally by a rise in air pressure.

Indeed, it is one of the time-honoured axioms of laryngeal physiology that the pitch of the voice rises when the subglottic air pressure and air flow are increased, all other factors being constant. But this concept has been challenged by Rubin (1963). In his investigations on dogs, he found that variations in air flow within physiological limits did not alter the resultant pitch, as determined by the intensity of contraction of the cricothyroid (external tensor) and thyro-arytenoid (internal tensor) muscles, although they did alter the volume (*see below*).

However, there is virtually unanimous agreement that the vocal cords elongate progressively as the pitch rises, and that this lengthening of the cords is a function of the cricothyroid muscle. During phonation, the cricoid cartilage rocks forward under the pull of the cricothyroid muscle. This, in its turn, increases the distance from the anterior to the posterior commissure and hence the glottis is elongated and the slack taken up. This powerful stretch tension of the external tensor provides a framework within which the internal tensor (the thyro-arytenoid muscle) can effect certain restricted variations in pitch. Slow-motion cinematographic studies have demonstrated other changes in the vocal cords with variation in pitch and, although there is no unanimity in the interpretation of these changes, there is much support for the following ideas. In the production of lower notes, for example, the whole length of the vocal cords (including the arytenoids) vibrates; the opposing surfaces of the cords present a 'thick' edge (*Figure 16.1*), and the period of approximation is prolonged. By

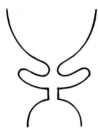

Figure 16.1 'Thick' cordal margins in low notes

contrast, in the production of higher notes, the membranous cords alone are permitted to vibrate while the arytenoids are held firmly together; the opposing edges of the vocal cords are definitely thinned and come into contact with one another only with a sharp-edged 'thin' margin (*Figure 16.2*); this contact is only momentary. In the

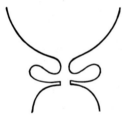

Figure 16.2 'Thin' cordal margins in high notes

'falsetto' voice, heard mainly in tenors, the vibrations are much faster and there is even less contact between the sharpened edges of the vocal cords; and in some voices only the anterior segments of the cords appear to move at very high pitches (*Figure 16.3*).

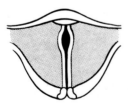

Figure 16.3 The 'falsetto' voice

In inexperienced singers, the whole larynx will often be seen to rise as the pitch of the voice rises, but most experienced singers and teachers of singing believe that this is undesirable and indeed, in some celebrated singers, the larynx is known to descend as the pitch is raised. It is probable that the disadvantage of allowing the larynx to

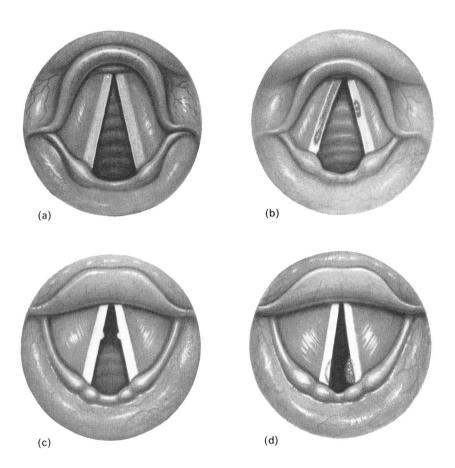

Plate 8 (a) Non-infective laryngitis; (b) submucosal haemorrhages of the vocal cords;
(c) singer's nodules; (d) contact ulcer

ascend as pitch rises is due in part to an elongation of the subglottic air column, and in part to the fact that it entails activity on the part of the accessory muscles, with consequent reduction in the resonating properties of the supraglottic structures of the throat and mouth.

Although the breath pressure is under the conscious control of the singer, the action of the vocal cords is, or should be, entirely passive and is under the 'automatic' control of the mind. As Madame Puritz (1956) expressed it: 'The mind determines pitch of the voice. The vocal cords must respond passively to the combined agents, mind and breath'. The subglottic air pressure which governs the intensity and loudness of the tone has a very slight effect on the pitch, there being a tendency for the note to 'sharpen'. This is particularly noticeable in the production of the 'messa di voce' (the gradual *crescendo* and *decrescendo* on a held note); this tendency to 'sharpen' is corrected by a corresponding reduction in the tension of the cords in the well-trained singer.

Volume or loudness

The loudness (or volume or intensity) of the voice is determined largely by the air pressure from the 'bellows' of the lungs, and a progressive increase in the air flow at any given pitch is accompanied by progressively greater vocal loudness. But vocal intensity is not influenced by air flow alone. A trained singer, for example, can sustain a singing tone *forte* about as long as he can sustain it *pianissimo*; furthermore, as Rubin (1967) has said, 'he may be able to accomplish a maximal vocal effort without so much as causing the flame of a candle held before his open mouth to flicker'.

There must therefore be some other factor which also contributes to the determination of vocal loudness, and this is thought to be the intensity of contraction of the tensor muscles; that is to say, sound-pressure levels are greatly affected by the degree of glottic resistance above. Hence, vocal loudness is determined by the balance between the air flow from the lungs and the tension of the cricothyroid and thyro-arytenoid muscles.

Rubin's studies have emphasized the importance of correct breathing in speaking and singing. Since greater sound volume may be achieved by heightened tension of the vocal muscles alone, inadequate breath support and associated disturbances of the optimal relationships between air flow and glottal resistance will subject the vocal apparatus to undue and harmful stress (Rubin, 1963).

Timbre

The tonal quality of the voice is determined mainly by the relative amplitude of the harmonic partials, or overtones, generated in the resonating cavities.

The fundamental laryngeal frequency and the overtones caused by the segmental vibrations of the vocal cords are radiated from the larynx into the throat and mouth, and the harmonic structure of the voice sounds can thus be modified, by the singer or speaker, partly by the natural frequency and the resonance characteristics of the cavities themselves and partly by changes in the shape, dimensions and consistency of the 'resonators'.

It is possible that the 'richness' of the voice may also be determined, to some extent, by minimal changes in the 'thickness' of the cordal margins and by minor variations above and below the fundamental tone, similar to the *vibrato* effect produced by the violinist.

In experiments upon himself Donovan (1967), with many years of personal experience both as a singer and as a laryngologist, has also produced evidence that some at least of the tonal variations in singing have their origin in the larynx itself. By 'fixing' his own oropharynx with an acrylic mould (thus preventing any alterations in its resonating properties) and recording his own voice on a 'sonograph', he has found that an increase of laryngeal intensity associated with a rise of subglottic pressure will lead to a progressive increase in the relative amount of energy in the higher harmonics, especially when singing low notes.

The range of the human voice

Nadoleczny, as long ago as 1926, wrote that the newborn infant cries on a note of approximately 435 Hz and, as growth proceeds, the vocal range is extended until, at the end of the first year, it encompasses six half-tones; at the end of the fourth year it covers about an octave, and just before puberty an octave and a half.

At puberty the male larynx grows very rapidly and the vocal cords increase appreciably in length. This process of 'breaking' may take as little as six months or as long as two years to become complete; and the change may occur as early as the eighth year or be delayed as late as the eighteenth. The vocal pitch falls by one-sixth at its upper limit, and by an octave at its lower limit.

In girls the change is much less marked. It is more rapidly completed and results merely in a slight extension of the upper and lower limits.

In normal speech, the fundamental frequency of the adult larynx may range from as low as 80 Hz in men's voices to as high as 400 Hz in women's, with an average of 128 Hz in men and 256 Hz in women. The normal conversational range is rather less than one octave.

The vocal range in singing, however, is considerably wider, with an overall range (from bass to soprano) of about four octaves. But exceptional cases have been

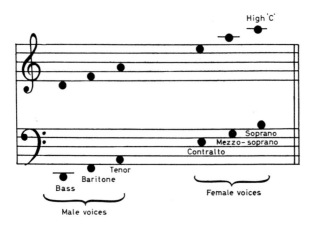

Figure 16.4 The range of adult singing voices

reported in which singers have been able to produce frequencies as low as 44 Hz and as high as 2048 Hz. The average range of each individual is about two octaves (*Figure 16.4*) but with training this may be extended to two (or even three) whole tones above and below this range.

The registers

A discerning listener is often conscious of a change in quality of the voice as a singer moves up and down a scale. Most singers recognize their voice as having distinct registers; the chest and head registers (and frequently a middle register). These terms really describe where the singer feels the maximum sensation of vibration as he moves from note to note in singing up and down a scale. Hence, in the chest register the singer experiences a maximum source of vibration in the thoracic cavity, while in the uppermost notes this appears to be experienced mainly in the head. The characteristic sound of a note in a particular register depends not only on the changes in the vocal cords but also on the resonators called into play. Physiologists and laryngologists use a different terminology which is based on their observations of changes which occur within the larynx itself. They usually refer to a 'thick' register and a 'thin' register which describes fairly accurately one of the changes which occur in the opposed edges of the vocal cords, which are 'thick' in approximately the lower octave of the singer's range, and 'thin' in singing the upper octave. Among singers and teachers of singing there is a generally held precept regarding these registers. The eminent soprano Emma Eames (1927), one of the famous pupils of Mathilda Marchesi states: 'Madame Marchesi trained the voice to have three distinct registers, instead of one perfectly even scale, in which the tones of the register melt into the tones of the next as do colours in a prism which is the only logical way of singing'. Dame Nellie Melba, perhaps the most famous Marchesi pupil, declares: 'There are three registers in a woman's voice. The chest registers should, in exceptional cases, end on the E above middle C. I myself occasionally sing F in chest, but that is not usually right, and for heavy voices it is very dangerous. The medium (or middle) register consists of the octave from F above middle C. The head register must begin on F sharp, above C on the third space'. When properly schooled in the blending of the registers by using 'mixed tones', the singer produces a 'seamless scale'. There are, however, some fortunate singers who have a completely 'natural' voice where nature has already blended the registers. Beniamino Gigli, Giacomo Lauri-Volpi and John McCormack (all tenors) are all well-known examples of the completely natural voice; whereas Fernando De Lucia, Alessandro Bonci, Enrico Caruso and Lauritz Melchior were products of schooling. All, however, studied for many years, to build up voice and art. The late lamented Maria Callas, a pupil of Elvira de Hidalgo, never fully achieved a seamless scale, but by the genius of her art used these very 'defects' to enhance the emotion and drama of her unforgettable characterizations in the roles she made her own.

As Guthrie (1938) said: 'it is not easy to describe an art in terms of science'.

Professional voice users such as singers, actors, public speakers, clergymen, teachers, barristers, and (I regret to add) general practitioners and other doctors who have to speak continuously for a fairly long time, are by the very nature of their occupations at greater risk of incurring laryngeal damage. Other people are also at risk of incurring these same conditions, but obviously the risk is much greater in the professional voice-using fraternity. These disabilities may best be discussed as those due to vocal abuse and misuse and those due to chronic inflammatory diseases, but it must be emphasized that these are not two complete and separate entities but are inter-dependent in the various aspects of vocal disability.

Non-infective laryngitis

This may be an acute condition or, in certain unfortunate cases due to prolongation of vocal abuse, chronic non-infective laryngitis. The symptom of these conditions as far as the throat is concerned usually consists of some degree of discomfort within the throat. The main symptom, however, is that of hoarseness with some degree of impairment of vocal range and quality. Even simple conversational speech may produce soreness in the throat, associated with a lowering of the pitch of the voice. In singers there is commonly difficulty in singing high notes with any degree of softness, the reason being that the thickened or irregular vocal cords of those with weakness of their muscle components cannot be stiffened and thinned, and so high notes can only be achieved by raising breath pressure and forcing the air through tightly opposed cords. These notes are therefore necessarily loud as well as shrill and lacking in the usual timbre of the voice. Resorting to that forced production, many singers can achieve the high notes, but when breath pressure is reduced and the opposing cordal-opening force lessened, the thickened or muscularly weak cords can only vibrate at slower rates resulting in the low notes being produced, but the singer often complains that he has difficulty with his middle range of notes.

Acute non-infective laryngitis

Acute non-infective laryngitis usually results from bouts of screaming or shouting, or other vocal excesses either in duration or loudness. It can also occur due to over-indulgence in coughing, smoking or drinking of alcohol, particularly spirits. The normal smooth, pearly glistening appearance of the vocal cords as seen by mirror examination is replaced by dull rough-looking pink vocal cords, the rest of the laryngeal mucosa often being diffusely injected or reddened (*Plate 8a, facing page 512*). It must, however, be understood that in professional voice users, particularly in baritones and basses, some degree of pinkness of the cords may be accepted as normal or at least physiological, even when their voices are at their very best. Punt (1968) describes this very vividly: 'the difference in appearance might be compared to that between fine white or faintly rose pink slipper satin and rather rubbed red velvet. All degrees of the condition are met with from slight cordal congestion and roughening to the well-marked state described. Many of the lower-pitched voices can disguise the condition if their technique is sound, but in the higher voices, particularly in tenors, the consequence is much more serious, the purity of the high notes being spoilt and distinctly clouded; this is particularly obvious in the category of so-called 'lyric' voices, where purity of tone is a greater attribute than mere loudness or power. Mirror examination will also show that there is usually an excess of rather sticky mucus around the larynx and particularly around the vocal cords. Treatment is primarily by vocal rest. A period of absolute silence is, if possible, the very best treatment that may be prescribed. If a singer continues to perform when suffering from this condition, he often risks the development of 'singer's nodes' and bleeding in the cords, with subsequent long-lasting changes in voice function and quality. Unfortunately, these cases are usually seen a few hours before a performance and, as the singer would be most loath to cancel a performance, it is the laryngologist's duty to sustain him through this period of acute vocal stress. Zilstorff (1968), of the Royal Theatre, Copenhagen, recommends that instillation of Bratt–Kagen's fluid may be helpful in such cases. This consists of two parts: (1) Argyrol solution (five per cent); (2) Basic cocaine (0.3 g menthol oil, eucalyptus oil, menthyl valeriana (each 1 g), and olive oil (5 g). 0.4 ml of the first component is mixed in the syringe with 0.1 ml of the second and the vocal cords are sprayed. Punt (1968) has devised a very effective solution for local application to the pharynx and larynx in such cases. It is a 0.5 per cent solution of diphenhydramine hydrochloride (Benadryl), preferably made up in a vehicle of liquor *pro guttae* to discourage contaminants. If there is much sticky mucus in the throat a tablet of Ascoxal (ascorbic acid 100 mg, sodium percarbonate 70 mg, copper sulphate 0.2 mg and menthol 2 mg) may be added with advantage as a mucolytic agent. This is an excellent vasoconstrictor and a mild and comforting analgesic. Alternatively, Solvellae borac Co. BPC, a helpful solution, may be applied first to the pharynx with a de Vilbis spray and then to the larynx with a curved laryngeal spray. These applications should never be made more than once a day and in any event should be reserved for just before a performance. It must be explained to the singer or actor that this is only a temporary procedure until such time as the artist has an opportunity of resting his voice. There is one serious drawback to this method of treatment in that the sensibility of the mucous membrane is reduced so that the singer no longer has his usual delicate sensation of vocal function and perhaps may be more apt to over-strain the voice. A singer should never be forced to carry through a performance if he feels himself physically unable to do so. If the singer is to carry on with a performance it is essential that the laryngologist be at hand and available for consultation if necessary.

Chronic non-infective laryngitis

The chronic non-infective type of laryngitis is a fairly common condition. There is usually a long history, often dating back to childhood, of vocal abuse. In addition, over-indulgence in smoking and alcohol are particular contributing factors in the development of this condition. Some degree of hoarseness and lowering of the pitch of the speaking voice is to be expected as a result of the cordal thickening and roughening. The hoarseness is often so characteristic that it has come to be named the 'gin and midnight voice'. It may be met with in all professional voice users with varying degrees of severity, but particularly so in actors. Often the characteristic hoarseness is turned to good account, making the actor instantly recognizable vocally. In singers, however, it is another question altogether. In high voices in particular, loss of clarity of production almost invariably indicates a decline in the singer's ability and probably his career. Every effort must be made to reduce excessive consumption of alcohol and tobacco and to minimize vocal abuse, but these subjects are often so habituated to such indulgences and to constant talking that they may find these restrictions intolerable. Many of these cases are of long standing and a complete and permanent cure cannot be expected. The voice can occasionally be restored for a particularly important performance by the use of laryngeal sprays but the performance will tend to leave the voice hoarser than before and subsequent rest will be all the more necessary.

Submucosal haemorrhages of the vocal cords

These are almost always due to a submucosal extravasation of blood following a sudden severe vocal strain. They are characterized by a sudden onset of hoarseness and local pain following immediately upon an intense vocal strain. Further, the performer may notice vocal fatigue on speaking. Some degree of myasthenia of the larynx usually accompanies such an acute episode. Examination of the larynx on or near the edge of the cord (*Plate 8b, facing page 512*). Treated properly – which means complete vocal rest – the haemorrhages usually disappear entirely within a few weeks, leaving no scar or other visible trace of their presence, the voice being restored to normal. If absolute vocal rest is not adhered to strictly, the haemorrhages may become organized into vocal nodules. Recurrent submucosal haemorrhages often leave the singer with dilated blood vessels of a rather prominent character seen on the upper surfaces of one or both vocal cords. If these changes persist despite perfect vocal rest and careful treatment, they will require to be removed by micro-dissection under the operating microscope. Prevention of a recurrence of this condition involves careful explanation by the laryngologist and a full realization of the degree of vocal abuse in which the subject has been indulging. The singer may often have to rethink his approach or technique in producing certain tones.

Singer's nodules

This condition is almost exclusively a disease of professional voice users, particularly singers of the pop variety. It may, of course, also occur in teachers and actors. Among singers it is particularly seen in sopranos and tenors, especially so in those singers who are attracted to roles which lie well above their normal vocal ranges or where the general tessitura of the music lies above that which is most comfortable for the voice. It must always be kept in mind that the alleged soprano or tenor voice is, in fact, better suited for the mezzo-soprano or high baritone range.

Singer's nodules are usually bilateral and symmetrical. They are white or greyish white and occur characteristically at the junction of the anterior and middle thirds of the cords (*Plate 8c, facing page 512*). They are much more likely to occur in singers who practise the so-called 'coup de glotte' (a forceful attack on the vocal cords akin to a cough but distinguished from it by the fact that the arytenoids remain together to prepare the vocal cords for phonation). 'Before the onset of tone the air accumulates under the tightly-closed vocal cords, being released by a sharp opening and closing of the glottis' (Husler and Rodd-Marling, 1965). When correctly performed 'the glottis is opened and closed without movement of the arytenoids' (Goesttler, 1950). This technique has in the past been taught as a necessity for the acquisition of the staccato in singing technique by many a famous vocal coach and teacher. If the mechanism is not clearly understood by the singer this method can cause severe damage with resultant formation of singer's nodules.

Nodules may result from the organization of submucosal haemorrhages; but nodules are usually symmetrical while haemorrhages are not. It would therefore seem more likely that in most cases the nodules are due to a hyperkeratosis; that is to say, that the vocal cords respond to the excessive strain by producing 'corns' the same way as the skin of the feet produces 'corns' in response to the constant pressure of tight shoes. Uncommonly, only one cord may show a nodule but Punt (1968) states that in such a case the other cord will usually develop one very shortly if steps are not taken to prevent it. They also occur in noisy children who have a tendency to shout, and are frequently seen in child vocalists. The present writer has often seen these in the case of children who are avid football fans. Initially the subject with vocal nodules may notice only a slight roughness of the voice, usually in the higher notes, especially when these have to be sung *pianissimo*. Indeed, it has been said that ideally a singer who cannot sing high notes softly should not sing them at all. The singer often declares that he or she can still reach a high note which usually implies that they were always forced. Eventually he finds that the vocal quality of his middle notes have also come to suffer and eventually the voice may only be used within a very limited range above which the note cracks.

The essence of treatment in these cases is vocal rest. Added to this the subject must be made aware that vocal misuse or abuse has been the prime factor in the causation of the nodules. Whenever possible it is advisable that the subject should have complete vocal rest amounting to total silence for at least 2–3 weeks. It must be stressed that whispering will often cause more damage than speaking in a proper voice. The intelligent singer will soon realize what the original mistakes causing the condition were, and he should be encouraged to visit a singing teacher to have these misuses corrected. Gentle speaking and eventual gentle vocal exercises can be resumed once laryngeal examination has determined that the nodules have disappeared. In advanced chronic cases a period of silence may be necessary for several months. Any septic focus in the teeth, sinuses or tonsils should be treated before any local surgery on the vocal cords is undertaken. The eminent and distinguished soprano, Lucrezia Bori, developed such a condition in the second decade of this century. Treatment in her case was by surgical removal followed by enforced silence over a number of years. Fortunately, to the delight of all lovers of good singing, Madame Bori restarted on a second and immensely successful career after the First World War. The great tenor, Enrico Caruso, developed a similar condition between 1908 and 1909 and this required excision of the nodules under direct vision by Professor della Vedova of Milan. This was probably the result of his taking on increasingly dramatic roles which his basically lyric voice (coupled with a period of great emotional distress) could not cope with. Fortunately for the world, removal of the nodules by careful dissection and enforced vocal rest enabled the great man to continue with his career until his untimely death in 1921. Sprays and other local applications to the larynx may be of help in enabling the singer to carry on for a few days while arrangements are made for a rest period. If conservative methods of treatment fail, then resort may have to be made to local surgery. Nodules may have to be removed by direct laryngoscopy using the micro-surgical technique. Great care must be taken that only the nodule is removed. It is vitally important not to damage the underlying tissues of the cord. Surgery should only be undertaken with the very greatest reluctance in those cases where all possible conservative treatment has been tried and failed, and never without allowing for a generous period of vocal rest post-operatively.

Following a period of rest it is essential that vocal re-education be carried out under the supervision of a good singing teacher or speech therapist, as a return to the previous habits of vocal abuse will only result in the formation of further nodules. It must, however, be stated that small vocal nodules may be found on routine laryngeal examination without any obvious change in the vocal quality of the subject. In fact, many a serious (as well as pop) singer's particular quality of slight huskiness in the voice has been responsible for an immensely successful career. The present writer knows of at least two mezzo-soprano singers who have very tiny vocal nodules present on their vocal cords but these have in no way affected their very successful careers as recitalists.

Contact ulcers

Contact ulcers on the vocal cords are fortunately uncommon and they occur almost exclusively in male adults. The problem is largely a mechanical one due to the hammering of the vocal processes of the arytenoids against each other. Vocal abuse, particularly the 'coup de glotte', is an important contributory factor. The symptoms may range from a mild discomfort and slight hoarseness to persistent pain, sometimes with referred otalgia, and persistent huskiness with vocal fatigue. Ulceration is of slow onset and progression, and consequently it may be associated with granulations, as seen in any slowly healing wound. In many cases the ulcer crater on one side is occupied by a granuloma (which may become very large) arising from the other side, the prominence of the granuloma fitting into the cup of the ulcer on the opposite side (*Plate 8d, facing page 512*).

Complete vocal abstinence must be practised, ideally for two or three weeks, followed by a period of vocal rehabilitation. The majority of these ulcers will heal within 2–3 months with conservative treatment but a persistent granuloma must be removed by direct micro-laryngoscopic dissection. Post-operative rehabilitation is of prime importance. Peacher (1961) has reported that contact ulcers heal far better and more quickly with vocal therapy than with surgery, but agrees that surgery may have to be resorted to when a large granuloma is present. Surgery is best done before vocal therapy is started. If surgical intervention has to be repeated the healing process takes much longer. Persistent cough, or irritation in the throat causing a cough, would naturally have to be treated by appropriate medication, as persistence of such a symptom may otherwise lead to reformation of the contact ulcer.

Myasthenia of the larynx (phonasthenia)

This is the name given to weakness of the phonatory muscles of the larynx. It may occur either in an acute form, or occasionally in a chronic form which usually occurs in ageing singers and voice users. Myasthenia is caused by vocal abuse and by misuse of the vocal organ. This in effect constitutes a form of trauma to the muscles of phonation. The muscles within the vocal cord itself are those which are the most used during the act of singing or speaking. The thyro-arytenoid muscles are the most affected, but the interarytenoid muscles are also affected to some degree depending on the severity of the case. It is a generalized weakening of these groups of muscle which leads to an inability to produce the voice properly. Myasthenia of the larynx should always be suspected when the singing voice actually sounds worse than the appearance of the vocal cords would suggest. In this condition the voice is very easily tired and the singer cannot maintain a constant pitch, particularly in the higher notes. There is a definite impairment of intonation, and in an attempt to correct this the singer invariably forces his voice. This further strain leads to some degree of hoarseness of the voice itself. Some degree of myasthenia of the larynx is commonly encountered in other laryngeal disabilities in singers, and in both the non-infective and infective types of laryngitis. The singer with laryngitis may be inadvisedly allowed to continue singing, and hence throws a greater strain on the internal tensor muscles of the larynx. Acute myasthenia usually follows a period of intense vocal abuse; the cords themselves may be severely engorged and occasionally a blood vessel may rupture, producing a submucosal haemorrhage in the vocal cord. The same condition may occur if the singer insists on singing when he is suffering from infective laryngitis. A subacute variety of myasthenia is often seen following weeks or months of continuous vocal abuse, particularly if the singer (and usually this involves tenors and sopranos) insists on singing roles to which his vocal equipment is unsuited. In singers with vocal nodules, some degree of myasthenia is almost invariably found.

It is generally accepted amongst singers that after a period of prolonged rest from singing, as after a holiday or lack of engagements, singing should be re-instituted gradually, to 'train' the internal muscles of the larynx to their previous normal degree of activity. In these cases, the resumption of major roles (which are, in any event, tiring for the singer) very often produce subacute myasthenia. Endocrine factors also play a part in these subacute cases, particularly during menstruation and on approaching the menopause. Certain opera houses in Europe actually provide a clause in the contracts of female singers allowing them to withdraw from performances during the menses. With ageing, both physical and vocal (that is, when a singer has sung consistently over a great number of years), some degree of weakening of the laryngeal muscles tends to develop if the subject has been prone to misuse or abuse of his voice. When this occurs it usually determines his age of retirement. Many a physically young singer has had to decide on premature retirement due to a chronic myasthenia of the larynx.

Myasthenia is often accompanied by corditis marginitus in which there is hyperaemia of the vocal cords, particularly along their free edges. Examination of the vocal cords by indirect laryngoscopy shows a characteristic appearance depending on which muscles are most involved. When the internal tensors (i.e. the thyro-arytenoid muscles alone) are involved, the vocal cords come together on phonation but leave an elliptical space between them (*Figure 16.5a*). When the interarytenoid muscles alone are affected, the anterior two-thirds of the vocal cords approximate on phonation but a triangular space is seen on the posterior commissure (*Figure 16.5b*). When both these groups of muscles are affected, the glottis presents a characteristic keyhole shape on phonation (*Figure 16.5c*).

Many singers unwisely accept a very heavy programme of professional engagements which might constitute full performances of operas or recitals with a great many 'one-

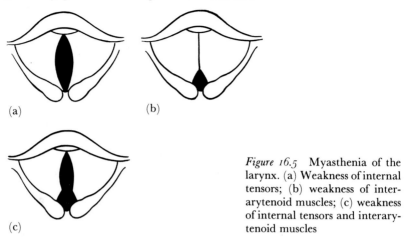

(a)

(b)

(c)

Figure 16.5 Myasthenia of the larynx. (a) Weakness of internal tensors; (b) weakness of inter-arytenoid muscles; (c) weakness of internal tensors and interary-tenoid muscles

night stands'. There is a natural reluctance on the part of the singer to cancel an engagement, particularly if he or she is due to appear with a prestigious orchestra, and despite the advice of the laryngologist, he or she may insist on continuing the tour. The laryngologist is often faced with the problem of having to assist a singer in this difficult position. Although it is his duty to advise the singer against singing under these conditions, he is duty-bound to help the singer if the performance cannot be cancelled. Under those circumstances the laryngologist may unwillingly have to refer the patient for a short exposure to ultra-shortwave diathermy, but it must be impressed upon the singer that this must be done not less than 10–12 hours before the performance. The application of sprays to the larynx is of doubtful value, but the Benadryl spray may often prove effective. The charmingly-named Melba spray, which was devised by the late Milsom Reece, is also frequently used. Its composition is as follows:

Menthol	0.3 g
Spiritus vini rectificatus	12 ml
Amylocaine	0.3 g
Tinct. ferri perchlor	2 ml
Glycerine	12 ml
Aqua. Dest.	30 ml

This preparation may be used up to twice a day but never more than this, and it must not be employed unless the performer can have vocal rest at least until the following day. Singers, by their very nature, are extremely anxious about the condition of their vocal cords and it is important that the laryngologist impresses upon them that, after the cords have been sprayed, absolute vocal rest is imperative. This advice is almost invariably followed. The correct treatment of myasthenia is vocal rest. In acute cases, 24–48 hours of absolute silence must be advised. The present writer invariably asks the subject to carry a pad of paper and a pencil and to communicate this way only. In subacute cases approaching some degree of chronicity, some weeks or even months of silence are essential. The patient often asks for a general fortifying tonic, and the intramuscular injection of vitamin B_{12} (cyanocobalamin 0.1 per cent) has been shown empirically to have an excellent tonic effect. Active singing should be resumed only when the appearance of the cords has returned to normal, and then only very gradually and never to the full compass of the voice. Rest – not vocal exercises – is the keynote of success in the treatment of myasthenia. Around the age of 45–50 a critical period is often encountered, in lyric tenors and sopranos, as they tend to start losing 'height' in their voices. A sensible singer will accept this as a natural change occurring with age and the constant use of his voice, and he will be prepared to change to less demanding roles. Leading tenors or sopranos might often have to step down to comprimario roles. There are, however, a few exceptional singers who maintain the power and height of their voices into fairly advanced age. The great English baritone, Sir Charles Santley, was a particular case in point as were Mattia Battistini, Lillie Lehman, Kirsten Flagstad, Elizabeth Schumann, and the amazing tenor Giacomo Lauri-Volpi. The wise artist, if financial considerations permit, would prefer to end his or her professional career with dignity rather than continue a losing fight until all beauty has left the once admired tones (Punt, 1968).

Ventricular band voice (dysphonia plicae ventricularis or psychogenic ventricular dysphonia)

Fortunately this condition rarely occurs in the trained singer but is usually found in street traders (such as newspaper vendors) who shout out the virtues of their wares, although the present writer has seen two well-known actors with similar trouble. Ventricular band voice is produced by the opposition of the ventricular folds or false vocal cords in an attempt to produce a voice. The normal action of the ventricular bands is that of a closing sphincter, as in straining with the breath held; but they may be used to some extent in phonation, in an attempt to compensate for myasthenia of the larynx or other laryngeal disorders. The voice is extremely unpleasant, gruff and 'gravelly'. The treatment is by vocal rest and speech therapy but unfortunately, once the condition is well established, the prognosis is extremely poor.

Mogiphonia

This is a psychoneurotic form of phonic spasm which occurs in professional voice users, particularly when they have to appear in public. Teachers, lecturers and clergymen are particularly prone to this. At the inception of speech the voice appears to be normal but the vocal cords soon become firmly pressed together and no further sound can be emitted. Characteristically, the voice is quite normal when speaking at home or among friends socially. Vocal therapy is of prime importance in the treatment of this condition, and a general understanding of the psychoneurotic problem is also of help to the subject. Ironically enough the present writer has come across this condition in two consultant psychiatrists. Treatment by drugs has no place whatsoever in people who suffer from mogiphonia.

The great majority of laryngeal problems of a non-infective nature are due to the sufferer's lack of insight into his own vocal mechanism, with subsequent vocal abuse and strain. A certain share of the blame must be laid at the door of inefficient singing teachers who often have very little insight into the vocal mechanism themselves but have drifted into their profession by way of other musical activities or a love of singing. Many famous singers take to the teaching of voice production when they retire but a good singer, no matter how famous he may have been in his time, is not necessarily a good vocal teacher. It is often advisable for a singer who runs frequently into vocal problems to move to another teacher who has a better understanding of his vocal technique and problems. Unfortunately, this often produces bad feelings and considerable emotional distress, both to the subject and to the previous teacher; but it is essential that the singer work under the constant supervision of a trusted teacher who understands his vocal failings and is able to correct them. Many a teacher's reputation is built upon the professional success of his or her pupils, but it can be said that a number of singers have successful careers despite the teacher with whom they have studied.

Many local laryngeal conditions may cause vocal stress but there are a few absolute contra-indications to singing a dramatic performance, the chief among them being uncontrolled asthma, severe acute laryngitis, acute myasthenia and the presence of singer's nodules or acute submucosal haemorrhages of the vocal cords. Any artist who insists on undertaking a performance in the presence of an acute infective laryngitis against the advice of his laryngologist runs a very strong risk of developing a permanent chronic laryngeal disability with a considerable alteration in the quality of the voice which would invariably curtail or affect the success of his career. Not infrequently a naturally beautiful voice in a young child may give hope of a promising career in singing, but proper vocal training should not be instituted until the voice has settled down, well after the natural 'break' during puberty. If there is any doubt as to whether a voice has the natural range of a mezzo-soprano or that of a soprano, of a baritone or that of a tenor, it is wise that the teacher should opt for the lower voice, at least in the first instance. For, as the voice is used and exercised under guidance, it will naturally and automatically develop upwards into its full range without any excessive strain on the vocal mechanism. The finished product will invariably have a far greater richness and modulation than if the initial training had been instituted in the higher category of voice.

Lubrication of the larynx

Frequent and constant appearances in over-dry and over-heated theatres and concert halls often leads to an uncomfortable sensation of dryness in the throat. This dryness may be exaggerated by some degree of stage fright. 'When one considers the nature of vocal cord vibrations during singing or dramatic speaking it is clear that the cords can only be expected to withstand such exercise if they are lubricated with an adequate amount of thin mucus, especially from the glands in the laryngeal ventricles. Stimulating these glands in cases where their secretion is insufficient or inspissated may be difficult. A useful preparation is Organidin tablets, two 30 mg tablets (q.i.d.), for a week or so and the course repeated when necessary is always worth trying' (Punt, 1968). The drug Eraldin has recently come into some prominence, and an article in the *Lancet* mentions a trial of Eraldin for treating cases of 'stage fright'. It must, however, be made clear that all the subjects used in this trial were instrumentalists. The present author feels that Eraldin (as a drug for the treatment of stage fright) should be treated with extreme caution; in fact, it is best avoided altogether if possible. Most singers and actors find that some degree of stage fright helps them, if anything, to give a better performance and puts them 'on their toes'. Once the opening lines or (in the case of singers) the opening aria has been delivered, the performer invariably settles down and gives a steadily improving performance if he is an artist of merit. When the dryness in the throat is accompanied by some degree of post-nasal drip, it is best to refrain from prescribing decongestants, as most of them contain a mucus-drying agent which will in fact increase the sense of discomfort in the throat.

Upper respiratory infections

Prevention of upper respiratory infections is obviously of prime importance to singers and professional voice users. Such subjects should be advised against the over-use of tobacco and alcohol, or working in dusty atmospheres. It is wise to avoid home decorating, as the inhalation of paint fumes is distinctly harmful to the throat. The artist must also be warned against exposure to cold or wet weather, and particularly against sudden extreme changes in temperature, as when moving out of doors on a cold evening from an over-heated, dry room. Some singers go so far as to make a point of wrapping up their throats with a scarf, as protection against a cold wet atmosphere. The famous tenor Aureliano Pertile made a point of never speaking when he was out of doors, particularly if he was on his way to a performance. Mild upper respiratory infections, such as the common cold, need not necessitate the cancellation of a performance, so long as it is uncomplicated by further infection, his general condition is good and his technique secure. Under these circumstances it may be helpful to spray an obstructed nose with a simple vasoconstrictor, and the pharynx and larynx with a Benadryl solution (such as that used in non-infective laryngitis) or with a dilute five per cent solution of Argyrol an hour or so before the performance. Decongestant tablets should definitely be discouraged under such circumstances, but vitamin C in the form of Redoxon tablets, taken three or four times a day, may help to shorten the duration of colds in some instances.

Antibiotics may shorten the course of an acute upper respiratory illness when secondary bacterial infection has supervened. If there is a non-productive cough, the act of constant coughing is positively harmful and can be suppressed by the use of Physeptone (methadone hydrochloride), one 5 mg tablet by mouth up to three times a day, for three or four days. If repeated attacks of tonsillitis are a problem, the laryngologist may face the problem of having to advise the singer regarding tonsillectomy. The indications are generally the same as with any other category of individual, but the greatest care and caution is necessary in performing tonsillectomy in a singer. The slightest injury to, or straining of, the velum of the faucial pillars must be avoided. Between the 14th and the 18th day after surgery, phonetic treatment should be commenced, in order to avoid cicatricial contractions and thickenings of the connective tissue. In nervous singers or those with a distinctly poor technique, the surgeon should refuse to carry out a tonsillectomy unless the general health is endangered, for such people will often blame the surgery for their own inherent defects in technique or for later deterioration of their voices, however excellently the operation may have been performed. When tonsillitis presents a problem in a young artist at the beginning of his or her career, a tonsillectomy done at this stage will be beneficial, as it will prevent repeated infections which at some time in the future may necessitate the cancellation of performances from which the artist can then be less readily spared.

General supportive measures

The use of stimulants should generally be condemned but very occasionally an exhausted singer or actor may be given a 10 mg tablet of methyliphenidate hydrochloride (Ritalin) half-an-hour before a performance. It is the general practice in many European and American centres to use vitamin B_{12} by intramuscular injection, either during an infection or in general asthenic conditions. An injection of ascorbic acid combined with an aqueous solution of vitamin A appears to have a favourable effect on acute infections, and tonics may be given on an empirical basis. Strychnine is perhaps the most rational one as it strengthens the tonus of the muscles, including those of the vocal cords. Zilstorff (1968) advocates its use, 0.5–1.0 mg subcutaneously, half-an-hour before a performance.

Hormonal preparations and anabolic steroids should generally be avoided, particularly in women, as voice changes have been reported in some subjects after the use of these preparations. Contraceptive pills have been observed to produce vocal changes in sopranos, with a loss of the higher tones and a general deepening of the voice. These changes disappear spontaneously after withdrawal of the drug (Zilstorff, 1965). A mild degree of oedema and reddening of the vocal cords often occurs before and during the menses, but if the technique is correct this need not prevent a good performance. The use of hormonal preparations to delay a menstrual period should be undertaken with extreme caution.

An understanding of the vocal problems of singers puts the laryngologist in a position of advantage, particularly if the artist has lost confidence in his ability to see a performance through. The very presence of his laryngologist will usually suffice to comfort the patient. Active treatment is very rarely asked for, and almost never once the first intermission has been reached. This is particularly so in the case of a rather demanding first night. Alcohol, however, should be forbidden in these cases, particularly if there have been previous episodes of inflammation or vocal disability, as it is particularly harmful to the throat. Gargles are similarly contra-indicated, as they will not reach the affected laryngeal tissues and will only strain the throat further.

References

Baker, D. C. Jr. (1962). 'Laryngeal problems in singers', *Laryngoscope*, **72,** 902.

Ballantyne, J. C. (1968). 'Vocal disabilities of singers', *Proceedings of the Royal Society of Medicine*, **61,** 1156

Caesari, E. Herbert (1951). *The Voice of the Mind*; Robert Hale Ltd, London

Donovan, R. (1967). Personal communication

Eames, Emma (1927). *Some Memories and Reflections*; D. Appleton

Erbstein, M. (1929). 'Vokalexpertise und objective Bestimmung des Charakters der Singstimme', *III Kongress der Internationalen Gesellschaft für Logopaedic und Phoniatric*;

Deuticke, Leipzig and Vienna

Garcia, M. (1847). *Traité Complet de L'Art du Chant*; Paris

Gatti-Casazza, Giulio (1977). *Memories of the Opera*; John Calder Ltd, London

Goesttler, K. (1950). *Die Anordung, Histologie und Histogenese der quergestreiften Muskulatur im menschlichen Stimmband*; Leipzig

Greene, M. C. L. (1968). 'Vocal disabilities of singers', *Proceedings of the Royal Society of Medicine*, **61,** 1150

Guthrie, D. (1938). 'Physiology of the vocal mechanism', *British Medical Journal*, **2,** 1189

Husler, F. and Rodd-Marling, Y. (1965). *Singing. The Physical Nature of the Vocal Organ*; Faber and Faber, London

Husson, R. (1950). 'Étude des phenomenes physiologiques et acoustiques fondamentaux de la vox chantée', *Thesis*; Faculty of Science, Paris

Leden, H. von (1960). 'Laryngeal physiology', *Journal of Laryngology*, **74,** 705

Leden, H. von and Moore, P. (1960). 'Contact ulcer of the larynx – experimental observations', *Archives of Otolaryngology*, **72,** 746

Melba, Dame Nellie (1926). *Melba Method*, Chapell, London and Sydney

Nadoleczny, M. (1926). *Lehrbuch der Sprach- und stimmheilkunde*; Vogel, Leipzig

Negus, V. (1929). *The Mechanism of the Larynx*; Heinemann, London

Negus, V. (1949). *Comparative Anatomy and Physiology of the Larynx*; Heinemann, London

Negus, V. (1962). Article on 'Voice', *Encyclopaedia Britannica*

Peacher, Georgiana M. (1961). 'Vocal therapy for contact ulcer of the larynx', *Laryngoscope*, **71,** 37

Pressman, J. J. (1938). *Proceedings of the Royal Society of Medicine*, **31,** 1179

Punt, N. A. (1952). *The Singer's and Actor's Throat*; Heinemann, London

Punt, N. A. (1968). 'Applied laryngology – singers and actors', *Proceedings of the Royal Society of Medicine*, **61,** 1152

Puritz, Elizabeth (1956). *The Teaching of Elisabeth Schumann*; Methuen, London

Rubin, H. J. (1963). 'Experimental studies on vocal pitch and intensity in phonation', *Laryngoscope*, **73,** 973

Rubin, H. J. (1967). 'Vocal intensity, subglottic pressure and airflow in relationship to singers', *Folio Phoniatrica*, **19,** 393

Simpson, J. F., Robin, I. G., Ballantyne, J. and Groves, J. (1960). *Synopsis of Otolaryngology*; John Wright, Bristol

Stein, L. (1942). *Speech and Voice*; Methuen, London

Zilstorff, K. (1965). *Nordisk Medicin*, **74,** 724

Zilstorff, K. (1968). *Proceedings of the Royal Society of Medicine*, **61,** 1147

17 Neurological affections of the larynx and pharynx
Peter McKelvie

The separation of the air and food passages in the region of the larynx and pharynx is, self-evidently, a vulnerable area as regards neural control. Fortunately, great reserves of accommodation to such failures exist so that swallowing and breathing may be carried out despite quite extensive damage; by the same token it seems probable that many minor defects which produce symptoms referable to the region, go undetected clinically, despite earnest and sometimes sophisticated search, coupled with bitter complaint on the part of the patient. Cortical control arises from Betz cells in the lower part of the pre-central gyrus as well as some frontal and parietal areas of the cortex which give rise to fibres passing down the cerebral peduncles, the main bulk remaining in the pyramidal tracts with partial decussation at the upper border of the medulla. These fibres reach the nucleus ambiguus.

This pattern means that only a bilateral symmetrical lesion of the cortex produces laryngeal palsy; rarely, unilateral cortical lesions may produce isolated palsies, so variable is the decussation. Because of the sheer size of the nucleus ambiguus, small lesions in it may produce isolated laryngeal and pharyngeal motor losses.

Pharyngeal and cricothyroid muscles are served by fibres existing in the vagus while the cranial portion of the accessory nerve contains the bulk of the fibres destined for the intrinsic muscles of the larynx. The superior laryngeal nerve parts from the vagus just below the inferior vagal ganglion. It contains sensory innervation of the supraglottis and motor fibres of the cricothyroid, passes medial to the carotid tree and enters its final distribution zone via the thyrohyoid membrane. Debate persists about its possible innervation of the interarytenoideus which could therefore have a double (as well as bilateral) nerve supply from superior and recurrent nerves. It is doubtful indeed that the superior nerve is extensively involved in this function, since stimulation of it produces no interarytenoid contracture.

Laryngeal sensation is provided with at least three different types of receptor. They are those in the capsules of the crico-arytenoid joints, those in the laryngeal mucosa itself and stretch receptors in the laryngeal musculature. These are discussed in great detail by Wyke and Kirschner (1976). As regards regional receptors, both tactile and pain, the sensitivity is of a high degree, particularly in the supraglottic mucosa. Large fibres are the afferent loop of the reflex initiating laryngeal response, a reflex which is bilateral. The chemoreceptors in the larynx have unknown functions. The subglottis has a similar receptor, being routed this time by the recurrent laryngeal nerve, though a little area under the anterior commissure has sensory nerves routed through the external laryngeal nerve (not a pure motor nerve). The subglottic chemoreceptors apparently modify breathing, since some chemical stimuli applied to them initiate slow deep breathing, as does carbon dioxide applied to this part of the respiratory tract when it is isolated. The articular joint afferents are particularly well developed, giving a very rapidly responsive, highly sensitive monitoring response. Some reflexes which control respiration and phonation may arise from stretch receptors in the musculature of the larynx demonstrable both histologically and by electrophysiology; their role in laryngeal function is to date highly debatable.

Some of the disorders of sensation of the larynx are trivial, due to low-grade irritation in the upper-air and food passages caused by sinus suppuration, smoking and vocal misuse; and local measures, re-assurance and advice from a speech therapist may suffice to give relief. While it is unwise to invite the menopausal, depressed, introverted patient with conversion symptoms to concentrate overmuch on the pharynx and larynx, a benign though unattractive lozenge such as potassium chlorate commonly helps. Minor defects in sensation in the supraglottis in particular, but in the larynx and pharynx in general, may be caused by central nervous system lesions, notably infarcts, demyelinating diseases and syringobulbia as well as posterior fossa tumours. Ultimately a tracheostomy/gastrostomy life is reached, despite the best intentions; the patient tends to drown in his own food and saliva, and occasionally laryngectomy itself has been proposed as a way of separating this part of the air and food passages. The sheer unpredictability of the neural defect is such as to preclude this in most cases, spontaneous improvement being possible, while in the long term, neurosurgery or new medication may restore some of the losses. Perhaps a novel method of circumventing this unhappy situation lies in using the epiglottis, the laryngeal surface bared to occlude the supraglottis, on to which it is sutured through a lateral pharyngotomy approach. A tiny posterior defect may prevent overspill and yet allow speech to take place, with the aid of a valved tracheostomy tube, the valve cusp being partially fenestrated. The operation can be reversed should the neurological losses improve, as recorded by Stuart (1965), Svien, Baker and Rivers (1963) and Vernet (1918).

Laryngeal spasm occurring in infants is far from being the simple matter presented traditionally. Many cases are not neural but are due to respiratory suppuration. Calcium deficiency (laryngismus stridulus) is a rare cause today and the defects caused by poliomyelitis, tetanus and rabies will, one hopes, become ever more rare.

In adults the majority of choking attacks are similarly of local origin, mainly in the plethoric and obese, rarely amounting to major lasting disability and are predominantly connected with disorders of the involved sensory innervation of the region revealed by Wyke and Kirschner (1976). The panic associated with some of these attacks may, coupled with the choking, often amount to massive 'functional overlay'. The part played by this and concomitant vasovagal activity may proceed to 'laryngeal vertigo' or a frank faint.

Paralyses of the larynx may be grouped as being central or peripheral. Those arising at the cortex are rare and the lesions 'spastic'. This is not to be confused with the spastic larynx treated by Dedo, Urrea and Lawson (1973) with assaults on the recurrent laryngeal nerve and which appear to resemble bizarre hysterical dysphonia with interarytenoid overaction against which the patient battles to produce a flow of speech, syllable by syllable. Brain-stem palsies are, by contrast, flaccid, commonly with isolated losses of small groups of muscles and some sensory losses. Peripheral damage to the laryngeal innervation is of three main types: that to the vagal trunk above the nodose ganglion, the origin of the superior laryngeal nerve; that to the vagus below that level, or to the recurrent laryngeal nerves; and finally, that to the superior laryngeal nerve.

Relevant lesions in the region of the base of the skull may arise from a wide range of diseases. Infections include jugular bulb thrombophlebitis of aural origin, a range of granulomata including TB and meningitides, skull fractures, neuropathies, neoplasms in the temporal bone and post-nasal space, as well as the para-pharyngeal structures, e.g. neurofibromata of the vagal ganglia themselves. These may all halt transmission through this giant nerve system.

In the cervical region, penetrating injuries, surgery of the thyroid gland and regional lymph nodes, as well as locally arising tumours in the upper oesophagus, carotid body and thyroid gland, commonly damage this innervation. As the vagus proceeds into the chest, additional features emerge; the left side is most vulnerable to cardiothoracic surgery, carcinoma of the bronchus, TB and lymphadenopathies. The right side is more vulnerable to the thyroid surgeon, the recurrent laryngeal nerve being rather laterally placed at the inferior pole of the thyroid gland rather than being deeply protected in the groove between oesophagus and trachea. The exhaustive list is impossible to compile and a substantial proportion of all laryngeal neural losses are 'idiopathic'.

A number of named pharyngolaryngeal palsies have been recorded; many are associated with other losses in the tongue, palate, trapezius or diaphragm.

Posterior fossa syndromes

Wallenburg: this consists of total vocal cord losses plus glossopharyngeal and Horner's syndrome. Nageotte adds to this a hypoglossal loss. The *Avellis* (1891) syndrome is similar, with sensory losses much to the fore while *Schmidt and Jackson* syndromes consist predominantly of laryngeal and trapezius paralyses, Jackson having a hemilingual loss of motor function. *Colet Sicard's* syndrome consists of trapezius, whole hemilarynx, tongue and palatal losses, while *Vernet's* syndrome of the jugular bulb adds loss of the hemilingual musculature.

Some lateral pharyngeal space infections and injuries may cause a massive loss in *Villaret's* syndrome, whose features are Horner's syndrome, and losses in tongue, palate, larynx and pharyngeal musculature. Isolated laryngeal and pharyngeal losses may arise from similarly located lesions. Pancoast tumours, for instance, in the lung apex or thoracic inlet may induce brachial plexus pain, recurrent nerve palsy and Horner's syndrome. Essentially these fine neurological distinctions serve moderately well as locators of lesions, directions for biopsy assaults and radiotherapeutic or other measures. The nomenclature is largely of historical interest.

Superior laryngeal nerve injuries produce a typical lesion, with an anaesthetic supraglottis and cricothyroid palsy; the larynx is askew, the thyroid cartilages being rotated over the cricoid ring, with one long vocal cord (on the palsied side) and arytenoid movements appearing to be unimpaired. The long vocal cord, deprived of one of its tensors, is flabby, the voice weak and tiring easily.

Damage to the recurrent nerve in thyroid surgery may be only temporary and due to oedema, developing in the post-operative week rather than immediately. A few are permanent even though the recurrent nerve is not divided and presumably the cause is fibrosis. Direct visualization of the nerve at operation is a worthwhile measure of protection. Hall-Allen (1967) is among many who are pressing on with the development of rescue attempts on these compromised nerves, as did Ogura (1961). While nerve regeneration is unlikely to innervate in the normal manner, mass action of the laryngeal musculature with a separation of the vocal cords is worthwhile and vastly preferable to the flaccid, palsied cord in the median position.

Minuck (1976) observes that unilateral vocal cord paralysis may follow intubation with an endotracheal tube, the top of which inflates irregularly, in which the cuff is inflated within the larynx rather than the trachea. Then hyper-inflation takes place. He postulates that terminal branches of the recurrent laryngeal nerve may be palsied by such instrumentation; Harn *et al.* (*see* Minuck, 1976) showed that the mechanism was possible. It took a full six months before cord movement began to be restored.

No more contentious subject exists than vocal cord palsy, and positions of the cord in such states, since they can come to rest in any position between full abduction and adduction. Fully or partly abducted positions are recognized, as are intermediate, paramedian and median positions. Probably the glottic chink, measured in millimetres, is most meaningful. Semon's law recounted the insidiously damaged recurrent nerve producing a palsy initially of the abductor mechanism and later of the adductor mechanism, resulting in an initially adducted cord with a slow retreat to an intermediate position.

Negus proposed that the larynx, phylogenetically first a sphincter for airway protection, acquired later an opening mechanism, which was relatively vulnerable to neuromuscular damage. Other explanations include the poor mechanical advantage of the crico-arytenoideus posterior versus the sheer bulk of the closing musculature; the passage of time may move the cord laterally, when fibrosis of the palsied musculature with contraction sets in. The presence of flaccid or tonic palsy may become a major feature and the persistence or loss of the cricothyroid musculature develops, as more important and degenerative changes take place in joints or major membranes and rigid structures of the larynx. Wyke and Kirschner (1976) are among many who would dispense with Semon's law, since the innervation of the muscle groups cannot be separated, either in myelination features or in separate nerve fibre bundles in the recurrent nerve, right up to the terminal branches. Despite these academic frustrations, a thriving and developing industry in surgery to separate palsied vocal cords, fixed uncomfortably in adduction with consequent respiratory obstruction, exists.

There are doubters convinced of the inadequacies of Semon's law and who hold that the position of the palsied cord is much more fortuitous than Semon suggested. The slow changes and retreat to a paramedian position may be due to denervated muscle contracture in the denervated hemilarynx.

The management of the single, flaccid, palsied cord depends very much on the causative lesion and the defect that it causes. Some patients are left with well-nigh perfect voices, only the timbre being altered and typical of the lesion. 'Idiopathic' defects may recover up to three years after onset and a number of these will be caused by apical, old tuberculous fibrosis. Most commonly these are at the right lung apex and never become clinically apparent, apart from the cord palsy.

Other cord palsies, e.g. those in carcinoma of the lung, are the more trivial elements of the disease and are overshadowed by the tragedy of the major condition which is almost, by definition, inoperable as soon as it or its nodal metastases cause left recurrent nerve damage in the mediastinum or root of the neck. Neck surgery for benign goitre and some slowly progressive, well-irradiated and controlled neoplasms remain in which a cord palsied well in abduction is associated with a voice reduced to a breathy whisper which tires easily. If faced with such for a prolonged period, a patient may be dramatically helped by restoring bulk and rigidity to the vocal cord with intracordal injection of teflon paste. This procedure has largely replaced the laryngofissure approaches of the past in which slivers of cartilage were inserted into the anterior end of the vocal cord at open operation via a laryngofissure-thyrotomy approach. Under general anaesthesia, with fine polythene intubation, and micro-laryngoscopy applied, a Bruening's syringe is loaded with teflon paste (Polytef shredded teflon very finely divided, particle size 7–100 μm in glycerine) and is injected, 3 mm clear of the vocal cord margin into the bulk of the cord. The injection should cause a gently fusiform enlargement; if too bowed it should be straightened with an injection of a lesser amount further forward or backward along the cord. Care needs to be taken to avoid placing the paste in Reinke's space, or alternatively too far laterally in the ventricle floor or into the perichondrium on the medial wall of the thyroid cartilage. The paste migrates minimally, in tissue planes, does not appear in the lymph nodes and appears to be totally inert. Dedo, Urrea and Lawson (1973) summarized the situation succinctly.

There is no question that teflon implantation of a cord palsied by total vagal loss or upper motor neurone disease is much less satisfactory than that in the case of isolated recurrent nerve palsy.

It may well be that the bulked, rigid implanted cord still requires the cricothyroid to tense it for the functioning vocal cord to occlude adequately and produce improved phonation.

Some enfeebled patients with carcinoma of the bronchus, virtually speechless, value the prompt restoration of the voice by this relatively trivial procedure, as do those who survive major cardiothoracic surgery with similar recurrent nerve losses. Awaiting the slow development of a restored voice is, under such circumstances, not so justifiable and the procedure may be done without delay.

These patients will have to be watched over the years in case, despite its very inert nature, teflon has unsuspected carcinogenic features. Post-operatively there is the development of a granuloma, with slow resorption of the suspending glycerol, and a slight reduction in cord bulk as the granuloma resolves. As the oedema abates, a very fine post-operative voice may at this point deteriorate a little, and the area is sore. Methods with the patient seated, larynx locally anaesthetized, and the injection done with the patient phonating under indirect laryngoscopy, are idealistic and tolerated by too small a minority of patients for general usage. Moreover, the ability to assess the right amount of teflon paste, should not be too highly regarded, since the depot size is unpredictable due to granuloma, oedema and glycerol resorption in the post-operative weeks. No gross over-injections causing laryngeal obstruction should occur at micro-laryngoscopy, under general anaesthesia, when the basic requirements are observed. These are that the other cord should be fully functional and that the injected cord should not be pushed right up to the midline. Bilateral injections (e.g. to close the larynx to overspill in the flaccid, bilaterally palsied larynx with a valved tracheostomy tube below, and yet to allow speech) have yielded rather unpredictable effects and have not been used extensively enough to be assessed.

Bilateral cord palsy results predominantly from thyroid surgery or thyroid disease; growing numbers come from bilateral, increasingly ambitious neck dissection operations. Palsy of the cords in adduction may be sudden post-operatively and it prompts either intubation or more properly tracheostomy. Some palsies may not so result and the airway is inadequate. Spontaneous restoration, at least in part, of the airway may ensue after a delay of even two years. A tracheostomy life of one year is justifiable in many cases. If recovery does not ensue, then a range of procedures is available to separate the cords.

Tracheostomy remains an option for the very aged, those who have had one for many years and cope well with it, the obese and frail, those who accept the obvious crippledom of tracheostomite life with no wish to swim, those with a brief but vital need to talk via a valved tracheostomy tube, and those who have had extensive but failed attempts at cordopexy. The newly tracheostomized patient must be patient, and await the hoped-for improvement; the final unrushed decision must be left to the well-informed patient.

Operations for separating the vocal cords palsied in adduction coupled with dyspnoea, stridor or tracheostomy abound and are largely of historical interest. Hoover (1932) started the matter but developed the procedure substantially. Essentially he developed the laryngofissure approach with incisions 1 mm above and below the cord margin. He removed the whole contents of the vocal cord, muscle, fat and fibrous tissue by this approach and also the arytenoid cartilage. Received opinion is that one 'trades one's voice for one's airway'. In fact the airway (and freedom from tracheostomy) is a major asset, while voice is at a premium only for a minority. Hence the former is a prize of great value. The tracheostomite is for ever at risk, falling into water or facing respiratory infection.

King (1939) used one of the lateral approaches to gain access to the larynx via the inferior constrictor, suturing the arytenoid to the ala of the thyroid cartilage. This was awkward and too simplistic. Kelly (1941) cut a hole through the thyroid cartilage, thence through this 1 cm aperture sutured the arytenoid laterally.

The result of this series was the procedure of Woodman (1946). This works well and is done as follows: a preliminary tracheostomy, a lateral approach and arytenoidectomy via the extramucosal route in the bed of the pyriform fossa. The vocal process is retained (indeed it is hard to remove without mucosal breach), and the process sutured to the inferior cornu of the thyroid cartilage.

For what it is worth, it seems probable that the anterior, laryngofissure approaches will retain their ascendancy. The notion that one is in a position to offer voice or airway is largely fanciful. The latter is a massive prize, the defects of voice nebulous and wide separation of the cords a worthwhile target. Decompression of the recurrent laryngeal nerve may well be followed by recovery, with mass movement of the musculature, but it is a procedure retained for known post-thyroidectomy damage without nerve division.

Hall-Allan (1967) noted that electrical stimulation cannot readily detect recurrent laryngeal nerve damage at the time of thyroid operation. He has collected some 51 cases of recurrent nerve paralysis associated with benign thyroid disease. The 50 per cent recovery and the time taken to recover corresponded with the distance from the larynx to the lesion. He discussed the subject of nerve resuture, to obtain mass movement from this 90 per cent motor nerve and to dispense with permanent tracheostomy.

The chapter by Wyke and Kirschner (1976) warrants full study, as it describes the enormous strides forward in the matters of fine laryngeal innervation, control and scientific investigation, and gives a good foundation of basic anatomy and physiology. Von Leyden (1976) follows on laryngeal function and Lund (1976) on deglutition in a detailed manner which deserves study in the original.

Pharyngeal palsies

Many of these are of sudden onset, and despite the patient's protestations about the absence of a precipitating emotional factor, are superficial enough and often reflect an intractable life problem. Recovery may be overnight. Speech therapists commonly manage this ailment extremely well; the more emotionally crippled should, however, be directed at once for psychiatric care. These are some of the more threatening of conversion symptoms in terms of serious psychiatric disease.

The cricopharyngeus muscle has been studied by O'Connor and Ardran (1976), who point out that its defects in performance have to be studied by physical, radiological, neurological and endoscopic examination. Kaplan (1951) pointed out that isolated pharyngeal palsies are not easy to detect and the patient's story is not very lucid. Moreover, the activity of swallowing is so rapid a performance as to be rather elusive, even though the symptoms are complicated with overspill. Videotape facilities are probably the best possible mechanism for recording these features which may identify those persons needing myotomy. Sullivan (1974) investigated pharyngeal pressures and recommend that we cease using the term 'globus hystericus' and call it 'idiopathic globus'. The matter is probably hair-splitting but they noted that the plane of contraction of the cricopharyngeus was mainly in the apical rather than the lateral plane, and they think that 'cricopharyngeal hypertonicity' is a better term than 'globus'.

Patients with dysphagia

A careful history with physical, radiological, endoscopic and neurological investigations is mandatory. The hypopharynx is a difficult target because of the involved nature of its musculature, and its function is coupled with the ability to compensate for any slowly developing disability. Spectacular dysphagia results from quite minor neurological impairment. Fluorography reported by Ardran, Kemp and Wegelius (1957) and by O'Connor and Ardran (1976) who exposed film at 7.8 m/s noted tongue, palate, hyoid elevation, bolus deflection and epiglottis movements. Videotape recording may make this a much more straightforward affair.

A number of disorganized cricopharyngeal functions are improved by cricopharyngeal myotomy in a wide range of functional dysphagias including old poliomyelitis, vascular accidents and systemic lupus erythematosus.

O'Connor and Ardran (1976) could detect no difference on manometry between those afflicted with globus and a wide range of controls.

The usual type of pharyngeal pouch (or hypopharyngeal diverticulum) is a posterior pulsion diverticulum between the lower cricopharyngeal fibres and the upper thyropharyngeal fibres of the inferior constrictor muscle, through a weak area known as Killian's dehiscence. The lower fibres (that is, the cricopharyngeus) surround the pharynx without a median raphe at the back, are normally closed and are alleged to prevent aspiration of air going into the oesophagus during breathing. Hair-splitting abounds in the theories concerned with the development of these pouches. There may be neuromuscular incoordination causing a delay or failure of relaxation of the cricopharyngeal sphincter, with second-stage swallowing which may represent an achalasia rather than a spasm. Negus believed it to be different, the descending wave of peristalsis being too rapid or forceful for the sphincter to relax adequately. There is no great doubt that it is of neuromuscular origin. A number of gross oesophageal obstructions do, as a result, arise in pharyngeal pouches. These pouches do not apparently recur after removal, especially when a myotomy on the cricopharyngeal sphincter has been performed (Lund, 1976). The barium radiographs of these patients show a larger pharynx than normal and a residue of barium after swallowing is completed. A second swallow has to take place to express this and it may be that it is the second swallow which causes the herniation. Earlan (1976) discusses the mechanism of the incoordination coupled with this second swallow by examining very early pouches which they visualize during the first swallow and not during the second obstructive swallow. One of the most instructive activities in which to engage while excising one of these pouches is to pass the finger into the pouch and then down into the oesophagus. The usual experience is to detect a tight band, not just muscular, giving access to the upper oesophagus through a very firm and narrow opening. A myotomy in several vertical parallel lines relieves this. Any healing of musculature is not really such as to produce a linear scar with similar stenosis afterwards but gross relaxation of large widths of denervated atrophic muscle.

Dohlman and Mattson (1959) initiated endoscopic methods for diathermizing the party wall between the oesophagus and the pouch, so as to throw them into one large chamber. This results, of course, in a cricopharyngeal myotomy (*see* Chapter 9).

In an age of 'chronic electronic implants' it appears possible that the neurological defects of this area may be made good by means of such devices. The central nervous system implants for Parkinson's disease, appliances such as pacemakers and those for neuromuscular losses in the region (e.g. for incontinence) may reach the laryngopharynx within the decade. Ready of access, the innervation of our region is ripe for such development.

Special investigations

Cineradiology and cinefluorography with videotape facility

Progress in this field is summarized by O'Connor and Ardran (1976). Difficult to diagnose pharyngeal palsies, acute or insidious in onset, may be missed in ordinary projections. Cinefluorography may reveal the defects, head-positioning in defective swallowing of a unilateral nature is important and a totally palsied lateral food channel may be symptomless. Improvements are to be expected, especially with videotape.

Stroboscopy and micro-stroboscopy of the pharynx

Stroboscopy via fibre-optic devices has been investigated. (McKelvie, 1944; McKelvie, Grey and North, 1970). Minor changes in cord motility are eminently observable with stroboscopy. Throat microphones, coupled either with fibre-optic or microscopic visualization, show best of all asymmetrical cord loading, loss of the ripple movement of the vocal cords and the sequence of changes associated with resolution of voice after favourable cord surgery, radiotherapy, or steroid antibiotic treatments.

Sonograms and colour sonograms

'Voice prints', whereby time is plotted horizontally on a trace, frequency and volume in density and vertical trace are difficult to interpret through changes with therapy or advancing disease. Trans-figuration of the trace into colour density patterns helps analyses, although to date they help the laryngologist minimally.

It is proper in this connection to re-assess the alleged psychogenic ailments afflicting the area. While there is good overall evidence that it is a much-favoured target zone for hysterical conversion symptoms (hysterical or functional dysphonia, globus hystericus, functional laryngeal cough for example) there is a current vogue for super-sophisticated investigation of these conditions, some of which do reveal minor structural or functional abnormalities.

References

Ardran, M., Kemp, F. H. and Wegelius, C. (1957). *British Journal of Radiology*, **30**, 169

Avellis, G. (1891). 'Klinische Beiträge zur halbseitigen Kehlkopflamungen', *Klinische Wochenschrift*, **40**, 1

Dedo, H. H., Urrea, R. and Lawson, L. (1973). 'Intracordial injection of teflon in the treatment of 135 patients with dysphonia', *Annals of Otology*, **82**, 661

Dohlman, G. and Mattson, I. O. (1959). 'The role of the cricopharyngeal muscle in cases of hypopharyngeal diverticulae', *American Journal of Roentgenology*, **94**, 299

Earlam, R. (1976). In: *Clinical tests of oesphageal function* (Eds Crosby and Lockwood) pp. 73–92; Staples, London

Hall-Allen, R. T. J. (1967). 'Laryngeal nerve and thyroid disease', *Archives of Otolaryngology*, **85**, 335

Hoover, W. B. (1932). 'Bilateral abductor paralysis. Operative treatment by submucous resection of the vocal cords', *Archives of Otolaryngology*, **15**, 339

Kaplan, S. (1951). *Annals of Surgery*, **133**, 572

Kelly, J. D. (1941). 'Surgical treatment of bilateral paralysis of the abductor muscles', *Archives of Otolaryngology*, **33**, 293

King, B. T. (1939). 'New and function-restoring operation for bilateral abductor cord paralysis', *Journal of the American Medical Association*, **112**, 814

Leyden, von H. (1976). In: *Scientific Foundations of Otolaryngology*; Heinemann, London

Lund, W. S. (1976). In: *Scientific Foundations of*

Otolaryngology; Heinemann, London

McKelvie, W. B. (1944). 'A stroboscope using a grid-controlled neon tube. The strobotron', *Journal of Laryngology*, **59**, 464

McKelvie, P., Grey, P. and North, C. (1970). 'Laryngeal strobomicroscope', *Lancet*, **ii**, 503

Minuck, M. (1976). 'Unilateral vocal cord paralysis following endotracheal intubation', *Anaesthesiology*, **45**, 448

O'Connor, A. F. F. and Ardran, G. M. (1976). 'Cinefluorography in the diagnosis of pharyngeal palsies', *Journal of Laryngology*, **76**, 1015

Ogura, J. H. (1961). 'Surgical decompression of the recurrent laryngeal nerve in idiopathic unilateral vocal cord paresis', *Annals of Otology*, **70**, 451

Stuart, D. W. (1965). 'The otolaryngologic aspects of myasthenia gravis', *Laryngoscope*, **75**, 112

Sullivan, W. C. (1974). *Lancet*, **2**, 1417

Svien, H. J., Baker, H. L. and Rivers, M. H. (1963). 'Jugular foramen syndrome and allied syndromes', *Neurology*, **13**, 797

Vernet, M. (1918). 'The classification of syndromes of associated paralysis', *Journal of Laryngology*, **33**, 354

Woodman, de Graafe (1946). 'Modification of extralaryngeal approach to arytenoidectomy for bilateral abductor paralysis', *Archives of Otolaryngology*, **43**, 63

Wyke, B. D. and Kirschner, J. A. (1976). In: *Scientific Foundations of Otolaryngology*, ch. 40, pp. 546–574; Heinemann, London

18 Disorders of speech

F Clifford Rose and Gaye Murrills

Introduction

Speech is the skill that most clearly separates humanity from the rest of the animal kingdom. It is an effective and expeditious system for communication and has been defined as an 'integrated function, involving the reception of words by the ear or the eye, their interpretation and synthesis as language within the brain and the expression of this language response in further written or spoken words' (Morley, 1967).

Despite the complex mental and physical processes involved, speech is a skill often taken for granted and, only when breakdown occurs, either as a developmental or acquired disorder, is its influence and value recognized.

The study of speech disorders and their therapy is concerned with all levels of activity, both developmental and acquired, so that physical, psychological, physiological and linguistic factors may all come under scrutiny. The scope of the subject is therefore extensive but this chapter must limit its attention to speech disorders related primarily to the interests of the otorhinolaryngologist.

The development of speech

Communicative sounds are vocalized in a baby long before the establishment of verbalization. Spectrographic analysis (Wasz-Höckert *et al.*, 1968) has demonstrated the different cries of a baby, each indicating another type of message. The cry of the newborn infant can be distinguished from its fellow by the mother as are the meanings of later purposive cries which may signify hunger or pain. During the first two years of life the cry pattern changes, probably correlating with anatomical changes in the oropharyngeal structures (Karelitz, Karelitz and Rosenfelt, 1960).

Within the first month or two, the infant will be heard to coo with pleasure and make reflex noises, such as a hiccup. Even different types of cooing can be recognized by the family, e.g. of repletion or that of mounting irritation preceding a cry (Murphy, 1964). The non-verbal vocalizations of cooing and gurgling are made with the mouth open; it is of interest that they are similar in babies of different races even though the languages later learned will be entirely different.

By the age of three or four months these vocalizations become repetitive to begin the babbling stage, an essential part in the development of speech and soon lost if the child is deaf. It is assumed that during this phase there is an auditory feedback, the infant listening to the noises it makes; certainly, if spoken to, the infant will stop babbling.

It is about the sixth month of life that the greatest variability in learning speech occurs, some children learning to repeat words (echolalia). It is easy to see how the same word, repeated often enough, will become associated with the object in view. For this reason, children without sufficient stimulation will have delayed development of speech (Rheingold, 1960). Echolalia that persists without the recognition that the words used have significance can be an early sign of mental retardation.

By the age of a year a child will be saying 'ma-ma' and 'da-da'. Again, these consonants and vowels are among the earliest to be learned, no matter in which part of the world the child is born. Within another two months, one or two recognizable words will be added, and by 15 months the average child could have up to six words. Reception is more advanced than expression and the child will understand simple commands at this stage and be able to point to familiar objects and persons.

By the age of 18 months the child will be able to join in nursery rhymes, point to objects in pictures and indulge in pretend play.

Although the average age for a child to say the first words is one year, the range of normality varies from eight months to two-and-a-half years. The same wide variability occurs with the construction of simple phrases, the average being 18 months but the range varying from 10 months to $3\frac{1}{2}$ years. Although speech is intelligible to family and friends by the age of two years, a third of children pass through a phase of unintelligible jargon speech at the age of three or four years. Development of speech, as with development of other neurological functions, does not take place at a steady rate; there may be periods, worrying to uninformed parents, where no progress is made and words known may be temporarily lost. Normal children can speak simple sentences by the age of three and if delayed beyond this, the child should be fully assessed.

Childhood speech disorders

Normal speech and language development is dependent on numerous complex interacting processes. It requires intact neurological and physiological systems for perception, recognition and gradual association of speech sounds and further central and peripheral processes to allow imitation, recall and reproduction of these within the developing language code. In addition, general intelligence, levels of neuromuscular maturation, environment, emotional stability and motivation all play their part in the process. For these reasons, a child presenting in the ENT clinic with what appears to be a straightforward speech defect may in fact turn out to have a very different diagnosis.

Examination of hearing, as well as structure and function of the articulators, is a vital aspect of investigation as is a comprehensive assessment by a speech therapist to cover both receptive and expressive language levels, even when there is only a suspicion of simple delay or when the disorder is mild. The advice 'he will grow out of it', apart from often being untrue, provides no assistance to anxious parents, who need guidance regarding normal patterns of language development and information to encourage progress along correct lines. Advice and management at the optimal time may ensure maximum development, and screening for potential problems as a 'prophylactic' service is important.

Structural abnormalities

Articulation is the process by which words are expressed through muscular movements controlled by nervous activity, with the production of vocal sounds (Morley, 1967). When in the presence of adequate neurological maturation and suitable environmental stimuli, articulatory development is hindered, this may be due to structural deformities.

Abnormalities of teeth, tongue, tonsils and adenoids can each contribute to defective articulation, but one of the most serious and common problems affecting this process is the incompetent palatopharyngeal sphincter. This inadequacy may be related to a cleft palate or submucous cleft; it may also occur (sometimes only temporarily) after adenoidectomy, where a congenitally short palate and deep nasopharynx become evident. Other causes are disorders of mobility rather than structural abnormalities, where there is mild paresis, or incoordination in the absence of true paralysis.

Cleft palate

The specialized field of cleft palate surgery and rehabilitation is a continuously developing one. Early surgery to lip and palate, primarily geared to facilitate feeding and prevent the development of abnormal muscular patterns of coordination in palate and pharynx, relate directly to developing patterns of speech. Similarly, adequate nasopharyngeal closure providing a means of separating nasal and oral airways, assisting control of the vocal air stream and creating intra-oral pressure for speech sounds, is basic to the necessary functions of sucking and swallowing in the young child.

Consonant sounds of speech may appear in a baby's babble by four months of age and, because of the normal early absorption of environmental stimuli, routine ENT examination and hearing assessment is advisable at the earliest feasible time. This is because of the high likelihood of fluctuating conductive deafness in this particular group of children as a result of eustachian tube dysfunction secondary to the palatal problems. Even when the child is too young for accurate hearing assessment, examination of the tympanic membranes may reveal features indicating that the middle ear is full of secretions causing conductive deafness. If hearing is significantly reduced, it may be restored by the insertion of grommets into the tympanic membranes to allow temporary ventilation of the middle-ear cavity pending return of normal eustachian function as the child grows older.

Referral to speech therapy should be automatic by the time the child is six months old. Since tremendous progress is being made on the surgical front, the speech therapist's role may now in many cases be primarily that of assessment. Early contact with parents to discuss normal speech development patterns can prove of great value. Not only does the therapist check on progress, but she is particularly aware of other factors which may adversely influence speech development until more detailed language assessment can be made at approximately two years. Regular hearing assessment should be continued and information obtained from the parents regarding response to sounds in the home. Regular speech and hearing reviews at six-monthly or yearly intervals are then advisable, the therapist investigating not only receptive and expressive levels of speech and language, but also voice resonance and prosody. Continuing support and advice should be provided to the parents regarding language acquisition and their role in encouraging this. If palatopharyngeal incompetence is suspected of giving a generalized hypernasal quality to speech and/or articulation substitutions, this will merit the earliest close investigation. Once deviant, compensatory sounds are established firmly in the speech pattern, e.g. glossopharyngeal fricatives and glottal stops, even if later palatopharyngeal competence is achieved, eradication will prove difficult. Quite apart from the speech therapist's report, investigations undertaken will depend on facilities available but may include lateral skull cinefluorography, radiography, palatography and nasendoscopy in addition to measurements with a nasal anenometer.

With the problem viewed from all aspects, the course of action to be followed usually becomes clear. Pharyngoplasty, palatoplasty or the use of an obturator may well be indicated but, where adequate palatal closure is inconsistent or lacking in coordination, speech therapy may be the chosen course of treatment. The results of audiometric testing should be known before therapy is attempted as the child's ability to self-monitor and develop useful auditory discriminative skills and so control nasal escape will be hampered by hearing deficit.

Therapy can be provided regularly over a period of time or perhaps in intensive blocks to produce optimal results, the full cooperation of both parents and child being basic necessities for success. The general approach by family members to the child's communication skills will also be carefully monitored, for an anxious child under pressure from even more anxious parents is unlikely to make great strides.

Even where true palatopharyngeal incompetence remains, if a discriminatory ear and good sense of kinaesthetics and coordination are developed, acceptable speech may well be possible. Greene (1972) advocates the cultivation of 'a quiet voice, and slow speech, free from all tension and stridency'. This basic approach is re-inforced by van den Berg (1962): 'Speech which is free from tension, produced without excessive air pressure with open-mouthed articulation so that more air-waves escape through the mouth than down the nose, may be so harmonically balanced that it is perceived as normal although nasal cues are clearly discernible in the spectrograph'.

In addition to the speech therapist's approach designed to develop adequate control of the expiratory air stream and involving attention to relaxation, auditory training and some articulation work, the dentist and therapist may also provide a child with a dental plate having an attached 'stimulator', consisting of a loop of wire just making contact with the relaxed palate (Tudor and Selley, 1974). Continual wearing of this alone may bring about some degree of improvement in function but it may also be used in conjunction with an Electrical Visual Speech Aid which provides the child with motivating visual feedback on the movement of his soft palate (*see* Tudor and Selley [1974] for detailed description of device).

The aim will be to have the child speaking intelligibly, at least by the time he reaches school age, to minimize pressure and distress caused by continuing frustration with communication. After this time, it may be necessary for the child to undergo further completion or revision surgery from the plastic surgeon and he may receive oral surgery for malocclusion or as part of orthodontic management. Speech progress, if requiring no further direct attention, may be reviewed at combined clinics, with ENT, plastic and orofacial surgeons who will arrange repeated assessments of hearing and eustachian tube function.

Tonsils and adenoids

The decision to perform an adenoidectomy operation in a cleft-palate child is a sensitive one, as the pad of tissue may be assisting with nasopharyngeal closure by reducing the dimensions of the nasopharynx. This may avoid adenoidectomy and its attendant complications in cleft-palate children.

Similarly, in a normal child it may unmask underlying palatopharyngeal incompetence. A congenitally short palate may become evident once the adenoid bulk has been removed and many children without this condition may also suffer temporary nasopharyngeal insufficiency post-operatively. A referral to the speech therapist may be worthwhile during this transient phase to provide re-assurance to both parent and child and prevent any build-up of nasal grimace or abnormal compensatory movements.

Enlarged tonsils and adenoids will not in themselves cause a true defect of articulation. Resonance can be distorted and may improve after adenotonsillectomy but, if a genuine developmental disorder of speech is present, operation will effect no change.

Dental abnormalities

Malocclusion, whether in a normal or a cleft-palate child, may contribute to defective articulation but will rarely be the single causal factor. In the absence of dysarthria or articulatory dyspraxia, i.e. the impairment of voluntary movement in the absence of paresis, a healthy mobile tongue will usually compensate for dental or other structural disorders.

Tongue tie

Normal speech development is possible in the presence of a fairly severe degree of tongue tie and, if defective articulation is present and persistent, the likelihood of another contributory factor is high. The possibility of mild paresis or articulatory dyspraxia, i.e. the impairment of voluntary movement in the absence of paresis, will need consideration, in addition to other factors which can influence normal speech acquisition.

Childhood voice disorders

Childhood dysphonia is particularly common in boys between the ages of 5 and 10 years (Ellis, 1952). A full ENT assessment will have excluded factors such as sinus and catarrhal problems or recurring tonsillitis. Laryngoscopy generally reveals symptoms directly related to vocal hyperfunction e.g. thickening of the vocal folds and 'singer's nodules' although, in slightly older children, hoarse, husky voices may be more directly the result of pre-pubertal laryngeal changes. Surgical removal of vocal nodules or cord stripping in children is not recommended as these conditions often respond well to the simpler forms of voice training.

There is disagreement regarding the management of dysphonia in children related to vocal abuse. One view is that the problems are likely to right themselves by the age of 11 years as, by this time, screaming and shouting should be naturally lessened and, for this reason, voice therapy should be avoided until after this age (Greene, 1972). Another view is that considerable improvement can be achieved in a 3–6 months' period by concentrating on reducing vocal abuse, intensity of voice, and habitual pitch level (Wilson, 1961). Boone suggests a therapy programme isolating situations in which the child is really abusive, with 'yelling charts' to plot and evaluate episodes and map progress (Boone, 1971). Although total voice rest will be almost impossible, when the child and parents are receptive and are able to grasp explanations, they can in time take up responsibility for the problem and success follows. The speech therapist will need to spend time involving other individuals in contact with the child, particularly in school, as well as providing incentives and enjoyable goals to be reached. In this positive way she develops the child's consciousness towards voice usage without increasing anxiety or pressurizing developing communication abilities.

Stuttering

The literature on the complex disorder of stuttering – the term in the United Kingdom is used synonymously with stammering – is large and cannot be fully reviewed here but, since many patients with fluency disorders are referred to the ENT surgeon, it is necessary briefly to discuss the disorder here.

Theories suggesting an organic basis of stuttering have concentrated on possible abnormalities in the nervous system, especially aspects of cerebral dominance such as bilateral representation for speech or incomplete cerebral dominance. Although recently refuted, there is some evidence that the stutterer *could* have some 'minimal disorder of the nervous system' (Beech and Fransella, 1968).

The question of impaired auditory and/or other feedback systems for speech has also received considerable attention in relation to the aetiology and treatment of stuttering. Experiments with normal speakers found fluency to be disturbed by Delayed Auditory Feedback (DAF) (Lee, 1951) and much work has been done on this aspect as well as on total masking of sound in stuttering subjects. Surprisingly good results have been achieved using both air- and bone-conduction masking, producing almost total fluency with elimination of concomitant movements – but this usually only lasts while the devices are *in situ*. Treatment programmes have been developed from these observations using in particular DAF which modifies speech output to produce an easier, prolonged pattern.

Stuttering can also be considered in terms of learning theory; for example, anticipation of certain words produces anxiety leading to an abnormal approach to the situation. Dysfluency occurs, the word is eventually communicated and the anxiety level falls, all of which may re-inforce the stuttering behaviour. Once expectancy and predictive ability are developed, the stutter becomes an habitual part of the speech behaviour, but it is difficult to be certain where the chain reaction begins. Wischner (1950) and Johnson (1959) both attributed the early stages of this learned behaviour to the anxiety of parents in response to stages of normal non-fluency during the development of speech. This stage of non-fluency coincides with a vulnerable period in language development when fuller use of connected speech is developing (Dalton and Hardcastle, 1977) and 'it hardly seems far-fetched to ask whether some children during this time are so sensitized by the difficulties they encounter in learning adult syntax that, especially if they are subject as well to communicative pressures, they tend to acquire the feelings that express themselves in tense and fragmented realizations of the grammatical structures of the language' (Bloodstein, 1974). Johnson (1959) was the first to focus attention on the damaging and powerful effects of actually labelling a child a stutterer – 'At the point of origin of the problem of stuttering, the most crucial single factor to be considered is that of the listener's sensitivity to the speaker's non-fluencies, his inclination to evaluate them as undesirable and distressing and particularly his tendency to classify them specifically as stuttering'. For these reasons the young child presenting in the ENT clinic with a normal non-fluency pattern of speech may well be at risk, particularly where there is a family history of stuttering and a heightened sensitivity towards hesitancy and delay.

Treatment

No one method of treatment will prove successful with every individual stutterer. There is little 'unequivocal evidence that stutterers as a group are more neurotic or maladjusted than non-stutterers but psychological aspects will certainly exacerbate and perpetuate a problem and much attention needs to be paid to this' (Beech and Fransella, 1968). For this reason, full assessment in planning a suitable individualized programme by a team approach of speech therapist and psychotherapist will often prove useful. Group therapy provides an excellent basis for a discussion of attitudes towards difficulties as well as an establishment of realistic aims. Psychotherapy may be run simultaneously with programmes geared towards modification of the abnormal speech pattern. These are divided into three categories (Dalton and Hardcastle, 1977):

(1) Those which seek to replace stuttering by an alternative pattern of speaking.
(2) Those which aim at reducing the stutter to an easier relaxed form.
(3) Those which attempt to eliminate dysfluencies by inhibition of disruptive elements.

Dysphasia

Dysphasia is the difficulty in the formulation, expression and understanding of acoustic symbols. The classical distinction is between motor dysphasia, which affects the expressive side, and sensory dysphasia, which affects the receptive aspects. It is very rare to have one without the other being affected, albeit slightly (Espir and Rose, 1976). Perhaps a better classification is in terms of fluency whereby non-fluent speech indicates expressive dysphasia, while fluent speech is that where the patient is able to produce jargon dysphasia but with normal articulation and rhythm. Expressive dysphasia may leave out prepositions and conjunctions (*telegrammatism*) and word output is reduced. There may be confusion of articulation and conjunctions with many grammatical errors (*paragrammatism*) (*see Table 18.1*).

Table 18.1   Clinical types of dysphasia

Expressive	*Receptive*
Motor	Sensory
Non-fluent	Fluent
Reduced word output	Logorrhoea, circumlocution
Dysarthria	Neologism
Dysprosody	
Broca's area,	Wernicke's area
(inferior frontal lobe)	(upper temporal lobe)

Dysarthria

Dysarthria is disordered articulation. This type of speech disorder may be due to non-neurological causes such as loose-fitting dentures or cleft palate (*see* above).

The neurological causes may be due to a lesion of:

(1) Muscle.
(2) Lower motor neurone.
(3) Upper motor neurone.
(4) Extrapyramidal system.
(5) Cerebellar system.

Dysarthria is often accompanied by dysphonia (*see* 'Dysarthrophonia', later in this chapter).

Muscle

Primary muscle disease

It is unlikely that any of the primary myopathies will present first to ENT specialists. Primary muscle disease is divided into: polymyositis, which is an inflammatory collagen affection; and muscular dystrophy, which is genetically determined. Both types of disease affect the proximal limb musculature but in each the muscles concerned with articulation can be affected, e.g. the palate in polymyositis and the facial musculature in facio-scapulo-humeral muscular dystrophy. The diagnosis can usually be made clinically but is confirmed by electromyography (EMG) and muscle biopsy.

Myasthenia

Perhaps more likely to be seen by the ENT surgeon is the increasing dysarthria and difficulty in mastication that is seen in myasthenia gravis, a biochemical disorder of the neuromuscular junction. In addition to dysarthria and dysphonia there may be dysphagia but the diagnosis can be confirmed by Tensilon injection.

Lower motor neurone lesions

The lesion in such cases may be anywhere from the anterior horn cell in the neuromuscular junction. The commonest disease of this sort seen by the ENT surgeon is Bell's palsy which produces paralysis, total or partial, of the facial musculature on one side. The slurred speech is due to the unilateral weakness of the muscles around the mouth.

Acute polyneuritis producing symmetrical weakness and changes in the distal part of the limbs can also produce dysarthria and dysphonia with a nasal voice (hyper-rhinolalia). If the lower cranial nerves are affected, paresis of the lips, palate, pharynx, larynx and tongue may occur. When the respiratory musculature is involved, tracheostomy and assistance in respiration may be necessary.

The lower cranial nerves seven, nine, ten, eleven and twelve may be affected by neoplasm, goitre, aneurysm of the aorta or trauma. Bulbar poliomyelitis may also affect the motor nuclei of these cranial nerves producing dysarthria and dysphonia but, with immunization, this is now rarely seen.

Motor neurone disease

Cases of motor neurone disease are not infrequently referred in the first instance to ENT surgeons. This is a condition which develops in middle age with progressive deterioration resulting in death within five years. There is progressive bulbar palsy with wasting and fasciculation of the tongue, as well as limb musculature. Articulation becomes more indistinct, the labials being particularly affected because of weakness of the lips. The dental and velar sounds are also impaired because of progressive weakness of the tongue, and weakness of the soft palate causes nasal tone and dysphonia. The diagnosis is usually made clinically but can be confirmed by EMG (Rose, 1977).

Another rare condition that may produce dysarthria and dysphonia is syringo-bulbia, a developmental disorder producing cystic degeneration around the 4th ventricle and central canal of the spinal cord. The symptoms usually begin after the age of 20 years and are slowly progressive. Nowadays surgical decompression is often indicated.

Progressive involvement of the cranial nerve nuclei produces dysarthria and dysphonia which may also be seen in brain-stem lesions, e.g. pontine glioma, which tends to occur in children.

Bulbar palsy

Bulbar palsy indicates paralysis of the cranial nerves coming from the bulb or hind brain. In addition to dysarthria and dysphonia, there is dysphagia and, in addition to hyper-rhinolalia, there is nasal regurgitation, particularly of fluids.

Upper motor neurone lesions

The site may be anywhere from the frontal cortex to the anterior horn cell. When bilateral, it may produce the syndrome of pseudobulbar palsy and, in addition to dysarthria, dysphagia and dysphonia, there may be pathological laughter and crying (emotional lability). This can be caused by cerebrovascular lesions, motor neurone disease, bilateral neoplasm (e.g. metastases), or widespread disease such as severe brain injury or encephalitis.

Extra-pyramidal lesions

The commonest of these is Parkinson's disease in which the voice is monotonous and feeble due to rigidity of the laryngeal musculature. There may be dysarthria due to involvement of the articulatory muscles and sometimes a phrase may be repeated (palilalia). In addition there is excessive salivation.

Cerebellar lesions

Cerebellar lesions will also produce dysarthria. The commonest of these is in multiple sclerosis where the dysarthria is of a scanning type, that is, each syllable is pronounced as if it were a separate word. The emphasis is occasionally put on the wrong syllable to produce staccato speech.

Dysphonia

This can be classified as follows:

(1) Organic.
    (a) Neurological.
    (b) Endocrine.

(c) Due to vocal abuse.

(2) Functional.

Accurate classification of dysphonia in terms of a functional/organic dichotomy may prove difficult in practice and is not always necessary in terms of therapy.

In addition to fairly exhaustive information on environmental and emotional influences on the voice, evaluation of respiration, phonation, resonance and articulation may need to be carried out.

Respiration

Faulty patterns of posture, breath control and air-flow may all adversely influence voice production. Generally, investigations are based on subjective assessment of habitual patterns of respiration, vital capacity and expiratory control. Although frequently effective and adequate, these can now be advantageously supplemented with numerical measurements on air-flow rates, control and phonatory capability. Such investigations are not entirely new, but the simple scoring systems devised provide an assessment measure which can now be of immediate benefit in the clinical situation.

Quality

Description of voice quality has also been, and generally still remains, a question of subjective assessment. Numerous attempts have been made to clear the confusion surrounding the vague labels used, including studies into the feasibility of a numerical scoring system, e.g. one imaginative study has proposed a descriptive model of voice quality, utilizing general phonetic theory (Laver, 1968). The sound spectograph (Potter, Kopp and Green, 1947), originally invented to throw a display of 'visible speech', although of use to phoneticians and acoustic physicists, is of little benefit to the practising clinician. Speech scientists are now developing visual displays of 'speech pattern features' which can have important assessment and therapeutic applications for hearing-impaired patients as well as those with voice disorders.

For example, the Electrolaryngograph measures the changing resistance across the vocal folds as they vibrate. This is done by means of two superficially applied electrodes providing a method of 'measuring vocal fold closure without inconvenience to the speaker and without disturbance to his phonation' (Fourcin and Abberton, 1972, 1976). The laryngograph signal can be displayed on an oscilloscope in two ways:

(1) As a wave-form showing frequency and regularity of vocal fold vibration; the shape of the wave-form is related to voice quality. The normally sharp upward gradient corresponds to vocal fold closure and the positive peak to maximum vocal fold contact. The detailed pattern of the wave-form will be influenced in physical terms by: 'the mechanical stiffness of the folds, their distributed masses, the presence of non-linearities and the effects of damping' (Fourcin and Abberton, 1976, which *see* for full details).

(2) The laryngograph signal may also be displayed as a single trace across the screen, the height of which is a function of the frequency of vocal fold vibration. This trace can display a complete phrase or short sentence and also gives information on timing, intonation and, to some extent, voice quality in addition to overall pitch. These functions are particularly useful for assessment and therapeutic techniques with the deaf (*see later* in this chapter).

Pitch

Although laryngographic analysis of frequency distribution and its perceptual correlate, pitch, is certainly advantageous, the final discriminator and detector may still be the trained human ear.

Inappropriate pitch usage can contribute significantly to voice disorder so that a patient's total range, habitual pitch and optimal pitch (the level at which the thyroarytenoids and other intrinsic muscles of the larynx can produce adduction with minimal effort) will be carefully assessed in addition to the patient's ability to discriminate pitch changes and imitate patterns.

Resonance

The pharyngeal, oral and nasal cavities are the primary sites of vocal resonance so that, for the voice to sound 'normal', a certain amount of resonance must occur at each of these sites.

Structural abnormalities will clearly influence the facility for resonant speech – an undesirable amount of nasal cavity resonance may be the result of palatopharyngeal incompetence, possibly requiring further investigation through cinefluorography or nasendoscopy. Conversely, insufficient nasal cavity resonance causing dull, muffled quality (if not due to a geographical/dialectal variation) may be associated with nasal obstruction, catarrh or deviated nasal septum.

If reasonably normal relations between intact structures exist, the trained ear should be able to assess the necessary compensatory muscular movements which will help vary the shape and size of the resonating cavities and modify the harmonic structure of the voice produced.

Organic dysphonia

Neurological

Paralysis

Surgery to the thyroid gland resulting in recurrent laryngeal nerve damage is a not infrequent cause of unilateral vocal cord palsy. The left recurrent nerve is also particularly vulnerable to pressure from tumours, the commonest being carcinoma of the lung. It is occasionally due to a virus mononeuropathy of the vagus or recurrent laryngeal nerve. The clinical features of neurological dysphonia will depend on the mode of onset, the position of the paralysed vocal cord and on structural changes, anatomical variations in the larynx, e.g. position of the arytenoids, the shape of the glottis, and the compensation of the non-paralysed cord (*see* Chapter 17).

In cases where natural recovery is limited, more structured help to assist compensation will be indicated. With relaxation and resonance work as a basis for therapy, pushing exercises based on encouraging brisk glottal closure can be instigated which result in extra compensatory excursion of the unaffected cord over the midline. There are no studies which validate this assumption (Luchsinger and Arnold, 1965) but, under these exercise conditions, the air-flow rate is definitely increased, resulting in better vibration of the paralysed cord. Once a plateau is reached, which may be over a year after the original paralysis, consideration of a teflon implant may be advisable.

Dysarthrophonia

Dysarthria denotes defective articulation due to lesions in the nervous system causing motor disorders of the muscles involved. Dysarthrophonia (dysarthria plus dysphonia), a term coined by Peacher (1950), refers to voice disorders due to neurological lesions. Symptoms will depend on the type, severity and site of lesion and may occur in association with central language disorders of reception and/or expression, i.e. receptive and expressive dysphasia.

Disorders of lower motor neurones involving damage to cranial nerves and motor nuclei of the brain stem – e.g. polyneuritis or motor neurone disease – may cause dysarthrophonia characterized by slurred speech, indistinct articulation and hypernasal voice, with likely paresis of lips, palate, pharynx and tongue. Voice quality may also be hoarse with limited intensity and pitch variation. Some articulation and vocal therapy may assist in cases where the medical prognosis is encouraging. A 'Proprioceptive Neuromuscular Facilitative' (PNF) approach based on stimulation by ice, brushing or resistance therapy is often useful, and palatal training appliances may be indicated for certain patients (Tudor and Selley, 1974).

Pseudobulbar palsy

Lasting pseudobulbar palsy resulting from bilateral involvement of the upper motor neurone will present a slightly different picture of dysarthrophonia. It may be the result of cerebral vascular lesions, neoplasm or motor neurone disease with involvement of the upper motor neurones and will show a spastic type of dysarthria and dysphonia (dysphasia may be present where the dominant cerebral hemisphere is affected). Articulation will be slurred, voice quality hyper-nasal and hoarse, with weak intensity. Respiratory control may also be affected and the dysarthria may be staccato or explosive in nature.

Many patients may have in addition dysphagia. Palatal function may be assisted again by a Palatal Training Appliance (Tudor and Selley, 1974) and a rigorous programme of exercises and PNF may be instigated. Prosody, i.e. intonation, rhythm and tempo of speech may also benefit from attention, for those aspects may influence a patient's overall speech intelligibility.

Suprabulbar palsy in congenital disorders (e.g. cerebral palsy) may be accompanied by mental defect, hearing loss or specific language disorder, and for these reasons speech may also be very severely affected.

Dysarthrophonia resulting from disorders of the extra-pyramidal system demonstrates a different speech pattern. A patient with Parkinson's disease may suffer from an increasingly festinant speech pattern and poverty of movement in the muscles of articulation. Vocal intensity and flexibility may gradually deteriorate and resonance become increasingly hyper-nasal, with a husky quality.

Athetosis may be the result of congenital extra-pyramidal disorder. This 'type' of cerebral palsy may cause speech to be explosive and indistinct with facial grimace and involuntary movements of the lips. Voice production may be 'jerky' owing to irregular, spasmodic contractions of the diaphragm and other respiratory muscles. For these children, speech therapy will usually proceed alongside physiotherapy.

Disorders of the cerebellum may result in a slurring, scanning, staccato dysarthrophonia, with some abnormalities of coordination between respiration, phonation and articulation.

Spastic dysphonia

Spastic dysphonia has been defined as a 'disorder of phonation characterized by a strained, creaking and choked vocal attack, a tense, squeezed voice sound accompanied by extreme tension of the entire phonatory system' (Berendes, 1959). This 'stuttering' of the vocal cords is often associated with spastic or grimacing contractions of the neck and facial muscles.

Voice therapy and psychotherapy have for many years proved singularly ineffective with this disorder. Spastic dysphonia has remained generally accepted as an expression of psychoneurosis or hysterical conversion symptoms, although others have suggested an organic pathology of the nervous system (Aronson, Peterson and Litin, 1966; Robe, Brunlik and Moore, 1960). More recent work describes exploratory, temporary paralysis of the recurrent laryngeal nerve followed, where indicated, by surgical section (Dedo, 1976). This resulted in loss of spasticity in the voice and decrease or disappearance of associated tics and grimaces, although several patients initially complained of husky vocal quality and reduced intensity. These residual aspects were generally improved with speech therapy which ranged from a few days to several weeks. Of 34 patients with surgically sectioned recurrent laryngeal nerves, none reverted to the severe pre-operative spastic dysphonia and there were no hysterical conversions. Patients who had already been undergoing psychotherapy were reported to be doing much better, as the disability of spastic dysphonia had been causing or increasing their emotional disturbances, rather than the reverse which had generally been the explanation (Dedo, 1976).

Endocrine

Hypothyroidism/myxoedema

This condition may result in a gradual deepening of the voice which becomes husky and blurred. Vocal symptoms can be the first sign of hypothyroidism requiring treatment with thyroxin.

Menopause

Hormonal imbalance during this period may be troublesome, particularly to the professional voice user as, in addition to emotional upset, irritability and depression, the vocal cords can become oedematous causing a pitch drop and a husky quality. Short courses of hormone-replacement treatment may greatly alleviate the symptoms but can damage the voice if administered for long periods. Some counselling help and advice to family members to tide over the difficult time may be beneficial.

Trans-sexualism

The majority of trans-sexual patients make the transition from male to female 'gender'. Hormone treatment appears to have little, if any, effect on the pitch register with this group and therefore many patients will experience great difficulty in producing acceptable feminine voices. Surgical attempts to shorten the vibrating length of the vocal cords at Charing Cross Hospital (Holden, personal communication) have had some limited success, although pitch is clearly dependent on additional factors such as bulk which remain unaffected by this form of surgery.

Voice therapy is symptomatic and supportive. Emphasis is placed on optimal relaxed usage of the upper pitch registers and resonators through auditory training and vocal exercises, with encouragement to produce light, clearly articulated speech.

Organic dysphonia as the result of vocal dysfunction

Professional voice users who have received adequate training rarely develop serious vocal disorders unless commitments become excessive. (Detailed discussion of this particular group appears in Chapter 16.)

Prolonged misuse and abuse, in the presence of various irritants, may result in pathological changes taking place in the larynx requiring surgical assistance or speech therapy; many patients are most successfully treated by a combination of these two approaches.

Vocal nodules

These are among the most common disorders resulting directly from continued trauma to the vocal folds. If small and recently acquired, they may be eliminated by voice rest and therapy alone, although larger, more established lesions are optimally treated by surgery followed by rest and therapy. Ideally, the therapist should be able to visit the patient pre-operatively, both for assessment and to build a working relationship. There are constitutional and personality factors common to these individuals – 'being mostly energetic, active, hard-working and anxious besides being talkative' (Greene, 1972) – which may limit cooperation once they are back into daily living activities again.

Vocal cord polyps

These are not always the result of voice misuse but therapy post-operatively is again indicated. Otherwise, during this period of altered voice production, attempts to 'normalize' the sound can become incorrect and habitual, so that surgery may not result in immediate cure. Symptomatic voice therapy is usually effective in restoring voice.

Contact ulcers

These are not commonly diagnosed in the British Isles but are generally found in male individuals with 'perfectionist personalities who are compulsive hard workers, make demands on themselves and tend to build up inner tensions without relaxation or exteriorized discharge' (Luchsinger and Arnold, 1965). Vocal rehabilitation is the preferred treatment for all but the most severe ulceration, once the epithelium has grown over mucosal defects. Voice rest alone will be inadequate and ineffective.

Chronic laryngitis

This can be the result of abuse alone and may be treated effectively in the early stages by 'vocal rest' therapy, and elimination of other contributing, aggravating factors. Once the condition is prolonged by chronic misuse or infection, actual tissue changes may indicate the need for surgical treatment of cord thickening, nodules or polyps. This, by itself, without attempts to remove the abusive causes, will not lead to a permanent solution of the voice disorder.

Functional aphonia and dysphonia

(Also known as psychogenic aphonia, pseudoparalytic dysphonia, hysterical aphonia.)

The majority of these patients fall within the age range of 18–34 years and the disorder is much more common in women than men, 7:1 (Greene, 1972). In these cases the relative influence of vocal misuse, emotional aspects, tension and environmental features need to be evaluated. An example from the author's clinical experience was a menopausal housewife doing a part-time teaching job, with a lively family, deaf mother-in-law and unsympathetic husband.

Management

It is possible for patients with total functional aphonia to regain their voices within the first session of treatment, practically any tactic succeeding if put into effect with sufficient aplomb (Greene, 1972). Tactics alone are not sufficient since recovery of voice is not the sole aim in therapy as, without insight into the aetiology of the vocal symptom and solution of conflicts involved, prognosis must remain guarded.

Use of the term 'hysterical' is not advised in the management of these patients, for a psychiatric dimension may not exist, and a social stigma is still attached to the description. Once ENT examination confirms normal adductor ability in swallowing and coughing, referral to a speech therapist as early as possible is strongly recommended. The voice may be totally aphonic or demonstrate a breathy or grating quality and, on occasions, the ventricular bands may also contribute to phonation. If these symptoms are allowed to remain, they are likely to become increasingly intractable.

Full case history information will be basic to understanding of the situation which, although often associated with an event of acute stress (Aronson, Peterson and Litin, 1968), can be the result of a combination of relatively minor problems, the relevance of which may not be fully appreciated by the patient. Voice loss is often treated successfully with a direct symptom-modification approach. Through explanation, verbal suggestion, sometimes using coughing, sighing, or an auditory masker, the vocal cords can usually be persuaded to adduct again. Non-verbal phonations will generally be used first, leading gradually into 'nonsense syllables' and eventually into real speech communication again. Allusion is not made to the fact that the patient could vocalize if desired and maximum opportunity will be provided for discussion – 'the catharsis of talking things over is real' (Greene, 1972). With sympathetic but firm and encouraging support, the patient should gradually re-assume responsibility for the voice production and, with insight, be in a stronger position not to suffer a recurrence.

If a trial period of therapy fails, this usually indicates more deep-seated emotional disturbance, indicating referral for psychiatric help. Most often, the emotional factors in cases of functional dysphonia are not deep-seated – attention to these, elimination of abuse and a search for the best, most appropriate, voice production will usually be successful.

Puberphonia/'maturational falsetto'

Endocrine imbalance may influence the progress of sexual maturity in males resulting in failure to develop secondary sexual characteristics. Most maturational disturbances in young men are not of organic origin, although this would clearly need full examination. A high voice in itself may serve as proof that sexual development has taken place, as the falsetto voice is different from the voice of a young boy, usually being characterized by weak quality and small dynamic range.

Generally, normal sexual development has been followed by abnormal functional adaptation and, once diagnosed, referral to speech therapy may be indicated. Although some cases may prove intractable and are related to deep-seated psychological problems, requiring psychiatric help, many can be treated successfully by speech therapy alone.

Freudian psychology interprets persistence of immature voice in those able to produce normal 'chest voice' as due either to an Oedipal or Narcissus complex, but several rather more practical factors may predispose an individual to the condition (Greene, 1972):

(1) Unusually early breaking of the voice may make a boy self-conscious, leading him to favour the boy's voice until it becomes so habitual that it is impossible to achieve normal voice (West, Ansberry and Carr, 1957).
(2) A desire to retain a successful soprano voice which has brought distinction and loss of which will bring loss of limelight (Seth and Guthrie, 1935).
(3) Fear of assuming a full share of adult responsibility or of losing maternal protection, so that there is consequent unconscious assertion of immaturity by means of prolongation of the child's voice.
(4) Hero worship of an older boy or man by a boy with strong feminine tendencies which, if encouraged, may also result in rejection of masculine voice.
(5) The possession of a natural tenor voice, small larynx or short vocal folds – any of which may perpetuate this condition.

(Factors such as deafness, congenital laryngeal abnormalities or delayed pubertal development may provide an organic basis for puberphonia.)

Speech therapy of puberphonia with auditory training, 'pitch work' and elimination of possible symptoms of abuse, will also include an assessment of the individual's immature emotional attitude and make-up. Many patients will respond to common-sense explanations and a sympathetic, understanding approach.

Laryngeal carcinoma

Conservative radiotherapy may effect a total cure for cancer of the larynx with dryness, slight discomfort and hoarseness being probably the only symptoms of which the patient is aware. Complete recovery of vocal function is also frequent although during the periods of dysphonia and anxiety, abusive patterns of voice production may well develop which will require the attention of a speech therapist. A prophylactic, counselling approach as soon as radiotherapy commences has generally been found a satisfactory way of managing the problem, for even those patients with no obvious signs of abuse may need assistance in obtaining optimal voice recovery some time after treatment and the effects of treatment die away.

Partial laryngectomy/laryngofissure

Partial laryngectomy (by laryngofissure) is seldom practised in Great Britain, where total laryngectomy is usually undertaken when radiotherapy has failed to effect a total cure. In this unusual situation, results for speech can be adequate. The position of the substitute cicatricial fibrous band is of great importance, the recovering voice developing more successfully if the healthy cord does not have to cross over the midline in order to meet it. Speech therapy plays an important role in the rehabilitation of this small group of patients and will be based on resonance, relaxation and pushing exercises similar to those used in therapy in cases of unilateral vocal cord palsy.

Laryngectomy

Laryngectomy, although frequently life-saving, results in the crippling loss of voice, the means of expressing personality, thoughts and emotions through the vocal symbols of speech. Physiological changes which not only prevent verbal communication but cause disfigurement of neck structures, alteration of respiration channels and loss of other capabilities previously taken for granted, provide a basis for emotional and psychological problems. For these reasons, successful rehabilitation of the laryngectomee, can be a complex and difficult process requiring an organized multidisciplinary approach, thorough pre-operative counselling being a crucial preliminary aspect. Close liaison between members of the team will be imperative to ensure that consistent and realistic information is transmitted and, unless surgery is an emergency measure with limited time schedules, the speech therapist should spend several pre-operative sessions with the patient and spouse.

Prior to surgery, an individual's capacity to receive and comprehend information may be hampered by fear, leading to misconceptions and sometimes dangerous misunderstandings; the prospective laryngectomee is no different in this respect: the resulting shock and depression in these patients may severely inhibit not only physical recovery, but also alaryngeal speech and total psychological rehabilitation.

Given sufficient time, the speech therapist will assess in detail the circumstances of each individual – his family, social contacts and occupation – in order to evaluate personality, reliance on verbal communication and attitude towards the challenge which will face him post-operatively. Any evidence of hearing loss should be immediately investigated (in spouse as well as patient); presbyacusis is common in older males, and this has a significant effect on the ability to learn new methods of communication. Speech discrimination, in addition to pure tone testing, in diagnostic evaluation of hearing can be particularly useful.

During counselling, information regarding speech rehabilitation is of paramount importance to most individuals, and may be given with the help of diagrams and demonstration. Decisions about artificial larynges and aids may rest with the individual therapist, but all the patients should be supplied with information on all methods of alaryngeal communication; pneumatic and electronic devices, in addition to oesophageal voice, should be available for proficient demonstration. In addition, should it be deemed desirable by the surgeon, therapist and patient, a successfully rehabilitated laryngectomee, carefully selected (with spouse if possible) may be called upon to visit. Early contact with another couple can be tremendously beneficial and supportive for some individuals, but are wisely postponed for others, since this experience can increase already high levels of anxiety, and lead to possible rejection of surgical measures.

Following operation, the speech therapist maintains close contact with the patient, attempting to maximize ease of communication between him, his family and nursing staff. Attempts at lip-reading may be more useful in the long term than frantic scribbled messages, as clarity of articulation, which can be encouraged even before tubes are removed, will provide a good basis for later intelligible speech patterns. Some patients, particularly those with whom healing is slow, may also successfully use an aid to assist communication at these early stages. Pneumatic devices, or electronic neck devices, may be contra-indicated because of unhealed tissues or tubes *in situ*. The electronic-mouth Cooper–Rand artificial larynx may be used to great benefit as, without necessary contact with neck tissue, it could be utilized within one or two days after surgery.

No one aid is suitable for every patient, and any device involving a mouthpiece, whether pneumatic or electronic, can prove unpalatable for some, who may be much happier writing notes. Whatever immediate post-operative method is chosen, the opportunity and time to talk and ask questions will be vital for patients, as this is the optimal time for relieving fears and anxieties not previously expressed. Once healing has progressed to a satisfactory point, the therapist may then approach the problems of communication in a more comprehensive way, the specific needs of each individual being carefully borne in mind. Many therapists have opted in the past for instant work on oesophageal voice, but a revived interest in artificial larynges appears to be altering the emphasis towards a more combined approach.

There are no research statistics to prove that use of an aid will hinder any individual's acquisition of voice or make him 'lazy'. Recent practice appears to indicate the opposite, for provision of an early and relatively simple means of communication during the crucial stages of post-operative recovery (and depression) may predispose individuals more favourably towards learning the more challenging new skill of oesophageal voice. Use of an aid also facilitates verbal discussion and allows exploration of anxieties. Early attention to articulation may positively influence later speech intelligibility and the sad statistic, that over a third of all laryngectomees fail to acquire functionally useful oesophageal voice, gives even stronger support for its early use; it may also, in the long term save valuable therapy time. Patient and therapist will need to experiment with several different larynges to select the one which provides the most intelligible speech. As mentioned above, a patient with a tube *in situ* may be unable to cope easily with a pneumatic mouth device unless alterations can be made to the 'cup' covering the stoma. Emphysema or other chronic respiratory disorder may also contra-indicate use of such a lung-powered device. Some patients may find articulation 'around' the tube which transmits the sound into the oral cavity an insurmountable problem or may find its use simply unpleasant. For these patients an electronic neck device may be indicated.

The three most commonly used electronic larynges in Great Britain are the German Servox, the American Bell Western Electric No. 5 (male or female version) and the British 'Bart's Vibrator'. Each requires firm contact of the electronically powered vibrating head against tissues of the neck to transmit sound into the oropharyngeal resonating system over which the patient articulates clearly. Extensive surgery or radiotherapy may either over- or under-sensitize the tissues, or harden them considerably, reducing the possibility of efficient use. There are also certain limitations inherent in each of the designs. The Bell Western Electric, for example, has a large vibrating head unsuitable for small neck areas and rather excessive volume. The Servox, although having the best quality production, has no real facility for producing intonational variations during connected speech. Each of the devices provides intelligible, usable communication (over the telephone as well) and must be seriously considered, not only as a preliminary means of verbal expression but as a viable and acceptable alternative to oesophageal voice.

Production of oesophageal voice appears to provide the greatest area for misinterpretation and misunderstanding for patients and medical staff alike. This is confirmed by a report on 50 interviews with pre-operative (counselled) laryngectomy patients who had been asked how they would be able to talk without their voice-box (Duguay, 1975). One or more of the following misconceptions were common in most of the patients interviewed. They believed they would:

(1) Have to swallow air all the way down to the stomach in order to speak.
(2) Speak from the stomach.
(3) Speak from the diaphragm.
(4) Speak from the lungs.
(5) Speak through the tracheal stoma.
(6) Have to cover the hole in the neck in order to speak.
(7) Speak from some kind of voice-box 'put in' by the surgeon.

None of these are of course correct, as oesophageal voice is produced by the injection or inhalation of air down into the oesophagus to just below the point of the pharyngo-oesophageal sphincter at approximately the level of the fifth and sixth cervical vertebrae (C5 and C6). This air is then expelled from its 'reservoir' up through the PE segment consisting of the cricopharyngeus muscle, inferior pharyngeal constrictor muscles and/or upper oesophageal muscles, which vibrate – these being the muscles which form the neoglottis for oesophageal voice. The speech therapist working with a newly laryngectomized patient obviously will not explain voice production in these terms. It may be possible to utilize and develop incipient spontaneous sounds; alternatively, demonstration and informal experimentation, designed to be assured of at least some success, can be undertaken. The therapist may encourage exercises leading to the inhalation technique of voice production; in this, air is drawn into the oesophagus by keeping airways patent, using the increase in negative air pressure produced by normal inspiration, which eventually breaks through the resistive pressure at the PE segment and into the oesophagus.

The injection technique is probably more widely used by proficient laryngectomy speakers, although many use a combination of methods. It involves a build-up of pressure above the PE segment, which is encouraged by lip and palatopharyngeal closure and backward pumping movement of the tongue against the roof of the mouth; this pressure gradually overcomes resistance in the PE segment and air moves into the oesophagus. This may be associated with a 'Consonant Injection' technique, which relies on the increased oral breath pressure employed in the articulation of certain voiceless consonants. Well-articulated speech may spontaneously produce oesophageal voice in this way. Once the first sounds have been produced, therapy will concentrate on developing consistency of production and, for this, the facility for producing voice by several methods may be advantageous. Early and lengthy attempts at voice in conversation may be discouraged by the therapist in order to prevent the possibility of 'bad habits' developing, e.g. excessive stoma noise, or 'audible klunk', which may be perceived as a patient attempts to take too much air in too quickly. Here again, the artificial larynx can be a valuable asset, enabling the patient to communicate at will. Therapy will also encourage extended voice production (which will be vital for later phrasing) paying attention to articulation rate and general communication skills. Only when voice is well established and progressing favourably will considerations of pitch or volume be introduced.

Successful social rehabilitation does not always accompany the developing oesophageal voice proficiency, and the psychological aspect requires considerable attention. Laryngectomee Clubs provide a useful bridge between the sheltered speech therapy environment and the outside world, in which the patient may continue to feel isolated and lacking in confidence. Assistance and motivating support can frequently be gained from those who have suffered similar experiences, and the clubs provide a positive social atmosphere where independence and total rehabilitation can be encouraged.

Glossectomee speech rehabilitation

Although the laryngectomized patient has received an increasing amount of attention in terms of pre- and post-operative speech rehabilitation, there has been a neglect of research and clinical endeavour with another group of patients undergoing head and neck surgery affecting communication, *viz.* the glossectomee.

Surgery, which may involve not only partial or total removal of the tongue but possibly also laryngectomy or hemimandiblectomy, may cause severe disability to the mechanisms of mastication, deglutition, phonation and articulation. Perhaps because the radical treatment appears to be irreversible, or because prognosis may be generally poor, few of these patients appear to have received adequate help to achieve usable oral communication again.

There are two widely divergent views regarding the re-acquisition of intelligible speech post-operatively:

(1) Intelligible speech is totally impossible after glossectomy.
(2) Intelligible speech develops spontaneously as a consequence of passage of time, and exercise on the part of the patient.

Explanation of these divergent views depends on the definition of intelligibility and whether patients have undergone total or only partial glossectomy. Skelly (1973), in her study of 25 patients, used an 'objective, realistic panel of listeners' to evaluate speech and defined the patients on admission to her programme as having speech not intelligible in the everyday situation.

There is certainly a relationship between the extent of surgery involved and achieved intelligibility and these differences in performance will be discussed later. However, *any* patient who is likely to suffer defective functioning of the speech mechanism following head and neck surgery should be referred routinely to the speech therapist in time for pre-operative consultation and assessment. This will allow the therapist to establish contact and rapport so that case history details, pertinent to communication needs, can be taken, facilitating later interaction. When desirable, a description of post-operative speech therapy procedures, in terms of assistance with feeding as well as speech, can be given and early support and encouragement provided to patient, spouse and family.

Post-operatively, the following day if possible, rehabilitation in communication may be started. When the larynx remains intact, two or three intelligible phrases may be elicited later by covering the tracheostome with a gloved hand and, most importantly, contact can be re-established with the patient. Since these patients with communication problems may, even after the recovery period, also experience swallowing difficulties, nasogastric feeding may be vital. Clearly the mechanisms of chewing, sucking and swallowing are closely involved with those of speech, and swallowing competence is a necessary pre-requisite of speech rehabilitation. For these reasons it is useful to call in the speech therapist as early as possible since her detailed knowledge of oropharyngeal structure and function will assist in treating this problem.

In cooperation with the surgeon, physiotherapist and nursing staff, the therapist will need to know which nerves and muscles have been sacrificed during surgery and, using imagery, visual cues, tactile sensation and kinaesthetic awareness, will encourage return of specific functions. With suctioning facilities and medical help on hand if required, the therapist will generally use semisolids or soft foods as the most effective initial agent, rather than liquids which lack texture, with less control for the patient; in addition, the therapist will spend considerable time talking with the patient and re-assuring him, as many achieve an adequate stage of physical recovery but remain anxious and convinced that they are unable to swallow. As swallowing skills develop and salivary incontinence, which is acutely embarrassing socially, improves, concomitant changes will be observed in articulation and overall speech intelligibility.

Once the patient is recovered sufficiently to attend to, and willingly cooperate with, the therapist, a full speech assessment can be carried out. With the medical data, the speech therapist will add her own evaluations of oral structure and function, a detailed analysis of the returning accurate and deviant sounds of speech, in addition to a functional assessment as far as this is possible in the confines of a hospital environment.

With cinefluorographic analysis, the definite differences between compensatory movements in total and partial glossectomees can be clearly seen today. Depending on the extent of surgery and the spontaneous progress being made, programmes of communication therapy can be designed which are geared to the specific needs of each individual patient.

Speech in total glossectomy

This group of patients, often with a less favourable prognosis, may commence therapy by improving non-speech communication; this provides an effective back-up and alternative to oral speech, particularly in the early stages.

Skelly (1973) advocates work on 'telegraphic writing', making this as efficient and rapid as possible by reducing all sentences to minimal numbers of 'information-carrying' words and by increasing sensitivity to 'reader' reactions so that writing ceases as soon as decoding has taken place. Advice on re-organization of verbal output may also be advantageous so that rephrasing of an utterance, rather than pure repetition, becomes the natural response when communication fails. The total glossectomee will need a structured programme of exercises aimed to improve the mobility, control and excursion of the articulators as well as intelligibility drills for vowels, non-glossal consonants, glossal consonants and combinations of each, in addition to a systematic exploration of potential compensatory articulations for each of the glossal sounds. The emphasis should be on 'effective communication rather than meticulous articulation', with as much attention paid to aspects of voice quality, resonance, tonal patterns and stress as to specific speech sounds. These elements of spoken communication contribute much to overall intelligibility and will assist greatly in the planning of realistic, achievable goals.

Speech in partial glossectomy

Those undergoing partial glossectomy may only need articulation assistance for a few deviant phonemes, although this will again be influenced by personality and situational needs. Unlike the total glossectomee, these patients' goals may well coincide with their pre-operative speech intelligibility as they are able to make marked use of the residual tongue stump; flexibility of this is a critical factor. The type and extent of tongue section is also related closely to achieved speech clarity; for example, those with right or left hemiglossectomies will need to make fewer speech adaptations than those with excisions involving only the tongue tip.

Speech therapy in the deaf and partially hearing

Although speech therapists are not usually involved with the management of the deaf and partially hearing, since the Quirk Report (Speech Therapy Services, 1972), which discussed the possible contribution of the speech therapist in this field, gradual changes in the situation have occurred. This area of expertise is a highly specialized one, requiring additional training. Experience in the field also gives insight into the educational issues such as the continuing discussions on the 'natural *v.* structured' approach in managing deaf children and the controversy of 'oralism *v.* signing' (Schmitt, 1966).

The speech therapist may be employed with the deaf and partially hearing:

(1) As a member of a diagnostic team; in conjunction with the ENT surgeon and teacher of the deaf she may be able to assist in diagnosis, particularly as deafness and other developmental language disorders may present with very similar patterns of behaviour. Once a diagnosis of hearing loss has been made, the pre-school child will become the responsibility of the peripatetic teacher of the deaf, who may, at a later stage, request assistance for speech problems from the speech therapist.

(2) In schools for the deaf or Partially Hearing Units, where the therapist's role may vary from working with teachers in the assessment and treatment of speech and language problems which are a direct result of the hearing loss, to the management of other factors contributing to a language and speech problem, e.g. cerebral palsy.

(3) With the congenitally deaf adult and those with problems of acquired deafness. These groups are very different since the latter will have had an opportunity to acquire full and secure patterns of language. If communication with other people can be maintained, spoken language may, with help, be preserved. The continuous effort to understand speech and monitor their own, without the acoustic clues relied upon for so long, may result in acute depression, distress and social withdrawal. The vital skills of lip-reading will be taught by teachers of the deaf or speech therapists who may also assist with speech conservation programmes. Recordings of speech (ideally before any deterioration becomes evident) are required as a basis for planning treatment programmes and assessing progress; this is followed by work on articulatory and prosodic difficulties in addition to self-monitoring exercises.

Current research

Visual displays of 'speech pattern features' may be derived instantaneously from live speech. These displays can have important therapeutic applications with hearing-impaired patients as well as those with voice disorders (*see* section on 'Assessment of vocal disorder').

The Electrolaryngograph provides objective measurements of prosodic features and along with subjective assessment of speech, gives a sounder basis for planning therapy. In addition, the display is also useful therapeutically in that it gives immediate visual feedback of prosodic features, often abnormal in hearing-impaired speakers; improvements in perception and control of these features can contribute greatly to increased intelligibility of speech. In speech work with hearing-impaired children, using a visual display as an adjunct to auditory input can lead to improved auditory discrimination of speech patterns (King and Parker, 1978). Research is also progressing into the use of a 'vocal-trace like' display from a linear prediction analysis of the acoustic speech signal (Crichton, 1974).

References

Aronson, A. E., Brown, J. R. and Litin, E. M. (1968). 'Spastic dysphonia. I. Voice, neurologic and psychiatric aspects', *Journal of Speech and Hearing Disorders*, **33,** 203, 218

Aronson, A. E., Peterson, H. W. and Litin, E. M. (1966). 'Psychiatric symptomatology in functional dysphonia and aphonia', *Journal of Speech and Hearing Disorders*, **31,** 115

Beech, H. R. and Fransella, F. (1968). *Research and Experiment in Stuttering*; Pergamon Press, Oxford

Berendes (1959). Cited by Arnold, G. E., 'Spastic dysphonia; changing interpretations of a persistent affliction', *Logos*, **2,** 3

Berry, M. F. and Eisenson, J. (1967). *Speech Disorders*; Peter Owen Ltd, Kendrick Mews,

Kendrick Place, London

Bloodstein, O. (1974). 'The rules of early stuttering', *Journal of Speech and Hearing Disorders*, **39,** 379

Boone, Daniel R. (1971). *The Voice and Voice Therapy*; Prentice Hall, Englewood Cliffs, New Jersey

Bull, T. R. and Cook, J. L. (1976). *Speech Therapy and ENT Surgery*; Blackwell Scientific, Oxford

Cooper, R. L. and Rosenstein, J. (1966). 'Language acquisition of deaf children', *Volta Review*, **68,** 58–67, 125

Crichton, R. G. (1974). 'Linear prediction model of speech production with applications to the deaf and speech training', *Proceedings of the Institution of Electrical Engineers*, **121,** 865

Dalton, P. and Hardcastle, W. J. (1977). *Disorders of Fluency*; Edward Arnold, London

Damste, P. H. and Lerman, J. W. (1975). *An Introduction to Voice Pathology*; C. C. Thomas, Springfield

Darley, F. L. (1964). *Diagnosis and Appraisal of Communication Disorders*; Prentice Hall, Englewood Cliffs, New Jersey

Dedo, H. H. (1976). 'Recurrent laryngeal nerve section for spastic dysphonia', *Annals of Otology, Rhinology and Laryngology*, **85,** 451

Diedrich, W. M. and Youngstrom, K. A. (1966). *Alaryngeal Speech*; C. C. Thomas, Springfield

Duguay, M. (1975). *Proceedings of the Laryngectomee Rehabilitation Seminar*; Mayo Clinic, Rochester, Minnesota

Ellis, M. (1952). 'Acute diseases of the larynx', in: *Diseases of the Ear, Nose and Throat* (Ed. W. G. Scott-Brown), Vol. 1, pp. 570–589; Butterworths, London and Boston

Espir, M. L. E. and Rose, F. C. (1976). *The Basic Neurology of Speech*, 2nd edn; Blackwell, Oxford

Fourcin, A. J. and Abberton, E., (1972). 'First applications of a new laryngograph', *Volta Review*, **74,** 161

Fourcin, A. J. and Abberton, E. (1976). 'The laryngograph and the voice-scope in speech therapy', *XVIth International Congress of Logopedics and Phoniatrics*, 116

Greene, M. C. L. (1972). *The Voice and its Disorders*; Pitman, London

Guthrie, S. G. (1935). *Speech in Childhood*; Oxford University Press, Oxford

John, J. E. J. and Howarth, J. (1965). 'The effect of time distortions on the intelligibility of deaf children's speech; *Language and Speech*, **8,** 127

Johnson, W. (1959). *The Onset of Stuttering: Research Findings and Implications*; University of Minnesota Press, Minneapolis

Karelitz, S., Karelitz, R. and Rosenfelt, L. (1960). 'Infant vocalisations and their significance', in: *Mental Retardation* (Eds P. Bowman, and H. Mautner); Grune and Stratton, New York [Mental retardation: proceedings of the First International Medical Conference]

King, A. and Parker, A. (1978). *Speech and Hearing Work in Progress*; University College, London, Dept Phonetics and Linguistics

Laver, J. D. M. (1968). 'Voice quality and indexical information', *British Journal of Disorders of Communication*, **3,** 43

Lee, B. S. (1951). 'Artificial stutter', *Journal of Speech and Hearing Disorders*, **16,** 53

Luchsinger, R. and Arnold, G. E. (1965). *Voice, Speech, Language; Clinical Communicology: Its Physiology and Pathology*; Wadsworth Publishing Co., Belmont, California

Morley, M. E. (1954). *Cleft Palate and Speech*, 3rd edn.; Churchill-Livingstone, Edinburgh

Morley, M. E. (1967). *The Development and Disorders of Speech in Childhood*; Churchill-Livingstone, Edinburgh

Murphy, K. (1964). 'Development of normal vocalisation and speech', in: *The Child who does not Talk* (Eds C. Renfrew and K. Murphy), Clinics in Developmental Medicine; Heinemann, London

Negus, V. E. (1950). 'Radiotherapy in cancer of the larynx', *Journal of Laryngology and Otology*, **64,** 731

Parker, A. (1974). 'The laryngograph', *Hearing*, **29,** 256

Peacher, W. G. (1950). 'The aetiology and differential diagnosis of dysarthria', *Journal of Speech and Hearing Disorders*, **15,** 252

Potter, R. J., Kopp, G. A. and Green, H. C. (1947). *Visible Speech*; van Nostrand, New York

Rheingold, H. L. (1960). 'The measurement of maternal care, *Child Development*, **31,** 565

Robe, E., Brunlik, J. and Moore, P. (1960). 'A study of spastic dysphonia. Neurologic and electroencephalographic abnormalities', *Laryngoscope*, **70,** 219

Rose, F. C. (1977). 'Clinical aspects', in: *Motor Neurone Disease* (Ed. F. C. Rose); Pitman, London

Schmitt, P. J. (1966). 'Language instruction for the deaf', *Volta Review*, **68,** 85–105, 123

Seth, G. and Guthrie, D. (1935). *Speech in Childhood: Its Development and Disorders*; Oxford University Press, Oxford

Sheehan, J. (1970). *Stuttering Research and Therapy*; Harper and Row, New York and London

Skelly, M., (1973). *Glossectomee Speech Rehabilitation*; C. C. Thomas, Springfield

Speech Therapy Services (1972). Report for Dept of Education and Science. (Prof. R. Quirk – chairman), pp. 1–135; HMSO, London

Living with Deafness; BBC Publications, London

Tudor, C. and Selley, W. G. (1974). 'A palatal training appliance and a visual aid for use in the treatment of hypernasal speech: a preliminary report'; *British Journal of Diseases in Communication*, **9,** 117

van den Berg, J. W. (1962). 'Modern research in experimental phoniatrics. 12th International Congress of Logopedics and Paediatrics report', *Folio Phoniatrica*, **14,** 81

Wasz-Höckert, O., Lind, J., Vuorenkoski, V.,

Portamen, T. and Volonne, E. (1968). *The Infant Cry*, Clinics in Developmental Medicine, Vol. 29; Heinemann, London

West, R. W. Ansberry, M. and Carr, A. (1957). *The Rehabilitation of Speech*; Part 1, 3rd edn; Harper and Row, New York and London

Wilson, D. K. (1961). 'Children with vocal nodules', *Journal of Speech and Hearing Disorders*, **26,** 19

Wischner, G. J. (1950). 'Stuttering behaviour and learning: preliminary theoretical formulation', *Journal of Speech and Hearing Disorders*, **15,** 324

19 Intubation of the larynx, laryngotomy and tracheostomy

R Pracy

This chapter is concerned with the establishment of artificial airways and their management. Before the principles involved can be discussed it is necessary to state in a general way the anatomical and physiological basis which affects the transport of air to and from the lungs. Unless this is understood, complications may occur when an artificial airway is made.

Air enters the body physiologically through the nose. It is filtered by vibrissae in the anterior nares, moistened and humidified by the mucous glands in the nasal mucosa and warmed to near-body temperature by contact with the extremely vascular membrane lining the nose. It passes into the lower respiratory tract through the larynx. This is the narrowest part of the airway and, since air passes through it and food over and around it, there is an extremely efficient sphincter to guard the lower respiratory tract, triggered by a highly sensitive sensory nerve supply.

On the way to the lungs the air spends a relatively short time in the trachea. However, after oxygen and carbon dioxide exchange has taken place at the pulmonary interface, the air is expelled from the lungs and with it any particles of debris which may be small enough to move in the tracheobronchial mucus. Thus, when an artificial airway is established, not only is it absolutely essential to bear in mind that a free airway must be provided, but thought also must always be given to the mucus transport on the tracheal wall. This is effected by the ciliated lining, and its propulsion is assisted by the expiratory thrust of expired air. Cine studies show that the mucus is propelled out of the larynx only in the expiratory tide. Thus, the introduction of an artificial airway may provide for adequate oxygenation but it is bound to interfere with mucus transport. It is this interference which leads in many cases to the complications which are seen. Finally, it should be appreciated that in the adult when a tracheostomy is required there is an immediate reduction of the 'dead-space' from $150\,\mathrm{cm}^3$ to about $50\,\mathrm{cm}^3$, and a corresponding reduction in the child.

Indications for tracheostomy and intubation

The commonest indication for a temporary artificial airway is in general anaesthesia. A very considerable percentage of general anaesthetics is administered through endotracheal tubes. The anaesthetist has therefore an advantage in experience and in the passage of endotracheal tubes and this should be borne in mind in the semi-urgent situation. Furthermore, he has additional knowledge and experience of tracheo-pulmonary physiology and in intubation his help and advice should be sought where possible. On the other hand tracheostomy lies in the province of the surgeon and while he should certainly be skilled in the passage of endotracheal tubes he should be absolutely confident about the technique of establishing and maintaining a tracheostomy. Failure of confidence may jeopardize the patient's safety.

Basically the indications for intubation and for tracheostomy are complementary. For the short-term airway obstruction intubation is ideal, provided that the tube can be passed with no trauma to the larynx. It can be maintained *in situ* for several days and provides an adequate means for aspiration of mucus from the lower respiratory tract and for the administration, if necessary, of intermittent positive pressure ventilation. Aspiration may be made more efficient if combined with physiotherapy. The disadvantage of intubation is that, however smooth and non-irritant the tube may be, the larynx must move over it on swallowing and the vocal cords and subglottic region may be traumatized. Furthermore, if an airtight seal is to be obtained by the passage of a tube which fits the larynx comfortably, then the laryngeal trauma will be absolutely assured. In practice, therefore, it is customary to pass a tube which is one size smaller than that which would fit comfortably. Even after a relatively short period some evidence of laryngeal irritation may be seen. Tracheostomy, on the other hand, does not have the disadvantage of intubation. Its disadvantage lies in the fact that it requires a surgical procedure, that it makes super-added lower respiratory tract infection and complications more certain, that it reduces the dead-space and, finally, that it may lead to problems in the surrounding structures following operation and at the time of de-cannulation.

Both procedures may increase respiratory efficiency in a wide variety of diseases. In general these may be summarized as:

(1) Respiratory obstruction.
(2) Retained secretions in the lower respiratory tract.
(3) Inhalation of fluid into the trachea.
(4) Respiratory insufficiency from exogenous and endogenous causes.

These will now be considered in more detail.

Acute laryngeal or tracheal obstruction

This may be either sudden or gradual in onset. Examples of sudden onset are the impaction of a foreign body, trauma such as laryngeal injury or the inhalation of burning gases, and inflammatory episodes which may be typified by acute laryngotracheobronchitis, or acute allergic obstruction such as angioneurotic oedema.

Causes of gradual onset include paralysis of the vocal cords, gradual increase in the size of laryngeal or peri-laryngeal cysts and neoplasms and, finally, the airway may be restricted as a result of pressure in or on surrounding structures. Examples of the latter are tracheal compression in thyroid enlargement, and tumours and inflammation of the floor of the mouth as in Ludwig's angina. Fracture of the mandible may lead to the tongue falling backwards and obstructing the airway.

Secretions retained in the lower respiratory tract

Secretions may be retained by reason of their exceptional viscosity or by the patient's inability to raise the expulsive forces required. From whatever cause, retained secretions impose a barrier between the in-coming oxygen and the alveolar epithelium. The effect of this is a build-up of carbon dioxide in the blood (high pCO_2) leading to changes in the alkali reserve, mental confusion and even loss of consciousness. If the secretions are not cleared rapidly they form an ideal culture medium for bacteria. This in turn leads to toxic absorption and further deterioration in the general condition. If the retained secretions have accumulated over a short period, intubation combined with physiotherapy, humidification to the in-coming air and aspiration will suffice. In rare cases bronchoscopy may be all that is required. However, when the patient is weak and the cause is likely to persist, tracheostomy offers the most effective treatment. Aspiration through a tracheostomy is on the whole easier than via an endotracheal tube.

Fluid in the trachea

Always provided that the possibility of inhalation of blood, pus or other fluid is borne in mind, steps can be taken to make this less likely to occur. However, in unusual circumstances such as an unexpected pharyngeal or laryngeal haemorrhage or discharge of pus into the lower airway, it may be necessary to by-pass temporarily the physiological channel. Bulbar paralysis may lead to overspill into the tracheobronchial tree. Normally the cough reflex itself provides a useful first line of defence, but when this fails an artificial airway may be necessary to preserve life.

Respiratory insufficiency

The causes of respiratory insufficiency may lie within the lung itself, may be cardiovascular or neurological, or occasioned by actual trauma to the chest wall. This may be deemed to be functional lower respiratory obstruction. Mechanical ventilation of the lungs may be needed to overcome this for, in several cases, the effective dead-space of $150 \, cm^3$ may rise to $500 \, cm^3$ or more.

The particular circumstances which obtain at the time that the airway relief is called for will determine which method is applicable. However, when there is any doubt about the availability of staff specially trained in the supervision and management of endotracheal intubation, it is wiser to make a tracheostomy. Whenever possible, unless the tracheostomy is made as a dire emergency, a preliminary endotracheal intubation should be employed while the tracheostome is being made.

Clinical applications

It is not possible to deal with every situation which may call for tracheostomy. Groups of conditions therefore will be dealt with.

Upper respiratory obstruction

One cannot lay down *rules* for emergency conditions arising outside hospital. Where full facilities are available peroral intubation using a laryngoscope clearly offers the opportunity of most rapid relief of symptoms. However, if the laryngeal inlet is obstructed by inflammatory swelling or by a foreign body, tracheostomy or laryngotomy followed by tracheostomy may be required. If there is any obvious distortion of the laryngeal architecture tracheostomy is a life-saving procedure. Trismus, which of course makes intubation difficult or impossible, is also an indication for tracheostomy.

When the obstruction develops more slowly there is greater time available for assessment. However, it should be appreciated that the slower the obstruction is in developing the longer it is likely to take to recover and it is therefore more probable that tracheostomy is the safest procedure. Thus it is obvious that the patient who has an increasing upper respiratory obstruction, with no rapid solution available, is the subject for a tracheostomy before there is any change in the serum electrolytes and a deterioration in the general condition. Under no circumstances should sedatives be administered before the airway has been safeguarded.

Coma

In comatose states secretions tend to accumulate in the bronchial tree. In many patients this can be prevented and the chest kept clear by posturing and by physiotherapy. However, in some patients these measures may prove inadequate or posturing may be prevented by the presence of other lesions. In such patients intubation or tracheostomy is indicated.

If, when the patient is first seen, it seems likely that the coma will persist and if it is evident that posturing will prove inadequate, then a tracheostomy should be made early before any degree of hypoxia can occur from obstructing secretions and before any infection can develop. This is of importance because hypoxia alone may produce a state of confusion and, later, coma which may be attributed to the original lesion, and a correct diagnosis and vital treatment may be overlooked.

Coma from head injuries may be complicated by damage to other structures such as a fractured femur which may prevent turning of the patient. These patients are best treated by tracheostomy at the outset. When coma occurs in patients suffering from chronic respiratory disease the problem of keeping the bronchial tree clear will greatly increase and a tracheostomy is likely to be required.

Chest injuries

Damage to the wall of the thorax may lead to totally inadequate respiratory exchange. If this damage is so severe as to produce suction pneumothorax, or there is a flail injury to the chest wall, it is imperative to establish intermittent positive pressure respiration immediately as a life-saving procedure. This is controlled most easily through a tracheostomy although, if the injury is not severe, intubation combined with intermittent positive pressure respiration may suffice.

Muscular spasm

Laryngeal spasm due either to toxin, as in tetanus, or to epileptic seizures can in some cases be managed by observation and sedation. However, in severe cases, controlled respiration by means of muscle relaxants and an artificial airway offer the most likely chance of a successful outcome.

Primary neurological disorders

Respiratory paralysis occurring in poliomyelitis or polyneuritis can in some cases be managed in a cuirass. However, this is a large and cumbersome piece of apparatus and, for the majority of any one 24-hour period, parts of the trunk are inaccessible to nursing care. Tracheostomy or intubation (rarely) allow of intermittent positive pressure respiration. Tracheostomy is to be preferred because of the length of time for which airway support is likely to be needed.

Localized lung disease

Any condition leading to stasis of secretions in the lungs may call for assisted airway control. Patients whose lung elasticity has diminished over the years, as in the case of emphysema and chronic bronchitis, react badly to super-added infection. Elderly and debilitated patients may succumb to stasis through inanition. Cough may be inhibited by the pain of an abdominal wound or multiple rib fractures. In any of these situations airway relief may be called for. Intubation in these cases is to be preferred.

Tracheostomy

From the time of the first tracheostomy, during or before the first century BC until about 1930, the operation was performed almost exclusively for laryngeal obstruction. Nowadays this is only one of several indications for the procedure (*see above*) and most patients who have the operation have no obstruction to the larynx or trachea. Whatever the indication, the operation is best performed as an elective procedure under endotracheal general anaesthesia in a properly equipped operating theatre. Even then, certain hazards can be encountered but the difficulties are greatly increased if the operation has to be carried out as a matter of urgency or if the facilities are inadequate. For these reasons, as has already been pointed out, intubation for a period before operation may offer an advantage.

Operative technique

The degree of urgency with which the operation has to be performed will determine many of the details of the operation. Therefore operative technique will be considered under three separate headings. Whenever possible the operation is best performed as an elective procedure in a non-obstructed patient.

Emergency operation

If the patient must have an airway established urgently because of complete or almost complete respiratory obstruction, and if it is impossible for some reason to relieve the obstruction in any other way such as by intubation or laryngotomy, then an emergency tracheostomy will be required. Under these circumstances all that can be done is to make whatever arrangements are feasible, for the head to be kept as steady as possible in the midline, to palpate the thyroid and cricoid cartilage with the finger of one hand – with a knife in the other – and to make a vertical incision downwards from the thyroid cartilage in the midline of the neck. At this stage the wound will fill with dark blood but time will not permit any steps to control the haemorrhage. However, if an assistant and a suction apparatus happen to be available these are an invaluable asset. At this stage, it should be possible to feel the cricoid cartilage and the cartilaginous rings of the trachea with the fingers of one hand in the wound, and the best that can be done then is to make a vertical incision through two or three rings of the trachea. A slight twist of the knife blade will open the trachea and the patient will usually then splutter and cough through the blood. A tube of some sort should be inserted into the trachea as soon as possible and the blood sucked out, if necessary by the operator applying oral suction to the end of the tube or a catheter introduced through it. Inflation of the lungs may be needed and in an emergency this can be carried out by mouth-to-trachea respiration. Once an airway has been established and the immediate emergency overcome, the tracheostomy must be refashioned, as in the elective operation described below.

Intermediate operation

In some patients there may not be quite the same need for haste in performing a tracheostomy and there might be time to transfer the patient to an operating theatre but it may be considered unwise to administer a general anaesthetic or to attempt intubation in case such procedures precipitate complete obstruction. Under these circumstances it will be necessary to carry out the operation under a local anaesthetic and under such conditions tracheostomy can of course be performed adequately in the way described below, but the difficulties for the patient and for the operator are much greater than if the procedure can be undertaken on a fully oxygenated and relaxed patient having a general anaesthetic administered through an endotracheal tube. This is the ideal which should be aimed for and practised unless conditions make it impossible.

Elective operation

When a tracheostomy is performed on an anaesthetized intubated patient the first step is to position the head correctly without any rotation and without too much extension. A little extension helps to keep the chin up and out of the way, but if the movement is excessive an undue length of trachea may be drawn upwards into the neck. This will not interfere with the operation and may even aid it a little, but it may increase the obstruction and the subsequent management of the patient will be rendered difficult unless the opening into the trachea is made to suit the position in which the patient will lie or sit post-operatively. In young patients it is sometimes possible to extend the neck to such a degree that an opening can be made so low in the trachea that it comes to lie behind the manubrium when the head is flexed. This must of course be avoided. Ideally the tracheal opening should be at the level of the third cartilaginous ring. Openings higher than this may give rise to subglottic stenosis while ones which are lower may prevent proper fitting of the tube and also allow an insufficient distance between the stoma and the tracheal bifurcation. This latter point is of special importance when a cuffed tube is to be used. In some patients tracheal rings are close together and portions of two of them will need to be excised; in such cases the third and fourth rings will usually be the most suitable but in patients with a short neck it may be necessary to make the opening through the second and third rings. The first ring should always be left intact, thus avoiding the risk of subglottic stenosis.

A vertical incision is still sometimes advocated because it is regarded as being easier and is said to allow better drainage of the wound. However, transverse incisions have the compelling advantage that they allow a more satisfactory closure of the skin edges to the tracheal opening and this makes the management of the patient after the operation safer and easier. For this reason a transverse incision should be used. Adequate drainage of the wound is not a problem; even if the operation is made fractionally more difficult this cannot outweigh the advantage of increased safety to the patient. The cosmetic advantage of a transverse incision is also of some importance, especially in women, although scarring after tracheostomy is caused mainly by the presence of the tracheostomy tube and this is independent of the incision used. The scar can be excised inconspicuously when the original incision has been transverse.

After a short collar incision has been made approximately 2 cm below the cricoid cartilage through the skin, subcutaneous fat and deep cervical fascia flaps are raised for a short distance and the infrahyoid muscles exposed. The interval between the right and left sternomastoid muscles is defined and the two muscles separated and retracted; the sternothyroid muscles on a deeper plane are dealt with in the same way. After these muscles have also been retracted the thyroid gland and trachea are visible. The anatomical variations at this stage are considerable. In some patients the lateral lobes of the thyroid are small and situated well to the sides of the trachea with only a very narrow isthmus crossing the trachea away from the position where the opening will be made. In the majority of patients, however, the thyroid isthmus is of such a size or in such an area that it will interfere with a tracheostomy and in that case it needs to be divided and retracted. Division of the thyroid isthmus is best carried out by means of a diathermy knife in order to prevent haemorrhage. The cut edges should also be oversewn, or simply ligated if the isthmus is narrow.

The trachea is now exposed and the third tracheal ring identified (*Figures 19.1* and *19.2*). It is necessary to make a circular opening into the trachea of the same size as the

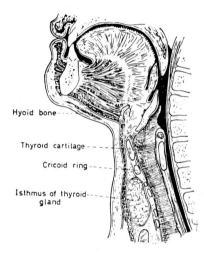

Hyoid bone

Thyroid cartilage

Cricoid ring

Isthmus of thyroid gland

Figure 19.1 Surgical anatomy of the trachea and larynx

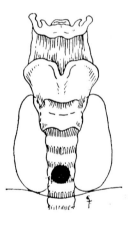

Figure 19.2 The incision in the trachea for tracheostomy

tracheostomy tube to be introduced. A simple vertical incision in the tracheal wall in adults is unsuitable because it makes it much more difficult to replace the tube that becomes dislodged in the early post-operative period and pressure of the tube on the tracheal ring can lead to necrosis of the cartilage. A circular opening which is too small will often result in the upper edge of the stoma being forced inwards by the tube and this will give rise to stenosis. An opening which is too large will allow blood from the wound to run easily into the trachea and also encourages surgical emphysema. However, if a cuffed tube is to be used, these dangers will be avoided and in such a case it is necessary to make an opening large enough to permit the easy passage of a cuff into the trachea. Attempts to force it through a narrow opening may lead to fracture or displacement of a cartilage, or to puncture of the thin-walled cuff.

At this stage before the trachea is opened all bleeding points must be dealt with and a tracheostomy tube of appropriate size selected for insertion. A sucker should be at hand to prevent any blood from the cut edges of the trachea from entering the lumen and to aspirate any retained secretions from the bronchial tree. A circular area the size of the tube is then excised from the anterior wall of the trachea, care being taken to retain the excised portion firmly with a pair of forceps before its final separation in order to prevent any possibility of it being inhaled. The skin edges are then sutured to the edges of the tracheal opening with fine catgut on an eyeless needle, and the tracheostomy tube inserted and, if necessary, the rest of the incision closed loosely with further sutures. The incision should not be tightly sutured because of the risk of air from the trachea being trapped in the wound giving rise to surgical emphysema which can dislodge the tube.

It is sometimes advocated that a window should be cut in the tracheal wall in such a way that a flap of tracheal wall is hinged inferiorly (Bjork, 1960); this flap is then sutured to the lower skin edge. However, if this flap of tracheal wall were to become detached from the skin and forced inward into the tracheal lumen, a fatal obstruction could occur and has been known to do so. It is therefore simpler and safer to excise completely a circular area of tracheal wall and then suture the skin edges around the opening (Hewlett and Ranger, 1961). This ensures faster healing, and prevents the risk of the tube being extruded from the trachea post-operatively and coming to lie in the pre-tracheal space. It reduces the risk of haemorrhage from the wound into the trachea and it reduces the risk of surgical emphysema in the tissues of the neck. The tube is retained in position by tapes around the neck. Any dressing around the tube must be so large that there is no possibility of the dressing becoming hidden under the flange of the tube or forced into the tracheal lumen if the tube becomes slightly extruded and then pushed back into position. Fatalities have occurred in this way. The safest method of all is to secure any dressings with a tape passed around the neck. If the secretions are coughed out of the tube it is often an advantage to fasten a bib of water-proof plastic material below the tracheostome but precautions must be taken to ensure that this plastic cannot flap over the opening on inspiration.

Differences between adult and child tracheostomy

There are fundamental differences between the operation which is carried out for the adult and that which is required in the child.

Anatomical differences

The space available in the child is smaller. The larynx lies higher in the neck and is not so easily palpable. The trachea is softer, smaller and relatively deeper beneath the skin. Furthermore, there is an impression of the trachea passing into the superior mediastinum at a deeper level. The head and neck articulation is more mobile and it is therefore essential constantly to check that the symphysis menti and the suprasternal notch lie in the same sagittal plane.

Differences in operative technique in children

It is neither necessary nor desirable to remove sections of tracheal rings when performing tracheostomy in children. The cartilages are soft and springy and can be distracted easily to permit the introduction of the cannula. There is no danger of necrosis of cartilage due to pressure on vessels. For this reason tracheal rings 2, 3 and 4 should be divided in the midline; this makes the insertion of the tube relatively easy. However, the space available is still limited and it is usually not possible to employ Trousseau's dilator to keep the cut surfaces of the rings apart while the tube is inserted; it may be found easier to compress a plastic tube's distal end in curved artery forceps and to insert both into the tracheal lumen, withdrawing the artery forceps when the surgeon is satisfied with the lie of the tube within the lumen of the trachea. The original incision should be left short in length so as to lessen unwanted exposure of unnecessary tissue planes. Sutures should be restricted to one at either end of the incision and no attempt is made to suture the skin edges to the tracheal opening. After 48 hours the plastic tube may be changed for a metal one if this appears to offer advantages.

Tracheostomy tubes

A bewildering variety of tubes confronts the surgeon, and an attempt is being made to standardize the tubes for use. Basically tubes are made of two materials: silver and plastic. Silver tubes are rigid and expensive and are not disposable; plastic tubes are relatively inexpensive, soft and disposable. If necessary plastic tubes may be fitted with an inflatable cuff or a valve. Tubes have to be made in varying sizes and they have been designed to have varying curves and angles. Current opinion is that a radial curve probably offers the most universally acceptable format for the tube design. However, it may be desirable to provide for variations in the position of the shield. Metal tubes can be fitted with an inner tube which projects beyond the distal end of the outer tube. This is safer because if the inner tube becomes obstructed it can be changed, leaving the outer tube to maintain a safe airway. Another advantage of the metal tube is that, when considered necessary, an expiratory valve may be fitted to restore physiological expiration. This allows for phonation and assists in the expulsion of mucus from the trachea. Plastic tubes have been fitted with valves but they are not as efficient (*see* the section on post-operative management of valved tubes).

Post-operative management

Tracheostomies are provided to give an adequate airway and to allow for aspiration of secretions. The management of the tracheostome is therefore of vital importance and should be thoroughly understood by both medical and nursing staff. In many hospitals a tracheostomy routine is printed and hung over the patient's bed. The following points should be observed with the closest attention.

(1) Unless the tube is valved the patient is unable to talk. In the case of the child this makes 24-hour supervision mandatory. In the unconscious patient constant

supervision is also necessary. The conscious adult must be provided with the means of summoning help, e.g. a bell.

(2) All suction apparatus introduced into the tube and trachea must be sterile and, having been used, must be destroyed or resterilized. This means that the person using it should wash and put on a mask before aspiration. The tube should be held in a sterile disposable glove.

(3) There is no fixed interval for aspiration. It should be carried out as soon as the patient appears to require it.

(4) Where inner tubes are fitted they should be removed, cleaned and sterilized at least twice daily.

(5) Where valved tubes are fitted the inner tube must be removed before aspiration is carried out.

(6) When secretions increase, swabs should be taken and sent for culture and sensitivity. It is a good practice to send swabs for culture twice weekly even if the secretions do not increase.

(7) Humidification is helpful in the early stages after a tracheostomy is established and at some period in every 24 hours for children. However, particle size is important and unless the significance is understood it can lead to over-humidification. Cold humidity is to be preferred for all patients. For children it is essential because of the danger of hyperthermia. Cold humidity is provided most efficiently by ultra-sound. Particles will then be less than 5 μm in diameter and the resulting vapour will not cause dampness of the bed clothes. However, the efficiency of this method can rapidly lead to hyper-humidification. For this reason it should be used in children for limited periods only and supplemented by bubbling oxygen through cold water.

Points requiring particular attention

Tube position

Little difficulty is anticipated if the tube is of the right size and is inserted through a correctly placed incision. In adults where the skin edges may be sutured to the tracheostome it is difficult to lodge the tube in the soft tissue of the neck anterior to the tracheostome. If it is felt that the tube is not lying in its optimum site this should be confirmed by lateral soft tissue x-ray of the neck. In all probability a different type of tube may be required.

Tube patency

The distal end of the tube may become obstructed either by dried secretions, granulations or by an over-inflated cuff which has moved distally. If detachable cuffs are used, they must be carefully positioned and very carefully inflated. The amount of air required is just that which is required to prevent a leak around the tube; if this amount is relatively large it is better to insert a larger tube.

Obstruction of the lumen by dried secretions is usually due to under-humidification or to insufficient tracheobronchial toilet. The inner tube should then be removed and cleaned and replaced. If the secretions remain viscid and difficult to aspirate they can be thinned with enzymes.

More difficulty may be encountered with plastic tubes. (Rubber tubes, although still available, are rough and cause abrasion of the track; their use is not to be recommended.) Plastic tubes have in most cases no inner tube and they tend to collect mucus and debris more readily than silver tubes. Once the track is well established it is desirable to change plastic tubes every three days or as often as its lumen becomes narrowed by secretions.

Figure 19.3   Inspiratory valve showing front and sectional views

The principal cause of drying of secretions is lack of exposure of inspired air to humidity; however, when the conditions are suitable, the use of an expiratory valve (de Santi) (*Figure 19.3*) will help to keep the expiratory tide in its physiological pathway. This reduces sedimentation of stagnant mucus down the tracheal wall and reduces the need for humidification. Their use is made more efficient if a hole is cut in the tracheal cannula in register with the tracheal lumen. Valves cannot ever be used with cuffed tubes and once again they must be removed before aspiration procedures are carried out. Failure to do this will result in amputation of the distal end of the suction tube.

Tracheal patency

Crusting may occur in the tube, and it may also occur on the tracheal wall. This is serious because it interferes with mucociliary transport; it may lead to loss of epithelial lining, and separating crusts may be inhaled and cause bronchial obstruction. When crusts form they should be removed by the passage of a tracheoscope or bronchoscope. Very occasionally the obstruction is so low in the respiratory pathway that the tube used is not long enough to pass the obstruction. This can be overcome by the use of Koenig's flexible tube with an olive-shaped end. However, this tube is exceptionally difficult to keep free from debris and secretions.

De-cannulation

Once the obstruction has been treated and the cannula is to be removed there may be no difficulty in the case of the adult who will welcome the return of physiological airway. This is more likely if the tracheostomy has been established for only a short time. However, after long-term cannulation and in most children, de-cannulation can present problems. In general it will be found useful first to employ an expiratory valve, thus restoring physiological expiratory thrust and stimulating the reflex for vocal cord abduction. Once this is tolerated well the cannula should be blocked and reduced in size. This permits the patient to breathe around the tube. In all but the most apprehensive adult it may then be removed.

In children more difficulty may be encountered. They come to trust their artificial airway and they are more sensitive to attempts to obstruct the tube. However, the early use of the respiratory valve followed by a blocker in a smaller tube (Alder Hey pattern) usually makes it possible to wean the patient off his tube. In some cases it will be found useful to trickle oxygen (1 l/min) through a soft catheter placed in the fistula by the tube for about 12 hours and then to remove the cannula leaving the catheter behind for a further 12 hours. This allows the tracheostome to narrow down and after 12 hours the cannula can be removed. The fistula heals quickly if a dry dressing is placed over it. Unsightly scars are unusual and can be excised at a later date.

Intubation

Intubation may be effected by either the oral or nasal route. The oral route is used only in an emergency and once homeostasis occurs it is replaced with a nasotracheal tube; the anaesthetist's laryngoscope (Mackintosh or Magill) is ideal for the purpose. A variety of tube sizes should be available together with suction tubing and Magill's forceps. Portex tubes should be used and if they are to remain for more than a few hours it is necessary to ensure that they are marked 'Z79'. This means that the composition of the plastic contains zinc and not tin which can cause biochemical irritant damage if the tube is sterilized in ethylene oxide. It is useful to have some guide as to the tube size which may be appropriate and the following formula will be found to be a useful guide:

$$\frac{\text{age in years}}{4} + 4.5$$

However, this is not an absolute guide. In the unobstructed larynx there is a variation of one size above and below these figures in one per cent of the population and of two sizes below and above in 1:1000 of the population. If difficulty is experienced in visualization of the larynx an assistant should stabilize the larynx by *gently* pressing it posteriorly while anchoring it in the midline between the index and middle fingers (*Figure 19.4*). If it is found impossible to pass the tube it may be possible to insert a bronchoscope; oxygen can then be fed down this while a tracheostomy is made.

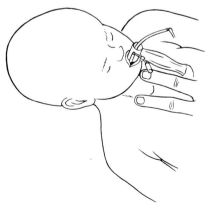

Figure 19.4 Digital pressure on either side of larynx while intubating in order to bring larynx into view

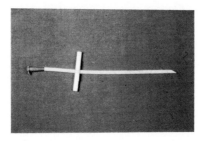

Figure 19.5   The Jackson-Rees nasotracheal tube

Once an airway is established by intubation the patient's condition can be brought under control and a second intubation carried out using a Jackson-Rees nasotracheal tube (Jackson-Rees and Owen-Thomas, 1965). This has ports for suction, for inspired and for expired air (*Figure 19.5*). This should be fixed *in situ* in a plaster headband and if the patient is restless it can be extended to a neck back slab.

Complications of intubation and tracheostomy

Apnoea

In patients who have had a laryngeal obstruction for a long time the sudden reduction of carbon dioxide tension consequent on intubation or tracheostomy may produce apnoea. The administration of five per cent carbon dioxide in oxygen for a few hours may be necessary.

Tracheitis and pulmonary infection

Infection may be present in the bronchial tree before a tube is introduced and may have been the precipitating factor which made the procedure necessary. Infection may also be introduced during aspiration and the need for adequate care and sterility during the procedure has already been stressed. Any pressure necrosis of the tracheal wall will predispose to infection while infection itself makes it more likely that ulceration may occur from pressure of the tube. Antibiotics will be required if infection is present before intubation or tracheostomy, or if it develops subsequently.

Blockage of the endotracheal tube

The majority of deaths associated with this procedure are due to obstruction of the lumen of the tube. For this reason it is essential to have a routine procedure which is carried out in every case of long-term endotracheal intubation.

(1)   *Monitoring.* Pulse rate and respirations of every intubated patient should be monitored. A rise in the pulse rate accompanied by irregular respiration or prolongation of either phase of the respiratory cycle should lead to an immediate

inspection of the circuit. When there is doubt about the patency of the tube this should be replaced using a sucker attached to the suspect tube as it is withdrawn in order to prevent retention of the obstruction within the trachea.

(2) *Routine aspiration* of the tube every 1–2 hours, preferably preceded by the insertion of 1.5 ml of sterile isotonic saline.

Tracheitis and pulmonary infection

Infection may have been the condition for which the intubation or tracheostomy was required. The infection will be brought under control by the administration of adequate doses of the appropriate antibacterial agent. If this does not happen a secondary infection is a possibility. In all cases of long-term intubation or tracheostomy for infection the secretions should be cultured every 48 hours in order to monitor the progress and to recognize secondary invasion at the earliest opportunity. If pressure from the tube or tube tip has been severe, ulceration of the mucosa and possibly necrosis of the cartilage may occur. A granuloma will develop on the ulcerated site and this may be followed later by fibrosis and stenosis.

Laryngotracheal trauma

The larynx and trachea are normally mobile in everyday life. It is neither possible nor desirable to render both completely immobile during treatment in which the airway has been by-passed. Any tube which is introduced into the airway is a foreign body. It may cause trauma to the walls of the respiratory passages and this may lead to both long-term and short-term problems. Furthermore, gross scarring was produced before it was appreciated that the stannous compounds, of which the plastics were made, gave rise to chemical irritation when the tubes were sterilized in ethylene oxide.

Initially it was felt that the largest tube which would fit comfortably at the time of intubation was the tube of choice. However, it is now obvious that the mechanical irritation produced adds to the oedema of the airway walls leading to pressure necrosis and to fibrosis.

Common sites for necrosis followed by fibrosis include the posterior commissure and interarytenoid region of the glottis. In the subglottis an anterior scar may be seen above the cricoid ring or there may be a circumferential stricture at the level of the cricoid ring. Below the cricoid, necrosis of the tracheal rings may lead to fibrotic stenosis of 2–6 tracheal rings and finally necrosis may occur where the tip of the tube abrades the anterior tracheal wall. This produces the condition known as 'tube tip stricture'.

Subglottic or circumferential stenosis may also occur if the tracheostomy is made through the first tracheal ring or if a laryngotomy is maintained for more than 2–3 hours. The question of laryngotracheal trauma is dealt with in a separate chapter; however, some attention should be given to possible iatrogenic causes and their avoidance. From the foregoing account it will be clear that scrupulous attention must be paid to the following matters:

(1) The size of the tube.
(2) The site of insertion.
(3) The position of the tube tip within the lumen.
(4) The sterility and frequency of toilet procedures.
(5) Regular decompression of cuffs, where fitted for 5–10 minutes every hour.
(6) The material of which the tube is made and the efficiency with which it is fixed *in situ*.

Another serious complication of tracheostomy is erosion of a major blood vessel. Fatal erosion of neck vessels is a well-recognized complication (Jarvis, 1964). The usual way in which this damage occurs is by pressure of the tracheostome tube either by the shield or the tube tip on the wall of the trachea or directly onto a major vessel. Provided the anatomical relationships are normal this can be avoided by limited exposure of para-tracheal tissue, by asepsis and by careful attention to the lie of the tube in the neck. When in doubt this should be checked radiologically. Two other complications of tracheostomy occur with sufficient frequency to merit description. These are post-operative surgical emphysema and haemorrhage.

Surgical emphysema

Surgical emphysema may be seen when the skin edges are sutured together rather than to the tracheal opening. The extension of air into the tissues of the neck may extend to the lower eyelids and down to the region of the nipples. The swelling produced may be so great as to dislodge the tube. Therefore only a limited closure of the wound should be carried out if the skin edges are not sutured to the tracheal opening.

Haemorrhage

In an urgent situation inadequate attention may be paid to haemostasis in hurrying to secure an airway. Wherever possible, great attention should be paid to trans-fixing and tying the sections of the thyroid isthmus even if this has been divided by cutting diathermy. If bleeding occurs in the immediate post-operative period a cuffed tube should be inserted and all bleeding points secured after the wound has been re-opened. Secondary haemorrhage must be treated with antibiotics and the great vessels protected by sewing the sternomastoid up to the strap muscles.

Laryngotomy

This operation is reserved for dire emergency, where immediate airway relief is required and where it is not possible to carry out endotracheal intubation or tracheostomy because the necessary apparatus is not available.

The operation

The instrument of choice for laryngotomy is Cawthorne's combined laryngotomy knife and tube (*Figure 19.6*). The patient's neck is extended. The interval between the

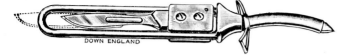

Figure 19.6 Cawthorne's (1964) instrument for emergency laryngotomy. (Reproduced by courtesy of Down Bros. and Meyer & Phelps Ltd)

thyroid and cricoid cartilages is palpated and an incision made in the skin in the midline over this interval. A horizontal incision is made through the cricothyroid ligament and the oval-section laryngotomy tube is introduced through the opening. Where Cawthorne's instrument is not available the incision may be made with a sharp knife or scissors; the incision must then be kept open by separation of the skin edges and introduction of any object with a hollow lumen. The patient should then be accompanied to hospital where a form of tracheostomy is carried out and the emergency opening closed in layers and carefully inspected to ensure that any possible damage which may have occurred has been corrected.

Non-iatrogenic tracheal trauma

Tracheal stenosis can follow external injury to the neck and is usually seen following road traffic accidents. This can result in stenosis of a considerable length of the trachea. This difficult condition can be reduced in incidence and in severity if an early open operation on the trachea is carried out following the accident. Fractured rings are identified and sutured back into register with other fragments over a stent. When this is done a tracheostomy should be established below the injured area. However, for long-standing post-traumatic stenosis a different approach is required. If the stenosis is severe and the damaged area extends over not more than 2.5 cm, Bryce (1976) recommends excision of the damaged area followed by end-to-end anastomosis of the airway accompanied by 'dropping of the larynx', and mobilization of the mediastinal trachea. The suspensory muscles of the larynx from the hyoid are divided, thus exposing the thyrohyoid membrane just at the level of the upper border of the thyroid ala. This prevents damage to the superior laryngeal nerve. The drop is completed by incision of the superior cornu of the thyroid cartilage and resection of fibres of the inferior constrictor muscle. Following 'laryngeal drop' the patient's head is flexed and the end-to-end anastomosis completed using stainless steel sutures. After closure a plaster back slab is applied to maintain the head in flexion during the healing period. Where the site of the resection is low it may not be possible to make the tracheostomy below the suture line. In these cases a tracheostomy is made above the line of the anastomosis and a small tube passed through the reconstructed lumen (*Figure 19.7*).

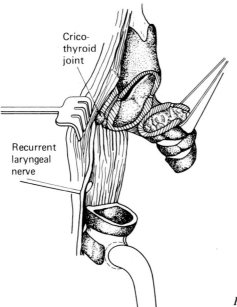

Crico-
thyroid
joint

Recurrent
laryngeal
nerve

Figure 19.7

Post-operative care and management

The immediate post-operative period should be spent in intensive-care facilities. Points which require special attention are:

(1) *Aspiration of accumulated saliva and food.* If this occurs feeding may have to be established via gastrostomy.
(2) *Airway difficulties.* Since the patient will be unable to talk easily a tracheostomy routine has to be maintained with stomal care, bronchial suction, and humidification to an adequate level.
(3) *Haemorrhage.* This can be prevented by careful haemostasis at the time of operation followed by attention to the airway which avoids obstructed breathing or straining. Since many of these cases follow open wounds of the neck as a result of traffic accident trauma, secondary haemorrhage is a possibility. If it occurs the wound should be opened, clots turned out and antibiotics given. The sterno-mastoid muscles should be sewn over the great vessels to the strap muscles.

Speech

Many patients have voice problems following this type of surgery. Stimulation and encouragement by the surgeon and intensive support from the speech therapist help to overcome these difficulties.

Late stenosis

Prolonged follow-up is advisable as some patients show a tendency to stenose again at the site of injury.

References

Bjork, V. O. (1960). *Journal of Thoracic, Cardiovascular Surgery,* **39,** 179

Bryce, D. P. (1976). *Operative Surgery: Nose and Throat,* 3rd edn, pp. 249–272; Butterworths, London and Boston

Cawthorne, T. (1964). *Lancet,* **1,** 1081

Hewlett, A. B. and Ranger, D. (1961). *Postgraduate Medical Journal,* **37,** 18

Jackson-Rees, G. and Owen-Thomas, J. B. (1965). *British Journal of Anaesthesia,* **35,** 901

Jarvis, J. F. (1964). *Journal of Laryngology,* **78,** 781

Lawrence, R. A. and Bailey, B. J. (1971). *Southern Medical Journal,* **64,** 1049

Reading, P. (1958). *Journal of Laryngology,* **72,** 785

20 Cervical node dissection
David Wright

It is not uncommon to find a reference to Crile (1905), who first described the operation of radical neck dissection, in any treatise on cervical node dissection. There is no doubt that this particular operation has constituted the major advance so far towards the control of metastatic neck cancer. The technique of the operation has remained virtually unchanged except for the development of alternative incisions for exposing structures to be removed. In most cases it is unwise to deviate from the classical operation (Ellis, 1971). New developments or variations of this operation have done little to improve the cure rate. Attempts have been made to exclude parts of the neck where metastatic nodes are thought unlikely to occur in specific cancers; for example, it has been suggested that in the absence of palpable submandibular or upper deep cervical nodes the contents of the submandibular triangle can be left undisturbed in a radical neck dissection for laryngeal cancer (Feldman and Applebaum, 1977). It has been the experience of most head and neck surgeons that any modification of the recognized standard radical neck dissection leads to poor results. This is especially so with cancer of the floor of the mouth (Shaw and Hardingham, 1977).

The technique of functional neck dissection has been described by Bocca (1975) who removes a 'package' of lymph nodes and their vessels but retains the internal jugular vein, accessory nerve and sternomastoid muscle. The weakness of this operation is emphasized by McKelvie (1976) who demonstrated the distribution of metastatic nodes in neck dissection by clearing the tissues with cedar-wood oil over a period of at least six weeks after preliminary preparation and then superimposing the specimen on a Rouvière's diagram (*Figure 20.1*). Microscopically involved nodes have been seen invading the adventitia of the jugular vein and it is clear that these would not have been removed in a functional neck operation. There is no evidence to demonstrate that microscopically positive nodes either recede or disappear, or that once the node is involved it is able to do anything other than grow into a larger cancerous node.

For most patients with a metastatic node in the neck, surgery gives better results than radiotherapy and it is probably true to say that treatment with radiotherapy is not helpful once nodes have developed, except in cases where the removal of fixed nodes is beyond the scope of surgery when palliative treatment may be indicated. Prophylactic treatment of the neck with radiotherapy is indicated in

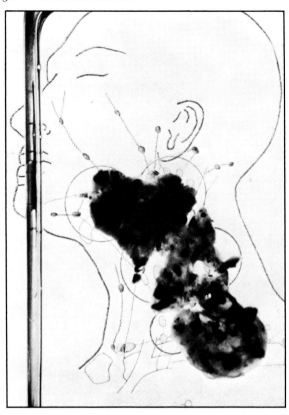

Figure 20.1   Metastatic nodes in a neck dissection specimen after clearing with cedar-wood oil, superimposed on a Rouvière's diagram. (Reproduced by courtesy of Mr. P. McKelvie)

tumours where the histology shows a highly cellular character, as may be found in tumours of the post-nasal space or tonsil. If chemotherapy is to be used as an adjunct to radiotherapy as a positive measure in the treatment of neck nodes, it is better to give it before the radiotherapy has had a chance to cause endarteritis within the smaller blood vessels.

Radical neck dissection can give good results when combined in continuity with excision of the primary tumour, as in laryngectomy (*Figure 20.2*). It can be combined with the use of replacement skin flaps, e.g. the deltopectoral flap as used in the reconstruction of the oropharynx during a combined operation for carcinoma of the tonsil. Large rotation flaps can be used with the Y-type incision to provide facial skin for replacement in the excision of parotid neoplasms (Smith, Black and Teachey, 1974).

The presentation of bilateral neck nodes (N3) usually indicates widespread permeation of the lymphatics of the neck by carcinoma and this is unlikely to be dealt with adequately by bilateral radical neck dissection and would explain why this procedure does not produce a significant improvement in the survival of patients with bilateral neck glands. The exception to this may be a patient with a supraglottic tumour. McKelvie (1976) has shown that such tumours spread by emboli to the nearest adjacent node where they tend to remain localized for long periods without further node involvement. In these cases bilateral neck dissection is worth considering.

Fixed glands in the neck (N3) usually offer a poor prognosis, but Stell (1976)

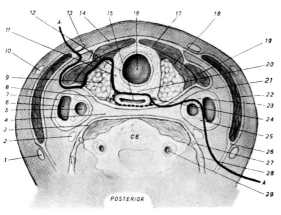

ANTERIOR

POSTERIOR

Figure 20.2   En bloc dissection of larynx with cervical lymph nodes

1 Posterior jugular vein	16 Trachea
2 Sympathetic trunk	17 Sternohyoid
3 Pre-vertebral fascia	18 Sternothyroid
4 Retro-oesophageal space	19 Omohyoid
5 Common carotid artery	20 Cricoid cartilage
6 Internal jugular vein	21 Lymph node area
7 Carotid sheath	22 Sternomastoid
8 Recurrent nerve	23 Descendens hypoglossi
9 Thyroid gland	24 Inferior thyroid artery
10 External jugular vein	25 Vagus
11 Crico-arytenoideus posticus	26 Investing fascia
12 First tracheal ring	27 Phrenic nerve
13 Anterior jugular vein	28 Brachial plexus
14 Pre-tracheal fascia	29 Vertebral dorsal vessels
15 Oesophagus	

showed that radical neck dissection could prolong the survival of these patients by many months and that in 12 per cent of cases actually cured the patient.

Removal of the external carotid artery with invading tumour usually presents little problem but it is doubtful whether resection and replacement of the internal or common carotid arteries is justifiable.

Scope of the operation

A block dissection consists of the removal of a single mass of all the lymph nodes in the anterior and posterior triangles of the neck, as well as their associated lymphatic vessels. To achieve this, all the cervical nodes and fasciae of the neck must be removed in a single block from the clavicle below, to the base of the skull and mandible above; and from the anterior border of the trapezius behind to beyond the midline in front. Anteriorly the dissection must extend to the anterior belly of the digastric muscle on the opposite side.

The sternomastoid muscle, the internal jugular vein, the submandibular salivary gland and the tail of the parotid gland are all included in the excision.

The operation can be carried out on both sides, and it is not essential to preserve either internal jugular vein; however, if both are removed there is a serious risk of producing venous congestion in the head resulting in cerebral oedema. This presents with severe headache and a raised blood pressure but may be controlled by an intravenous infusion of 200 ml of 25 per cent mannitol.

It is wise to separate the first from the second operation by at least six weeks or as many weeks as is safely possible. It is advisable to do a tracheostomy at the time of the second operation. The results of bilateral node dissection are of necessity extremely poor as it is only likely to be carried out in patients with advanced disease.

The limitations of the disease are clearly apparent when the nodes involved in the metastatic spread lie at the periphery of the operative field and in particular those nodes at the upper end of the internal jugular vein. Tumour arising from subglottic tumours may spread into the tracheo-oesophageal or jugulosubclavian lymph nodes and the incidence of stomal recurrence from retrograde spread may be improved by trans-sternal dissection of the mediastinum with removal of the clavicles and manubrium (Sissons, Bykell and Becker, 1977).

When radical neck dissection is combined with the removal of a primary tumour situated in the mouth, pharynx or larynx, as much as possible of the tissues joining these structures to the neck should be left in continuity. This is not difficult in laryngeal or pharyngeal cancers, but in oral cancers which drain to the sub-mandibular and upper deep cervical nodes, the specimen should be left attached along the lower border of the mandible and should include the inner layer of periosteum.

The skin incision

Martin, Del Valle and Erlich (1951), who did much to develop the radical neck

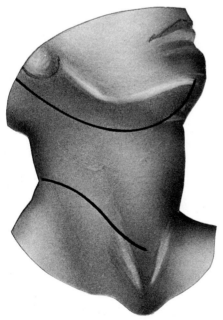

Figure 20.3   Double   horizontal incision

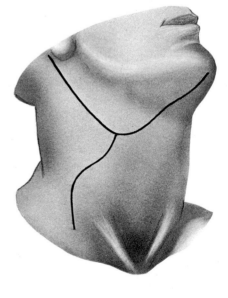

Figure 20.4 Y-Shaped incision

dissection on a sound scientific basis, gave a masterful description of the surgical technique and clarified the indications and contra-indications. The double Y-incision must now be considered obsolete because of the high incidence of flap necrosis that follows. There have been many incisions described since, but the most successful ones have been based on McFee's (1960) double horizontal incision (*Figure 20.3*), which is most suitable after preliminary irradiation, or the Y-type flap (*Figure 20.4*) which allows easier access to the structures of the neck. This was initially described by Schobinger (1957) as a T-shaped incision but was later modified by Babcock and Connelly (1966) by making the horizontal limb into a curve to join the vertical incision. It is important that the flaps are widely based with a good blood supply, especially if the area has previously been irradiated.

The platysma muscle is included in the skin flaps to increase the blood supply. If a local area of platysma has been invaded by growth, the overlying skin should be completely excised and replaced either with a flap rotated to close the defect, or by a split-skin graft.

Reflection of the skin flaps

The skin flaps, if the Y-type incision is used, are raised to expose the complete field from the clavicle and manubrium to the mastoid process and mandible, and from the anterior border of the trapezius to the lateral border of the opposite infrahyoid muscles (*Figure 20.5*). The double horizontal incision requires a bridge flap to be lifted

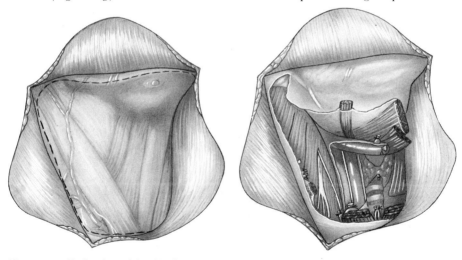

Figure 20.5 Reflection of the skin flaps

Figure 20.6 The inferior and lateral dissection

between the two incisions. The entire lower part of the dissection must be mobilized so that this part of the specimen can be passed under the flap to allow the remaining upper part of the dissection to be completed. In reflecting the superior flap, the mandibular branch of the facial nerve should be identified and preserved by making the incision through the fascia at the inferior border of the capsule of the submandibular gland. The fascia can then be elevated in continuity with the skin flap with the knowledge that the mandibular branch is safely preserved. The cervical branch is almost invariably divided.

The inferior and lateral dissection

The cervical fascia is incised over the clavicular origin of the sternomastoid muscle, along the clavicle to the anterior border of the trapezius muscle and then medially to the medial border of the opposite sternomastoid muscle (*Figure 20.6*). The sternal and clavicular heads of the sternomastoid muscle are divided close to their origins. The omohyoid muscle is divided where it passes deep to the trapezius.

The external jugular vein, the transverse scapular vein and the transverse cervical vein are encountered at the posterior border of the clavicular head of the sternomastoid, and must be identified and ligated. Care should be taken not to damage the thoracic duct on the left side where it lies medial to the internal jugular vein, as a troublesome chylous fistula can result if the duct is torn.

The internal jugular vein should be ligated as early as possible in the procedure to limit the possible spread of systemic metastatic emboli. The vein should be dissected out of the carotid sheath and completely freed for a length of about 2 cm as close as possible to the subclavian vein. The vagus nerve is identified in the carotid sheath and left undisturbed. Throughout the dissection it should be handled as little as possible and always very gently. The freed portion of the internal jugular vein is doubly ligated and, before division, the lower end is further secured with a transfixion suture.

The tissue thus separated inferiorly can now be swung upwards and medially, progressively easing the internal jugular veins out of the carotid sheath as the dissection proceeds superiorly along the border of the trapezius. The supraclavicular triangle is filled by fat and its floor is formed by pre-vertebral fascia overlying the phrenic nerve and brachial plexus. The plane of dissection is most easily identified by finger dissection beneath the layer of fat and this technique is unlikely to cause damage to the phrenic nerve or brachial plexus.

The fascia along the anterior border of the trapezius is incised and the dissection carried across the floor of the posterior triangle. The accessory nerve is divided for the first time as it enters the trapezius at the junction of the upper two-thirds and lower one-third of the anterior border of the muscle, and just below it the transverse cervical vessels are identified and ligated. The dissection is then carried medially exposing the scalenus medius muscle, the trunks of the brachial plexus and the scalenus anterior muscle, and preserving the phrenic nerve which runs downwards from lateral to medial on the surface of the scalenus anterior.

The superior dissection

The attachment of the cervical fascia is divided along the whole length of the exposure from the mastoid process to just beyond the midline of the mandible (*Figure 20.7*). The facial artery and vein are closely attached to it at the anterior border of the insertion of the masseter and must be ligated and divided. Beginning laterally, the levator scapulae and the splenius muscles are exposed in the apex of the posterior

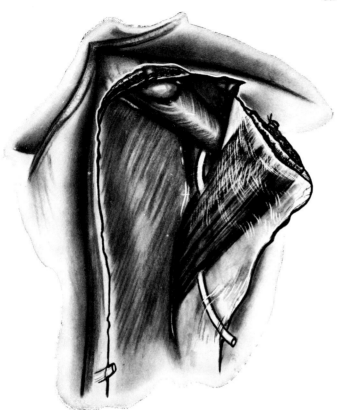

Figure 20.7   Division of the facial vessels and sternomastoid
muscle

triangle, and the sternomastoid muscle is divided as close as possible to its insertion on
the mastoid process and retracted medially.

The accessory nerve is then exposed for the second time as it passes under the
surface of the muscle but superficial to the internal jugular vein. It is again divided.

The dissection is next carried medially across the tail of the parotid gland, care
being taken not to damage the facial nerve. The posterior belly of the diagastric
muscle then comes into view (*Figure 20.8*). A large number of veins are encountered
and must be carefully isolated and ligated. The main trunks are the posterior
auricular vein, the posterior facial vein and its posterior and anterior divisions
inferiorly, the common facial vein and the external jugular vein. The posterior border
of the submandibular gland is then exposed.

The posterior belly of the digastric muscle is not divided but retracted to allow
ligation and division of the occipital artery running near its lower border, and the
posterior auricular artery near its upper border must also be found and ligated. The
internal jugular vein and the glossopharyngeal nerve are now exposed (*Figure 20.9*).
The glossopharyngeal nerve appears between the vein and the internal carotid artery
deep to the styloid process, while the larger hypoglossal nerve appears lower in the
neck, running downwards and then forwards superficially to the external artery, just
above the greater cornu of the hyoid bone and usually accompanied by large venae
communicantes.

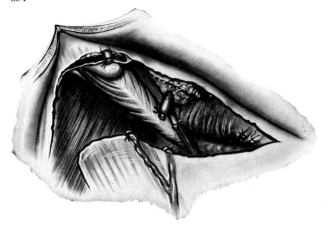

Figure 20.8 Dissection
across the parotid tail

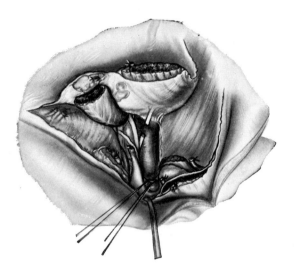

Figure 20.9 Ligation and division
of the internal jugular vein

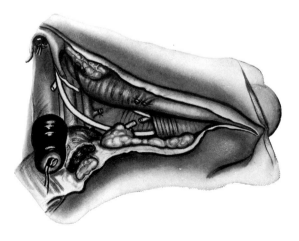

Figure 20.10 Dissection of the
submandibular salivary gland

The internal jugular vein, usually grossly distended following ligation of the lower end, is carefully isolated and doubly ligated and further secured with a fixation suture as near to the base of the skull as possible. The whole mass of tissue, comprising the fascia and cellular tissue of the posterior triangle, the omohyoid and the sterno-mastoid muscles, and the excised segment of the internal jugular vein can now be reflected medially to the line of the external and common carotid arteries.

The submandibular salivary gland, which is now fully exposed (*Figure 20.10*), is stripped forwards and downwards after the facial artery has been divided and ligated near its origin from the external carotid artery. The lingual artery sometimes loops into the field of dissection at the posterior border of the hyoglossus muscle, but it can usually be spared. The duct of the submandibular gland is separated from the lingual nerve and divided where it dips deeply between the hyoglossus and mylohyoid muscles.

Anterior dissection

The anterior belly of the digastric muscle is divided at its origin from the lower border of the mandible near the midline.

The fascia is now incised along the medial border of the opposite anterior digastric belly down to the greater cornu of the hyoid bone (*Figure 20.11*).

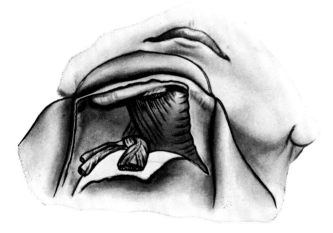

Figure 20.11 Division of the anterior belly of the digastric muscle

The fascia and submental nodes are cleared from the mylohyoid, and the anterior dissection is then continued downwards from this point to include the anterior belly of the omohyoid.

Lateral lobe of thyroid gland

The neck dissection should include the lateral lobe and isthmus of the thyroid gland. The superior thyroid artery is identified where it originates from the external carotid, just below the greater cornu of the hyoid bone where it is ligated and divided. The inferior thyroid artery is to be found behind the common carotid artery at the level of the cricoid cartilage curving medially before it breaks up into a number of branches. The artery is similarly ligated (*Figure 20.12*). Care must be taken not to damage the recurrent laryngeal nerve (if the larynx is to be retained).

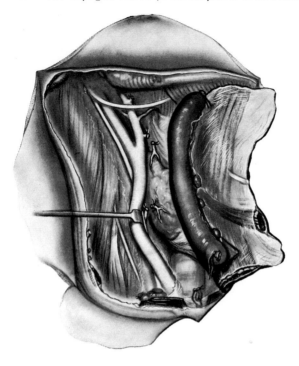

Figure 20.12 Ligation and division of the superior and inferior thyroid vessels; dissection of the lateral lobe of the thyroid gland

The isthmus of the thyroid gland is divided near its junction with the opposite lateral lobe, and the cut surfaces are trans-fixed with a thread suture, encircled and tied. The fascial plane behind the thyroid gland is now entered from above allowing dissection of the lateral lobe from the pharynx, larynx and trachea.

The complete block is now free to be removed and should be sent as a specimen for histological examination.

Closure

Before the wound is closed, it is of utmost importance to secure haemostasis. If hypotensive anaesthesia has been used it is advisable to allow the blood pressure to return to at least 100 mmHg before the end of the operation, to make sure that all bleeding points are well controlled.

The most satisfactory form of drainage is by continuous suction through two tubular drains that are inserted through separate stab incisions. The tubes should be joined by a Y-connection to a low-pressure pump providing continuous suction. The suture lines must be airtight to allqw the flaps to collapse, thus obliterating any deadspace. Suction should be continued for 4–5 days. Intravenous fluids are continued for 24 hours and then oral feeding can commence the following day. The sutures should be ready for removal between the sixth and eighth days.

Complications

Haemorrhage, chylous leak, nerve lesions to the phrenic, sympathetic trunk, brachial plexus, vagus, accessory, facial and hypoglossal nerves are not uncommon complications. The problems of cerebral oedema after bilateral neck dissection have already been discussed. Infection and wound breakdown may occur if the incisions have not been carefully planned in a heavily radiated neck. The most serious complication is that of rupture of the common or internal carotid arteries, either of which has a mortality rate of 90 per cent. It is most likely to occur in a patient who has undergone radiation to the neck or had a previous tracheostomy. The risk is also high if a pharyngeal fistula develops following necrosis of the skin flaps.

In order to avoid this formidable complication, attempts have been made to cover the artery when the risk of rupture is thought to be high. The levator scapulae can be swung forward on an anterior pedicle after being freed posteriorly so that the muscle can swing forward to cover the carotid artery.

The use of autogenous dermis for carotid-artery protection was first described by Corso and Gerold (1961). The early observations confirmed that the dermis once exposed would epithelialize, thereby affording some protection to an exposed carotid artery.

The efficacy of the dermal graft for carotid-artery protection continues to be investigated experimentally, but Dedo *et al.* (1975) reported from their series that the dermal graft had not substantially reduced the overall incidence of carotid catastrophies to date.

References

Babcock, W. W. and Connelly, J. (1966). *Archives of Otolaryngology*, **84,** 554
Bocca, V. (1975). *Laryngoscope*, **87,** 151
Corso, P. F. and Gerold, F. P. (1961). *Surgical Forum*, **12,** 487
Crile, G. (1905). *Journal of the American Medical Association*, **47,** 1780
Dedo, D. D., Sessions, D. G., Alonso, W. A. and Ogura, J. H. (1975). *Archives of Otolaryngology*, **101,** 649
Ellis, M. (1971). In: *Diseases of the Ear, Nose and Throat*, 3rd edn, Vol. 4, (Eds J. Ballantyne and J. Groves); Butterworths, London and Boston
Feldman, D. E. and Applebaum, E. L. (1977). *Archives of Otolaryngology*, **103,** 705

Martin, H., Del Valle, B. and Erlich, H. (1951). *Cancer*, **4,** 441
McFee, W. F. (1960). *Annals of Surgery*, **151,** 280
McKelvie, P. (1976). *Proceedings of the Royal Society of Medicine*, **69,** 409
Schobinger, R. (1957) *Annals of Surgery*, **146,** 221
Shaw, W. J. and Hardingham, M. (1977). *Journal of Laryngology and Otology*, **91,** 467
Sissons, G. A., Bykell, D. E. and Becker, S. P. (1977). *Laryngoscope*, **87,** 751
Smith, R., Black, F. D. and Teachey, W. S. (1974). *Archives of Otolaryngology*, **84,** 554
Stell, P. M. (1976). *Proceedings of the Royal Society of Medicine*, **69,** 411

21 Skin grafts in otolaryngology
P M Stell

Definitions

A *skin graft* is a transplant of epidermal and dermal tissue, surviving in the recipient bed by nourishment from the plasmatic circulation.

A *skin flap* is composed of skin and subcutaneous tissues, surviving in the recipient bed by nourishment from an intact and functioning arterial and venous circulation reaching it through its pedicle which is the stem or base of a flap.

The cutaneous blood vessels may be divided into 'musculo-cutaneous' and 'direct cutaneous' arteries. The small musculo-cutaneous arteries pierce the muscle layers immediately beneath the skin perpendicular to the skin surface and supply a small area of skin (*Figure 21.1*). The direct cutaneous arteries are entirely different: these are specific named vessels, such as the superficial temporal artery, which run within the

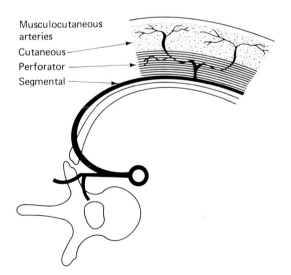

Musculocutaneous arteries
Cutaneous
Perforator
Segmental

Figure 21.1 Musculo-cutaneous blood supply to the skin. (Reproduced by courtesy of the Editor of *Annals of the Royal College of Surgeons* [1977], **59**, 237)

skin parallel to its surface and which supply a large area of skin (*Figure 21.2*). The venous drainage consists of superficial direct cutaneous veins and of the deeper venae comitantes which accompany the cutaneous arteries. It is possible to design skin flaps

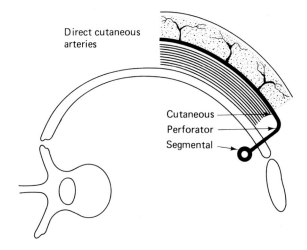

Direct cutaneous
arteries

Cutaneous
Perforator
Segmental

Figure 21.2   Direct cutaneous arteries. (Reproduced by courtesy of the Editor of *Annals of the Royal College of Surgeons* [1977], **59**, 236)

which are supplied by only one type of cutaneous artery, but their surviving lengths are dramatically different. It is therefore necessary to classify skin flaps on the basis of their supplying vessels into random or axial flaps.

Random (cutaneous) flaps

A random flap is based on the musculo-cutaneous arteries, and it is not designed to include a specific named vessel in its pedicle. The venous drainage passes through the subdermal venous plexuses, the paired venae comitantes, and (occasionally) a direct cutaneous vein. Most of the clinically used skin flaps are of this type, ranging from the triangular flaps of the familiar Z-plasty to the abdominal tubed flaps with their long pedicles.

Axial (arterial) flaps

An axial flap is deliberately designed to include a named direct cutaneous artery within its longitudinal axis and pedicle. Venous drainage consists of the associated direct cutaneous vein, the paired venae comitantes, and the subdermal venous plexuses. Clinical examples include the delto-pectoral, the groin and the temporal flaps.

Island flaps

An island flap is a flap whose maintained pedicle consists only of the nutrient vessels (*Figure 21.3*). The arterial supply is provided continuously by an anatomically recognized direct cutaneous artery, with venous drainage through its paired venae comitantes.

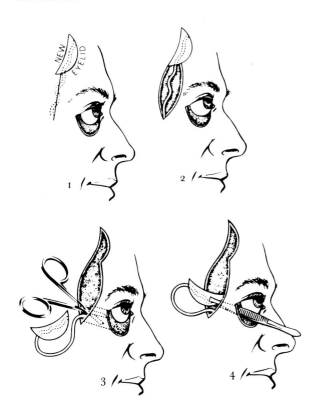

Figure 21.3 An island flap

Free flaps

A free flap is an island flap which has been completely detached from the body and transferred to a distant recipient site, where micro-vascular anastomoses are done to re-establish its essential intravascular circulation. The arterial supply may be through either direct cutaneous or musculo-cutaneous arteries, with the venous drainage provided by venae comitantes and/or direct cutaneous veins. Clinically, the ilio-femoral, the delto-pectoral and the dorsalis pedis flaps have been successfully transferred to distant sites.

A *local flap* is a term used to describe any flap, be it random or axial, which is moved either by rotation or lateral transposition into a defect which is immediately adjacent to the donor area.

A *distant flap* is any flap, be it axial or random, which is moved to a distant site with an intervening area of normal tissue between the donor and recipient sites.

Delay is a term used to describe a technique whereby the vascularity of a random flap may be increased. An area of skin receives its blood supply through the small musculo-cutaneous vessels which pierce it perpendicularly from the underlying layers and from each side; with the exception of specific axial flaps such an arrangement will in general only sustain a flap which is not longer than the width of its base. However, if a bipedicled flap is marked out which is twice as long as the width of its base, but is left attached at each end (hence the term 'bipedicled') in some way not clearly understood the blood vessels become aligned along the flap and dilate so that the blood supply to the flap is increased; 2–3 weeks after the flap was first raised the distal end can then be divided and the entire flap moved in comparative safety. Such bipedicled flaps can be shown to have a dominant and a non-dominant end depending on which end provides the major blood supply and it is obviously preferable to divide the non-dominant end. A laterally based thoraco-acromial bipedicled flap was until recently a very popular flap in head and neck surgery; but its dominant end is medial so that logically such a flap should not be based laterally. This is one of the reasons that this flap has been abandoned in favour of the medially based delto-pectoral flap.

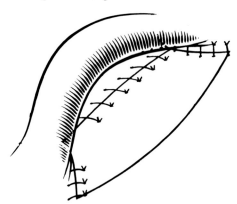

Figure 21.4   Tubed pedicle flap (From *Head and Neck Surgery*. Eds P. M. Stell and A. G. D. Maran. Heinemann, London. Reproduced by permission of the publishers)

Tubing is a technique used to protect the pedicle of a distant flap. If a flap is to be moved over intervening tissue to its recipient site either immediately or after a period of delay, its pedicle should be protected from infection by tubing the skin with the skin surface outwards (*Figure 21.4*).

Viability of skin flaps

In 1920 Gillies stated that the base of a flap should usually be at least as wide as any other part of the flap apart from flaps containing a definite artery, such as the superficial temporal. He also stated that the viability of flaps varies greatly in different regions of the body and may be compromised by scar tissue.

The amount of skin which can normally be moved by a flap is severely limited, and over the following 50 years several techniques were developed for increasing the length of a flap which could be moved safely, the main technique being that of delayed flaps. It gradually became appreciated, however, that a flap with an artery in its base was entirely different from a flap without such an artery, and in 1973 McGregor and Morgan divided flaps into two types: random and axial, as defined above.

A random flap, as its name implies, can be raised anywhere on the body and can run in any direction; its blood supply is dependent on the subdermal plexus in the neighbourhood of its base and this is supplied by small musculo-cutaneous arteries which pierce the underlying muscle layers perpendicular to the skin surface (*see Figure 21.1*). An axial flap is specific in design, its boundaries are determined by specific anatomical landmarks and it is supplied by large named vessels running in the skin parallel to its surface and superficial to the underlying muscle layer (*see Figure 21.2*).

Gillies originally stated that a flap should in general not be longer than the width of its base and this has been confirmed by later research work on the pig (Stell, 1977). In the true random flap the surviving length does increase with increasing size of base but there is an upper limit to this and it is probable that random flaps cannot be raised in safety beyond a length of about 12 cm irrespective of the size of their base.

Other factors which are known to affect the survival pattern of random flaps are previous operations, previous radiotherapy, the position of the flap on the body (flaps on the face survive to a greater length than flaps elsewhere) the direction of the flap (a flap based superiorly on the leg survives to a greater length than a flap based inferiorly), and generalized diseases such as diabetes and peripheral vascular disease. Random flaps are used in the head and neck in Z-plasty; as an outer lining in the closure of small fistulae; for reconstructing the defect remaining after excision of skin cancer on the face and for reconstruction within the mouth including lateral and median cervical flaps and naso-labial flaps.

Axial flaps have only been developed within the last ten years. Their principle is entirely different from that of a random flap; the cutaneous vessel supplying them is always a large named artery so that the flap has a very good blood supply and will survive to a much greater length than a random flap. The boundaries of such a flap are dictated by the anatomical area of the vascular territory of the vessel supplying the flap. Axial flaps are thus specific in their design, blood supply and uses. The following axial flaps are important in head and neck surgery:

The delto-pectoral flap (Bakamjian, 1965).
The temporal flap (McGregor, 1963).
The nape or occipito-mastoid flap (Mütter, 1842).

The delto-pectoral flap (*Figure 21.5*)

This flap was first described in England in 1917 by Aymard for reconstruction of the nose, but its use was entirely forgotten and it was not popularized until 1965 by Bakamjian.

The flap is based medially on the upper part of the chest on the upper three or four perforating branches of the internal mammary artery which emerge through the medial end of the intercostal spaces. Its boundaries are the clavicle superiorly, the acromion laterally, and a line running through the anterior axillary fold, superior to the nipple, inferiorly. It will reach any site on the neck and the face up to the level of the zygoma; this is partly explained by the fact that this flap retracts from side to side after it has been elevated but does not retract from end to end and may indeed

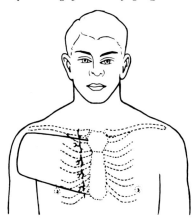

Figure 21.5   The delto-pectoral flap (From *Operative Surgery, Nose and Throat*, Eds C. Rob and R. Smith, Butterworths, London)

elongate slightly, particularly in patients over the age of 60 (Stell and Green, 1976). This flap is used for:

(1) Replacement of the pharynx after pharyngo-laryngectomy.
(2) Replacement of the lateral wall of the pharynx after resection of a tonsillar carcinoma.
(3) Replacement of the tongue after glossectomy.
(4) Replacement of the skin of the neck and of the face after extensive excision for a carcinoma arising primarily in the skin or extending secondarily into the skin.
(5) For the closure of pharyngo-cutaneous fistulae.

The temporal flap (*Figure 21.6*)

This flap is based on the superficial temporal vessels which provide an excellent blood supply so that the entire forehead can be moved in one stage without previous delay providing that the external carotid artery and the superficial temporal artery have not been divided. Either half or the entire forehead may be used; surprisingly it is better to use the entire forehead since the defect is less noticeable than if only half the forehead is used. The temporal flap is used mainly in the following circumstances:

(1) For reconstruction within the mouth after resection of a carcinoma.
(2) For reconstruction of the lateral wall of the oropharynx after removal of a tonsillar carcinoma.

The occipital flap (*Figure 21.7*)

The occipital flap or nape flap is based superiorly on the occipital vessels and posterior auricular vessels. It is usually thick and should be used without delay particularly if a neck dissection has been done. Furthermore, the patient has to be turned on his side to raise the flap which is thus tedious to use.

The flap is based superiorly on a line joining the mastoid process to the external

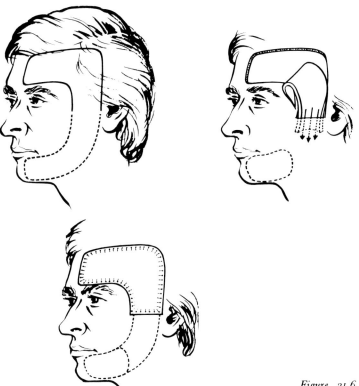

Figure 21.6 The temporal flap. (Reproduced by kind permission of the Editor of the *British Journal of Plastic Surgery*)

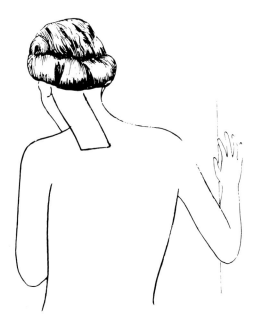

Figure 21.7 The occipital flap

occipital protuberance. It is usually raised in an oblique direction running towards the shoulder. This flap has few uses, the commonest being the replacement of the skin of the lower part of the centre of the neck.

Free flaps

Although it is very unlikely that the ear, nose and throat surgeon will use this technique, at the present time micro-vascular anastomosis must be mentioned. In this method a flap is detached entirely from its bed and undergoes free flap transfer to a new site at which its artery and vein are re-anastomosed. Readers are referred to some of the original papers such as those of O'Brien *et al.* (1974). Very few free flaps have been used in the head and neck, but free delto-pectoral flaps have been used to replace facial and scalp skin (Harii, Ohmori and Ohmori, 1974).

Reconstruction at specific sites will now be discussed.

Mouth and oropharynx

This section will be concerned with the use of grafts in reconstruction within the mouth and oropharynx after resection of cancer. Reconstruction of the mandible will not be considered nor will reconstruction of the lip, an organ which strictly speaking is within the mouth but whose reconstruction forms a separate subject which is seldom relevant to the ENT surgeon.

A free skin graft may be used to cover defects remaining after excision of a tumour in the mouth by one of several techniques:

(1) Epithelial inlay.
(2) Buried tubes of skin.
(3) Quilting.

An epithelial inlay is usually used to release a tongue which has been previously tethered after excision of a cancer in the mouth, or to form a new alveolar ridge so that the patient may wear dentures. The adhesions binding the tongue are divided or a gutter is formed at the point where it is wished to create a new alveolus, and split skin is then applied to the raw area both to epithelialize it and to prevent contraction. The split skin graft is applied, raw surface outwards, over a gutta percha bung which is held in place by a denture, the whole being wired in place usually by circumferential wires around the mandible. This device must be left in place for about ten days for healing to take place, and thereafter a denture must be worn, often with a special flange to keep the groove permanently open.

The burying technique is used either at the time of excision or later to provide mobility for the lateral part of the tongue when little of the bulk has been sacrificed. At the primary excision a gutter remains between the alveolus and the remaining part of the tongue; if this has been closed at a primary operation and it is required to restore mobility at a later operation, the gutter must be re-opened. A split skin graft is then taken and fixed either by sutures or with skin-glue, raw surface outwards, over a rubber tube of suitable size. The graft is then placed in the gutter, which must be closed completely by stitching the tongue to the remnants of the alveolar and buccal mucosa. The tongue and the graft must be immobilized by circumferential wires placed around the mandible (*Figure 21.8*). The principles of this operation are thus

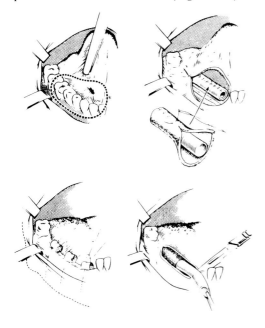

Figure 21.8 The burying technique. (Reproduced by courtesy of the Editor of *American Journal of Surgery* [1962], **104**, 727)

that immobility is guaranteed by the wires and the graft is protected from saliva by closing the tunnel completely over it. The pre-requisites for primary healing are thus fulfilled. Ten days after the original operation the tunnel is re-opened by dividing down on to it through the tongue, or by re-opening the previous incision, and the rubber tube is removed, hopefully leaving the split skin graft securely healed in position (Corson and Gerold, 1962).

Much the easiest and most successful technique of applying split skin in the mouth is the quilting technique described by McGregor (1975). The main pre-requisites for the 'take' of a split skin graft in the mouth are the following:

(1) The graft must be completely immobile over its bed during the healing phase.
(2) Blood should not be allowed to collect between the graft and its bed.
(3) The technique must be as comfortable as possible for the patient, and bolsters and other devices which are uncomfortable and which become infected should be avoided.

In the quilting technique a piece of split skin is sewn into the defect on the tongue or on the buccal mucosa after achieving absolute haemostasis of the bed. The graft is sutured at approximately 5 mm intervals around its edges and tacking sutures are placed through the graft into the bed at approximately 5 mm intervals over the entire graft. Small slits are then cut in the graft between some of the sutures to allow any accumulations of blood to escape. No dressings are necessary and because of the proximity of the sutures the graft is completely immobilized on its bed.

Although it is possible after removal of a small tumour (less than 2 cm in diameter) to close the defect primarily or to repair it with a split skin graft, as described above, the vast majority of tumours are much greater than this and once they have been resected with the recommended margin of 3–4 cm, the tongue is involved and the amount of tongue remaining is small. While it is technically possible to close the defect in the mouth by suturing the remnant of the tongue to the cheek this results in a very crippled tongue, particularly in two circumstances: in resection of a carcinoma of the lateral border of the tongue, much the commonest site; and secondly in resection of tumours involving the anterior part of the floor of the mouth. In the first case loss of the greater part of the bulk of the tongue leads to severe crippling if the small remnant is sewn down; and in the second place, if the tongue is sewn to the internal surface of the lower lip to close the defect of the anterior part of the floor of the mouth, the tip of the tongue is immobilized leading to an unsightly swelling of the lip and more particularly to immobility of the tongue so that it becomes difficult or impossible to articulate dento-labial consonants. The result can be improved by a later epithelial inlay (Slanet and Rankow, 1962), but for the last 20 years or so it has been widely agreed that the defect remaining in the mouth after a partial glossectomy or after resection of a tumour involving the anterior part of the floor of the mouth (a pelvimandibulectomy) requires reconstruction of the soft-tissue defect, with local or distant flaps.

The principles of reconstruction within the mouth are as follows (Myers, 1972):

(1) The reconstructive techniques should neither interfere with nor limit the excisional surgery.
(2) Form and function should be quickly restored.
(3) The morbidity and mortality should not be increased by the reconstructive phase.
(4) A secondary cosmetic deformity should not be produced.
(5) The reconstructive phase should be completed as quickly and as simply as possible, especially if cure is doubtful.
(6) Prolonged reconstructive procedures should not ordinarily be carried out on patients for whom a prosthesis would provide satisfactory rehabilitation.

Local mucosal flaps

The following local flaps for reconstruction within the mouth have been described: *lingual* flaps and *buccal* flaps. The tongue has a very rich vascular supply from the lingual artery (*Figure 21.9*); there is unfortunately little cross-over at the midline but one small artery crosses the midline in the tip of the tongue on which thin bipedicled flaps can occasionally be raised. The lingual flap is, however, usually based posteriorly.

The lingual flap is mainly used for reconstruction of the lateral part of the floor of the mouth and alveolus (Chambers, Jaques and Mahoney, 1969; Papaioannou and Farr, 1966) and of the soft palate and tonsillar area (Klopp and Schuster, 1956); all or virtually all of the tongue must have been preserved. The tongue flap is outlined by marking a line lengthwise on the tongue, of about 20–40 per cent of the width of the tongue (*Figure 21.10*). The lingual flap is then rotated into the defect of the floor of the

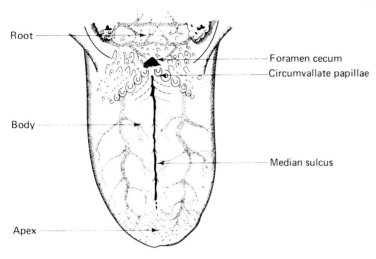

Root

Foramen cecum

Circumvallate papillae

Body

Median sulcus

Apex

Figure 21.9 Dorsum of the tongue. (Reproduced by courtesy of the Editor of *American Journal of Surgery* [1969], **118**, 783; article by C. T. Klopp)

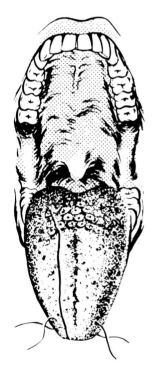

Figure 21.10 Incision for lingual flaps. (Reproduced by courtesy of the Editor of *American Journal of Surgery* [1969], **118,** 783; article by C. T. Klopp)

mouth or of the oropharynx. The edges of the anterior one-third or free portion of the tongue are then closed primarily, avoiding production of a pointed tip of the tongue (*Figure 21.11*). The raw edges of the remaining part of the donor site are usually covered by a split skin graft to prevent the mobile portion of the tongue adhering to the flap.

The tongue flap has also been used to line defects of the buccal mucosa. This flap may also be used for lining the lateral floor of the mouth and the lateral part of the tongue, by using a flap based anteriorly on the *opposite* side of the tongue (the median transit tongue flap). The flap is passed from the donor site to the defect through a defect in the centre of the tongue; the pedicle is divided and returned three weeks later (Calamel, 1973).

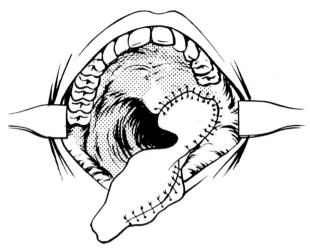

figure 21.11   Reconstruction of the palate with lingual flap, and repair of the tongue. (Reproduced by courtesy of the Editor of *Cancer* [1956], **9,** 1239; article by C. T. Klopp and M. Schurter)

Buccal flaps, consisting of the mucosa of the internal surface of the cheek and the lip have been described for reconstruction of the tonsillar area and the mouth (Craft, 1961). Such a mucosal flap has certain advantages, notably its vascular supply and its physical characteristics, providing an elastic pliable lining for motion and deglutition; it also serves as a sounding board in speech and, because it is provided with minor salivary glands which secrete mucus, it facilitates the movement of food. Nevertheless, this type of flap is very much less successful than the lingual flap which generally gives very good results.

Regional random flaps

The following regional random flaps have been described for repair of defects within the mouth: nasolabial flaps, median cervical flaps based superiorly, and lateral cervical flaps; the latter may be used as compound flaps in which case the sternomastoid muscle is included within them to increase the blood supply (Littlewood, 1967).

It is particularly important to reconstruct the anterior part of the floor of the mouth since a simple closure of the remaining part of the tongue to the lip binds the tongue, makes speech and the fitting of a denture difficult and causes salivary incompetence. At the end of the resection, inferiorly-based flaps are raised from the naso-labial fold (*Figure 21.12*). A tunnel is then developed beneath the mucosa of the cheek and the linguo-alveolar sulcus so that the flap can be turned downwards to be passed through the tunnel into the floor of the mouth. The point at which the flap appears in the

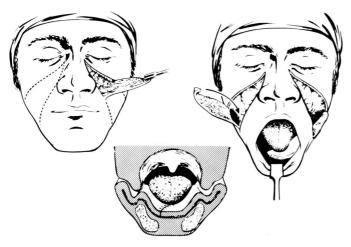

Figure 21.12   Raising inferiorly-based flap from the naso-labial fold.
(Reproduced by courtesy of the Editor of *American Journal of Surgery*
[1975], **130**, 479; article by I. K. Cohen)

mouth is marked by methylene blue, the flap is taken out again and the epidermis is
removed with an electric dermatome. The flaps are then re-introduced into the
mouth and are sewn in place one behind the other, the one placed anteriorly being
sewn to the edge of the incision in the lip and the posterior one being sewn to the edge
of the defect in the tongue. If the pedicle is denuded in this way the flaps can be
regarded as subcutaneous pedicle flaps, as first described by Barron and Emmett
(1965), and the defect can be closed primarily so that it is not necessary to divide the
pedicle and return it. Alternatively, a small oro-cutaneous fistula can be left as
originally described; the flap is then divided, the pedicle returned and the fistula
closed three weeks later (Cohen and Edgerton, 1971). The defect in the naso-labial
area is easily closed by primary suture and the scar rapidly becomes inconspicuous
since it is placed in a skin crease. Indeed, the enthusiasts for this operation claim that
the patient derives a bonus since he gets a face lift at the same time!

Lateral cervical flaps *(Figure 21.13)*

These flaps were mainly designed to be turned into the mouth and oropharynx after
resection of a tumour at this site, but could also be used as a compound flap which
included the sternocleidomastoid muscle to provide bulk to the flap and also to
improve its blood supply for reconstruction of the palate immediately after a radical
maxillectomy for an antral carcinoma (Bakamjian and Littlewood, 1964). The flap is
raised at the end of the excisional phase and is sewn into the defect, leaving a
temporary oro-cutaneous fistula which must be closed three weeks later after the flap
has been divided and its pedicle returned. The lateral cervical compound flap
including the sternomastoid muscle may be used for reconstruction of the hard palate
after maxillectomy. At the end of the resection the flap is passed through a
subcutaneous tunnel dissected superficial to the ramus and angle of the mandible; the
edges of the flap are then sutured to the cut edge of the mucoperiosteum of the

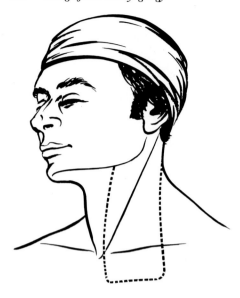

Figure 21.13 Lateral cervical flaps. (Reproduced by courtesy of the Editor of *British Journal of Plastic Surgery* [1967], **20,** 403)

remaining hard palate in front and to the soft palate behind; the divided end of the sternomastoid muscle is then anchored to the remnants of the pterygoid muscle to relieve tension on the distal portion. The upper surface of the flap is now covered by cheek skin, septal mucosa from the contralateral side of the nasal septum or by a free skin graft. The defect in the neck is resurfaced by a split skin graft; the temporary oro-cervical fistula is closed in the customary fashion three weeks later.

Median cervical flaps (apron flap)

This flap was first described in 1951 by Edgerton; its principle is shown in *Figure 21.14*. At the end of the excisional phase the flap is raised, rotated in to the floor of the mouth and its end sutured to the inner surface of the labial mucosa; the flap is thus used to reconstruct the anterior part of the floor of the mouth and can also be used to cover a bone graft of the mandible at this site. As originally described, an oro-cervical fistula

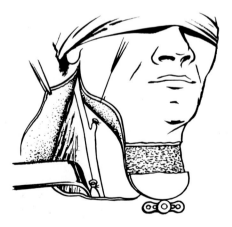

Figure 21.14 Principle of the median cervical flap. (From *Modern Trends in Plastic Surgery*, Ed. Tom Gibson; Butterworths, London)

was left which required to be closed at a later date by division and return of the pedicle flap, but if the flap is converted into a subcutaneous pedicle by denuding it of its epidermis, the wound can be closed primarily leaving the island of skin in place in the floor of the mouth.

Distant axial flaps

Two axial flaps have proved extremely useful for reconstruction of large defects in the mouth and the oropharynx: the temporal flap and the delto-pectoral flap.

The use of the temporal flap in filling a defect in the mouth after resection of a carcinoma was popularized by McGregor in 1963. The temporal flap is a true axial flap based on the superficial temporal vessels; its use for filling an intra-oral defect is summarized in *Figure 21.15*. The flap is raised at the end of the excisional phase,

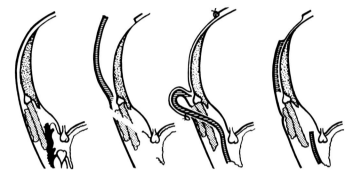

Figure 21.15 The temporal flap. (Reproduced by courtesy of the Editor of *British Journal of Plastic Surgery* [1963], **16**, 318)

turned into the mouth through a tunnel in the substance of the cheek and sewn into the intra-oral defect. Three weeks later the temporary fistula is closed by division or return of the pedicle. Although only just over half of the forehead is required to resurface most defects within the mouth, the cosmetic defect on the forehead is less if the entire forehead is removed and replaced by a split skin graft which is placed over the pericranium which must be carefully preserved.

This flap can be used for reconstructing any defect in the mouth or oropharynx, and indeed is a very successful flap which rarely if ever undergoes necrosis. Facial palsy is a potential but uncommon hazard which usually recovers spontaneously. The external salivary fistula is not a real complication since it is placed high in the mouth. A persisting external fistula after the second stage is very uncommon. The skin of the flap is difficult to keep clean at first but it settles rapidly and softens, and then behaves like a free skin graft within the mouth. This is a very successful flap which has enjoyed great popularity, but its main disadvantage is the very obvious cosmetic defect on the forehead (Myers, 1972).

The delto-pectoral flap may also be used for reconstruction of large defects of the mouth or oropharynx. The flap may be used in several ways but in the original description by Bakamjian, Long and Rigg (1971) it was passed upwards beneath the cervical skin, the distal end was sewn into the defect in the oropharynx with its skin surface facing into the pharynx, and the rest of the flap was formed into a tube, skin surface inwards, running beneath the cervical skin. At a second stage, three weeks later, the pedicle was divided and the oro-cutaneous fistula closed.

Alternatively, the flap can be passed through the defect below the mandible and the distal end of the flap is sewn to the remnant of the tongue. The remainder of the flap is tubed, skin surface outwards (*Figure 21.16*). Three weeks later the tube is divided, the distal part is threaded into the mouth, opened and spread over the remaining part of the defect (*Figure 21.17*). The base of the flap is returned to the chest and the fistula in the neck is closed.

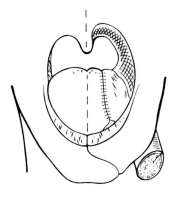

Figure 21.16 Delto-pectoral flap in repairing floor of mouth defect: first stage. (From *Operative Surgery, Nose and Throat*, Eds C. Rob and R. Smith; Butterworths, London)

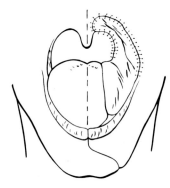

Figure 21.17 Delto-pectoral flap in repairing floor of mouth defect: final stage, with pedicle returned to donor site. (From *Operative Surgery, Nose and Throat*, Eds C. Rob and R. Smith; Butterworths, London)

As a rough guide the best policy at the moment can be summarized as follows:

(1) Small defects (less than 2 cm in diameter) can be closed primarily or by the quilting technique with split skin.

(2) Larger defects (2–4 cm) which involve less than half the bulk of the tongue can be closed primarily by split skin, again using the quilting technique, to preserve mobility. However, defects of the anterior part of the floor of the mouth should be filled by naso-labial flaps to preserve the mobility of the tongue. It may also be advisable to fill defects of the lateral part of the floor of the mouth or the tonsil with a lingual flap for the same reason.

(3) Larger defects involving more than half of the bulk of the tongue must be filled by a large distant flap, either a temporal flap or a delto-pectoral flap, to provide bulk to the tongue and to restore mobility.

Closure of fistulae

The causes of fistulae occurring after head and neck surgery are shown in *Table 21.1*.

The incidence of fistulae obviously varies according to several factors: the experience of the surgeon, previous radiotherapy, and surgical technique including the incision used. An oro-cutaneous fistula occurs after about 30 per cent of commando procedures (Yonemoto *et al.*, 1972); the incidence of pharyngo-cutaneous fistulae after total laryngectomy varies between 10 and 40 per cent (Lavelle and Maw, 1972). The predisposing factors include principally radiotherapy and a low haemoglobin level after the operation.

Table 21.1

Pharyngo-cutaneous fistulae
Total laryngectomy
Supraglottic laryngectomy
Vertical hemi-laryngectomy
Lateral pharyngotomy
Commando procedure
Pharyngo-laryngectomy and pharyngeal replacement by either skin repair or visceral repair

Oro-cutaneous fistulae
Resection of buccal tumours
(1) Squamous carcinoma
(2) Salivary carcinoma – the majority of which are of the adenoid cystic variety

A fistula may basically be due to one of two processes: disruption of the suture line, or loss of tissue. In the former case, particularly if the patient has not been irradiated, the fistula will almost always heal spontaneously since there has been no loss of tissue. In the latter case, particularly if the patient has been irradiated, a period of about 60 days is required for local infection to be overcome and for the edges of the wound to become clean and established. Thereafter, the fistula must be closed, in such a way that epithelial surfaces are supplied both inside to line the pharynx, and outside to replace the lost skin. Depending on the availability of tissue, fistulae can thus be classified as shown in *Table 21.2*.

Table 21.2

Type I fistula:	Both tissue surfaces can be provided locally
Type II fistula:	One tissue surface can be provided locally and one must be provided from a distance
Type III fistula:	Both surfaces must be provided from a distance

Using the classification shown in *Table 21.2* fistulae can be closed as follows.

Closure of type I fistula

In this type, the inner layer is provided by two ellipses of skin turned inwards. A crescentic flap is marked out on each side of the fistula, each being the same width, at its widest point, as the fistula (*Figure 21.18*). The ends of each ellipse are close to the margin of the fistula to avoid bunching of excess tissue.

The flaps are elevated (*Figure 21.19*) and suturing begins at one end (*Figure 21.20*); the inner layer of sutures should be of the Connell inverting type. It is preferable to begin suturing from each end of the defect and to tie the knot in the middle to ensure that the skin at each end of the defect is inverted into the lumen (*Figure 21.21*). After suturing the flaps, the resultant pressure of the excess tissue forces the edges of the flaps down into the lumen, producing good apposition of their edges. A second layer and preferably a third layer of subcutaneous sutures is inserted to strengthen the closure.

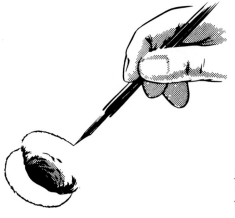

Figure 21.18   (From *Operative Surgery, Nose and Throat*, Eds C. Rob and R. Smith; Butterworths, London)

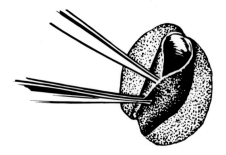

Figure 21.19   (From *Operative Surgery, Nose and Throat*, Eds C. Rob and R. Smith; Butterworths, London)

The resulting raw surface must be covered by a local flap, nearly always a rotation flap fashioned in accordance with the basic principles of plastic surgery, as follows. An isosceles triangle is drawn around the defect with pen and ink (*Figure 21.22*), the sides of the triangle adjacent to angle X being equal. The triangle then forms a wedge of an exaggerated semicircle which is used as a rotation flap. The flap is raised, rotated into the defect and sutured in place (*Figures 21.23* and *21.24*). Split skin is then used to cover any defect resulting from mobilization of this flap. These steps are shown in cross-section in *Figure 21.25*.

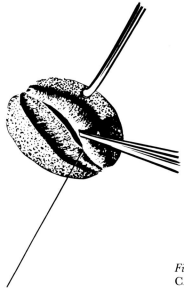

Figure 21.20   (From *Operative Surgery, Nose and Throat*, Eds
C. Rob and R. Smith; Butterworths, London)

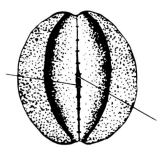

Figure 21.21   (From *Operative Surgery, Nose and Throat*, Eds C.
Rob and R. Smith; Butterworths, London)

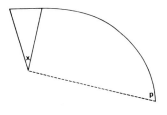

Figure 21.22   (From *Operative Surgery, Nose and Throat*,
Eds C. Rob and R. Smith; Butterworths, London)

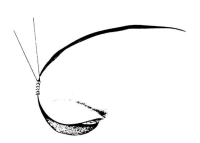

Figure 21.23   (From *Operative Surgery, Nose and Throat*,
Eds C. Rob and R. Smith; Butterworths, London)

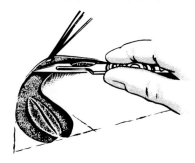

Figure 21.24 (From *Operative Surgery, Nose and Throat*, Eds C. Rob and R. Smith; Butterworths, London)

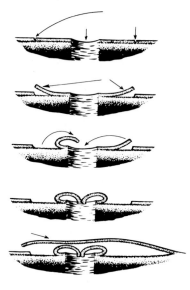

Figure 21.25 (From *Operative Surgery, Nose and Throat*, Eds C. Rob and R. Smith; Butterworths, London)

Closure of type II fistula

For most situations the best flap for external cover is the delto-pectoral flap. Experience has shown that this can be used for skin cover of the neck and of the face

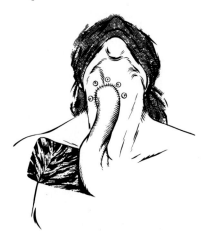

Figure 21.26 (From *Operative Surgery, Nose and Throat*, Eds C. Rob and R. Smith; Butterworths, London)

up to the level of the zygoma. Examples of the use of other flaps include the closure of a fistula at the inner canthus after a lateral rhinotomy by local flaps turned in and covered by midline forehead flaps based inferiorly, and the closure of a fistula at the angle of the jaw after a commando procedure using a nape flap. To close a type II pharyngeal fistula local flaps are turned in as shown in *Figures 21.18* to *21.21*. The resulting raw area must be filled, preferably by a delto-pectoral flap (*Figure 21.26*). The technique is shown in cross-section in *Figure 21.27*.

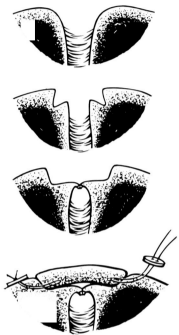

Figure 21.27   (From *Operative Surgery, Nose and Throat*, Eds C. Rob and R. Smith; Butterworths, London)

Closure of type III fistula

Such a fistula may be closed by a lined flap or by two flaps. A lined nape flap (Zovickian, 1957), a laterally-based lined acromial thoracic tube (Conley, 1956), a delto-pectoral flap lined by turning in a tab of skin three weeks before the definitive operation (Stell and Cooney, 1974), or two non-delayed laterally-based acromio-pectoral flaps may be used to provide inner and outer lining (Ogura and Dedo, 1965).

For a very large post-laryngectomy fistula, the commonest problem for the ENT surgeon, the method suggested by Bryce (personal communication) appears to be the best. In this method a midline gutter, connecting the orostome to the oesophagostome is covered with a delto-pectoral flap, as follows: a flap is raised, tubed, and set into the submental skin immediately anterior to the orostome (*Figure 21.28*).

Three weeks later the tubed flap is divided just below the oesophagostome (*Figure 21.29*) and the proximal part of the flap returned to the chest wall.

The skin immediately below the oesophagostome is then incised in a semicircular fashion (*Figure 21.30*) and the distal end of the tube is inset into this incision.

Once the flap has taken, the patient is left with two lateral slits (*Figure 21.31*) which

620

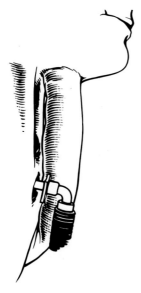

Figure 21.28 (From *Operative Surgery, Nose and Throat*, Eds C. Rob and R. Smith; Butterworths, London)

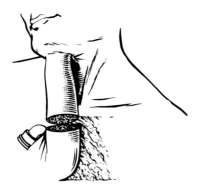

Figure 21.29 (From *Operative Surgery, Nose and Throat*, Eds C. Rob and R. Smith; Butterworths, London)

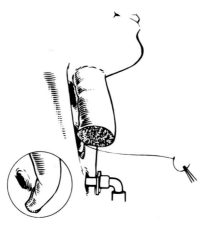

Figure 21.30 (From *Operative Surgery, Nose and Throat*, Eds C. Rob and R. Smith; Butterworths, London)

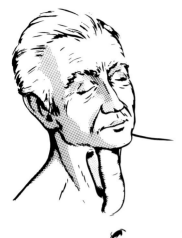

Figure 21.31 (From *Operative Surgery, Nose and Throat*, Eds C. Rob and R. Smith; Butterworths, London)

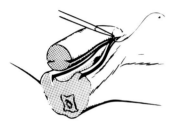

Figure 21.32 (From *Operative Surgery, Nose and Throat*, Eds C. Rob and R. Smith; Butterworths, London)

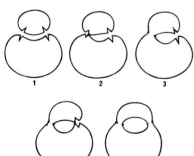

Figure 21.33 (From *Operative Surgery, Nose and Throat*, Eds C. Rob and R. Smith; Butterworths, London)

must be closed. Two weeks later the lateral edges of the gutter are incised and the edges undermined. Similarly, the lateral borders of the tube are also incised and undermined (*Figure 21.32*). The corresponding edges are then sutured as shown in cross-section in *Figure 21.33* to complete closure of the new pharynx.

Replacement of the skin of the neck and face

Only those situations which the ENT surgeon is likely to encounter will be dealt with here. Replacement of the skin of the face after resection of primary tumours of the skin is a vast, complex topic which seldom concerns the ENT surgeon.

Occasionally it is necessary to resect the skin of the neck in continuity with a malignancy, particularly a lymph node which has invaded the skin. A melanoma of the skin of the neck, particularly if associated with cervical lymphadenopathy, may also require resection of the skin of the neck and its subsequent replacement. Other indications include squamous carcinoma of the skin of the neck, extensive squamous carcinoma involving the auricle, carcinomas of the parotid gland involving the overlying skin and tumours within the mouth involving the cheek, the angle of the mouth and the chin and the lip. At all of these sites the skin can be replaced using the delto-pectoral flap.

Nape flaps, scalp flaps and a laterally-based flap from the anterior chest wall may be used to cover deficiencies of the neck skin after radical surgery for fungating metastases or severe post-irradiation damage of the skin (Conley, 1960). The laterally-based anterior chest flap (Conley, 1967) (*Figure 21.34*) receives its blood

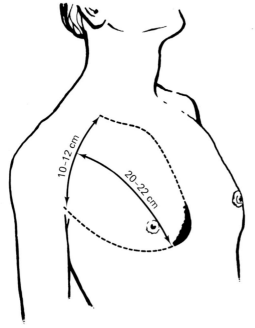

Figure 21.34   The laterally-based anterior chest flap. (Reproduced by courtesy of the Editor of *Archives of Surgery* [1967], **94,** 413)

supply from the branches of the axillary artery and it can be used non-delayed, but like a delto-pectoral flap may undergo partial necrosis in ten per cent of cases. This flap does not appear to have become popular and in all probability has been displaced by the delto-pectoral flap. The skin of the lower part of the centre of the neck may also be replaced by the nape flap as first described by Mütter in 1842.

Replacement of the hypopharynx

The first recorded case of resection of the cervical oesophagus is that by Czerny in 1877. Czerny sutured the lower end of the oesophagus to the wound in the neck and discharged the patient home 'healed' five weeks later. Although there were occasional sporadic attempts made in the early part of the 20th century to reconstruct the pharynx, surgery for carcinoma of the hypopharynx and upper oesophagus only became established in the 1940s by Wookey. Wookey (1942) described a staged operation in which the pharynx was repaired with a laterally-based neck flap in stages. The steps are shown in *Figures 21.35* to *21.38*. In an attempt to preserve neck

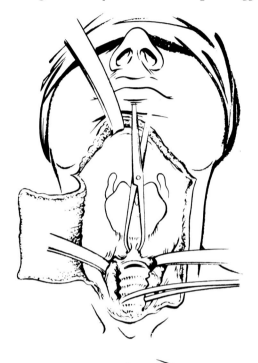

Figure 21.35 Pharyngolaryngectomy with Wookey flaps: stage 1. (Reproduced by courtesy of the Editor of *British Journal of Surgery* [1948], **35,** 249)

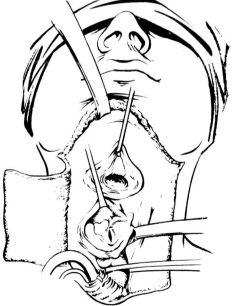

Figure 21.36 Pharyngolaryngectomy with Wookey flaps: stage 2. (Reproduced by courtesy of the Editor of *British Journal of Surgery* [1948], **35,** 249)

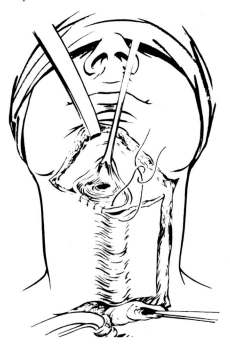

Figure 21.37 Pharyngolaryngectomy with Wookey flaps: stage 3. (Reproduced by courtesy of the Editor of *British Journal of Surgery* [1948], **35**, 249)

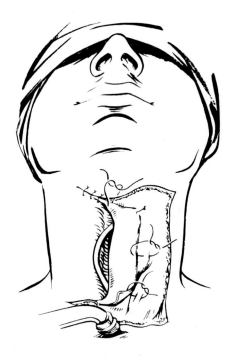

Figure 21.38 Pharyngolaryngectomy with Wookey flaps: stage 4. (Reproduced by courtesy of the Editor of *British Journal of Surgery* [1948], **35**, 249)

skin other forms of reconstruction have been devised: autogenous split skin wrapped round a prosthesis has been recommended.

This approach to the problem had several disadvantages – healing by first intention is unusual so that fistulae often occur; as these heal, stenosis is left in their wake. Furthermore, the patient is in hospital for months because of the staged operations; Ranger (1969) has shown that the one-year survival in this disease treated by these methods is less than 50 per cent so that many patients are dead before normal swallowing is restored by these methods. Accordingly, surgeons have sought methods of immediate restoration of gullet continuity.

Prostheses of varying types, eg. Stuart's (1966) tube, have been used, but many surgeons feel uneasy about using foreign materials in a situation where anastomotic leaks can be fatal, and an alternative method of primary repair has been attempted using other parts of the alimentary tract: pedicled colon and pedicled jejunum, jejunum as a free transplant with vascular anastomosis, revascularized colon, revascularized gastric antrum and transposed stomach. Rather unusual methods have been published using a tube of penile skin, the larynx, a tube of laryngeal mucosa, a free autogenous tracheal graft and aortic grafts.

Of these latter methods, pedicled colon and stomach are the only two in common use in this country now. Although the originally high morbidity and mortality has fallen with improving technique, there can be little doubt that these operations place stress of a high order both on the patient and on the surgeon; visceral replacement still remains attractive, however, because it gives immediate restoration of pharyngeal continuity, but the five-year survival is of the order of ten per cent. The technique using the medially-based chest flap (the delto-pectoral flap) appears to give a satisfactory primary skin repair of the pharynx but at the expense of a longer stay in hospital (Bakamjian, 1965).

After the pharynx and larynx have been removed at the excisional operation, the flap is raised and tubed with its skin surface inwards; the end of the tube is then anastomosed to the orostome (*Figure 21.39*) and the oesophageal stump is anastomosed, end to side, to the lower part of the tube (*Figures 21.40* and *21.41*). A temporary

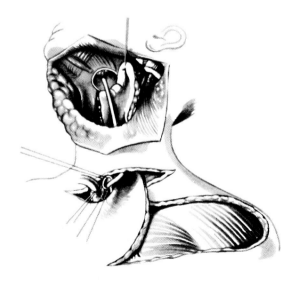

Figure 21.39 Pharyngolaryngectomy with delto-pectoral flap: stage 1. (From *Operative Surgery, Nose and Throat*, Eds C. Rob and R. Smith; Butterworths, London)

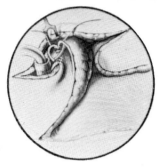

Figure 21.40 Pharyngolaryngectomy with delto-pectoral flap: stage 2. (From *Operative Surgery, Nose and Throat*, Eds C. Rob and R. Smith; Butterworths, London)

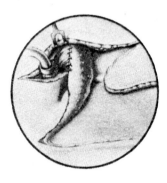

Figure 21.41 Pharyngolaryngectomy with delto-pectoral flap: stage 3. (From *Operative Surgery, Nose and Throat*, Eds C. Rob and R. Smith; Butterworths, London)

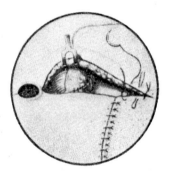

Figure 21.42 Pharyngolaryngectomy with delto-pectoral flap: stage 4. (From *Operative Surgery, Nose and Throat*, Eds C. Rob and R. Smith; Butterworths, London)

fistula is left where the pedicle emerges from the neck and is closed three weeks later by division and return of the flap (*Figure 21.42*).

This technique is tedious, and the patient is in hospital for much longer (on average three months) than after repair using a viscus. Furthermore, fistulae are common, but they almost always heal spontaneously; strictures also occur, as after any other form of repair using skin, in ten per cent of patients requiring repeated dilatation. This method has two enormous advantages over visceral repair: a very much lower operative mortality and a much higher long-term survival (35–40 per cent at five years).

References

Aymard, J. L. (1917). 'Nasal reconstruction', *Lancet*, **i,** 888–891

Bakamjian, V. Y. (1965). 'A two staged method for pharyngo-oesophageal reconstruction with a primary pectoral skin flap', *Plastic and Reconstructive Surgery*, **36,** 173–184

Bakamjian, V. Y. and Littlewood, M. (1964). 'Cervical skin flaps for intra-oral and pharyngeal repair following cancer; surgery', *British Journal of Plastic Surgery*, **17,** 191–210

Bakamjian, V. Y., Long, M. and Rigg, B. (1971). 'Experience with the medially based delto-pectoral flap in reconstructive surgery of the head and neck', *British Journal of Plastic Surgery*, **24,** 174–183

Barron, J. N. and Emmett, A. J. J., (1965). 'Subcutaneous pedicle flaps', *British Journal of Plastic Surgery*, **18,** 51–78

Calamel, P. M. (1973). 'The median transit tongue flap', *Plastic and Reconstructive Surgery*, **51,** 315–318

Chambers, R. G., Jaques, D. A. and Mahoney, W. D. (1969). 'Tongue flaps for intra-oral reconstruction', *American Journal of Surgery*, **118,** 783–786

Cohen, I. K. and Edgerton, M. T. (1971). 'Transbuccal flaps for reconstruction of the floor of the mouth', *Plastic and Reconstructive Surgery*, **48,** 8–10

Conley, J. J. (1956). 'Management of pharyngostome, oesophagostome and associated fistulae', *Annals of Otology, Rhinology and Laryngology*, **65,** 76–79

Conley, J. J. (1960). 'The use of regional flaps in head and neck surgery', *Annals of Otology, Rhinology and Laryngology*, **69,** 1223–1234

Conley, J. J. (1967). 'The chest flap in ablative surgery about the mouth and gullet', *Archives of Surgery*, **24,** 413

Corson, P. F. and Gerold, F. P. (1962). 'Immediate and secondary reconstruction of the floor of the mouth and mobilisation of the tongue by a new technique', *American Journal of Surgery*, **104,** 727–731

Craft, J. W. (1961). 'Immediate reconstruction of the pharynx using rotated mucous membrane flaps', *Plastic and Reconstructive Surgery*, **28,** 26–42

Czerny, V. V. (1877). 'Neue operationen: Vorlaufige Mittheilung', *Zentralblatt zur Chirurgie*, **4,** 433–434

Edgerton, M. T. (1951). 'Replacement of lining to oral cavity following surgery', *Cancer*, **41,** 110–119

Gillies, H. (1920). *Plastic Surgery of the Face*, p. 22; Hodder and Stoughton, London

Harii, K., Ohmori, K. and Ohmori, S. (1974). 'Free delto-pectoral skin flaps', *British Journal of Plastic Surgery*, **27,** 231–239

Klopp, C. T. and Schurter, M. (1956). 'The surgical treatment of cancer of the soft palate and tonsil' *Cancer*, **9,** 1239–1243

Lavelle, R. J. and Maw, A. R. (1972). 'The aetiology of post-laryngectomy pharyngo-cutaneous fistulae', *Journal of Laryngology and Otology*, **86,** 785–793

Littlewood, M. (1967). 'Compound skin and sternomastoid flaps for repair in extensive carcinoma of the head and neck', *British Journal of Plastic Surgery*, **20,** 403–419

McGregor, I. A. (1963). 'The temporal flap in intra-oral cancer. Its use in repairing the post-excisional defect', *British Journal of Plastic Surgery*, **16,** 318–335

McGregor, I. A. (1975). 'Quilted skin grafting in the mouth', *British Journal of Plastic Surgery*, **28,** 100–102

McGregor, I. A. and Morgan, G. (1973). 'Axial and random pattern flaps', *British Journal of Plastic Surgery*, **26,** 202–213

Mütter, T. D. (1842). 'Cases of deformity from burns, relieved by operation. Mütter's cases of deformity from burns', *American Journal of the Medical Sciences*, **4,** 66–80

Myers, E. N. (1972). 'Reconstruction of the oral cavity', *Otolaryngologic Clinics of North America*, **5,** 413–433

O'Brien, B. M., Morrison, W. A., Ishida, H., Macleod, A. M. and Gilbert, A. (1974). 'Free flap transfers with microvascular anastomoses', *British Journal of Plastic Surgery*, **27,** 220–230

Ogura, J. H. and Dedo, H. H. (1965). 'Repair of large pharyngostoma utilizing bilateral non-delayed regional pedicle flaps', *Laryngoscope*, **75,** 588–600

Papaioannou, A. N. and Farr, H. W. (1966). 'Reconstruction of the floor of the mouth by a pedicle tongue flap', *Surgery, Gynecology and Obstetrics*, **122,** 807–810

Ranger, D. (1969). 'The problems of repair after pharyngolaryngectomy', *Proceedings of the Royal Society of Medicine*, **57,** 1099–1103

Slanet, C. A. and Rankow, R. M. (1962). 'The intra-oral use of split-thickness skin grafts in head and neck surgery', *American Journal of Surgery*, **104,** 721–726

Stell, P. M. (1977). 'The pig as an experimental model for skin flap behaviour: A reappraisal of previous studies', *British Journal of Plastic Surgery*, **30,** 1–8

Stell, P. M. and Cooney, T. C. (1974). 'Management of the fistulae of the head and neck after radical surgery', *Journal of Laryngology and Otology*, **88,** 819–834

Stell, P. M. and Green, J. R. (1976). 'The retraction of flaps: Clinical observations and design of experimental model', *Acta Otolaryngologica*, 161–166

Stuart, D. W. (1966). 'Surgery in cancer of the

cervical oesophagus: Plastic tube replacement', *Journal of Laryngology and Otology*, **80,** 382

Wookey, H. (1942). 'The surgical treatment of carcinoma of the pharynx and upper oesophagus', *Surgery, Gynecology and Obstetrics*, **75,** 499

Yonemoto, R. H., Ching, P. T., Byron, R. L. and Riihimaki, D. U. (1972). 'The composite operation in cancer of the head and neck (commando procedure)', *Archives of Surgery*, **104,** 809–813

Zovickian, A. (1957). 'Pharyngeal fistulas: Repair and prevention using mastoid-occiput based shoulder flaps', *Plastic and Reconstructive Surgery*, **19,** 355–372

22 Lower respiratory conditions in otolaryngology
Stewart W Clarke

Introduction

In the previous edition this chapter was written by an ear, nose and throat surgeon. The present chapter is written by a chest physician and the topic is therefore discussed from a different angle. Many of the diseases which bring the two specialties together in modern practice are concerned with nasal and bronchial allergy, respiratory infection – so-called sinobronchitis – and bronchial neoplasms, presenting with hoarseness due to recurrent laryngeal nerve paresis, for instance. In the author's experience post-operative lung complications of ear, nose and throat practice are now uncommon with modern anaesthesia and techniques. Inhaled foreign bodies, at least in the United Kingdom, also appear to be less frequent than in the past, though it would seem that their incidence varies widely from country to country.

Some of the otolaryngological practice described in this chapter is based on that in the previous volume, while that dealing with the chest and lungs is the author's own work. The aim of the chapter is to highlight what the author considers to be the important aspects linking upper and lower respiratory conditions, a subject not well-covered in the literature.

Nasal polyps and bronchial asthma

Hippocrates (460–370 B.C.) was well acquainted with both these conditions and the association between them is now accepted, though the precise nature of this association remains obscure (Moloney and Collins, 1977). The reported incidence of asthma in patients with nasal polyps has ranged from 2.9 to 72 per cent while the incidence of nasal polyps in asthmatics has varied from 23 to 42 per cent. From their review, Moloney and Collins note that a patient with nasal polyps or with asthma has a 25–30 per cent chance of developing both conditions.

The histological changes in the nasal and bronchial mucosa of patients with polyps and asthma are similar (Dunnill, 1960), showing thickening of the basement membrane, infiltration by eosinophils, oedema and epithelial hyperplasia. Possible aetiological factors common to both conditions include allergy, bacterial or viral infection, autonomic nerve dysfunction, hyper-sensitivity to aspirin, and in the case of asthma, psychological mechanisms (Cauna *et al.*, 1972; Turner-Warwick, 1971).

It is tempting to speculate that nasal polyposis and asthma may be a common allergic reaction to an extrinsic inhaled allergen. Certainly symptoms (rhinitis and wheezing) from both may present simultaneously when, for instance, the pollen count is high in the atopic patient with the triad of hay-fever, eczema and asthma and high levels of IgE antibodies in the serum. These patients have been termed 'extrinsic asthmatics'. However, in the other type of asthma – intrinsic asthma – no definite immunological mechanism has been identified; yet intrinsic asthmatics are also prone to develop nasal polyps.

The reported incidence of nasal polyps in extrinsic and intrinsic asthmatics varies widely. Some authors have found a predominance in extrinsic asthmatics (Samter and Lederer, 1958) while others have found the reverse (Caplin, Haynes and Spahn, 1971), noting nasal polyps in almost all their aspirin-sensitive intrinsic asthmatics, with an incidence of only 0.5 per cent in 3000 atopic subjects.

The relationship between aspirin and asthma and nasal polyps is worth noting. It has long been known that salicylates may cause acute hyper-sensitivity reactions with wheezing and collapse in susceptible persons. Between 2 and 4 per cent of asthmatics are sensitive to aspirin, most of these being of the intrinsic non-atopic type, and nasal polyps are present in most of them. It should be further noted that other drugs may cause a similar reaction; these are paracetamol, codeine, phenylbutazone, indomethacin (and related compounds, including mefenamic acid) morphine and morphine derivatives, and tartrazine used as food colouring. The mechanism of this reaction remains unknown, though inhibition of prostaglandin synthesis may be involved. The clinical development of aspirin-sensitivity varies but individual patients may develop nasal polyps followed by asthma and then sensitivity to aspirin. This should be borne in mind when advising such patients about the use of analgesics.

The effect of nasal polypectomy on asthma is also controversial. Improvement, deterioration and the initial appearance of asthma have all been noted after polypectomy. Nasobronchial neurogenic reflexes have been cited (Swineford, 1962) and, supporting this hypothesis, the stimulation of the maxillary sinuses with balloons may cause wheezing. However, the changes in asthma after operation may merely reflect spontaneous fluctuation in the severity of asthma.

Treatment

If nasal polyps are causing severe obstruction of the airway, polypectomy is indicated. Oral antihistamines may reduce mucosal congestion and secretion at the expense of some drowsiness. A warning about drinking alcohol and driving should be given. Adrenergic drugs in droplet- or spray-form reduce mucosal swelling in the short term but their long-term use is inadvisable. Beclomethasone diproprionate (Beconase) inhaled into each nostril four times daily may control symptoms. Correction of septal deviation by submucosal resection may be indicated.

Where allergic rhinitis is present without nasal polyps, as is usually the case with atopic subjects, disodium cromoglycate (Rynacrom) may block the allergic reaction at mucosal level and afford relief. Where individual specific allergens are incriminated by skin-prick allergy tests (Bencard Pharmaceuticals Limited) hyposensitization with increasing strength of specific vaccine may reduce symptoms. When multiple allergens are involved the results are less satisfactory.

The treatment of asthma is not curative but palliative. As far as possible known allergens should be avoided by the extrinsic asthmatic. The commonest allergens are house dust and house dust mite, pet dander from cats and dogs, and grass pollens. House dust and mite can be much reduced by scrupulous vacuum cleaning and dusting. Feather pillows and quilts are banned, and the mattress and synthetic pillow should be plastic-covered.

Desensitization or hypo-sensitization with aqueous or oily extracts may be attempted in the extrinsic asthmatic with ascending doses of the allergen involved. This must be done cautiously since acute allergic reactions are occasionally provoked. Unfortunately only a small percentage of patients benefit from this procedure, usually when the main allergens are pollens or house dust and mite.

There are three main types of drugs useful in treating asthma. The first are known as beta-adrenergic or sympathomimetic drugs. Adrenaline and isoprenaline have been largely superseded by more selective drugs having less stimulation on the heart; these include salbutamol, terbutaline, and orciprenaline. Their use by inhaler is favoured since adequate bronchodilation results from a small dose which avoids side-effects. Alternatively, they can be given in tablet-form and the first two by injection in emergencies. In severe status asthmaticus, where the patient is refractory to the usual treatment, salbutamol 0.5 per cent solution may be usefully given by intermittent positive pressure breathing (IPPB), using a Bird or Bennett respirator and 40 per cent oxygen. This group of drugs is the mainstay of day-to-day management in asthma.

The second type of drug is the group of theophyllines, the best known of which is aminophylline; a slow-release preparation (Phyllocontin) or choline theophyllinate (Choledyl) may be given orally and aminophylline suppositories rectally. Amino-phylline is most effective in acute asthma, however, given as a slow intravenous injection, 0.25–0.5 g in 10–20 ml over 2–10 minutes, or as an infusion.

The third group of drugs are the corticosteroids. Beclomethasone diproprionate (Becotide) or betamethasone valerate (Bextasol) is inhaled as a pressurized aerosol. These drugs have a long-term stabilizing effect on asthma, acting over a period of several days, and they are the equivalent of about 7.5 mg of prednisolone taken orally, but lacking the latter's side-effects. A short, sharp course of prednisolone, starting at 30–40 mg daily and reducing over 10–30 days depending on response, is used in acute asthma. Long-term low-dose prednisolone may be required in chronic asthma where the dose is titrated against severity as measured by forced expiratory volume in one second (FEV_1) or peak flow rate (PFR). Intravenous hydrocortisone is required in status asthmaticus.

A further drug which comes into none of the preceding categories is disodium cromoglycate or Intal, since it interferes with allergy. This is inhaled by spinhaler, .and has a prophylactic effect, mainly in extrinsic asthmatics.

In status asthmaticus the patient should be managed by an expert in a hospital with oxygen, steroids, aminophylline and salbutamol. For further information about treatment in general the reader is referred to the textbook by Crofton and Douglas (1975).

Sinusitis, bronchitis, and bronchiectasis

Upper respiratory infection accounts for some 50 per cent of working days lost per year from illness. Sinus infection develops in a significant number. The sinuses are kept sterile and swept clean by mucociliary action. Most paranasal sinus infection arises from nasal disease itself (e.g. deviated septum, polyps), infection (bacterial or viral), allergy, and rarely dental cause or trauma. When upper and lower airways are simultaneously inflamed, the condition has been termed 'sinobronchitis', or 'bronchosinusitis' (Wasson, 1929). Much of the descriptive work on this topic was done several decades ago. The interrelationship remains as indeterminate as that between nasal polyps and asthma.

Since Quinn and Meyer (1929) demonstrated iodized oil in the thorax after instillation into the nostrils of sleeping patients, it has been known that post-nasal drip may be aspirated into the trachea and bronchial tree during sleep, at which time clearance virtually ceases (Bateman, Pavia and Clarke, 1978). Thus, the secretions will fail to clear until a bout of early morning coughing. In the meantime they may lead to inflammatory changes in the bronchial tree, thereby perpetuating the cycle of cough and sputum. Clearly, the treatment for this condition is principally to clear the sinuses and to prevent post-nasal drip as far as is possible.

The converse situation may also arise with chronic bronchitis, defined by the MRC (1965) as chronic cough and sputum for at least three consecutive months of the year for two successive years, a disease for which Britain has the highest national mortality. Chronic contamination from sputum as well as irritation from the common aetiological factors, namely smoking and air pollution, may occur. However, Hodge (1935) was unable to give convincing evidence of sinus contamination using iodized oil. This field is ripe for further studies with modern techniques to settle this point.

The treatment of this condition is to control the chronic bronchitis, firstly by stopping smoking, ensuring no atmospheric pollution in general and at work, treating any super-added infection with suitable antibiotics (usually ampicillin, tetracycline or trimethoprim), and using adrenergic drugs, both for their bronchodilator action, should there be additional airways obstruction, and for their enhancement of mucociliary clearance.

More frequently sinusitis is related to bronchiectasis, occurring in 60.9 per cent of the cases described by Hogg (1950). Whether Hogg's figure remains as high now is not known, although clinical experience suggests it is lower.

The term 'bronchiectasis' means chronically dilated bronchi. The condition is important if it leads to chronic or recurrent cough with infected sputum, severe haemoptysis or airways obstruction. The incidence of bronchiectasis itself has fallen over the past three decades following the advent of antibiotics and immunization against predisposing childhood diseases such as measles and whooping cough. The best known but rarest cause is congenital, Kartagener's (1933) syndrome, in which bronchiectasis is associated with dextrocardia and sinusitis or absent frontal sinuses. Bronchial obstruction by mucus plug, foreign body or tumour may result in bronchiectasis if left untreated, and if accompanied by infection resulting in an area of lung fibrosis. Bronchiectasis may be post-tuberculous in origin, although here again the incidence has fallen. Bronchiectasis is a constant feature of patients with cystic fibrosis in whom chronic productive cough with impairment of pulmonary function is associated with fatty diarrhoea (Anderson and Goodchild, 1976). In these patients the incidence of sinusitis and nasal polyposis is increased. Finally, proximal bronchiectasis may occur in allergic bronchopulmonary aspergillosis, characterized by fleeting eosinophilic lung shadows in the asthmatic in whom skin-prick tests are positive and aspergillus precipitins in the serum are present. The common super-added infecting micro-organisms are *Haemophilus influenzae*, *Staphylococci* in cystic fibrosis, and *Pseudomonas pyocyaneus*.

Recently it has been found that sinobronchitis may be a manifestation of an underlying immuno-deficiency syndrome. Berdal *et al.* (1976) describe 18 such patients: ten had deficiency of the IgG, IgA or IgM classes; while seven had an isolated deficiency of IgA, the immunoglobulin found in sputum. Two patients had defects of the T-cell, and both T and B cells respectively. It is important, therefore, that immunoglobulins be checked in chronic sinobronchitis, since this may suggest a cause and require replacement therapy.

A further possible immunological link is seen in patients with rheumatoid arthritis in whom the incidence of bronchiectasis is increased, though the precise nature of this link is not clear (Walker, 1967).

Treatment

Both the sinuses and the bronchiectasis require coordinated treatment. Bronchiectasis is now mainly controlled medically with postural drainage and self-physiotherapy, appropriate antibiotics for super-added infection and bronchodilators for concomitant airways obstruction. Surgery for bronchiectasis is now rare. Previous results have often been unsatisfactory due to the diffuse nature of the condition leading to recurrent symptoms after surgery. However, if the bronchiectasis is demonstrably localized by bilateral bronchography, and if pulmonary function (vital capacity, FEV_1, and gas transfer) is good, then localized resection should be considered, particularly if medical treatment fails. In some patients with immuno-deficiency, substitution therapy with periodic gamma-globulin injections may be beneficial.

Lung abscess

This is usually the term used for a necrotic, suppurative, cavitated, lesion due to infection with pyogenic microorganisms. They may be bronchogenic, pneumonic, pyaemic (including infected pulmonary embolus), or subdiaphragmatic (including amoebic) in origin, and occasionally follow trauma. The general incidence has fallen steadily in recent years with improved chemotherapy and general anaesthesia. Previously almost 25 per cent of solitary lung abscesses were said to follow removal of tonsils or adenoids. This should be suspected in the post-operative patient with undue fever, leucocytosis, and a shadow on the chest x-ray. With modern methods this has now fallen to less than two per cent. Tartar and fragments of septic teeth may be aspirated during dental treatment. Other foreign bodies such as peanuts and gum may impact after accidental aspiration and cause abscess formation. However, carcinoma of the bronchus is currently the cause of at least 25 per cent of lung abscesses. A cavitating carcinoma may be recognized by its thick irregular wall visible on chest x-ray. Aspiration during alcoholic coma or after an overdose is not uncommon and occasionally staphylococcal abscesses are seen. With intravenous drug abuse septic embolus may result. Occasionally a tuberculous cavity may enter into the differential diagnosis.

The abscesses usually contain mixed aerobic and anaerobic flora.

Diagnosis and treatment

The diagnosis is confirmed by the typical radiographic features of the lung cavity with a horizontal air–fluid level. Tomography will give information as to the possible nature and extent of the abscess. Bronchoscopy plays an essential role in ruling out carcinoma, foreign body, or other obstruction, in obtaining pus for examination, and in establishing bronchial drainage.

Treatment consists of appropriate antibiotics often including high-dose penicillin, drainage and possible surgery if resolution is inadequate or if there is a resectable underlying carcinoma.

Inhaled foreign bodies

The otolaryngologist, the chest surgeon, or the chest pysician may be called upon to deal with an inhaled foreign body depending on its type, location, and available resources and expertise. The foreign bodies may be divided into exogenous or endogenous, organic or inorganic. Most are aspirated into the right lower lobe in the conscious patient for anatomical reasons. In the unconscious patient, they may be inhaled into the apical segment of the right lower lobe or the posterior segment of the right upper lobe, and again less frequently on the left.

Exogenous foreign bodies

Holinger and Holinger (1978) have reported their experience in over 2000 patients with laryngeal, tracheal and bronchial foreign bodies. Of 534 of these patients seen between 1961 and 1975, 76 per cent were children below 4 years of age, 18 per cent were 4–14, and only 6 per cent were over 14 years of age. Peanuts, popcorn, or seeds were present in 60 per cent; hardware, pins and pens in 23 per cent; dental objects in 3 per cent; and a miscellany in 14 per cent. Vegetable matter, such as a peanut, excites a rapid, severe chemical bronchitis and is more noxious than inorganic non-vegetable matter.

Clinical picture

Episodes of choking, gagging and cyanosis are followed by unilateral wheezing if the object lodges in the bronchus or bilateral wheezing if in the trachea. Thereafter there may be a symptomless interval varying from hours to months depending on the nature of the foreign body, location and degree of bronchial obstruction.

Vegetable matter excites an early reaction leading to purulent bronchitis. Any foreign body may lead to obstructive emphysema seen on the expiration chest x-ray or to collapse with complete bronchial occlusion.

Diagnosis

The clinical history is usually suggestive but may be absent in infants who inhale tiny plastic toys, for instance, which are not radio-opaque. Unilateral wheezing is highly suggestive, particularly when associated with decreased chest movement, impaired percussion note, and reduced breath sounds distal to the foreign body.

Chest x-ray on expiration is essential, particularly if the foreign body is radio-lucent and cannot therefore be seen. Bronchoscopy is mandatory.

Removal of foreign bodies from the tracheobronchial tree

Foreign bodies should be promptly removed since only 2–4 per cent are coughed out spontaneously. In small children (below the age of ten years) general anaesthesia with rigid open-tube bronchoscopy is indicated. This should be done by a bronchoscopist expert in using the variety of special forceps (*see* Chapter 10) now available. Thoracotomy with bronchotomy or segmental resection is rarely justified for removal of an endobronchial foreign body.

In older patients (over the age of ten years), in whom the larynx and trachea are larger, fibre-optic bronchoscopy under local anaesthetic may be used. Rapid strides have been made in the past few years with this technique and Cunenan (1978) has reported his experience in 300 cases of which 89 per cent were performed with a fibre-optic bronchoscope alone, the remaining 11 per cent being done with a rigid bronchoscope. He was able to remove the same range of foreign bodies as above with special forceps. He mentioned a significant drop in mortality and morbidity from 12 per cent in the previous five years to 1 per cent in the last five years on switching to the fibre-optic bronchoscope. He attributed this fall in part to the avoidance of general anaesthesia in patients with complicating illnesses. Again it must be stressed that the bronchoscopist must be experienced and have the appropriate forceps. A point in favour of fibre-optic bronchoscopy is that the technique is simple enough to allow visual inspection to assess the situation without necessarily attempting immediate removal.

Endogenous foreign bodies

Saliva and mucopus may be inhaled by patients in coma from whatever cause and in those with neuromuscular disorders such as bulbar palsy. In some such cases a cuffed endotracheal tube with a floppy, low-pressure cuff released at regular intervals may be indicated. Releasing the cuff pressure periodically avoids tracheal trauma and subsequent stenosis. In protracted cases, tracheostomy may be necessary.

During ear, nose and throat surgery, blood and debris may be aspirated into the lungs, although modern anaesthesia with tracheal intubation has largely eradicated this complication.

Post-operative pulmonary collapse

This is now rare. It can be guarded against by postponing operation if a respiratory tract infection, such as the common cold, is present. Routine history and physical examination are important; smoking history should be appraised, and smoking discontinued for several days pre-operatively. Depending on the clinical examination, a chest x-ray may be required, together with pulmonary function tests, to establish whether or not the patient has airways obstruction for instance. Patients with chronic obstructive lung disease are more prone to develop respiratory infection post-operatively, and intensive physiotherapy should always be given both before and after operation.

The cardinal features of post-operative pulmonary collapse are fever, cough, sputum, and dyspnoea, depending on the degree. Dullness to percussion, with diminished breath sounds, and added sounds, crackles and wheezes in the affected area are found, and chest x-ray will confirm the extent. Broad-spectrum antibiotics (ampicillin, tetracycline, or trimethoprim) are indicated together with chest physiotherapy. Fibre-optic bronchoscopy under local anaesthesia should be kept under consideration, since selective aspiration may speed up resolution. Pain must be carefully controlled, and coughing encouraged.

Bleeding may still occasionally occur after adenotonsillectomy and, if unrecognized, occasionally leads to death from asphyxia. Emergency measures with bronchoscopy may be necessary.

Inhalation of gastric contents leads to severe lung damage. This occurs in ill-prepared patients who vomit at the time of anaesthesia or operation, and particularly in obstetric and dental cases and in those undergoing out-patient procedures; this is known as Mendelson's syndrome (1946). In cases where alveolar flooding with acid gastric juice (pH < 3.5) occurs the patient develops progressive respiratory failure over several days. The clinical signs are those of tachypnoea, cyanosis, fever, and widespread lung crackles (synonym: râles or crepitations). Arterial blood gases show a progressive fall in pO_2, with a low pCO_2 (reduced by the tachypnoea) and the pO_2 eventually failing to respond to increasing levels of inspired oxygen. This is due to alveolar damage with impairment of oxygen diffusion and imbalance of ventilation perfusion ($\dot{V}/\dot{Q}$) probably reflecting alveolar instability following loss of surfactant. The chest x-ray shows diffuse shadowing of alveolar type.

Initially the patient may appear reasonably well after the acute episode of aspiration. However, progressive deterioration over the succeeding few days can be predicted. Treatment in an Intensive Care Unit is indicated with oxygen, assisted ventilation, intravenous hydrocortisone, appropriate antibiotics, and possible lung lavage with hydrocortisone. Even so, the prognosis is poor.

The risk from a full stomach can be reduced in three ways; by prior aspiration, by neutralizing the acid with magnesium trisilicate (30 ml), or by inserting a cuffed endotracheal tube which should be left in place until the laryngeal reflexes have returned. Gastric aspiration may be safely carried out during this time.

Finally, mention should be made of the syndrome of choking, usually in elderly subjects chewing a large bolus of meat which impacts in the larynx leading to asphyxia. This is common in the USA and can be rapidly relieved by the Heimlich (1975) manoeuvre, where sudden direct pressure is applied to the stomach by the encircling arms of the attendant, with expulsion of the bolus.

Tumours of the tracheobronchial tree

Benign tumours (hamartoma, chondroma, lipoma) are greatly exceeded in incidence by carcinoma which is related to cigarette smoking.

Benign tumours

Hamartoma is the most common tumour being composed of mixed elements of lung tissue. It gives rise to a slow-growing peripheral shadow on chest x-ray which usually shows speckled calcification. Biopsy and occasional resection may be necessary to confirm its nature.

Tumours which may become malignant

Bronchial adenoma

This tumour may become malignant and metastasize in about ten per cent of cases. Lawson *et al.* (1976) found an actuarially assessed survival of 75 per cent at 15 years, in 71 patients undergoing surgery for this condition.

About 90 per cent are carcinoid in histological type, the remainder being adenoid cystic carcinoma (cylindroma). Their incidence in a series of lung tumours ranges from one to six per cent. The mean age of presentation is lower (about 45 years) than for carcinoma itself.

The commonest presenting symptoms are haemoptysis, cough, sputum, repeated chest infections, and wheezing – usually misdiagnosed as asthma. The chest x-ray shows abnormal shadowing in most patients, but is occasionally clear. Bronchoscopy and biopsy are necessary to confirm the diagnosis. These tumours, being highly vascular, have a reputation for bleeding on biopsy.

Treatment is surgical removal, usually by lobectomy; endoscopic removal is rarely successful. Careful follow-up is required, particularly in patients with atypical or metastatic carcinoid, and especially in those with adenoid cystic carcinoma in whom late recurrence is common.

Carcinoma of the bronchus (Crofton and Douglas, 1975)

This tumour is now the commonest in the western world, and has the highest national incidence in Britain. In 1974 in England and Wales it led to 40 per cent of all deaths from all cancers in males. The mortality in women is rising with the increased prevalence of women smokers. The evidence incriminating cigarette smoking is incontrovertible. Other factors such as exposure to asbestos and atmospheric pollution are important.

The main types are: squamous cell carcinoma (56 per cent); anaplastic, including oat cell carcinoma (37 per cent); adenocarcinoma (6 per cent); and others, including alveolar cell carcinoma (1 per cent).

Clinical features

Most patients present with respiratory symptoms (68 per cent), including cough, haemoptysis, and often unresolved pneumonia. Up to 27 per cent may present either with evidence of metastases or the non-metastatic extra-pulmonary manifestations, which include weight loss, endocrine disorder (Cushing's syndrome; inappropriate ADH secretion), neurological disorder (neuropathy, encephalopathy, myopathy), muscular, vascular (thrombophlebitis migrans), skeletal (finger clubbing and hypertrophic osteo-arthropathy), skin and blood disorders. Finally, five per cent may present without symptoms but with an abnormality on chest x-ray.

The diagnosis is made by the finding of a typical mass on chest x-ray; by positive sputum cytology in about 50 per cent of cases; and by bronchoscopy, now often with the fibre-optic bronchoscope, which yields a positive result in 80 per cent or more of cases. Percutaneous aspiration lung biopsy may be required for peripheral lesions larger than about 2 cm in diameter.

Treatment

Resection gives the best hope of cure, and should be considered in patients below the age of 70 years with local disease and good lung function. Contra-indications include the anaplastic oat cell type of tumour which is not amenable to surgery. The five-year survival rate for those selected and treated with lobectomy is about 30 per cent at five years; only five per cent of all the patients who present, however, survive five years.

Radiotherapy is essentially palliative, for symptoms such as cough, chest pain, and haemoptysis. Cytotoxic drugs may be effective initially, particularly in oat cell tumours. Immunotherapy with BCG is under investigation, although early reports show only marginal benefit.

Bronchial carcinoma may be seen in otolaryngological practice in three ways: first, when enlarged metastatic cervical lymph nodes are the presenting feature; secondly, when hoarseness of voice betrays left recurrent laryngeal nerve palsy due to hilar carcinoma. The latter is usually visible on x-ray with tomography and, if not, bronchoscopy should be undertaken to ascertain the diagnosis. With superior mediastinal lesions, either mediastinoscopy or limited thoracotomy may be required. The third is when stridor due to upper airways narrowing is the presenting complaint. This may be confused by the unwary with asthma, and in these cases bronchoscopy is again mandatory.

Tracheal stenosis of non-malignant origin may rarely be congenital, in which case early repair is advisable. More often tracheal stenosis follows tracheostomy in the unconscious ventilated patients, or prolonged intubation with inadequate control of the endotracheal tube cuff, which should be of low-pressure, floppy type, periodically deflated. Meticulous repair technique is required to avoid recurrent stenosis (Pearson *et al.*, 1975).

Finally, tracheal stenosis with stridor may indicate tumour, cystic adenoid carcinoma being the commonest type. If possible it should be removed. Tracheal reconstruction is a highly specialized task, and may require the use of various synthetic stents. (*See also* Chapter 12.)

References

Anderson, C. M. and Goodchild, M. C. (1976). *Cystic Fibrosis, Manual of Diagnosis and Management*; Blackwell Scientific, Oxford

Bateman, J. R. M., Pavia, D. and Clarke, S. W. (1978). 'The retention of lung secretions during the night in normal subjects', *Clinical Science and Molecular Medicine*, **55,** 523

Berdal, P., Brandtzaeg, P., Frøland, S. S., Henriksen, S. D. and Skrede, S. (1976). 'Immunodeficiency syndromes with otorhinolaryngological manifestations', *Acta Otolarlygologica*, **82,** 185

Caplin I., Haynes, J. T. and Spahn, J. (1971). 'Are nasal polyps an allergic phenomenon?' *Annals of Allergy*, **29,** 631

Cauna, N., Manzetti, G. W., Hinderer, K. H. and Swanson, E. W. (1972). 'Fine structure of nasal polyps', *Annals of Otology, Rhinology and Laryngology*, **81,** 41

Crofton, J. and Douglas, A. (1975). *Respiratory Diseases*, 2nd edn; Blackwell Scientific, Oxford

Cunenan, O. S. (1978). 'The flexible fibreoptic bronchoscope in foreign body removal. Experience in 300 cases', *Chest* (Supplement), **73,** 725

Dunnill, M. S. (1960). 'The pathology of asthma with special reference to changes in the bronchial mucosa', *Journal of Clinical Pathology*, **13,** 27

Heimlich, H. J. (1975). 'A life-saving manoeuvre to prevent food-choking', *Journal of the American Medical Association*, **234,** 398

Hodge, G. E. (1935). 'Relation of bronchiectasis to infection of the paranasal sinuses', *Archives of Otolaryngology*, **22,** 537

Hogg, J. C. (1950). 'Discussion on the role of sinusitis in bronchiectasis', *Proceedings of the Royal Society of Medicine*, **43,** 1089

Holinger, P. H. and Holinger, L. D. (1978). 'Use of the open tube bronchoscope in the extraction of foreign bodies', *Chest* (Supplement), **73,** 721

Kartagener, M. (1933). 'Zur pathogenese der bronchiektasien: I. Bronchiektasien bei situs viscerum inversus', *Beitrage zur Klinik der Tuberkulose*, **83,** 489

Lawson, R. L., Ramanathan, L., Hurley, G., Hinson, K. W. and Lennox, S. C. (1976). 'Bronchial adenoma: Review of an 18 year experience at the Brompton Hospital', *Thorax*, **31,** 245

Medical Research Council (1965). 'Definition – classification of chronic bronchitis for clinical and epidemiological purposes', *Lancet*, **1,** 776

Mendelson, C. L. (1946). 'Aspiration of stomach contents into lungs during obstetric anaesthesia', *American Journal of Obstetrics and Gynaecology*, **52,** 191

Moloney, J. R. and Collins, J. (1977). 'Nasal polyps and bronchial asthma', *British Journal of Diseases of the Chest*, **71,** 1

Quinn, L. H. and Meyer, O. O. (1929). 'The relation of sinusitis and bronchiectasis', *Archives of Otolaryngology*, **10,** 152

Samter, M. and Lederer, F. L. (1958). 'Nasal polyps: Their relationship to allergy and particularly to bronchial asthma, *Medical Clinics of North America*, **42,** 175

Swineford, O. (1962). 'The asthma problem', *Annals of International Medicine*, **57,** 145

Turner-Warwick, M. (1971). 'Provoking factors in asthma', *British Journal of Diseases of the Chest*, **65,** 1

Walker, W. C. (1967). 'Pulmonary infections and rheumatoid arthritis', *Quarterly Journal of Medicine*, **36,** 239

Wasson, W. W. (1929). 'Bronchosinusitis disease', *Journal of the American Medical Association*, **93,** 2018

Index